HANDBOOK OF EXPERIMENTAL NEUROLOGY

T0155719

Basic relevant information on methodologies used in neurological disease models can be extremely hard to find. The *Handbook of Experimental Neurology* contains 30 chapters from over 60 internationally recognized scientists and covers every major methodology and disease model in the neurosciences. The book is divided into two major sections: Part I deals with general methodologies in neuroscience research covering topics from animal welfare and ethical issues to surgical procedures, postoperative care, and behavioral testing, while Part II covers every major disease model from traumatic brain injury, ischemia and stroke, to CNS tumors, hydrocephalus, demyelinating disease, Parkinson's, motor neuron disease, epilepsy, bacterial infection, and sleep disorders. Delivering critical, up-to-the-minute, methodological information and describing small-animal models for almost all major neurological diseases, this book is written specifically for beginners and young scientists in neurosciences. It will also serve as a cutting-edge reference for more experienced researchers.

DR. TATLISUMAK received his neurology training in the Helsinki University Central Hospital. His Ph.D. was gained in experimental brain ischemia and magnetic resonance imaging at the University of Massachusetts. His research field is clinical and experimental stroke and magnetic resonance imaging. He holds board certificates in neurology and healthcare administration in Finland. He is currently an associate professor and Vice-Chairman at the Department of Neurology, Helsinki University Central Hospital and the director of the Experimental Magnetic Resonance Imaging Laboratory. Dr. Tatlisumak is a Fellow of the American Heart Association. He is an awarded teacher and holds a degree in teaching sciences.

DR. FISHER received his medical degree from the State University of New York at Syracuse and then trained in medicine at the University of

Wisconsin and neurology at the Medical Center of Vermont. He has been at the University of Massachusetts Medical School since 1978 and currently holds the position of Professor and Vice-Chairman in the neurology department. He performs clinical activities approximately 50% of the time with a special emphasis on patients with cerebrovascular disorders and multiple sclerosis. He has directed an animal stroke research laboratory for more than 15 years that has emphasized the use of novel magnetic resonance imaging techniques to evaluate stroke evolution and to assess therapeutic interventions in vivo. He has participated in many clinical stroke trials as a member of the steering committee. He has published extensively in both of these areas with 190 peer-reviewed publications, and he has edited 10 textbooks. He has worked closely with the pharmaceutical industry in the development of novel stroke therapies as well as in designing and implementing clinical trials for acute stroke therapies.

HANDBOOK OF EXPERIMENTAL NEUROLOGY

Methods and Techniques in Animal Research

edited by

TURGUT TATLISUMAK
Helsinki University Central Hospital

and

MARC FISHER
University of Massachusetts

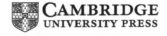
CAMBRIDGE
UNIVERSITY PRESS

CAMBRIDGE UNIVERSITY PRESS
Cambridge, New York, Melbourne, Madrid, Cape Town, Singapore,
São Paulo, Delhi, Dubai, Tokyo, Mexico City

Cambridge University Press
The Edinburgh Building, Cambridge CB2 8RU, UK

Published in the United States of America by Cambridge University Press, New York

www.cambridge.org
Information on this title: www.cambridge.org/9780521184205

First published 2006
First paperback edition 2010

A catalogue record for this publication is available from the British Library

ISBN 978-0-521-83814-6 Hardback
ISBN 978-0-521-18420-5 Paperback

Contents

Contributors

Ricardo M. Arida
Laboratory of Experimental
Neurology
Departments of Neurology and
Neurosurgery
Faculty of Medicine
Federal University of São Paulo
Rvo Botucatu 862
04023 São Paulo
Brazil

Joshua B. Bederson
Department of Neurosurgery
Mount Sinai School of Medicine
1 Gustave L. Levy Place
Box 1136
New York, NY 10029
USA

Erica Butti
Neuroimmunology Unit
San Raffaella Scientific
Institute–DIBIT
Via Olgettina 58
20132 Milano
Italy

Esper A. Cavalheiro
Laboratory of Experimental
Neurology
Departments of Neurology and
Neurosurgery
Faculty of Medicine
Federal University of São Paulo
Rvo Botucatu 862
04023 São Paulo
Brazil

Pak H. Chan
Department of Neurosurgery and
Neurosciences
Stanford University Medical Center
Palo Alto, CA 93304
USA

Zhao Zhong Chong
Departments of Neurology and
Anatomy and Cell Biology
Centers for Molecular Medicine and
Institute for Environmental Health
Sciences

Wayne State University School of
Medicine
8C-1 UHC
4201 St. Antoine
Detroit, MI 48201
USA

Shlomi Constantini
Department of Pediatric
Neurosurgery
Dana Children's Hospital
Tel Aviv Medical Center
Tel Aviv 64239
Israel

Ruth Danzeisen
Department of Neurology
University of Ulm
Albert Einstein-Allee 11 (025)
89081 Ulm
Germany

Marc R. Del Bigio
Department of Pathology
(Neuropathology)
University of Manitoba
D212 – 770 Bannatyne Avenue
Winnipeg MB R3E 0W3
Canada

Stephen B. Dunnett
School of Biosciences
Cardiff University
Museum Avenue
P.O. Box 911
Cardiff CF10 3US
UK

Marc Fisher
Department of Neurology
University of Massachusetts Medical
School
UMASS/Memorial Health Care
119 Belmont Street
Worcester, MA 01605
USA

Rosemary A. Fricker-Gates
School of Biosciences
Cardiff University
Museum Avenue
P.O. Box 911
Cardiff CF10 3US
UK

Nobuhiro Fujiki
Center for Narcolepsy
Stanford University School of
Medicine
701B Welch Road
Palo Alto, CA 93304
USA

Roberto Furlan
Neuroimmunology Unit
San Raffaele Scientific
Institute–DIBIT
Via Olgettina 58
20132 Milan
Italy

Monte A. Gates
School of Biosciences
Cardiff University
Museum Avenue
P.O. Box 911
Cardiff CF10 3US
UK

Larry B. Goldstein
Department of Neurology
Duke Center for Cerebrovascular
Disease
Duke University Medical Center
P.O. Box 3651
Durham, NC 27710
USA

Lilly Hsieh
Department of Neurosurgery and
Neurological Sciences
Stanford University Medical School
1201 Welch Rd MSLS P357
Stanford, CA 94305
USA

Taichang Jang
Department of Neurology and
Clinical Neurosciences
Stanford University Medical Center
Palo Alto, CA 93304
USA

Richard E. Jones
Portland Veterans Affairs Medical
Center
Oregon Health and Science
University
R&D-31
3710 SW US Veterans Hospital Rd
Portland, OR 97239
USA

Anumantha G. Kanthasamy
Department of Biomedical Sciences
2062 Veterinary Medicine Building
Iowa State University
Ames, IA 50011
USA

Siddharth Kaul
Department of Biomedical Sciences
2062 Veterinary Medicine Building
Iowa State University
Ames, IA 50011
USA

Robert W. Kemp
AstraZeneca Inc.
Alderley Park
Macclesfield SK10 4TF
UK

Osaama H. Khan
Department of Pathology
(Neuropathology)
University of Manitoba
D212 – 770 Bannatyne Avenue
Winnipeg MB R3E 0W3
Canada

Tammy Kielian
Department of Neurobiology and
Developmental Sciences
University of Arkansas for Medical
Sciences College of Medicine
Room 110B Biomedical Research
Center
4301 W. Markham St, Slot 510
Little Rock, AR 72205
USA

Julia Kofler
Department of Anesthesiology and
Peri-Operative Medicine
Oregon Health and Science
University
3181 SW Sam Jackson Park Rd
Mail Code L335
Portland, OR 97239
USA

Tarja Kohila
University of Helsinki
00014 Helsinki
Finland

Ronen R. Leker
Laboratory of Molecular Biology
Bldg 36, Room 3c12
National Institute for Neurological
Disorders and Stroke
National Institutes of Health
Bethesda, MD 20892
USA

Michael Lev
Department of Radiology
Harvard Medical School
Boston, MA 02115
USA

Faqi Li
Departments of Neurology and
Anatomy and Cell Biology
Centers for Molecular Medicine and
Institute for Environmental Health
Sciences
Wayne State University School of
Medicine
8C-1 UHC
4201 St. Antoine
Detroit, MI 48201
USA

Fuhai Li
Department of Neurology
Duke University Medical Center
P.O. Box 3651
Durham, NC 27710
USA

Päivi Liesi
Department of Biosciences
University of Helsinki
P.O. Box 65
Viikinkaari 1
00014 Helsinki
Finland

Hans Link
Department of Neurology
Karolinska Institute and Huddinge
University Hospital
M 98, 14186 Huddinge
Stockholm
Sweden

Jason M. Link
Portland Veterans Affairs Medical
Center
Oregon Health and Science
University
R&D-31
3710 SW US Veterans Hospital Rd
Portland, OR 97239
USA

Eng H. Lo
Departments of Neurology and
Radiology
Harvard Medical School
Boston, MA 02115
USA

Albert C. Ludolph
Department of Neurology
University of Ulm
Oberer Eselsberg 45
89081 Ulm
Germany

Carolina M. Maier
Department of Neurosurgery and
Neurological Sciences
Stanford University Medical School
1201 Welch Rd MSLS P357
Stanford, CA 94305
USA

Kenneth Maiese
Departments of Neurology and
Anatomy and Cell Biology
Centers for Molecular Medicine and
Institute for Environmental Health
Sciences
Wayne State University School of
Medicine
8C-1 UHC
4201 St. Antoine
Detroit, MI 48201
USA

Gianvito Martino
Neuroimmunology Unit
San Raffaele Scientific
Institute–DIBIT
Via Olgettina 58
20132 Milano
Italy

Naoya Masutomi
Toxicology Laboratory
Mitsubishi Pharma Corporation
1-1-1 Kazusakamatari
Kisarazu, Chiba 292-0818
Japan

Seiji Nishino
Center for Narcolepsy
Stanford University School of
Medicine
701B Welch Rd, RM 142
Palo Alto, CA 94304
USA

Halina Offner
Portland Veterans Affairs Medical
Center
Oregon Health and Science
University
R&D-31
3710 SW US Veterans Hospital Rd
Portland, OR 97239
USA

Anders Paetau
Department of Pathology
Helsinki University Central Hospital
Haartmaninkatu 3
00290 Helsinki
Finland

Katja E. Peltola Mjosund
Programme of Neurosciences and
Department of Neurology
University of Helsinki and Helsinki
University
Central Hospital
Biomedicum Helsinki
Haartmaninkatu 8
00290 Helsinki
Finland

Margareth R. Priel
Laboratory of Experimental
Neurology
Departments of Neurology and
Neurosurgery
Faculty of Medicine
Federal University of São Paulo
Rvo Botucatu 862
04023 São Paulo
Brazil

Lawrence Recht
Department of Neurology and
Clinical Neurosciences
University of Stanford Medical
School
Palo Alto, CA 93304
USA

René Remie
Department of Biomonitoring and
Sensoring
University Center for Pharmacy
Groningen University
Antonius Deusinglaan 1
9714 AW Groningen
The Netherlands

Birgitta Schwalenstöcker
Department of Neurology
University of Ulm
Albert Einstein-Allee 11 (025)
89081 Ulm
Germany

Fatima A. Sehba
Department of Neurosurgery
Mount Sinai School of Medicine
1 Gustave L. Levy Place
Box 1136
New York, NY 10029
USA

Makoto Shibutani
Division of Neuropathology
National Institute of Health Sciences
1-18-1 Kamiyoga, Setagayu-ku
Tokyo 158-8501
Japan

Alexandre V. Silva
Laboratory of Experimental
Neurology
Departments of Neurology and
Neurosurgery
Faculty of Medicine
Federal University of São Paulo
Rvo Botucatu 862
04023 São Paulo
Brazil

Daniel Strbian
Department of Neurology
Helsinki University Central Hospital
Haartmaninkatu 4
00290 Helsinki
Finland

Anu Suomalainen
Department of Neurology
Helsinki University Central Hospital
Haartmaninkatu 4
00290 Helsinki
Finland

Turgut Tatlisumak
Department of Neurology
Helsinki University Central Hospital
Haartmaninkatu 4
00290 Helsinki
Finland

George T. Taylor
Behavioral Neuroscience Group
University of Missouri – St. Louis
8001 Natural Bridge Rd.
St. Louis, MO 63121
USA

Eduardo M. Torres
School of Biosciences
Cardiff University
Museum Avenue
P.O. Box 911
Cardiff CF10 3US
UK

Richard J. Traystman
Department of Anesthesiology and
Peri-Operative Medicine
Oregon Health and Science
University
3181 SW Sam Jackson Park Rd
Mail Code L335
Portland, OR 97239
USA

Arthur A. Vandenbark
Department of Neurology
Tykeson Multiple Sclerosis Research
Laboratory
Veterans Affairs Medical Center
Oregon Health and Science
University
Portland, OR 97239
USA

Carina Wallgren-Pettersson
Department of Medical Genetics
University of Helsinki and
Folkhälsan Institute of Genetics
Haartmaninkatu 8
00290 Helsinki
Finland

David Whittaker
Huntingdon Life Sciences Ltd
Woolley Road
Alconbury
Huntingdon PE28 4HS
UK

Juergen Weiss
Center for Biomedicine
University of Heidelberg
INF 347
D-69120 Heidelberg
Germany

Bao-Guo Xiao
Department of Neurology
Karolinska Institute and Huddinge
University Hospital
M 98, 14186 Huddinge
Stockholm
Sweden

Frank Zimmermann
Center for Biomedicine
University of Heidelberg
INF 347
D-69120 Heidelberg
Germany

Part I

Principles and general methods

1

Introduction: Animal modeling – a precious tool for developing remedies to neurological diseases

TURGUT TATLISUMAK AND MARC FISHER

Human beings owe a great deal to animals. From the earliest periods of history of mankind, animals have been used by humans for food, clothing, tool making, and for several other purposes. Primitive artists painted animal figures onto stone surfaces; animal figures became parts of religions and tribal identities. Over time, some animals were domesticated, serving as regular sources of meat and milk; additionally, animals were used in farmwork and for transport. Dogs were used to defend property and were trained for rescue missions. Cats were used as pets as early as the ancient Egyptian Kingdom. Interesting additional missions have been given to animals such as searching for illicit drugs, explosives, and mushrooms. Some areas where we are still strictly dependent on animals include the drug industry (e.g., insulin isolated from swine pancreas), but there are also areas subject to intense debate (e.g., fur farming, fox hunting, and the cosmetics industry).

We are very much dependent on animals in medical research and in clinical surgery training. Neurological diseases comprise a major health problem all over the world and their importance continues to grow as the population ages and as neurology moves from being largely a diagnostic field to one with more therapeutic approaches. Neurological diseases already absorb approximately one-fourth of health budgets in industrialized countries. It is urgent to develop novel effective therapies for neurological diseases: the aging of the population will increase the number of neurological patients whereas the labor force available in the health sector appears to be decreasing. Additionally, the burden of the neurological disease to the individual patient and their relatives is more dramatic than diseases of other organs. Many critically important discoveries regarding disease mechanisms and most therapies that are currently being used for neurological diseases have been developed in animal models, and the need for animal models is expanding.

Use of animals for scientific purposes has a long history. One animal dies for scientific reasons every second in the USA and every three seconds in the

Handbook of Experimental Neurology, ed. Turgut Tatlisumak and Marc Fisher. Published by Cambridge University Press. © Cambridge University Press 2006.

European Union. Whereas total medical research has expanded several-fold over recent decades, the number of animals used for scientific purposes has remained the same or even slightly decreased in absolute terms, and substantially decreased in relative terms. A Medline search with the word "rat" gave 1 100 000 hits and "mouse" gave 770 000 hits (March 2005). It is easy to understand why the rat and the mouse are so popular in medical research. They breed easily, profusely, and continuously, have a short gestational period, are relatively inexpensive, and can be housed in large numbers in relatively small spaces; and their anatomy, physiology, biochemistry, genetical properties, and behavior are well described. Rats and mice are easy to handle and the size of their organs is suitable for staining, antibody generation, and many other research activities. Specimens from rats and mice can easily be stored for later studies. Furthermore, the rat and mouse are not generally considered as pets and their experimental use is more acceptable than other animals.

The "3 R" rule (Reduce, Refine, Replace) refers to the efforts to reduce the number of animals used in scientific experiments, to plan and perform the experiments in a way that decreases the suffering of animals, and to develop alternative methods to replace the use of live animals. Even though the aim is ethically well established, it is difficult to develop alternative approaches and some are unreliable. Although the ethics of using animals in research is not a new issue, standards remain to be established. It must be remembered that the very early ethical principles regarding the use of animals in scientific research were written with efforts initiated by scientists themselves in the 1830s, not by animal activists. Furthermore, animal experimentation is rather expensive. If alternative approaches were available, most researchers would readily abandon the use of animals. Interestingly, possessing a pet animal does not require any training, while fishing or shooting animals does not require more than a permit. Scientific use is strictly controlled, suitable facilities are required, extensive training is a must, and permission must be obtained. Anyone can take a pet animal to a veterinary physician for castration without permission of regulatory authorities, despite the fact that this is not necessary for the animal's health, alters its natural life course, and causes pain. To carry out a similar procedure for scientific reasons would require regulatory approval. The final target of animal experimenting is to develop remedies to cure human diseases. Therefore, it is never unnecessary to mention the importance of treating the experimental animals humanely as the source of scientific research is humane and it must be accomplished in a humane way.

We felt frustrated with the difficulty of finding even the most fundamental information in a centralized source for animal experimentation and to collect information from a large number of articles some of which were published in journals that were difficult to access and was time-consuming. Therefore, we decided to centralize the joint effort of over 60 universally well-recognized scientists and cover most major issues about neurological animal methodology under one cover. This is a first-of-its-kind book in its comprehensiveness. The methods included in this book may improve animal welfare, decrease the number of animals required, and may increase the quality of experiments. Success in animal experiments and the reliability of the results largely depend on the proper use of techniques including proper handling of the animals, suitable anesthesia and analgesia, clean and least-damaging surgery, and use of most appropriate models and techniques. Failure in following the crucial steps in animal experimenting will lead to unreliable results and unnecessary suffering of animals and sometimes of the researcher when he/she is bitten.

This book comprises 30 chapters and is divided into two parts. The first part of this book deals with general principles and methodology, whereas the second part delivers comprehensive data on animal models of individual neurological disorders. In each disease chapter, the authors first discuss the magnitude of the problem in epidemiologic and economic dimensions followed by detailed and critical information on present models. References are generally limited and readers who are interested in more in-depth knowledge are encouraged to further explore the references listed in each chapter or directly contact experts in that field. This book is planned to deliver a broad view to young neuroscientists, but may even be useful to more experienced scientists. Animal modeling deals mostly with rodents and with other animal species where appropriate.

We are grateful to all the authors for their contributions and the time spent in preparing them. Even though we engendered our best to cover all major neurological experimental issues in this book, space limitations led to compromises. We hope that scientists will benefit from this book. Feedback from readers is most welcome. It is of our mutual interest that, in the long run, these animal models can be replaced with novel technologies that are at the same time ethically more acceptable and scientifically more reliable, making new editions of this book unnecessary.

2

Ethical issues, welfare laws, and regulations

DAVID WHITTAKER

2.1 Introduction

The ethics, morals, and laws of any culture or nation are intimately interwoven and dependent upon each other for their continuation within that society. At the same time most cultures are under continual evolution, change, and development due to many factors, but usually due to ingress, influences, and pressures from other external factors and cultures. This is best illustrated by the notion that "developed" nations frequently bring about cultural changes in very old "traditional societies" through their presence and financial impact. Once there is cultural change, then almost certainly it will be followed by changes in the ethical and moral stances taken. Ultimately the laws and regulations will no longer reflect or uphold the current "values" of that society and will need modification.

This point is made to emphasize the fact that ethics and morals are not only diverse in a global sense but also dynamic. What was once ethically acceptable in history (e.g., slavery) may now be locally or globally seen as morally wrong and laws enacted to reflect those views.

With regard to laws it must also be acknowledged that as the "global village" becomes an increasing reality so does a meeting of minds on points of ethics and morals. As the meeting of minds becomes a reality, then it is possible to develop and implement international laws and regulations. This is particularly pertinent when considering the European position with regard to the Council of Europe (CoE) and the European Union (EU).

Finally in this introduction it must be emphasized that the roots of ethics and moral principles lie in the considerations and writings of the great philosophers. It is not the intention of this paper to concentrate on the history and theories which consider the rights and wrongs of animal experimentation. However, consideration will be given to the more practical and pragmatic ethical considerations surrounding animal use.

Handbook of Experimental Neurology, ed. Turgut Tatlisumak and Marc Fisher. Published by Cambridge University Press. © Cambridge University Press 2006.

2.1.1 Ethical issues and considerations

There are probably three simple categories for those practically considering the ethical rights and wrongs of animal experimentation. They are:

- *All* animal experimentation (indeed man's use and killing of all animals) is wrong and therefore should be stopped, absolutely. This is the position of the abolitionists.
- It is ethically wrong to use animals for some *types* of experimentation. Easy examples here are the use of animals for testing cosmetics, alcohol, tobacco, and for offensive weapons research.
- It is ethically wrong to use certain *species* of animals for research, e.g., the great apes, lower-order primates, and perhaps dogs and cats.
- There is a fourth perspective, which is that of complete dominion over animals where any treatment of animals is acceptable without moral guilt. I believe that such a category of ethical consideration for all uses of animals is largely redundant.

In considering these views we can postulate that those falling within the first category do believe that all animals have equal rights to humans and should not be "exploited," simply because we have the physical and mental capacity to do so. People holding this view frequently draw analogies of animal exploitation with slavery or the possibility of using babies or mentally handicapped people for research.

People holding the second view probably do so more on their moral values and ethical view of the research topic in question, e.g., it is wrong to drink alcohol or smoke in the first place, and therefore animals should not die to help save people from their self-inflicted disease, or to prosecute war.

Those people holding the third ("speciesist") view may be more concerned about the cognitive ability or neurophysiological sensitivity of the animals being used, i.e., their "closeness" to humans, and perhaps more commonly are more concerned with "animal welfare" than they are with "animal rights."

Should the "burden of guilt" (if any exists) be spread amongst those who benefit from animal experimentation and not laid fully on those who conduct it? In short, currently societies around the world welcome the benefits of animal research whilst largely remaining ambivalent to the work itself and will probably choose to remain ignorant of the issues for as long as possible. Is the guilt of benefiting from a medicine any the less because it was developed using animals (perhaps chimpanzees) in another country?

What about animal welfare? So much is said about animal welfare, so little is understood! Many aspects of animal welfare are tangible, indeed often quantitative. Body weights can be measured and disease is detectable by the veterinary clinician, as is malnutrition. Extremes of behavioral abnormalities can be observed (e.g., stereotypic behavior). Fear is readily detected through the "fight or flight" responses. All of these characteristics contribute to measuring animal welfare. Perhaps the area of greatest interest and of most conflict is currently that of measuring behavioral "needs/drivers" and assessing whether containment in laboratory conditions allows animals to sufficiently satisfy these needs.

The UK Farm Animal Welfare Council (1993) defined the "five freedoms" that should be given to every farm animal. They are:

Freedom from malnutrition
Freedom from injury and disease
Freedom from thermal and physical discomfort
Freedom from fear and stress
Freedom to express most normal patterns of behaviour.

These five freedoms (of welfare) are equally applicable to laboratory animals and serve as an excellent measuring template. It is clear however, that thankfully many of these markers of freedoms are now taken for granted in our animals, specifically freedom from hunger, thirst, malnutrition, (incidental) pain, injury, and disease. Therefore if we were to simply draw up a welfare-scoring template and compare our laboratory animals' lives to those of the average farm animal, they would probably compare very favorably.

However, we are, when using these freedoms to measure welfare, left with some challenges for some laboratory animals. As already considered, the freedom to express normal behavior perhaps remains the greatest concern of the challenging but responsible animal welfare groups. Within the research community we refer to this aspect of welfare as social and environmental enrichment. Whilst there still remain elements of the unknown and doubt regarding suitable and appropriate enrichments, a large degree of the concern surrounds sufficient funding for their implementation and overcoming concerns that they do not prejudice the scientific integrity and regulatory validity of experiments.

The scientific community as a whole frequently broadcasts that the "inflicted" discomfort, pain, suffering, distress, and lasting harm to animals in experiments is mostly minimal. However, there are still opportunities using refinements to reduce these further, thereby better fulfilling this freedom.

Finally a challenge for every laboratory animal-user and handler is to provide totally the freedom from fear and distress. So much of providing this freedom centers on the staff and on policies and procedures regarding both staff and animal training.

To summarize and conclude this review of animal rights and welfare it is probably best to give a quotation. It is taken from *Animal Welfare: A Cool Eye towards Eden*: "It is not what you think of the animal that matters. It is what you do to it that counts!"[1]

As an example, the rabbit kept for meat production, for experimental purposes, or as a pet has still the same basic welfare needs and knows not (nor cares) why it is there, or what its fate is to be, nor what its carer thinks of it. But the consequences of negligence and neglect on each of the three rabbits will be the same!

2.2 Laboratory animal welfare laws and regulations

National laws and regulations tend to reflect the ethics and moral attitudes of the prevailing culture. I believe it therefore inappropriate to take any piece of national legislation in isolation of a nation's cultural position or in context of its total legislative framework and decide on its "value" or "worth" in achieving what that law sets out to do. Often it is as important to reflect on the cultural attitude to and interpretation of law enforcement within a country as it is to simply evaluate the words.

It must also be remembered that in most countries statute law is frequently supplemented with further "regulations" in the form of guidelines and codes of practice.

I believe in and work to three fundamental concepts, or objectives, of the laws governing animal experimentation. Those concepts or objectives are:

- To bestow a privilege on individuals to conduct research on live animals, which may cause pain, suffering, distress, or lasting harm.
- To provide the opportunity and ability to advance science for the overall benefit of mankind.
- To secure as far as possible the highest welfare standards compatible with the research objectives.

2.2.1 Council of Europe (CoE) and Convention ETS/123

The Council of Europe (CoE) is the continent's oldest political organization, founded in 1949, and currently has 46 Member States.

The CoE was set up with primary aims:

- To defend human rights, parliamentary democracy, and the rule of law.
- To develop continent-wide agreements to standardize Member States' social and legal practices.
- To promote awareness of a European identity based on shared values and cutting across different cultures.

In summary the CoE was established to harmoniously bring Europe back together after the war, and as such it works through mutual understanding, handshakes, and gentlemen's agreements, in contrast to the European Union which keeps order through legal enforcement.

The CoE uses Conventions as instruments of harmonization, and Member States of the CoE can choose to respond to a Convention in one of three ways. They can refuse to recognize a Convention and in doing so make no obligation to comply in whole or part. They can "sign" a Convention and in doing so acknowledge the existence of the Convention but again make no binding obligations in respect of compliance. Finally a Member State can "ratify" a Convention and on ratification acknowledge a "moral" obligation to comply. In reality should a Member State which has ratified the Convention fail to comply, then there is little the CoE can do to enforce compliance short of dismissing the state from the CoE.

Clearly such a method of implementation combined with a historical picture of enrolment to the CoE (many Eastern states joining in very recent times) leads to significant variations in the degree of compliance between Member States.

The relevant Convention regarding animal experimentation in the CoE is titled the European Convention for the Protection of Vertebrate Animals Used for Experimental and other Scientific Purposes 1986 and is commonly referred to as Convention ETS/123 (1986).[2] This Convention is one of five relating to animal welfare.

Of most relevance today is Article 30 of the Convention which requires multilateral consultations by the parties within 5 years of its enforcement and every 5 years thereafter. The first multilateral consultation took place in 1993 and since then they have been held regularly, involving not only the competent authorities responsible for its implementation at national level but also all interested European and global stakeholder organizations including user groups, animal welfare organizations, and animal rights representatives. In such a way the CoE attempts to progress the Convention in terms of meeting current needs of all stakeholder organizations through consensus.

The multilateral consultations have addressed many issues over the last 14 years or so including the introduction of new technologies such as transgenic manipulation, as well as topics such as education, training, and the collection of statistics.

Most recently and for the last 5 years or so the multilateral consultation has concentrated on reviewing and revising Appendix A to the Convention wherever possible basing any modifications on scientific evidence. Appendix A of the Convention provides guidance on the care, housing, and husbandry of the species commonly used in experimentation.

Ratification by the Council of Europe of the revised version of Appendix A can be expected in 2005. It will then be for Member States to decide on individual implementation plans. Of most concern will be the changes of recommended minimum cage sizes and stocking densities, which almost certainly will result in most users across the CoE having to commit to extensive and expensive upgrading programs.[3]

In concluding a short consideration of the Convention it must be emphasized that whilst enforcement is difficult within the CoE, we will go on to see how it is closely mirrored within the European Union and where enforcement at national level is much more closely monitored and applied.

2.2.2 European Union (EU) and Directive 86/609

The European Union is a much smaller (25 Member States in 2004) but is also a growing community. The EU Directive 86/609[4] is a Council Directive on "The approximation of laws, regulations, and administrative provisions of the Member States regarding the protection of animals used for experimental and other scientific purposes."

The CoE Convention and the EU Directive were implemented in the same year (1986) and given the two groups had Member States in common it is not surprising their contents mirror each other closely in format and content. However, they differ in two significant ways:

(1) Their aims are different. The primary aims of the Convention (for the author at least) appear to be directed to the protection of the animals through the "3 Rs" (Refine, Reduce, Replace) with a desire to make this protection common across Member States. The Directive on the other hand places much more emphasis on the aim for the adoption of approximated laws, regulations, and provisions so as to avoid affecting the establishment and functioning of the common market, in particular by distortions of competition or barriers to trade. It seems to the author that the Directive is more concerned with having a level playing field of conditions than it is with the welfare of the animals it covers.
(2) The second major difference, as alluded to earlier, is the "enforceability" of the Directive through national legislation compared with the Directive. It is a mandatory requirement of the EU that national legislation exists in each Member State to cover all Directives. Compare this to the "gentleman's handshake" of the Convention. Sticks and carrots come to mind!

A project carried out for the Eurogroup for Animal Welfare in 1992[5] reported how slowly some Member States were implementing the Directive either through ongoing lack of national legislation or poor administrative support.

Finally as this chapter is written the Directive is under extensive review and revision with consultation being undertaken with a broad and comprehensive group of stakeholders. The extent of the exercise is too great to consider in this chapter but readers should ensure that when referring specifically to the Directive they have the most current edition. The implementation of any revision is unlikely before 2006.

Before looking at how animal experimentation is controlled in detail, it is useful to briefly review the legislation, regulations, and controls in the USA before directly comparing specific aspects of control. Within the USA basic animal welfare provision is implemented through the Animal Welfare Act (AWA) of 1966 (with subsequent amendments) and the Animal Welfare Regulations (AWR) of 1985. The AWA and AWR set out to protect animal welfare in a number of situations including pet and exhibition animals, as well as animals used in research. Part 2 of the AWR specifically addresses those elements of research, testing, or teaching procedures that involve the care and use of animals.

Regulatory authority under the AWA and AWR is vested in the US Department of Agriculture (USDA) and implemented by the USDA's Animal and Plant Health Inspection Service (APHIS). However, in addition to this broad level of animal welfare control and on a much more active basis users of laboratory animals in the USA use the Institute of Laboratory Animal Resources (ILAR) *Guide for the Care and Use of Laboratory Animals.*[6] The *Guide* was first published in 1963 with several later editions. ILAR is part of the US National Research Council. The *Guide* provides comprehensive advice on the care and use of laboratory animals and is used as the performance standard by the Association for the Assessment and Accreditation of Laboratory Animal Care (International), often referred to as AAALAC. AAALAC is an independent, non-profit-making organization which validates the quality of animal care programs and verifies that they meet or exceed national, European, and international standards. It offers a voluntary, confidential peer-review accreditation process which serves as a valuable adjunct to other quality initiatives and legislation. In reality all publicly funded US laboratories must have AAALAC accreditation in order to obtain funds, and most peer-review journals accepting papers involving the use of live animals insist on accreditation also.

In many ways AAALAC seeks to deliver, in conjunction with the Institutional Animal Care and Use Committee (IACUC), self-regulation with only periodic inspection (annual) of facilities by APHIS. This is in stark contrast to the UK for example where there is intensive pro-active control of animal experimentation by the competent authority (Home Office) with little opportunity for self-regulation.

2.3 Scope of legislation

Whichever country you are in, the legislation controlling the use of animals for experimental and other scientific purposes has a common approach in so much as it covers four categories:

- The work
- The facilities
- The people
- The administration.

2.3.1 The work

Whilst regulations covering the scope of work is a common theme across international legislation there are differences (marked and subtle) in what is "included" and what is "excluded." Some areas such as practising of veterinary medicine, use of animals in teaching or other scientific work (e.g., raising of antibodies), and husbandry procedures on farm animals (e.g., castration) are commonly excluded. Others such as veterinary clinical trials and wildlife investigations requiring the catching, tagging, and release of animals (e.g., birds) may be included in some (national) circumstances, as may be the catching and bleeding and rerelease of semi-domesticated animals. It is essential therefore that when working across international boundaries note is taken of this point and checks are made before embarking on any live animal work.

Next under the heading of the work we must consider the authorization process of work. Whilst again there are too many variations on how each study or experiment is authorized there is, nevertheless, a broadly common approach on how that authorization is considered. This can broadly be called the cost–benefit analysis, i.e., a weighing of the harm to the animal against both the possible benefit resulting from the work and indeed the likelihood of that benefit being materialized.

This weighing of cost–benefit is often referred to as the ethical review. In the USA it is the duty of the IACUC on an experiment-by-experiment basis to authorize work. IACUCs are balanced by having both internal and external lay members as well as interested parties such as a scientist and attending veterinarian. European law is not very specific with regard to the process for authorizing work, leaving individual Member States to incorporate this in national legislation. Hence there is currently wide variation, though this is a specific area likely to come under close scrutiny during the review and revision of the Directive.

I believe there is international consensus on certain considerations of the authorization, that being the consideration of the 3 Rs. I believe there is now universal regard to the principles of the 3 Rs and all authorization processes require some attention to be paid to them.

When giving consideration to authorization, the legal framework must first and foremost define the minimal pain, suffering, distress, or lasting harm which if likely to be inflicted upon the animal will bring it under the controls of the legislation. There are two potential harms to be considered here: first, the potential harm of the procedure itself, e.g., taking a blood sample; second, the potential harm resulting from the procedure, e.g., administration of toxic substances or removal of vital organs. Within Europe at least and partly through the multilateral consultations there is a broad understanding developing on what constitutes the minimal "harm threshold" and it is that "which may cause pain, suffering, distress, or lasting harm equal to, or greater than the insertion of a hollow needle through the integument." It is my belief that in practice this definition is broadly upheld in the USA.

A major consideration under authorization must also be the species to be used. Two points need to be emphasized here. In the USA, rats, mice, and birds are explicitly excluded from the AWA and AWR, which in theory therefore provide them with little or no welfare protection. However, things are nowhere near as bad as this situation may seem. The *Guide* and indeed the AAALAC program explicitly include all birds and rodents, thus ensuring protection for the vast majority of these animals.

The second important point around species selection is that of the use of primates. Whilst in the USA, there is clearly a moral obligation to justify the use of primates, I believe it to be more explicit in European law.

Under the Directive and under the UK's Animals (Scientific Procedures) Act 1986[7] there is a requirement to use the species with the lowest degree of neurophysiological sensitivity, thus implying that primates should be avoided if possible. A fuller description of this requirement can be found in Article 7.3 of the Directive.

Before leaving authorization of work I would like to make two more points. First, with regard to euthanasia. It is my understanding that personal or "project authorizations" of euthanasia are not required under either European or US law. However, in the USA, the *Guide* is explicit in requiring that all methods of euthanasia be consistent with the 1993 *Report of the American Veterinary Medical Association Panel on Euthanasia*.[8] With regard to Europe a similar guide has been published under the EU Commission umbrella.[9] In the UK, the requirements and control of euthanasia is more explicit.[10] All animals must be killed using a Schedule 1 method unless specifically authorized on both project and personal licence.[11]

Finally it is worth noting that there is no international or national law that I am aware of that controls the use of animals for ex vivo tissue experiments over and above the method of killing as described above.

2.3.2 The facilities

With regard to both Europe and the USA three types of facilities are generally recognized with regard to the holding of laboratory animals:

- Breeding establishments
- Supplying establishments
- User establishments.

There is probably good understanding of both breeding and use establishments. With regard to supplying establishments, these are establishments that act as intermediary holding facilities between source and final destination. Such establishments exist for the holding and supply of wild-caught animals and strays (pound animals). Whilst the use of both wild-caught and pound animals is declining, it still does occur.

All types of facilities generally require some form of registration or designation under both European law and the AWA. Such registration is usually consequent to meeting certain conditions and standards. These conditions are then subsequently monitored through an inspection process. The process in the USA is two-tiered with both USDA approval and annual inspections and AAALAC accreditation reapproved every 3 years. Standards and frequency of inspections throughout the EU Member States is generally considered to be extremely variable. In all cases there are published guidelines and codes on the minimal standards of husbandry, housing, and care expected. In the USA it is the *Guide*, in Europe it is Appendix A of the Convention and Annex 1 of the Directive. Within Europe it is common for Member States to have national guidelines or codes of practice based on but not necessarily limited to the provisions of Appendix A/Annex 1.

2.3.3 The people

Generally across all legislation a standard list of roles can be identified:

- Management
- Scientific

- Veterinary
- Technical.

Under management it suffices to say that both European and US law requires the appointment and naming of a senior individual responsible for administering, implementing and resourcing the regulations. In the US this individual is referred to as the Institutional Official, whose primary duty is to appoint an IACUC and oversee its effective operation. The Directive (and Convention) state under Article 16 and 20 respectively that:

The approval or the registration provided in Article 15 shall specify the competent person responsible for the establishment entrusted with the task of administering, or arranging for the administration of, appropriate care to the animals bred or kept in the establishment and of ensuring compliance with the requirements of Article 5 and 14.

Scientific staff includes those individuals responsible for designing, supervising, and reporting experiments but not necessarily personally carrying out the procedures upon the animals. Interestingly in both European and US legislation these individuals are apportioned no specific responsibilities though both the Convention and Directive as well as the US *Guide* make reference to ensuring these people have adequate education and training to ensure they have attained a level of knowledge sufficient for carrying out their tasks.

Veterinary supervision or advice is again explicitly required in both the European legislation and the US *Guide*. Great emphasis is placed upon such supervision within the *Guide* and within the operation of the IACUCs. As a side comment and with regard to veterinary supervision it is very advisable that such professional input is sought from veterinarians with appropriate specialist expertise. This may not always be traditional postgraduate qualifications in laboratory animal medicine, especially when "minority" species are being cared for such as fish, farm animals, or birds, or indeed exotic species such as amphibians and reptiles.

Technical staff refers to those people directly caring for the animals and frequently performing the actual procedures. It is surprising that there is little harmonization either across Europe or between Europe and the USA on a common understanding of the job titles for people engaged in this area of work. As such it is difficult to draw direct comparisons, but at least one can say that the laws and regulations and guidance on both sides of the Atlantic focus upon a requirement to ensure these people have adequate education and training to ensure they can perform their duties and tasks competently.

In closing this consideration of the people aspect I would reinforce the point that the direction and focus of the legislation and regulations are upon ensuring competence through education and training. In this respect I would draw the readers attention to recent recommendations from the Federation of European Laboratory Animal Science Associations (FELASA) with regard to the education and training of the various roles defined within the legislation.[12,13,14]

2.3.4 Administration

We have already touched on the governmental bodies (or competent authorities) responsible for implementing the legislation. Almost universally this falls either to the Ministry of Health (or equivalent) or the Ministry of Agriculture (or equivalent).

Turning to the collection of statistical data with regard to the use of animals, again there are significant differences. Within Europe these differences are being rapidly harmonized with the development of a single collection format. US figures are dramatically biased by the non-collection of rodent and bird use. One area which has yet to be settled between the Convention and the Directive is the frequency of collecting data on animal use. Whilst the Convention requires annual statistical returns the Directive only requires them to be collected every 3 years. This is another area likely to be revised during the review and revision of the Directive.

2.4 Conclusion

In concluding the chapter it is important to emphasize that in formulating, developing and implementing legislation controlling both whether and how animals can be used for scientific purposes it is vital that the underpinning principles discussed earlier continue to applied.

Finally it is essential that everyone before embarking on animal experiments in any given country, ensures they are fully complying with the appropriate laws and regulations.

References

1. Webster J. *Animal Welfare: A Cool Eye Towards Eden.* Oxford, UK: Blackwell Sciences, 1994.
2. *European Convention for the Protection of Vertebrate Animals Used for Experimental and Other Scientific Purposes*, ETS 123. Strasbourg, France: Council of Europe, 1986.
3. Whittaker D. Revision of Appendix A: the process and a cost/benefit analysis – winners and losers? *B&K Science Now* 2002, **11**: 1–5.
4. *Council Directive (86/609/EEC of 24 November 1986) on the approximation of laws, regulations and administrative provisions of the Member States regarding the*

protection of animals used for experimental and other scientific purposes. OJ L358/ 29, 18 December 1986.

5. Nab J, Blom HJM. (1993). *Implementation and Enforcement of EC Directive 86/609 on Animal Experimentation in Portugal, Italy, Greece and Spain*, Final Report of a project initiated by Eurogroup for Animal Welfare and supported by the European Commission. Brussels: Eurogroup for Animal Welfare.

6. National Research Council. *Guide for the Care and Use of Laboratory Animals*. Washington, DC: National Academy Press, 1996.

7. *Animals (Scientific Procedures) Act 1986*. Contained in the *Guidance on the Operation of the Animals (Scientific Procedures) Act 1986*, 2nd edn. London: The Stationary Office, 2002.

8. *Report of the American Veterinary Medical Association (AVMA) Panel on Euthanasia (1993 and later editions)*. *J. Am. Vet. Med. Assoc.* 2000, **202**: 229–249.

9. Recommendations for the Euthanasia of Experimental Animals: Working Party Report for DGX1 of the European Commission to be used with Directive 86/609. *Lab. Anim.* 1996, **30**: 293–316.

10. Recommendations for the Euthanasia of Experimental Animals: Working Party Report for DGX1 of the European Commission to be used with Directive 86/609. *Lab. Anim.* 1997, **31**: 1–32.

11. *The Humane Killing of Animals under Schedule 1 to the Animals (Scientific Procedures) Act 1986: Code of Practice*. London: The Stationary Office, 1997.

12. FELAS recommendations on the education and training of persons working with laboratory animals: Category A & C. *Lab. Anim.* 1995, **29**: 121–131.

13. FELAS recommendations on the education and training of persons working with laboratory animals: Category B. *Lab. Anim.* 2000, **34**: 229–235.

14. FELAS recommendations on the education and training of persons working with laboratory animals: Category D. *Lab. Anim.* 1999, **33**: 1–15.

3

Housing, feeding, and maintenance of rodents

ROBERT W. KEMP

3.1 Introduction

Article 5 in Directive 86/609[1] of the Council of the European Communities
states:

All experimental animals shall be provided with housing, an environment, at least
some freedom of movement, food, water and care which are appropriate to their
health and well being:
   any restriction on the extent to which an experimental animal can satisfy its
physiological and ethological needs shall be limited to the absolute minimum; ...

Animal needs are summarized in a report on farm animals by the Brambell
Committee which referred to the provision of "Five Freedoms."[2] These were
reported as:

   Freedom from malnutrition;
   Freedom from injury and disease;
   Freedom from thermal and physical discomfort;
   Freedom from fear and stress;
   Freedom to express most normal patterns of behaviour.

These freedoms are not confined solely to farm animals but are applicable
to all animals maintained in captivity, including those kept within laboratories
as breeding stock or for experimental use.

The scientist and the animal technician must be constantly aware that
animals housed in the laboratory either for breeding or scientific studies lack
the self-sufficiency of their wild counterparts. They are completely dependent
on him, or her, for all these physiological and ethological needs; they have a
limited ability to vary or improve their environmental conditions by seeking
warmer or cooler areas, are unable to vary their food or seek out additional
supplies should they become depleted, and have no control over access to
liquid as this is usually from a single source; and the space in which they
exercise, mate, and socialize is controlled and confined. Careful and regular

Handbook of Experimental Neurology, ed. Turgut Tatlisumak and Marc Fisher. Published by Cambridge
University Press. © Cambridge University Press 2006.

observation and attention to detail are essential, and remaining up to date with current practices and thinking on the care and use of laboratory animals is vital if we are to ensure that they receive the best possible care.

This chapter is confined to the use of rodents as experimental animals and will concentrate on mice (*Mus musculus*), rats (*Rattus norvegicus*), guinea pigs (*Cavia porcellus*), Syrian hamsters (*Mesocricetus* sp.), and Mongolian gerbils (*Meriones* sp.) Rodents are by far the biggest group of animals used in scientific research. In the UK during the first 4 years of this millennium rodents accounted for around 90% of the total number of animals used for experimental procedures, representing just over 2 million animals per annum. A similar percentage is to be found in other countries producing reports of experimental animal usage.

3.2 Environmental enrichment

Over the last few years there have been major advancements in the design and implementation of improved cages or pens with the aim of providing captive animals with an environment in which they are able to practice their normal behavioral repertoire. The first animals to benefit from the introduction of this environmental enrichment were generally the higher species, kept in captivity in zoos or housed in experimental laboratories. In the latter case laboratory-held New and Old World primates, dogs, and cats are an obvious example. Being generally larger animals with strong links to the wild or, in the case of dogs and cats, a long history of domestication, it is not surprising that much of the early efforts at environmental enrichment were directed at these species. It is easier to observe the effects of social deprivation in the stereotypic behavior of larger animals than it is in the mouse or rat. There is no doubt, however, that rodents also need their surroundings enriched and there is a wealth of evidence and examples to support this – barren metal, mesh rodent cages are, thankfully, becoming a thing of the past.

One of the strongest forms of enrichments for rodents and other animals is the companionship of conspecifics. Unless there are strong compelling scientific reasons all rodents should be kept in stable and harmonious groups. Even hamsters, which have a reputation for preferring a solitary existence, will, if grouped at weaning, live amicably together and benefit from close contact with others. Cage-mates provide opportunities for play, grooming, and other social activities. Rats in particular are extremely gregarious animals and will exhibit marked changes in behavior if deprived of companionship. Aggression when being handled and destructive behavior are two traits which may be encountered. The writer has personal experience of singly housing rats in polypropylene cages as part of a 3-month toxicity study. Several animals developed the knack of gnawing the plastic cage at the point where the automatic drinking nipple entered, even though the edge of the hole was protected by a metal washer. The socially deprived animals simply chewed completely round the washer and escaped through the back of the cage. It was not long before we acceded to the animals' needs and group housing was swiftly introduced! Should individual housing be unavoidable, due to experimental constraints, the introduction of some form of shelter should be introduced to improve the animals' environment. Townsend reported increased exploratory behavior in singly housed rats when provided with an upturned mouse cage within their home cage and observed the rats to be less fearful when compared with the control group who had no such enrichment.[3] Some species/strains, however, may fail to live in harmony and segregation is necessary to avoid serious, if not fatal, consequences. Male mice, gerbils, and hamsters can sometimes fall into this category, particularly if groups are formed once they have reached adulthood.

If we study the normal behaviors of wild rodents, together with the behavior of laboratory rodents released into a quasi-wild environment it becomes quickly apparent that one of their main activities is that of seeking nourishment.[4] Unfortunately, hunting for food is not a behavior that can easily be provided for in the relatively close confines of the laboratory cage. Gnawing animals such as the rats, mice, and hamsters can be made to work for their food supply by offering it in a wire-mesh hopper at high level. Guinea pigs, however, are unable to feed in this manner and are usually fed in an open dish or trough and their food is, therefore, easily and quickly obtained. In both these cases animals will spend much less time hunting and eating food than those exposed to an outside environment and must, therefore, be offered some form of compensatory activity. Key proposed the introduction of forage grains or pellets in addition to the animals' normal pelleted diet.[5] He reports that some diet manufacturers are considering producing standard rodent diet in a much smaller pellet form. These may be mixed with clean bedding and placed in a container within the animal's cage. If this is not an option consideration should be given to the introduction of enrichment objects to satisfy the inherent gnawing behavior of rodents. These should be safe and hygienic for the animals, economical, and adequately stimulating, but should require little or no increase in the work load of the animal technicians.[6,7,8] Many different objects made of a variety of materials have been tried by a number of researchers but the ones that appears to be the most popular are wooden blocks or sticks. Small wooden blocks drilled with holes are chewed fairly rapidly before they can become significantly soiled.[9] Eskola and Kaliste-Korhonen recommended the use of aspen gnawing blocks especially for animals held in grid-floored cages.[10] These are available from many specia-lized laboratory suppliers and can be bought together with a full quality assurance certificate.

Different enrichment objects have been used to cater for other types of normal behavior. The European Commission's international workshop on the *Accommodation of Laboratory Animals in Accordance with Animal Welfare Requirements*[11] recommended "there should be room for hiding or escape from conspecifics within the cage." There was also reference made to breaking up the cage into "structural divisions," a point that was discussed in the UK Home Office *Code of Practice for the Housing and Care of Animals in Designated Breeding and Supplying Establishments.*[12] The provision of baffles, barriers, shelters, and retreats in mouse caging is recommended in the report of the Laboratory Animal Science Association on Rodent Refinement.[13] The inclusion of cardboard tubes, or "fun tunnels" as they have become known, or other structures of many differing materials, has become fairly widespread in both breeder and user establishments. As well as providing an area in which the animals can shelter from the unwanted attentions of fellow cage-mates, such objects have the added attraction that many also satisfy the rodent's gnawing behavior and, over a period of days or weeks, are gradually destroyed. Structures within the cage also increase the available floor area, providing opportunities for the animals to use both horizontal and vertical dimensions and to demonstrate a range of behaviors.

The provision of bedding material, such as wood flakes, shredded paper, or some other substrate, in a solid-bottom cage allows rodents the freedom to explore, burrow, and construct nests, all of which are behaviors demonstrated in the wild. Gerbils in particular have a strong burrowing instinct which has been developed in the wild to give protection from their predators. In the laboratory environment they require a greater depth of bedding than other rodents, as being deprived of the ability to practice this behavior leads to unwanted stereotypic digging. As gerbils spend much of their time sitting in an erect position they should be provided with ample space between the bed-ding and the top of the cage to allow them to assume this position. Normally 15 cm is seen to be adequate.

A variety of bedding and nesting materials are available and careful thought should be given in their selection to ensure the one chosen meets the needs of both scientist and the animals. It is advisable to carry out some form of preference testing, no matter how simple, to evaluate various materials before making a financial commitment. What the scientist perceives to be a suitable substrate may be viewed in a completely different light by the animals living in it! For instance Patterson-Kane *et al.* surprisingly reported a strong preference on the behalf of rats for shredded document paper over tissue paper,[14] which may be perceived by many of us to be softer and therefore, more comfortable. Guinea pigs should be given access to a regular source of good-quality, clean meadow hay. Anyone working with these animals will readily confirm the amount of pleasure this provides, something that is easily recognized by the amount of extra activity and vocalization seen and heard when the hay barrow enters the room. As well as providing an excellent source of enrichment hay has the additional benefit of supplying the animals with an extra source of fiber which can help to alleviate the risk of enteric problems.

Lighting levels within animal rooms are normally a compromise, between that which enables staff to easily and safely carry out their daily tasks and that which is tolerable by, and unlikely to cause harm to, the animals. Rodents are naturally crepuscular or nocturnal animals and the lighting levels within their rooms are normally set higher than that preferred by the animals. It is desirable to provide some sort of filter or shelter to reduce light exposure to a level which is not likely to cause any long-term physiological damage, particularly to albino animals.[15] Provision of tinted plastic cages, or the inclusion of free-standing or fixed shelters, are aimed at reducing light intensity within the cage, or parts of it, without adversely affecting the ability of staff to observe the animals. Wadsworth and Priest reported greater utilization of the floor area of tinted polycarbonate cages by rats due to the lower lighting levels when compared with rats housed in similar-sized transparent plastic cages where the rear of the cage was favored.[16] Key and Hewitt described the introduction of a red-tinted plastic cage insert to provide a dark shelter area. This, they hoped, would reduce the aggression amongst mice that had been reported when transparent pipes had been used as enrichment objects. Inclusion of the "mouse house" resulted in significant increases in a number of positive behaviors and significant reductions in several negative behaviors.[17]

It is worth giving a word of caution regarding the introduction of environmental enrichment objects, indiscriminately or otherwise, into the cages of experimental animals. Applebee suggests an assessment of environmental enrichment using five criteria: (1) does it frustrate the research; (2) does it increase positive behavior; (3) does it increase adverse behavior; (4) is it practical; (5) is it affordable?[18] Great care must be taken not to compromise the scientific integrity of any study which could ultimately lead to an unacceptable wastage of animals. There is now a good supply of well-tested and validated enrichment objects obtainable from a number of reputable laboratory animal supply establishments. Many of these are deemed to be Good Laboratory Practice (GLP) compliant and are available with certificates of analysis. However Eskola *et al.* introduced a word of caution by showing the introduction of environmental objects, namely aspen blocks and a tube of dried aspen board, seemed to increase within-group variation, mainly of enzyme parameters. This could result in the need to increase the number of animals used in order to obtain statistically significant results.[19]

3.3 Caging

Traditionally, rodents are normally housed in plastic polycarbonate or polypropylene solid-floored cages or in stainless steel caging with a mesh floor. There is much evidence to suggest that solid-floored caging is favored by the animals, and when rats are housed within such cages they are less troubled with injuries and sores of the feet.[20] Until recently mesh-floored rodent cages were strongly favored, particularly by toxicologists, as they allowed easy observation of abnormal urine and feces, enabled food wastage measurements, and minimized interference with experimental results caused by the inclusion of bedding material in the cage. With the advent of cleaner, standardized, quality-assured and certificated bedding and nesting products, to exacting GLP standards, coupled with a better understanding of the welfare needs of laboratory rodents it is pleasing to see that even the strongest advocates of mesh flooring are being convinced that the welfare of animals can be improved, without compromising the integrity of the science. Preference testing studies clearly showed that given the choice between resting on a solid-floored area or a mesh floor laboratory rats had strong preference for the former.[21] A similar preference for solid floors has also been demonstrated in the Syrian hamster[22] and in mice.[23] Rodents in experimental studies should only be housed on mesh-floored cages when there are strong compelling scientific reasons for doing so and then only for the shortest time possible. Should it be necessary to house rodents in such cages, for example in a timed mating program during which identification of vaginal plugs is necessary, consideration should be given to providing some solid-floored area, in the form of a cage insert or shelf, which the animals may use as a resting area.[24]

Overcrowding of animals within the cage must be avoided as this may influence many physiological and behavioral systems. Increased stress leading to aggression, reduction in body weight, reduced food intake, decreased fertility, and higher mortality have all been attributed to restricted living conditions. Although there appears to be a paucity of scientific data on the ideal space allocation required for the various rodent species there are various guidance documents available providing information on amount of floor area and cage height that should be allowed for stock, experimental and breeding animals. The Council of Europe Convention ETS 123 Appendix A provides guidance on the care and accommodation of animals used for experimental or other scientific purposes.[25] Currently, this document is under review and it is expected the final version will be published later in the year. In the UK the Home Office publishes a code of practice for the housing and care of animals housed in experimental establishments which, together with comprehensive notes on the maintenance of a range of laboratory species, provides tables of the individual floor area required by animals at different body weights; a similar code is produced for animals housed in breeding or supplying establishments.[12] The Institute of Animal Resources in the USA has produced the *Guide for the Care and Use of Laboratory Animals*[26] and in Canada similar guidance is available from the Canadian Council on Animal Care.[27] It should be pointed out that it is not just the amount of space allocated to each animal that will result in their contentment. Animals kept in large cages with vast areas of space are just as likely to suffer and display stereotypic behaviors as their overcrowded counterparts. It is the quality of the space provided and the use it is put to by the animal that is all-important, not the quantity![28]

Height of the rodent cage is perhaps easier to define than their need for floor area. At all stages of the animal's life it should have sufficient headroom to rear up fully on its hind legs. Some designs of caging have internal shelves which not only provide the animals with the opportunity to climb and use vertical space but also add to the total floor area available to them. The guidance documents mentioned above provide details of minimum cage heights for rodent species together with the recommended floor area for individual animals and those that are group housed.

3.4 Environmental control

The environment within rodent rooms should be carefully controlled in order to provide conditions favorable to the animals during various stages of their lives whilst at the same time presenting the scientist with the stable milieu necessary for the experiment. The various guidance documents mentioned in the previous section provide information on the acceptable environmental parameters – temperature, relative humidity, ventilation, light intensity and duration, noise levels – for the commonly used rodent species, and there appears to be a great deal of correlation between them. The ranges listed in these documents are levels to be provided in the room itself (macroenvironment) and, in the case of some parameters, will differ considerably from those experienced by the animals within the confines of their cage (microenvironment). The magnitude of this difference will be dependent on the design and construction of housing employed, being generally greater for most of the environmental factors under discussion when cages or pens with solid sides and bottom are employed.

Clough demonstrated the considerable differences between room and cage conditions and how this was influenced by cage design, structure, and, for some parameters, position of the cage within the room or rack.[29]

3.4.1 Temperature

The temperature within rodent rooms should be carefully controlled within fairly narrow limits and monitored on, at least, a daily basis. Modern heating and ventilation plant and building construction materials should result in stable room temperatures easily maintained within a range of $\pm2\,°C$. This degree of control is often thought to be more important, for both the health of the animals and experimental consistency, than the optimum target temperature selected. Rodents, in general, appear to enjoy similar environmental temperature requirements and these are normally within the 19–23 °C range.

Temperatures outside of this range may, however, be needed in special circumstances. In particular animals recovering from major surgery or those bred for a lack of hair will demand higher temperatures as will, of course, neonates which are incapable of regulating their body temperature, although this may often be achieved by the addition of extra bedding material.

3.4.2 Relative humidity

It is not usually possible to maintain the relative humidity (RH) within the animal room with the same degree of precision as the temperature. Much wider fluctuations will be experienced though these will normally have no adverse effects on the animals. An acceptable range for rodents is 45–65%. Values outside this range can favor the proliferation of certain airborne pathogens resulting in health problems.[29] There is an increased incident of ringtail in rats when maintained in rooms with an RH of less than 40%.[30] This is prevalent in young newly weaned animals, particularly those recently transferred from the higher RH microenvironment of a breeding cage with solid walls and floor to a mesh caging system. The condition is easily recognizable as a series of constrictions that appear at the base of the animal's tail. In severe cases the complete tail may become necrotic and slough off.

3.4.3 Ventilation

The ventilation rate required in an animal room to distribute quality warm or, in summer, chilled air and to remove noxious vapors is related to the animal stocking density. An air change rate of 15–20 per hour is usually adequate, although it is acceptable to reduce this rate in partially stocked rooms. An important consideration in rodent rooms is that of laboratory animal allergy and all efforts should be made to reduce the airborne allergen burden in areas occupied by humans. In the animal room a directional flow of air, entering above the working environment, passing over the staff, through the animal cages before exhausting from the room may help to reduce staff exposure to these harmful allergens. The supply inlets and extract vents should be sized and positioned in such a way that drafts are avoided in all parts of the room.

3.4.4 Light

Two aspects of room lighting need to be considered: light duration (or photoperiod) and light intensity. Both are particularly important to the well-being of nocturnal or crepuscular species. Retinal damage can be caused by excessive light, measured either in length of exposure or in its intensity. Young reported renewal of both rods and cones during periods of darkness[31] and Weihe reported an increase in light-induced retinal damage in albino animals in which the dark recovery period was too short.[32] In rooms housing experimental rodents it is normal to operate a photoperiod of 12 hours light and 12 hours darkness whilst in breeding colonies the light period may be increased up to 14 hours.

Lighting intensity can often be a compromise between that which can be tolerated by the animals and that which is acceptable to the staff working with them. The lighting levels needed by staff to carry out their husbandry and experimental functions in a safe and effective manner are often much higher than that which can be tolerated by the animals without adverse effects. A level of 300–400 lux is required by the staff working within the animal room, whereas at the microenvironmental level this should be considerably lower to avoid harm to the animals, particularly albino strains. Clough tabulates references to harmful effects on rats and mice at lighting intensity in excess of 60 lux at the cage level.[29] Clough and Donnelly and Weihe *et al.* emphasize the wide variation in lighting levels within cages dependent on their position on the rack, closeness to the lighting source, and the material out of which the cages are constructed.[33,34] This variation can exceed an 80-fold difference at cage-floor level from the top to bottom of a rack of cages constructed from translucent polypropylene and a 13-fold difference in transparent polycarbonate cages.

3.4.5 Noise

There is a wealth of anecdotal evidence in support of the use of background music for animal rooms on the grounds that this will assist in masking other loud and/or unexpected sounds. Whereas this may be true for some species there does not appear to be any sound scientific evidence to support the use of sound systems within rodent rooms. In fact Pfaff and Stecken point out the usefulness of this constant artificial background noise, to the animals or the science, is severely limited as the majority of it occurs at a frequency imperceptible to the rodent ear.[35] The major benefits of this addition to the environment within the rodent animal room appears to be limited, therefore, to the scientific and technical staff! If it is deemed necessary to introduce a sound system it should, in the interests of standardization, be centrally controlled and certainly not within reach of those working in the animal rooms. Changes in the volume or type of music or the ability to turn it off should not be options.

The UK Home Office suggests there will be no damage to animals if the general background sound level within an empty animal room is kept below about 50 dB, below a noise rating curve of 25, and free from distinct tonal content.[12] Rodents can be affected by high-frequency noises, undetectable by the human ear. In determining the noise within the animal room it is, therefore, important to assess both intensity and frequency levels. Any source of unwanted ultrasound should be identified, and reduced or eliminated. Fire alarms are available for rodent units with an alarm tone pitched at a low frequency which, whilst audible to staff working in the area, is undetectable by the animals.

3.5 Husbandry provisions

3.5.1 *Feeding and watering*

There are many commercially produced rodent diets with a formula balanced so as to provide all a particular species needs, available in either an extruded cube or expanded form. Normally, for ease, these diets are fed on an ad libitum basis but this can, however, result in obesity in later life. Maintenance diets, in which protein levels are reduced, are available to combat this condition and may be considered for animals on long-term studies.

With the exception of the guinea pig rodents can be offered their diet in wire baskets. With their strong gnawing ability they can cope with all but the hardest of cubes. Guinea pigs, however, will require a much smaller cube or pellet and this should be presented in a gravity-fed hopper or an open dish or bowl. There is a tendency for guinea pigs to scratch diet out of the food receptacle leading to high wastage levels. This can be a problem in cages where there is little or no form of environmental enrichment. The addition of hay may help to alleviate this particular problem, or the food hopper may be modified with the addition of wire bars, which, whilst making it impossible for the guinea pig to scratch out the diet will not prevent it feeding. Guinea pigs are unusual amongst the rodents in that, like primates, they require a daily dietary source of vitamin C. This may be provided by dietary supplements of vegetables or fruit, addition of ascorbic acid to the drinking water, or inclusion by the manufacturer in the standard pelleted diet. If the latter option is selected it may result in this diet having a shorter shelf storage time than that of other rodent diets. The diet manufacturer should be consulted if there is an intention to autoclave the diet prior to use so that additional ascorbic acid can be included to counteract the losses resulting from the autoclaving process.

Rodents are coprophagic. Fecal pellets are removed directly from the anus and reingested, providing an additional source of B vitamins and improved utilization of protein.

Fluid requirements of rodents vary but it is essential that clean water is available at all times, supplied from either a bottle or an automatic supply. Hamsters and gerbils are, due to their desert origins, more adept at water conservation that other rodents. They can cope with less water intake and conserve fluids by producing very concentrated urine. The guinea pig on the other hand is extremely wasteful, allowing water to dribble away during drinking, or resting its body, obliviously, against the drinking nipple or bottle spout.

3.5.2 Cage cleaning

The frequency with which this task is carried out depends on a number of factors: the type of bedding material used; the number of animals in the cage; the species housed; the use of the animals. Some bedding materials will actively inhibit the release of ammonia and, as mentioned in the previous section, hamsters and gerbils produce drier feces and less urine than other rodents, leading to the possibility of a less frequent changing regime. Too frequent change cleaning can result in problems, particularly amongst mice. Pheromones are important in the mouse colony as they help to maintain stability within the cage. Their frequent removal can result in an increased incident of both fighting and "barbering" – a condition in which the dominant animals within the cage pluck hair from their subordinates. This appears to be a bigger problem in establishments that change both the bedding and the cage together, effectively removing all scent markers. The problem may be alleviated by retaining a small portion of soiled bedding, or transferring environmental enrichment objects from the soiled to the new cage.

3.6 Summary

Much has been said about the rights and wrongs of using animals in scientific
research and it is not within the remit of the author to expand on this or make
comment. Suffice it to say that failure to meet the needs of animals as listed in
the "five freedoms" would be a failure to exercise our ethical responsibilities
towards their use. It is worth quoting David Mellor, former Under Secretary
of State in the UK Home Office during the implementation of the Animals
(Scientific Procedures) Act 1986, who said at a British Veterinary Association
Congress: "The use of animals for experiments is a privilege, not a right. To
abuse this privilege or take it for granted is unforgivable." Although Mellor's
remark was confined to animals used in scientific procedures we can, and must,
extend it to encompass all animals used, bred, or held in readiness for use in the
laboratory or at the breeding establishment. Whilst our moral obligations to
the humane use of laboratory animals should always be our first priority it
should also be remembered that failing to satisfy both the physiological and
ethological needs of animals will result in their poor health which in turn may
well lead to poor experimental conclusions.

References

1. *Council Directive (86/609/EEC of 24 November 1986) on the approximation
   of laws, regulations and administrative provisions of the Member States regarding
   the protection of animals for experimental and other scientific purposes. OJ* L358/29,
   18 December 1986.
2. Harrison R. Special address. *Appl. Anim. Behav. Sci.* 1988, **20**: 21–27.
3. Townsend P. Use of in-cage shelters by laboratory rats. *Anim. Welfare* 1997,
   6: 95–103.
4. Berdoy M. *The Laboratory Rat: A Natural History.* (Film, 27 min.), 2002.
   Available online at http://www.ratlife.org
5. Key D. Environmental enrichment options for laboratory rats and mice. *Lab.
   Anim. Europe* 2004, **4**: 30–38.
6. Chamove AS. Environmental enrichment: a review. *Anim. Technol.* 1989,
   40: 155–178.
7. Cubitt S. Environmental enrichment for rats. *Reg. Anim. Technic.* 2, 1992.
8. Oruk-Edem E, Key D. Response of rats (*Rattus norvegicus*) to enrichment objects.
   Anim. Technol. 1994, **45**: 25–30.
9. Chmeil Jr D, Noonan M. Preference of laboratory rats for potentially enriching
   stimulus objects. *Lab. Anim.* 1996, **30**: 97–101.
10. Eskola S, Kaliste-Korhonen E. Effects of cage type and gnawing blocks on weight
    gain, organ weights and open-field behaviour in Wistar rats. *Scand. J. Anim. Sci.*
    1998, **25**: 180–193.
11. Brain PF. Rodents. In O'Donaghue PN (ed.) *International Workshop on the
    Accommodation of Laboratory Animals in Accordance with Animal Welfare*

Requirements, Berlin 17–19 May 1993. Bonn, Germany: Bundersministerium fur Erahrung, Landwirtschat und Forster, 1995, pp. 1–14.

12. Home Office. *Code of Practice for the Housing and Care of Animals in Designated Breeding and Supplying Establishments*. London: The Stationary Office, 1996.

13. Report of the rodent refinement working party. *Lab. Anim.* 1998, **32**: 233–239.

14. Patterson-Kane EC, Harper DN, Hunt M. The cage preferences of laboratory rats. *Lab. Anim.* 2001, **35**: 74–79.

15. Schlingmann F, De Rijk SHLM, Pereboom WJ, Remie R. Light intensity in animal rooms and cages in relation to the care and management of albino rats. *Anim. Technol.* 1993, **44**: 97–107.

16. Wadsworth M, Priest D. A comparison of conventional caging materials with respect to light level intensities. Poster at the Institute of Animal Technology Congress, Jersey, 1998.

17. Key D, Hewett A. Developing and testing a novel cage insert, the "Mouse House", designed to enrich the lives of laboratory mice without adversely affecting the science. *Anim. Technol.* 2002, **1**: 55–64.

18. Applebee K. Rodent environmental enrichment: animal welfare or human feel-good factor? *Anim. Technol.* 2002, **1**: 65 69.

19. Eskola S, Lauhikari M, Voipio H-M, Laitinen M, Nevalainen T. Environmental enrichment may alter the number of rats needed to achieve statistical significance. *Scand. J. Lab. Anim. Sci.* 1999, **26**: 134–144.

20. Manser CE, Morris TH, Broom DM. An investigation into the effects of solid or grid cage flooring on the welfare of laboratory rats. *Lab. Anim.* 1995, **29**: 353–363.

21. Manser CE, Elliot H, Morris TH, Broom DM. The use of a novel operant test to determine the strength of preference for flooring in laboratory rats. *Lab. Anim.* 1996, **30**: 1–6.

22. Arnold C, Gillaspy S. Assessing laboratory life for Golden Hamsters; social preference, caging, selection and human interaction. *Lab. Anim.* 1994, **23**: 34–37.

23. Schlingmann F, van de Weerd HA, Blom HJM, Baumanns V, van Zutphen LFM. Behavioural differentiation of mice housed on different cage floors. *5th FELAS Symposium: Welfare and Science*, 1993, pp. 355–357.

24. Olfert ED, Cross BM, McWilliam AA. *Guide to the Care and Use of Experimental Animals*. Ottawa, Ontario: Canadian Council on Animal Care, 1993.

25. Council of Europe *European Convention for the Protection of Vertebrate Animals used for Experimental or other Scientific Purposes*. Strasbourg, France: Council of Europe, 1986.

26. Institute of Laboratory Animal Resources. *Guide for the Care and Use of Laboratory Animals*. Washington, DC: National Academy Press, 1996.

27. Canadian Council on Animal Care. *Guide to the Care and Use of Experimental Animals*, 2nd edn, 2 vols. Ottawa, Ontario: Canadian Council on Animal Care, 1993.

28. Bantin GC, Sanders PD. Animal caging: is big necessarily better? *Anim. Technol.* 1989, **40**: 45–54.

29. Clough G. Environmental factors in relation to the comfort and well-being of laboratory rats and mice. In *Standards in Laboratory Animal Management*. Potters Bar, UK: Universities Federation for Animal Welfare, 1984, pp. 7–24.

30. Flynn RJ. Notes on ringtail in rats. In Conalty ML (ed.) *Husbandry of Laboratory Animals, 3rd International Symposium of the International Committee on Laboratory Animals*. London: Academic Press, 1967.

31. Young RW. Renewal systems in rods and cones. *Ann. Opthalmol.* 1973,
5: 843–854.

32. Weihe WH. The effect of light on animals. In: McSheehy T (ed.) *Control of the
Animal House Environment*. London: Laboratory Animals Ltd, 1976, pp. 63–76.

33. Clough G, Donnelly HT. Light intensity influences the oestrous cycle of LACA
mice. *Proceedings UFAW/LASA Joint Symposium on Standards in Laboratory
Animal Management*, 1983, p. 60.

34. Weihe WH, Schidlow J, Strittmatter J. The effect of lighting intensity on the
breeding and development of rats and golden hamsters. *Int. J. Biometeorol.* 1969,
13: 69–79.

35. Pfaff J, Stecker M. Loudness level and frequency content of noise in the animal
house. *Lab. Anim.* 1976, **10**: 111–117.

4

Identification of individual animals

TURGUT TATLISUMAK AND DANIEL STRBIAN

Most experiments necessitate the use of several animals simultaneously. Especially when the animals are randomized to different groups that receive different treatments, it becomes crucial to be able to recognize different animals at different time points all along the experiments. Just placing the animals in different cages alone or in groups with the cages numbered or posted otherwise is not a reliable enough procedure. It is always necessary to mark the individual animals in a reliable way. It is of utmost important that all researchers in the same laboratory or institution follow the same marking system to avoid confusion. Large amounts of work and animals may be lost if this issue is overlooked. Marking animals for later identification can be done with various methods as long as the researchers are familiar with the marking system, enabling the correct animals to be tracked until the end of the experiment. There are a number of commercially available instruments for this purpose.

4.1 Dyes

Waterproof pens (permanent markers) in various colors are available in most stationers and bookstores. Marking of the tail is easy even in awake animals. The dye lasts for several days but not longer. The dye should be applied all around the tail, thickly and widely to assure future identification and to avoid misinterpretation. The color and the mark can easily be seen in albino animals, but may be more difficult to interpret in wild-type animals. We have not observed any inter-observer difficulty. This method is very suitable for short-term experiments (a few days). If the experiment lasts longer, the mark should be redone at regular intervals. It is easy, inexpensive, and reliable. As it is a non-invasive marking method, it is completely stress-free for the animal. However, only up to 10 animals can be marked this way (Fig. 4.1), but using different colors for different groups or at different days of the week, the number of marked animals can be multiplied several-fold.

Coloration of hair with similar pens or with human hair dye is also a reliable marking method for short-term experiments (Fig. 4.2). Using different colors

Handbook of Experimental Neurology, ed. Turgut Tatlisumak and Marc Fisher. Published by Cambridge University Press. © Cambridge University Press 2006.

(a)

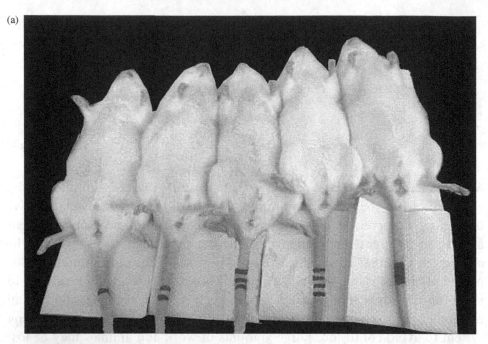

(b)

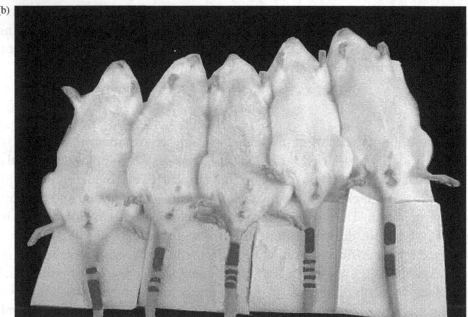

Figure 4.1. Tail-marking is the most commonly used marking method in albino rats. A simple 1 to 10 marking system is demonstrated. Use of various colors increases the number of animals in the same experiment. At least red, green, blue, and black colors are available.

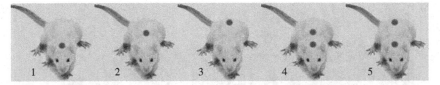

Figure 4.2. A quick and easy animal marking system that can be used in awake animals. Number 1 is on the top of the head, number 2 at the middle of the back, and number 3 is close to the root of the tail. Only a few animals can be marked with this method and the dye fades in days.

increases the number of animals that can be marked in an individual experiment, but red should not be used with green because of the likelihood of confusion by color-blind people. However, this method is again limited to albino animals.

4.2 Ear punching

Ear punching is a reliable method for the permanent marking of animals. This method is especially useful in long-term experiments and in wild-type animals in which hair- or tail-marking are not obvious because of the dark color of the skin and the fur. There are a number of commercially available ear punches in different sizes and shapes (Fig. 4.3). The ear punch can be wedge-shaped (triangular) or circular. Even though ear punching is believed to be painless, if the experiment necessitates anesthesia or sedation, it is recommended to make the punching during that time. The marking may not be easily recognizable later if the animal moves during the procedure. A cheap way is to use a pair of sharp scissors for marking the ears. This marking method is suitable for experiments with large numbers of animals, because depending on the side (left–right), location, and the number of punches, several hundreds of animals can be marked (Fig. 4.4). If the study protocol necessitates the use of both male and female animals, males can be numbered oddly and females can be numbered evenly. However, animals do fight with each other, especially mice. The marked ear might be torn during fights and recognition of the animal may be jeopardized.

4.3 Ear tags

Rats especially can be individually marked and identified using small metal ear tags. Because the metal tag will irritate the animal, many animals remove their tags. Tags contain individual numbers and therefore can be used to identify

Turgut Tatlisumak and Daniel Strbian

(a)

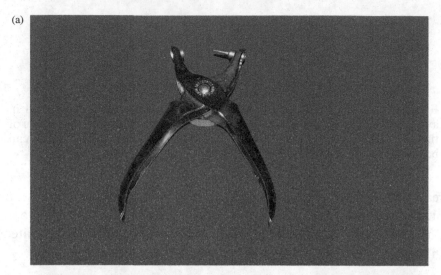

(b)

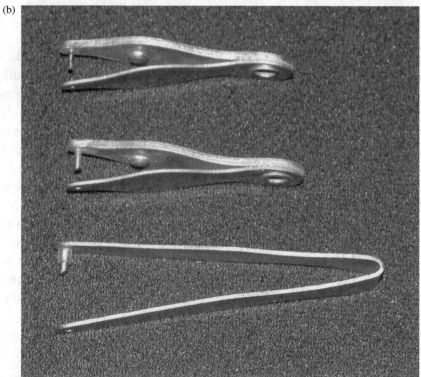

Figure 4.3. Ear punches in different shapes and sizes. They are all metallic in construction and very durable. They are available in different models so that the size and the shape of the punch vary. We have not experienced rusting. (Photographs courtesy of Dr Mara S Potter and Harvard Apparatus, Cambridge, MA.)

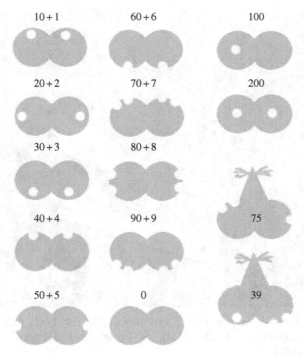

Figure 4.4. The most commonly used ear punch numbering system in the rat and mouse. No punches are "zero." Numbers 1 to 9 are marked on the left ear and tens are marked on the right ear. If necessary, males are numbered with odd and females with even numbers. This easy and low-cost system allows for marking to 299. There are some extensions of this numbering system, but they are seldom necessary.

several hundred animals. The size of ordinary tags is appropriate for rats, but not for mice or neonatal rats. Newer, smaller-sized tags have also recently been introduced and they can be used for mice and neonatal rats as well (Fig. 4.5). The weight of the tag should be taken into consideration. The animals might become sensitive to the metal used as most tags contain aluminum. The procedure is relatively simple: a hole is made in the animal's ear with an ear punch. The metal tag with or without a colored washer is inserted through the hole and the prongs of the ear tag are bent flat in opposite directions.

4.4 Removing digits

This procedure is used for neonatal rodents, especially for the wild-type animals, since alternative methods are lacking. One or more digits from one or more feet are removed using sharp scissors. The procedure is simple, but most likely painful. Albino neonates can be marked with coloring. Extensive

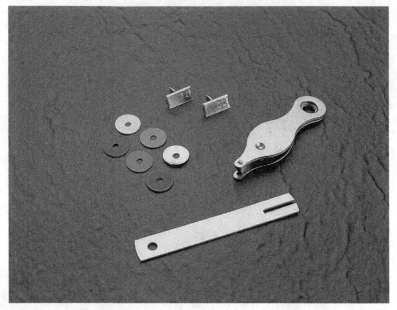

Figure 4.5. Ear tagging instrumentation suitable for both mice and rats. (Photograph courtesy of Dr Mara S Potter and Harvard Apparatus, Cambridge, MA.)

handling of neonatal animal may lead to rejection of the neonate by its mother and the mother might cannibalize her baby. This method is also used for later identification of wild rodents in field research. Alternative methods are either too expensive (electronic transponders) or not reliable (ear tags). Even if done under general anesthesia or sedation and local anesthesia, postoperative pain will still be considerably intense.

4.5 Tattooing

Permanent tattooing can be applied to ears or to the tail. There are manual and electronic tattooing methods. Tattooing ink comes in various colors. Tattooing pinchers are easy to use. The number or letter to be applied is selected, ink is applied to the surface, and the ear is squeezed with the pincher. Electronic tattooing sets offer more numbers, letters, and symbols. They also make it possible to mark other regions such as the tail.

4.6 Electronic tagging

Mice and rats can be tagged permanently with a subcutaneous microchip identification device. The microchip can be placed under the skin either by a relatively quick and limited surgical procedure or with a dedicated syringe system. The new chips are about 1 cm in size and can safely be applied to mice. The chip should always be placed in a standard region for recovering and reusing later. Each microchip has an individual number. When the reader device is placed close to the animal, the reader will identify the tag number. This method is currently used in larger-scale field research.

Acknowledgments

The authors thank Dr Mara S Potter and Harvard Apparatus (Massachusetts, USA) for providing some of the figures. This work was supported in part by the Helsinki University Central Hospital, the University of Helsinki, the Finnish Medical Foundation, the Sigrid Juselius Foundation, and the Maire Taponen Foundation, all located in Helsinki, Finland.

5

Analgesia, anesthesia, and postoperative care in laboratory animals

NAOYA MASUTOMI AND MAKOTO SHIBUTANI

5.1 Overview

Anesthesia in experimental animals is essential for both humane and scientific reasons to reduce or eliminate the pain and anxiety derived from physiological examinations or surgical treatments. Anesthesia also helps to immobilize animals to minimize the risk of injurious animal movements that could affect the outcome of experiments. Use of anesthesia should always be considered whenever experimental procedure accompanies the risk for animals to be caused pain or stress. Anesthetic agent is delivered either by injection or inhalation. Of those that are given by injection, the action may be local or systemic.

For clarity, the following terms are defined:

Sedation/tranquilization is a state of mild central depression in which the animal is awake and calm.

Analgesia refers to a temporal reduction of pain sensation accompanied by a trance-like neurolepsis, which is a state of depressed awareness of the surroundings.

Anesthesia is defined as a temporal and reversible reduction or elimination of feeling or sensation, often accompanied by loss of consciousness. When anesthesia is required, the purpose and extent of experimental procedure to be performed should be evaluated in order to determine if analgesia, sedation, or surgical anesthesia would be appropriate for a given procedure.

Many of the drugs used for anesthesia, such as opioids and barbiturates, are controlled and regulated by law. Information on controlled drug registration and also institutional/university policy should be obtained before starting to experiment. Licenses are needed to purchase these agents, and written records on purchase, storage, use, and disposal of them must be kept in a file.

To achieve a successful surgical treatment, appropriate management of preoperative medication, systemic anesthesia, monitoring of anesthesia, and

Handbook of Experimental Neurology, ed. Turgut Tatlisumak and Marc Fisher. Published by Cambridge University Press. © Cambridge University Press 2006.

postoperative care is essential. Guidance for each step is provided in the following sections. In addition, guidance for local anesthesia and fetal and neonatal anesthesia are provided in the latter sections.

5.2 Preoperative medication

Before anesthetic treatment, use of preanesthetic agents, such as anticholinergics and sedative agents, often serves beneficial effects to lessen the severity of side effects and to promote the anesthetic response. Representative preanesthetic agents and their recommended dosages in laboratory rodents and rabbits are listed in Table 5.1.[1–5]

Anticholinergics retain advantages for reducing the side effects induced by anesthetic treatment, such as vagal bradycardia and excess salivation or bronchial mucus secretion. Atropine sulfate is infrequently used in rodents and rabbits because of the rapid disappearance of the effect due to serum and tissue atropine esterases in these species.[6] Glycopyrrolate (Robinul®) would be preferred in these species.[7]

Sedative agents, such as diazepam (Valium®), and other benzodiazepines or phenothiazines including acepromazine, are often the choice to calm the animals. They have excellent sedative properties as well as muscle relaxation. They have no analgesic activity but reduce the catecholamine release and thus the anesthetic dose to promote a more successful induction of anesthesia.[8]

- Fentanyl-fluanisone (Hypnorm®), a neuroleptic opioid, would be the first choice for induction of sedation in rodents. The effect is mediated through the opiate receptor in the central nervous system (CNS). It also provides analgesia, to some extent, so that the skin biopsy or cardiac puncture can be performed.[9] This agent may repress respiration at high dose, and this repression can be antagonized by the administration of μ-opioid antagonist such as nalbuphine (Table 5.2).
- Medetomidine (Dormitor®) is a thiazine derivative to act as an α_2-adrenergic agonist. It induces a light to deep sedation to animals and loss of righting reflex at high dose. It also generates analgesia, but it is not enough for any invasive operation. Its sedative effect is helpful for procedures without accompanying pain including an X-ray exposure.[10] This agent is very useful in combination with other drugs, like ketamine for anesthesia in rodents. The effect of medetomidine can be reversed with yohimbine (0.2 mg/kg, i.v., 0.5 mg/kg, i.m.) or atipamezole (0.1–1 mg/kg, i.v./i.m./i.p./s.c.).

If the risk of postoperative infection is considered, antibiotics should be administered sufficiently in advance of a surgical procedure in order to obtain optimal blood levels. It is noteworthy that rodents are generally highly resistant to postoperative infection and may require only a single bolus dose of antibiotics.[11]

Table 5.1. *Representative preanesthetics and their recommended dosages in rodents and rabbits*

Agent	Dosage[a,b]	Species[c]
Tranquilizer/sedative agent		
Fentanyl-fluanisone	0.1–0.3 ml/kg, i.p	M
(Hypnorm®)	0.2–0.5 ml/kg, i.m., 0.3–0.6 ml/kg, i.p.	R
	0.5 ml/kg, i.p	H
	1.0 ml/kg, i.m./i.p.	G
	0.2–0.5 ml/kg, i.m	Rb
Medetomidine	30–100 μg/kg, s.c.	M
(Dormitor®)	30–100 μg/kg, i.p./s.c.	R
	100 μg/kg, i.p./s.c.	H
	0.25 mg/kg, i.m.	Rb
Diazepam (Valium®)	5 mg/kg, i.m./i.p.	M, H, G
	2.5–5 mg/kg, i.m./i.p.	R
	0.5–2 mg/kg, i.m./i.p./i.v.	Rb
Midazolam (Versed®)	1–5 mg/kg, i.m./i.p.	M, R, H, G
	1–5 mg/kg, i.m./i.v.	Rb
Acepromazine[d]	2–5 mg/kg, i.p./s.c.	M
	2.5 mg/kg, i.m./i.p	R
	5 mg/kg, i.p	H
	2.5–5 mg/kg, i.m.	G
	1–5 mg/kg, i.m./s.c.	Rb
Anticholinergic agent		
Atropine sulfate	0.4 mg/kg, i.m./s.c.	M, R, H, Gb
	0.1–0.2 mg/kg, i.m./s.c.	G
Glycopyrrolate	0.01–0.02 mg/kg, s.c.	M, R, H, G, Rb
(Robinul®)		

Notes:
[a] Values are derived from references 1–5.
[b] i.v., intravenous; i.p., intraperitoneal; i.m., intramuscular; s.c., subcutaneous.
[c] M, mouse; R, rat; H, hamster; G, guinea pig; Rb, rabbit; Gb, gerbil.
[d] Causes seizure in gerbil.

5.3 Analgesia

Analgesics are used to produce balanced anesthesia, neuroleptanalgesia, and relief of postoperative pain. Preoperative application should be performed to obtain greater analgesic effects especially for invasive surgical procedures. There are three major types of analgesics: (1) opioids, which act on the CNS via stimulation of opiate receptors; (2) peripherally acting compounds, such as antihistamines or local anesthetics, which block nociceptor impulses; and (3) non-steroidal anti-inflammatory drugs (NSAIDs), such as aspirin or

Table 5.2. *Representative analgesics and their recommended dosages in rodents and rabbits*

Agent	Dosage[a,b]	Species[c]
Opiates		
Buprenorphine	0.05–2.5 mg/kg, i.p./s.c. 6–12 hr	M
(Buprenex®)	0.1–0.5 mg/kg, i.p./i.v./s.c. 6–12 hr	R
	0.05–0.5 mg/kg, s.c. 8–12 hr	G
	0.5 mg/kg, s.c. 8 hr	H
	0.1–0.2 mg/kg, s.c. 8 hr	Gb
	0.01–0.05 mg/kg, i.v./s.c. 6–12 hr	Rb
Butorphanol	1–5 mg/kg, s.c. 2–4 hr	M, R, H
(Torbugesic®)	0.1–0.5 mg/kg, i.m./i.v./s.c. 2–4 hr	Rb
Nalbuphine	4–8 mg/kg, i.m. 3 hr	M, R, H, Gb
(Nubain®)	1–2 mg/kg, i.m. 3 hr	G
	1–2 mg/kg, i.m./i.v. 4–5 hr	Rb
Pentazocine	1–21 mg/kg, s.c.	M, R
	8–10 mg/kg, s.c.	Rb
Meperidine	20 mg/kg, i.m./s.c. 2–3 hr	M, R, G, H, Gb
(Demerol®)	10 mg/kg, i.m./s.c. 12 hr	Rb
Non-steroidal anti-inflammatory drugs (NSAIDs)		
Acetylsalicylic acid	120–300 mg/kg, p.o.	M
(Aspirin®)	100–150 mg/kg, p.o. 4 hr	R, H, Gb, Rb
	50–100 mg/kg, p.o. 4 hr	G
	20 mg/kg, s.c.	M, R, G
Acetaminophen	200 mg/kg, p.o.	M, R
	200–500 mg/kg, p.o.	Rb
Carprofen	4 mg/kg, s.c. 24 hr	R
(Zenecarp®, Rimadyl®)	2.2 mg/kg, p.o. 12 hr	Rb

Notes:
[a] Values are derived from references 1–5, 12.
[b] i.v., intravenous; i.p., intraperitoneal; i.m., intramuscular; s.c., subcutaneous; p.o., per os.
[c] M, mouse; R, rat; H, hamster; G, guinea pig; Rb, rabbit; Gb, gerbil.

acetaminophen, which inhibit the production of the chemical mediators that activate peripheral nociceptors. As a general rule, for maximal effectiveness for control of postoperative pain, analgesics should be first administered before the animal is fully recovered from anesthesia and should be continued for 2–3 days. However, even with a single postoperative dose, in many circumstances, recovery from surgical treatment would be greatly facilitated. Representative analgesics and their recommended dosages in laboratory rodents and rabbits are listed in Table 5.2.

Opioids, sometimes referred to as narcotics, are the most effective analgesics and can stimulate or depress the CNS, depending on the dose administered.

Depression of the CNS includes analgesia, respiratory depression, and sedation. Opioids and opioid agonist–antagonists have little effects on the myocardium, but may increase cerebrospinal fluid pressure, and overdosing causes excitement.[13] Therefore, they should be used with caution in craniotomy cases. The effects can be primarily analgesic, as with buprenorphine (Buprenex®), pentazocine (Talwin®), and nalbuphine, or a mixture of analgesia and euphoria with sedation as with butorphanol (Torbugesic®), fentanyl (Innovar-Vet®), morphine, meperidine (Demerol®), or oxymorphone (Numorphane®). The use of traditional parenterally administered opioid analgesics such as morphine, meperidine, and pentazocine is uncommon in rodents and rabbits because of their high metabolic rates.[13] As well as nalbuphine, naloxone is an opioid antagonist that can be used to reverse the effects of opioids (0.01–0.1 mg/kg, s.c./i.p. for all rodents; 0.01–0.1 mg/kg, i.v./i.m. for rabbits).

The NSAIDs, such as aspirin or acetaminophen, are generally less potent analgesics than are the opioids, but do not cause sedation nor are they addictive as are the opioids. In addition, they are more effective against pain caused by inflammation after surgery. However, they induce several side effects related to their pronounced antiprostaglandin activity, involving immune and platelet functions and sometimes causing gastric ulcers. Moreover, they all have the potential to cause nephro- and hepatotoxicity. Carprofen (Zenecarp®, Rimadyl®), on the other hand, has low cyclo-oxygenase 1 inhibitory effects resulting in a low potential for renal or gastric toxicity.[13] It is very effective when combined with opioids or buprenorphine and has a 24–48-hr duration of efficacy in most species.

5.4 Systemic anesthesia

Systemic anesthesia requires the state of unconsciousness with adequate analgesia and suppression of reflex activity and skeletal muscle tone to allow surgical procedure without pain or struggling. Systemic anesthesia can be achieved either by a single anesthetic dose or by balanced anesthesia, a combination of several different drugs, for example a sedative with an analgesic. Because many anesthetic drugs act synergistically on the CNS, balanced anesthesia permits a reduction of the dose of each agent (anesthetic potentiation), leading to reduction of the risk of toxic reactions and unwanted side effects.

The selection of anesthetic agents or techniques should be done considering the duration and depth of anesthesia needed, and the equipments and techniques available in the laboratory as well as the objectives of the study. Each anesthetic agent differs in its character in terms of the induction or recovery times, duration and degree of analgesia or muscle relaxation, metabolism, and excretion. The advantage of injectable anesthesia is in its simplicity; only a syringe and needle are required and anesthetic agents can be introduced into the animal's body by a simple procedure. The difficulty exists in controlling the depth of the anesthesia, since a relatively large dose should be administered at a time, which may lead to overdosing of the animals. Inhalation anesthesia has great advantages over the injectable anesthesia in the control of anesthesia including rapid induction and recovery or adjustment of depth or duration of anesthesia.

Skeletal muscle relaxants or neuromuscular blockers (e.g. succinylcholine, decamethonium, curare, gallamine, pancuronium) have no anesthetic or analgesic activity. They may only be used in conjunction with systemic anesthetics, and artificial ventilation must be provided for use.

Before surgery, fasting is not usually conducted in rats and mice unless gastrointestinal surgery is intended to be performed. Rabbits require fasting for approximately 6 hr before surgery. Water should not be restricted before anesthesia.

5.4.1 *Injectable anesthesia*

With respect to the control of the depth of anesthesia, intravenous (i.v.) injection is the preferable route of administration whenever the drug solution is feasible for this route. For irritating solutions such as a thiopental, the i.v. route must be selected. The lateral tail veins are usually used in rats and mice. For rabbits, a marginal ear vein may be used. Drugs with a wide safety margin are preferable when intraperitoneal (i.p.), intramuscular (i.m.), or subcutaneous (s.c.) injections are applied. The i.p. route is most common for injection in rats because of its simplicity that enables injection of relatively large volumes of solutions (typically up to 5 ml in rats). Injection by the i.p. route should be given lateral to the umbilicus in order to avoid injection into the cecum. The quadriceps or caudal thigh muscles may often be selected for i.m. injection, but the use of this method in rodents may be limited because of the limitation in injectable volume. The s.c. route allows large amounts of solutions to be dosed, but the absorption of the drug is relatively slow. The interscapular area is preferred for this route in both rodents and rabbits.

Injectable anesthetics are, in general, metabolized by the liver and excreted by the kidneys. Animals with liver or kidney dysfunction should not be anesthetized with these agents. In addition, the pharmacodynamic and pharmacokinetic characteristics of each agent should be taken into account when calculating doses. Barbiturates rapidly distribute to lipid-containing tissues such as the adipose tissue, leading to the rapid decrease of its blood concentration. Therefore, obese animals require higher doses to induce anesthesia. Once the adipose tissue becomes saturated with the agent, the elimination of the drug depends primarily on metabolism in the liver, which takes place much more slowly than the distribution of the drug to the adipose tissue, resulting in the sustained duration of anesthesia. Sex-related differences are also observed in anesthetic effects. For example, female rats are more susceptible to drugs like pentobarbital than male rats,[8] while in mice, narcosis induced by barbiturate lasts longer in males.[14] Some anesthetic agents, such as ketamine and pentobarbital, are known to induce drug-metabolizing enzymes in the liver.[15] Therefore, repeated use of these drugs may lead to the reduction of the drug effects. Table 5.3 summarizes the dosages and anesthetic time for representative anesthetic agents used in laboratory rodents and rabbits. For practice, the dosage should be best optimized by a preliminary dose test in a limited number of animals.

- Pentobarbital sodium (Nembutal®, Mebumal®), a short-acting oxybarbiturate, is usually used alone or supplemented with an analgesic. However, this drug shows a narrow dose-response range between surgical anesthesia and cardiovascular/respiratory depression,[16] as well as the poor analgesic effect. When given with i.v. route, approximately 50–75% of the calculated dose should be administered, and then the rest should be dosed with careful observation of the depth of anesthesia. If given i.p., usually the entire dose is given. After the confirmation of sufficient induction of anesthesia, intubation is recommended to perform before surgical procedure. The analgesic effect can be enhanced by balanced anesthesia with opioids, opioid agonist/antagonists, or ketamine (phenobarbital 20 mg/kg + ketamine 60 mg/kg in rats). Pentobarbital causes hypothermia in rats, and temperature control is always required when using this anesthetic.[17] In guinea pigs, hamsters, gerbils, and rabbits, pentobarbital can be highly lethal.
- Thiopental (Pentothal®) and thiamylal are classified as ultra-short-acting thiobarbiturates. Because of the extremely short duration of anesthesia effect, it is usually used as an anesthetic induction agent to allow intubation prior to inhalation anesthesia. Due to its alkaline nature, thiopental solution should strictly be administered i.v. Because of its highly lipid-soluble nature, a small amount injected rapidly produces a high concentration in the brain and an almost immediate state of deep narcosis. The agent, however, soon redistributes to the non-fat tissues of the body, resulting in a rapid decrease in the depth of narcosis.
- Propofol (Diprivan®, Rapinovet®) is an alkylphenol, presenting as a milky, oily suspension, and is virtually insoluble in water. This agent is chemically unrelated to barbiturates but with similar effects and should be given intravenously only for procedures involving little or no pain in rats and rabbits because of the poor analgesic activity in these species.[12] This agent exerts a rapid (30 s) anesthetic

Table 5.3. *Representative injectable anesthetics and their recommended dosages in rodents and rabbits*

Agent	Dosage[a,b]	Anesthesia time (min)	Species[c]
Pentobarbital (Nembutal®, Mebumal®)	50–90 mg/kg, i.p., 50–60 mg/kg, i.v.	10–300	M
	40–60 mg/kg, i.p.	80–95	R
	70–90 mg/kg, i.p.	60–75	H
	15–40 mg/kg, i.p.	60	G
	36–100 mg/kg, i.p.	50–60	Gb
	30–45 mg/kg, i.v.	20–30	Rb
Thiopental (Pentothal®)	25–50 mg/kg, i.v.	10	M, Rb
	20–40 mg/kg, i.v.	5–10	R
Propofol (Diprivan®, Rapinovet®)	12–26 mg/kg, i.v.	5–10	M
	7.5–15.0 mg/kg, i.v.	8–11	R
	10 mg/kg, i.v.	5–10	Rb
Fentanyl-fluanisone (Hypnorm®) + diazepam (Valium®)	0.4 ml/kg, i.p. + 5 mg/kg, i.p.	30–40	M
	0.6 ml/kg, i.p. + 2.5 mg/kg, i.p.	20–40	R
	1 ml/kg, i.p. + 5 mg/kg, i.p.	20–40	H
	1 ml/kg, i.p. + 2.5 mg/kg, i.p.	45–60	G
	1 ml/kg, i.p./i.m. + 5 mg/kg, i.p.	21	Gb
	0.3 ml/kg, i.m. + 1–2 mg/kg, i.m./i.p./i.v.	20–40	Rb
Fentanyl-fluanisone + medetomidine (Dormitor®)[a]	300 µg/kg + 300 µg/kg, i.p.	60–70	R
	50 µg/kg + 50 µg/kg, s.c.	72	Gb
	8 µg/kg + 330 µg/kg, i.v.	30–40	Rb
Chloral hydrate	400 mg/kg, i.p.	60–120	R
α-Chloralose	55–65 mg/kg, i.p.	480–600	R
	80–100 mg/kg, i.p.	–	H
	70 mg/kg, i.p.	180–600	G
	80–100 mg/kg, i.v.	360–600	Rb
Urethane	1000–1500 mg/kg, i.p.	360–480	M, R
	1000–2000 mg/kg, i.p.	360–480	H
	1500 mg/kg, i.v./i.p.	300–480	G
	1000–2000 mg/kg, i.v.	360–480	Rb

Table 5.3. (cont.)

Agent	Dosage[a,b]	Anesthesia time (min)	Species[c]
Ketamine (Ketaset®, Vetalar®) + diazepam[d]	100 mg/kg + 5 mg/kg, i.p.	20–30	M
	75 mg/kg + 5 mg/kg, i.p.	20–30	R
	70 mg/kg + 2 mg/kg, i.p.	30–45	H
	100 mg/kg + 5 mg/kg, i.m.	30–45	G
	25 mg/kg + 5 mg/kg, i.m.	20–30	Rb
Ketamine + medetomidine[d]	75 mg/kg + 1.0 mg/kg, i.p.	20–30	M
	75 mg/kg + 0.5 mg/kg, i.p.	20–30	R
	100 mg/kg + 0.25 mg/kg, i.p.	30–60	H
	40 mg/kg + 0.5 mg/kg, i.p.	30–40	G
	25 mg/kg + 0.5 mg/kg, i.m.	30–40	Rb
Ketamine + xylazine (Rompun®)[d]	100–200 mg/kg + 15 mg/kg, i.p.	20–30	M
	80–100 mg/kg + 10–20 mg/kg, i.p.	20–30	R
	200 mg/kg + 10 mg/kg, i.p.	30–60	H
	30–60 mg/kg + 5–8 mg/kg, i.p./s.c.	30	G
	30–40 mg/kg + 5–8 mg/kg, i.m./s.c.	25–40	Rb
Telazol® (Mixture of tiletamine and zolazepam)[e]	80 mg/kg, i.p.	–	M
	40 mg/kg, i.p.	15–25	R
Avertin® (2,2,2-tribromoethanol)	240 mg/kg, i.p.	15–45	M
	225–325 mg/kg, i.p.	10–35	Gb

Notes:
[a] Values are derived from references 1–5, 12.
[b] i.v., intravenous; i.p., intraperitoneal; i.m., intramuscular; s.c., subcutaneous.
[c] M, mouse; R, rat; H, hamster; G, guinea pig; Rb, rabbit; Gb, gerbil.
[d] Premix before injection.
[e] Induce renal tubular necrosis in rabbits.

induction; short duration (5–7 min); smooth recovery even after prolonged anesthesia through intermittent injections. Although it does not affect heart rate, it causes significant hypotension especially after bolus injection as well as severe respiratory depression after induction. Propofol may be used to induce anesthesia that will be maintained with an inhalant anesthetic.

- Neuroleptanalgesic combination of a neuroleptic opioid and a benzodiazepine provides an excellent full surgical anesthesia and muscle relaxation. Fentanyl-fluanisone or fentanyl-droperidol (Innovar-Vet®) in combination with diazepam offers an excellent anesthesia lasting 20–40 min. Diazepam should be given separately with fentanyl-fluanisone. Repeated dose of fentanyl-fluanisone (0.1 ml/kg, i.m.) every 30–40 min can prolong the duration of anesthesia. The anesthetic effect is antagonized with nalbuphine or buprenorphine after operation. A single dose of medetomidine/fentanyl cocktail provides good surgical anesthesia sustained for 60 min in rats,[18] but this combination is highly lethal to mice and contraindicated.[6]

- Chloral hydrate (trichloracetaldehyde monohydrate) produces a light anesthesia lasting 1–2 hr, but anesthetic induction is slow, which leads to an extended state of preanesthetic delirium which may be unpleasant for the animal, and it can cause gastric ulcers and adynamic ileus. Analgesia is adequate at 400 mg/kg, but there are unacceptable side effects such as hypotension and bradycardia with rapid and severe hypothermia. To prevent adynamic ileus, concentrations of working solution should be <50 mg/ml. Chloral hydrate must be refrigerated.

- Alpha-chloralose produces a mild hypnosis and muscle relaxation for a long period of time, but does not provide complete anesthesia because of its poor analgesic properties. Due to its extremely irritating nature to the gastrointestinal tracts, the drug should be administered only intravenously. The use of α-chloralose may be valuable in physiology studies that require stable cardiovascular parameters because this drug exhibits minimum effects on the cardiopulmonary performance.[19] This drug should only be used in experiments involving non-survival procedures.

- Urethane is a long-acting anesthetic that produces a minimal cardiovascular depression.[20] Urethane is a carcinogen,[21] and its use should be avoided as possible to prevent possible health risk to the personnel, and animals should be terminated after urethane anesthesia. This agent lengthens thrombin and activated partial thromboplastin times.

- Ketamine (Ketaset®, Vetalar®) is a dissociative anesthetic and can induce a catalepsy-like immobilization. With this agent, analgesic activity and muscle relaxation are poor. Ketamine induces a respiratory depression in rodents at a dose that is sufficient for anesthesia. Concomitant use of medetomidine, diazepam or xylazine (Rompun®) can reduce the dose of ketamine and can provide muscle relaxation without respiratory and cardiovascular depression and provides a sufficient surgical anesthesia in rabbits. They can be mixed with ketamine solution before application. Their analgesic effect varies among species. Ketamine with

diazepam does not exert enough analgesic effects in rodents. Ketamine with medetomidine or xylazine in combination may generally be good for surgery in rodents,
and reversal with yohimbine or atipamezole shorten recovery times. (For dosage
information, see Section 5.2 above).

- Telazol® is a combination of the dissociative anesthetic tiletamine and the benzodiazepine tranquilizer zolazepam. In rats and mice, this agent produces anesthesia
suitable for restraint, blood sampling, and minor manipulations. Analgesia is not
sufficient to permit surgical manipulations unless high dosages (60–100 mg/kg)
and/or combination with local anesthetics and/or tranquilizers are used.[12] For
recovery, several hours are required and hypothermia and occasional hyperacusia
may occur.[12] Telazol is not recommended for use in rabbits because of its nephro-
toxic effects and lack of analgesia.

- Avertin (2,2,2-tribromoethanol) is widely used in mice for embryo transfer, biopsy,
and vasectomy.[6] This agent is light sensitive and will decompose to toxic by-
products if not stored properly, and sensitizes some animals to subsequent exposure
to cause deaths (about 1% of naive mice). It also arguably has inflammatory
properties.[22]

5.4.2 Inhalation anesthesia

Inhalation anesthesia is superior to most injectable forms of anesthesia for the
advantage of real-time control of anesthetic depth by changing the exposure
level during each phase of induction, maintenance, and recovery. Since the
elimination of the agent is primarily conducted by exhalation, inhalation
anesthesia can be suitable for animals with retarded metabolism such as
those with liver or kidney dysfunction or obese animals. However, some agents
reveal significant effect on the drug metabolism in the liver, and therefore the
duration or frequency of the anesthesia should be determined considering the
type of agent used. The disadvantage of inhalation anesthesia is the complexity
of the equipment and the procedure for administration of anesthetic agents.
Another concern would be potential hazard to personnel.

An important concept in inhalation anesthesia is the minimum alveolar
concentration (MAC). MAC is the alveolar concentration of a given compound at a pressure of 1 atm, which will prevent response to painful stimuli in
50% of the animals/patients in a group. The lower the MAC, the more potent
the anesthetic drug. Generally, anesthetic maintenance requires 1.5–2.0 times
MAC. Vapor pressure is another factor that determines the potency of anesthetics. Agents with high vapor pressure are easily evaporated to reach fatal
concentration. They should be used under a controllable system using a
calibrated evaporator. On the other hand, agents with much less vapor pressure may be used safely in a conventional anesthetic chamber.

Anesthetic breathing systems

To provide very short-term anesthesia, a very simple 'open drop system' is applicable primarily to quick procedures. To achieve more controllable anesthesia, application of an anesthetic gas delivery system should be considered. The system requires the supply of O_2 to the lung alveolar membrane, the removal of CO_2 from the lungs, and the supply of anesthetic gas at a controlled pressure to the alveolar surface. In practice, there are two major anesthetic gas delivery systems for laboratory animals, i.e., non-rebreathing system suitable for rats and mice, and rebreathing system for animals as large as rabbits.

Open drop system The use of this system with an anesthetic chamber or bell jar gives only minimal control over anesthetic administration. The chamber consists of a large transparent container, anesthetic-absorbent material such as cotton or paper towels, and a wire mesh grid to prevent direct contact of animals with irritating anesthetic liquid (Fig. 5.1). The system involves placing the animals in an isolated environment where they become anesthetized as they inhale the volatized anesthetic that is absorbed in the paper materials. For this purpose, anesthetics with low vapor pressure, such as methoxyflurane, or with slow-acting drugs like diethyl ether have been traditionally used. Despite its

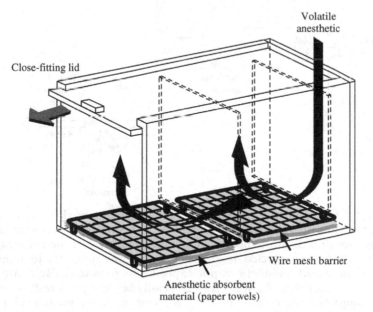

Figure 5.1. Anesthetic chamber in an open drop system, consisting of a transparent container, anesthetic-absorbent material (paper towels), and a wire mesh barrier between the animal and the liquid phase anesthetic.

simplicity, this method should be changed to any of the following methods because of the difficulty in controlling the depth of anesthesia and the risk to personnel by exposure to the anesthetic gas.

Non-rebreathing system In this system, previously exhaled gas from the animal is not rebreathed by the specific flows to prevent rebreathing. The basic system consists of a source of O_2, an O_2 flowmeter, a precision vaporizer, which produces a vapor from a volatile liquid anesthetic, a non-rebreathing circuit (tubing, connectors, and valves) and a scavenging device that removes any waste anesthetic gases (Figs. 5.2 and 5.3). The mixture of anesthetic vapor and O_2 is delivered to an animal. An induction chamber can be incorporated in the circuit to allow the animal to first be put under anesthetic in the chamber and then be maintained with a mask (Figs. 5.4 and 5.5). Because there is no

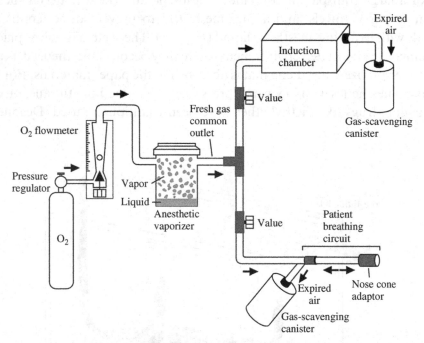

Figure 5.2. Components of the non-rebreathing system used for rodents. An evaporated anesthetic, adequately mixed with O_2 through a precision vaporizer, is introduced into either an induction chamber or a non-rebreathing circuit, which is connected to a mask (nose cone adaptor) to minimize risks of untoward anesthetic vapor exposure to personnel. By controlling the valves, direction of fresh gas flow can easily be changed. Fresh anesthetic gas coming in from the circuit is delivered to the mask and waste gas is pulled back through the circuit. The anesthetic gas remaining in the exhaust is scavenged in the canister filled with active charcoal that will filter out the gas waste and the clean oxygen in the air (F/Air® canister).

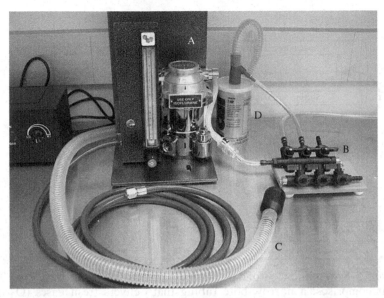

Figure 5.3. Typical setup of non-rebreathing system with a precision vaporizer (A), a manifold directing the flow of fresh gas to several anesthetic devices (B), a non-rebreathing circuit (C), and a gas scavenging F/Air® canister (D). (The devices are supplied from Harvard Apparatus, Cambridge, MA.)

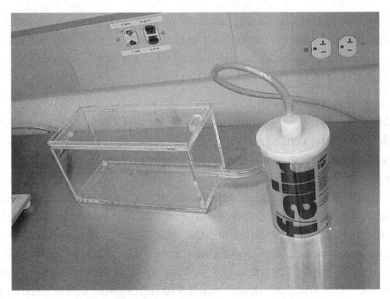

Figure 5.4. Anesthetic induction chamber in a non-rebreathing system consisting of a transparent container and equipped with two tubing connecters for introducing and exhausting the gas. (The devices are supplied from Harvard Apparatus, Cambridge, MA.)

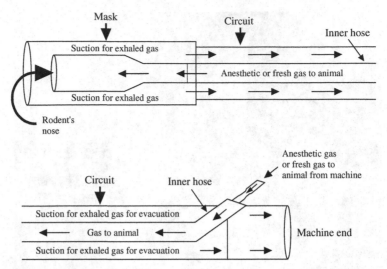

Figure 5.5. Schematic view of a non-rebreathing circuit used for rodents. The circuit comprises: a narrow-bore tubing that delivers fresh gases (O_2 and anesthetic) to the animal; a wide-bore tubing that collects exhaled gases; and its continuation into a corrugated tubing that leads to a scavenging activated charcoal canister. (This design is derived from "Rodent mask and C-pram circuit" supplied by Harvard Apparatus, Cambridge, MA.)

rebreathing, this system requires high flow of dry cool gas to the animal, which causes significant losses of body heat and humidity, and also brings a large waste of anesthetic gas to atmosphere which risks considerably to the personnel.

Rebreathing system This system incorporates a CO_2 absorber so that the anesthetic gas can be reused, leading to the reduction of anesthetics consumption, as well as the minimum loss of body temperature (Fig. 5.6). In this system, a breathing tube is communicated with the animal's airway, and the distal end of the breathing tube is connected with the expiratory ports via an adapter such as a Y-piece. The anesthetic circuit dead-space should be minimized by placing the adaptor close to the mouth, since the dead-space will result in the insufficient gas exchange which can cause suffocation. The exhaust gas breathed out is passed over to the CO_2 absorber system, then back into the system. An induction chamber and a mask can be used to supply anesthetic gas to animals. However, in case of respiratory arrest, assisted ventilation is difficult with this setup. An endotracheal intubation is needed to assist respiration by manually compressing the rebreathing bag or the introduction of a ventilator.

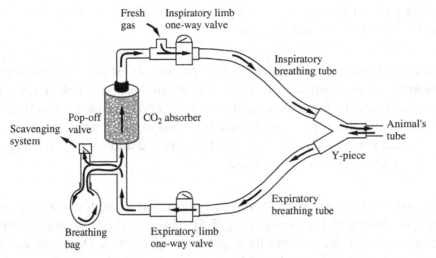

Figure 5.6. Air/gas flow in the rebreathing system. Fresh gas (O_2 and anesthetic) enters the circle from the common gas outlet of the anesthetic machine, and flows through the inspiratory limb one-way valve, inspiratory breathing tube, and then via the Y-piece to the animal. The exhaust gas breathed out from the animal enters through the expiratory breathing tube, expiratory limb one-way valve, breathing bag, CO_2 absorber where CO_2 is removed, and then back towards the animal. Excess gas is vented out through the pop-off valve to the scavenging system.

Anesthetic machine components

Non-rebreathing system consists of a source of O_2, an O_2 flowmeter, a precision vaporizer, a non-rebreathing circuit, and a gas scavenging device. In the rebreathing system, the CO_2 absorber should be incorporated in the circuit, and, whenever assisted ventilation is required, use of endotracheal catheter and ventilator is necessary.

O_2 supply O_2 can be provided by a central distribution system or by pressurized tanks (cylinders). Since cylinders store gas at very high pressure (15 MPa), a pressure-reducing valve or regulator is necessary to reduce the pressure to about 350 kPa, which is a level that can easily be handled by the flowmeter. Further reduction in pressure is achieved by O_2 flowmeter for safe delivery of gas to the animal. Central pipeline pressure is usually set at about 350 kPa of pressure for delivery. When the pressure reaches 3.5 MPa, the cylinder should be replaced with a new one.

O_2 flowmeter This device uses an adjustable valve to deliver the desired flow in ml/min or l/min to the patient circuit. Flows of around 0.5–2 l O_2/min are

commonly used with rodent anesthesia machines. Flowmeters should be individually calibrated for each gas supply.

Anesthetic vaporizer Precision vaporizers produce anesthetic gas and supply an accurate gas concentration from a volatile liquid anesthetic. Current types of vaporizers are accurate at oxygen flow rates and automatically adjust the anesthetic concentration to compensate for ambient temperature fluctuations. These precision items of equipment must be serviced and calibrated every 1–3 years, depending on the degree of use.

Non-rebreathing circuit The non-rebreathing circuit is the highway for anesthetic gas delivery to the animal (Fig. 5.5). This anesthetic breathing circuit is designed to: (1) deliver anesthetic properly mixed with O_2 to the animal, (2) remove CO_2 that is produced by the animal, and (3) provide a method for assisting or controlling ventilation, if needed.

CO₂ absorber In the rebreathing system, the CO_2 absorber is located on the exhalation side of the circle (Fig. 5.6). Exhaled gas goes through the canister which contains soda lime and the CO_2 is removed. Soda lime is a mixture containing about 94% calcium hydroxide, 5% sodium hydroxide, and 1% potassium hydroxide. Silica is included for granularity and the pH-sensitive dyeing is used to assess when to change the canister due to loss of CO_2 absorption capacity. Loss of capacity may be noted when the color changes from white to bloom (purple) or from pink to white, indicating that immediate change is required.

Intubation catheter In a procedure that utilizes an artificial ventilation system, endotracheal intubation is required. For rodents, intravenous polyethylene catheters with a flexible guide wire can be used as an intubation catheter.[23,24] Catheter sizes are different depending on the size of the rodents, being typically 14 gauge (60 mm in catheter length) for guinea pigs, 16 gauge (55 mm in length) for hamsters, and 14–20 gauges for various sizes of rats.[12] Before the intubation, animals should be deeply anesthetized, for example, by intravenous injection of thiopental. For intubation, rats should be put in a dorsal recumbence, while rabbits are placed in a ventral position. The animal's mouth can be kept open with the aid of an intubation speculum or laryngoscope,[25] and a guide wire can then be introduced into the trachea over the epiglottis. Then, an intubation catheter is threaded over the guide wire. While holding the catheter in place, the guide wire is removed and the catheter is attached to the anesthetic circuit. For non-survival procedure, tracheostomy can be applied. Illumination with a fiber-optic light is helpful for a successful intubation.

Ventilator Artificial ventilation is essential to maintain normal pO_2, pCO_2, and acid–base balance of the blood during the experiment and suitable for sequential analyses of biological parameters in physiological experiments. The function of a ventilator system includes control of the respiration by adjusting the respiration frequency, inspiratory/expiratory (I/E) ratio, and tidal volume. A basic system consists of a ventilator and a single breathing tube. The inspiratory fresh gas can be from any source, such as anesthetic gas, or air/O_2 mixture. This gas can be warmed and humidified before reaching the animal. Intrapulmonary exposure of some test chemical/compound is also possible when using a vaporizer unit.

When weaning an animal off artificial ventilation, the anesthetic agent should be eliminated from the respiratory gas flow until only oxygen is flowing; then the airway pressure or the frequency of ventilation should be gradually decreased. When spontaneous breathing starts, the airway pressure or frequency can be further reduced and then the ventilator can be disconnected. The endotracheal tube can be removed after confirmation of a few minutes of sustained spontaneous breathing.

Scavenging systems These systems are designed to absorb or eliminate waste anesthetic gases to prevent or minimize room pollution. Waste gas capture devices include direct exhaust to the outside through an outside wall, or a direct connection to the building exhaust system. Waste gases may be eliminated via an active (i.e., vacuum driven) or passive (outside wall, activated charcoal canister) system. Pollution may occur during chamber induction, maintenance of anesthesia by loose facemask or nose cone, discharge of waste gases from a breathing circuit into the room, and spillage or vapor escape when filling the vaporizer. To reduce pollution when using an induction chamber, scavenge the chamber adequately.

Activated charcoal canisters can be purchased (F/Air® Filter Canister; Harvard Apparatus Inc., Cambridge, MA). The weight of the F/Air® canister must be recorded upon installation and the canister should be replaced after a weight increase of 50 g; this indicates that its capacity to absorb halogenated anesthetics has been exhausted. Alternatively, the canister should be replaced after 12 hr of anesthesia time at an O_2 flow rate of 2 l/min. Halogenated anesthetics include isoflurane, halothane, enflurane, and methoxyflurane. It is important to note that F/Air® canisters do not absorb other anesthetic gases, such as nitrous oxide.

Inhalation anesthetics

Table 5.4 lists representative inhalation anesthetics used in laboratory animals.

- Halothane (Fluothane®), a halogenated halocarbon, is a clear, highly volatile liquid. Its vapor has relatively low blood/gas solubility and is neither irritating nor explosive. Animals can recover 10–20 min after removal of halothane. However, recovery may be delayed by the prolonged use of this anesthetic. It causes a significant respiratory depression and hypotension due to the decrease in cardiac output and increase in peripheral vasodilatation. It also induces microsomal enzymes in the liver[26] and sometimes causes hepatotoxicity, and therefore, is not recommended for drug metabolism/toxicity study.
- Enflurane (Ethrane®) is a chemically stable halogenated methyl ethyl ether with high vapor pressure. Its vapor is relatively insoluble and neither irritating nor explosive. It risks a cardiopulmonary depression like halothane. However, it is hardly metabolized in the liver and has an advantage over halothane in studies on drug metabolism and toxicity.
- Isoflurane (Aerrane®), chemically related to enflurane, has a high vapor pressure, resulting in faster anesthetic induction and recovery than halothane or enflurane. Its vapor is slightly irritating, but is neither flammable nor explosive in anesthetic concentration. This agent is even less well metabolized by the liver than enflurane, and most of what is inhaled is excreted by respiration, suggesting its suitability for the metabolism/toxicity studies. It causes a slightly more severe respiratory depression but less pronounced cardiovascular depression as compared with halothane.[27]
- Methoxyflurane is a halogenated ethyl methyl ether. It has a low vapor pressure, causing slow rate of induction, but has very potent analgesic properties. Its vapor is neither irritating nor explosive in anesthetic concentration, but induction of nephrotoxicity is potentiated by tetracyclines. This drug is not currently being manufactured in the USA.
- Diethyl ether is a colorless, highly volatile fluid. Its vapor is highly inflammable and much heavier than air resulting in accumulation on the floor, so that it should always be used in a well-ventilated area. It is highly soluble but the induction of anesthesia is slow. This agent is irritable to mucous membranes, and therefore, premedication with an anticholinergic may be necessary to reduce excessive respiratory secretions. It stimulates the release of catecholamine,[28] which results in both the maintenance of cardiovascular function and increase in the blood concentration of glucose. Although diethyl ether has been applied as an agent in an open drop system, its inflammable nature diminishes its usefulness.
- Nitrous oxide is a colorless gas with a sweet odor. The gas is neither irritating nor inflammable. It has a weak anesthetic potential itself but can be particularly useful when used with other anesthetic agents. It is usually used as a carrier gas, after mixture with O_2 at a ratio not exceeding 50%, of other inhalation anesthetics such as halothane or isoflurane. It causes minimum effect on respiratory or cardiovascular function.

Table 5.4. *Representative agents used for inhalation anesthesia*

Agent	Vapor pressure	Saturation at 22 °C (%)	Minimum alveolen concentration (v/v %)	Blood–gas partition coefficient	Percentage to be metabolized (human)	Vapor concentration (%) Induction	Vapor concentration (%) Maintenance	Induction/recovery
Halothane	242	32	0.9	2.3	20–25	4	1–2	Moderate
Enflurane	171	23	2.0	1.9	2.4	3–5	1–3	Fast
Isoflurane	240	32	1.5	1.3	0.17	4	1.5–3	Fast
Methoxyflurane	23	3	0.2	13	50	3	0.4–1	Slow
Diethyl ether	443	58	3.2	15	5–10	10–20	4–5	Slow
Nitrous oxide	39 500	100	180	0.4	0.004	–	–	Very fast

Source: References 2 and 11.

In rodents, use of isoflurane or halothane is often the choice and the anesthetic potency of these agents is similar to that in larger species. Between the two, isoflurane is safer than halothane and therefore most popularly used. Due to their high vapor pressure, these agents should be used with precision calibrated vaporizers. Low doses of these agents allow minor procedures, and opioids can be given to provide analgesia and reduce the anesthetic concentration during surgery. In rabbits, anesthetic induction with inhalation anesthetics is not recommended because these agents only give low anesthetic potency and sometimes produces fatal hypoxia.[29] A better approach for rabbits is to induce anesthesia with short-acting agents, such as propofol, and to maintain anesthesia with isoflurane or halothane. Rabbits require higher concentrations of these agents (10–20% increase) to obtain a similar degree of anesthetic depth with other animal species.[29]

5.5 Monitoring of anesthesia

Monitoring of anesthesia is essential to sufficiently remove pain from animals and to conduct a surgical procedure successfully without accidental deaths. If animals show signs of too light anesthesia, anesthetic supply should be increased by additional injection or increasing the anesthetic gas concentration. If anesthesia becomes too deep, the concentration of anesthetic vapor can be decreased. In case of injection anesthetics, care should be taken in advance to prevent excess anesthetization.

The depth of anesthesia can be assessed by reflex tests. The palpebral reflex (eye blinking after touching the eyelid) indicates that the anesthesia is not deep enough. On the other hand, loss of corneal reflex upon stimulation is generally the sign that the anesthesia is too deep. Withdrawal of the feet after pinching the toe or foot web indicates that the animal is sensing pain. Ear pinch would be more sensitive in rats and guinea pigs.

Physiological monitoring methods must also be applied to assess anesthetic depth, as normal reflex tests are less reliable. The following are suggestions from the American College of Veterinary Anesthesiology for monitoring anesthetized animals:[30]

Circulation: to ensure that blood flow to the tissues is adequate, heart rate, peripheral pulses, electrocardiogram (ECG), auscultation of heart beat, or blood pressure (non-invasive or invasive) should be examined or analyzed.

Oxygenation: to ensure adequate oxygen concentration in the animal's arterial blood, mucous membranes' color, pulse oximetry, or blood gas should be examined or analyzed.

Ventilation: to ensure that the animal's ventilation is adequately maintained, respiratory rate, movement of thoracic wall or breathing bag if animal is spontaneously breathing, auscultation of breath sounds, capnography, or blood gas should be examined or analyzed.

Recently, a wide range of veterinary monitors has been developed to cover parameters like ECG, pulse oximetry, and temperature in a single device that is suitable for use in small animals as well as in larger species.

Muscle tone can be tested by pulling the lower jaw or a limb; muscle tone decreases when the anesthetic depth increases unless a cataleptic agent like ketamine is used without a sedative treatment. The respiration should be deep and stable in the surgical plane of anesthesia. If the animal shows extremely decreased respiration, short, jerky, and gasping diaphragmatic movement, supportive cares including artificial ventilation should be performed. If the respiration is shallow and irregular, anesthesia is too light.

Because of the greater body surface area to body mass ratio in small experimental animals, thermal support becomes essential care during anesthesia. Anesthetized animals should be put on towels or heat pads, and never be placed directly on stainless steel tables. The use of a water blanket with circulating thermal water would be ideal. However, animals should not be put directly on the blanket to prevent thermal burns.

5.6 Postoperative care

Thermal control is one of the major components of postoperative procedures in rodents. Animals should be put on a water blanket with circulating thermal water to avoid hypothermia. An incandescent lamp may be useful to provide animals with supplemental heat. A temperature control unit or cabinet is commercially available. For rats, the optimum recovery temperature should be about 35 °C. The heat, whatever the source is, should not be so intensive as to cause thermal burns. S.c or i.p. administration of warmed sterile saline would compensate the volume loss during surgery and facilitate the animal's recovery; 1–2 ml for a mouse or 5 ml for a rat would be the typical dose. Whenever the animal is fasted prior to surgery, additional supply of calories by injecting a small volume of warmed 5% dextrose solution is recommended.[12]

During the recovery from anesthesia, animals may undergo a period of excitement at the transition between unconscious and conscious levels, which may itself result in self-inflicted injury if they are left unattended. Each anesthetized animal should be put in a separate cage until complete recovery is confirmed, otherwise the recovering animal may attack the unconscious animals causing accidental death.

If a surgical procedure includes penetration deeper than the skin or sub-cutaneous tissues, the use of analgesic agents should be considered unless reasonably justified by scientific reasons. Analgesics should be administered for the first 24 hr postoperatively and continued if necessary. On the other hand, administration of antibiotics is generally unnecessary, if the surgery is conducted under properly aseptic conditions. When needed, the treatment should be conducted preoperatively to obtain the desired effect. When animals are frequently anesthetized with injectable agents that inhibit blinking (e.g., ketamine), ocular lubrication is necessary to prevent corneal ulceration.[12]

5.7 Local anesthesia

Local anesthetics can be applied to block nerve depolarization and conduction in the area of interest for the performance of usually rather minor or rapid procedures. Normally, light sedation with some type of sedatives or tranquilizers is needed to restrain the animal to allow procedures to be performed. Depending on the purpose, any of the following methods of local anesthesia can be selected:

Topical anesthesia: topical application of a local anesthetic includes topical ophthalmic anesthetic, application to the skin before a procedure, or within an incision during a procedure. Generally, this method is only short-lived.

Regional anesthesia: this technique involves injection of an anesthetic to infuse an area with the anesthetic 10–15 min prior to the procedure. This may be used for small or large areas.

Spinal anesthesia: this technique involves an intrathecal or epidural injection of the drug to block sensation from a large part of the body. As well as the more traditional local anesthetics, xylazine has been used for this purpose. This technique is very useful for caudal abdominal, perineal, or hindlimb surgical procedures. The amount of anesthetic injected can be increased to increase the area that is anesthetized. Overdosing with this method can result in paralysis of the respiratory muscles, requiring mechanical ventilation until the drugs have worn off. Training should be needed for precise needle placement and drug dose calculations.

Nerve block: this technique involves injection of a relatively small volume of drug in the area of a peripheral nerve that distributes to the area of interest 10–15 min prior to the procedure. A precise knowledge of nerve locations is necessary for this technique.

For surgical purposes, local anesthetics are generally ineffective when applied topically either pre- or postoperatively.[6] Penetration of the agent is usually poor through intact skin, and in case of tissue inflammation, the acidic environment neutralizes the drug. Block of a surgical area by 0.5% lido-caine (Xylocaine®) will provide ~90 min of local anesthesia. To avoid cardiac arrhythmias, total dose should be <7 mg/kg. When the animal is under anal-gesia for hours, 0.25% bupivicaine (Marcaine®) is effective, but total local dose should be <8 mg/kg. Local anesthetic infusions can be performed to support anesthesia when systemic anesthesia induced by injection is not suffi-cient and additional injections may risk overdose.[6] Topical hypothermic sprays are useful for tail snips of young rodents.

5.8 Fetal and neonatal anesthesia

5.8.1 Fetal anesthesia

Fetuses can be anesthetized by anesthetizing the maternal animal to a suffi-ciently deep level. For this purpose, use of injectable anesthetics to the dam, such as ketamine + xylazine for rats or ketamine + xylazine + acepromazine for mice, is recommended. As well as a careful procedure to keep adequate ventilation, a preoperative dose of D5W (electrolytes with dextrose, i.p.) may provide some anesthetic support.[31]

5.8.2 Neonatal anesthesia

In neonatal rodents, use of inhalation anesthesia is recommended, because quick recovery from anesthesia that permits normal feeding is essential for these animals.[31] It is important to maintain body temperature during anes-thesia, because neonatal rodents have increased susceptibility to hypothermia. Care must be taken to maintain good ventilation and fluid balance.

Anesthesia using hypothermia

Hypothermia is the choice as neonatal rodent anesthesia because of low mortality, ease of use, safety, and low cost.[32-34] Newborn rodents are func-tionally poikilothermic and, with a relatively small body mass, are tolerable to rapid core cooling that causes "refrigeration analgesia" by blockage of nerve conduction. Neural conduction velocity is decreased by 75% when tissue is cooled below 20 °C and complete neural blockage occurs at about 9 °C. Loss of consciousness occurs by depression of neural conduction and synaptic trans-mission on the CNS. To induce hypothermia, pups (<14 postnatal days) are either (1) placed in a latex sleeve and submerged up to the neck in crushed ice and water (2–3 °C) for 3–4 min or (2) placed in a paper-lined test tube and packed in dry ice for 10–15 min.[6] Analgesia induced by these methods lasts approximately 10 min. Simply placing conscious animals in a cold room or on an ice pack are unacceptable as induction may take 30–45 min. The anesthetic state may be prolonged by placing the hypothermic pup on an ice pack (3–4 °C). Illumination of the surgical field should be fiber-optic in nature, because incandescent bulbs may cause inadvertent and uncontrollable warming. Pups should be recovered by rewarming slowly in an incubator at 33 °C or in a warm nest. Pups usually become active and responsive within 20–30 min, and when pups start crawling they can be returned to the dam. Recovery from hypothermia may be associated with pain, so postoperative analgesics should be considered. Successful use of neonatal anesthesia has been reported in the procedures such as castration, ovariectomy, lesioning the frontal cortex or hypothalamic area, olfactory bulbectomies, thymectomy, abdominal surgery, and vagotomy.[32–34]

References

1. Rossoff IS. *Handbook of Veterinary Drugs and Chemicals: A Compendium for Research and Clinical Use*, 2nd edn. Taylorville, IL: Pharmatox Publishing Co., 1994.
2. Flecknell PA. *Laboratory Animal Anaesthesia: An Introduction for Research Workers and Technicians*, 2nd edn. London: Academic Press, 1996.
3. Kohn DF, Wixson SK, White WJ, Benson GJ. *Anesthesia and Analgesia in Laboratory Animals*. Orlando, FL: Academic Press, 1997.
4. Hawk CT, Leary SL. *Formulary for Laboratory Animals*, 2nd edn. Ames, IA: Iowa State University Press, 1999.
5. Carpenter JW, Mashima TY, Rupiper DJ. *Exotic Animal Formulary*, 2nd edn. Philadelphia, PA: W. B. Saunders., 2001.
6. Huerkamp MJ. *Anesthetic Management of Rodents and Rabbits*. Available online at http://www.emory.edu/WHSC/MED/DAR/Anesthetic_drugs.htm, 2000.
7. Olson ME, Vizzutti D, Morck DW, Cox AK. The parasympatholytic effects of atropine sulphate and glycopyrrolate in rats and rabbits. *Can. J. Vet. Res.* 1994, **58**: 254–258.
8. Svendensen P. In Svendensen P, Hau J (eds.) *Handbook of Laboratory Animal Science*, vol. 1, *Selection and Handling of Animals in Biomedical Research*. Boca Raton, FL: CRC Press, 1994, pp. 311–337.
9. Green CJ. Neuroleptanalgesic drug combinations in the anaesthetic management of small laboratory animals. *Lab. Anim.* 1975, **9**: 161–178.
10. Virtanen R. Pharmacological profiles of medetomidine and its antagonist, atipamezole. *Acta Vet. Scand. Suppl.* 1989, **85**: 29–37.
11. Shibutani M. Anesthesia, artificial ventilation and perfusion fixation. In Krinke GJ (ed.) *Handbook of Experimental Animals Series: The Laboratory Rat*. London: Academic Press, 2000, pp. 511–521.
12. Rand MS. *Handling, Restraint, and Techniques of Laboratory Rodents*. Available online at http://www.ahsc.arizona.edu/uac/iacuc/rodents/handling.htm, 1996.

13. Huerkamp MJ. *The Use of Analgesics in Rodents and Rabbits.* Available online at http://www.emory.edu/WHSC/MED/DAR/Analgesic_drugs.htm, 2000.
14. Collins Jr TB, Lott DF. Stock and sex specificity in the response of rats to pentobarbital sodium. *Lab. Anim. Care* 1968, **18**: 192–194.
15. Marietta MP, White PF, Pudwill CR, Way WL, Trevor AJ. Biodisposition of ketamine in the rat: self-induction of metabolism. *J. Pharmacol. Exp. Ther.* 1976, **196**: 536–544.
16. Buelke-Sam J, Holson JF, Bazare JJ, Young JF. Comparative stability of physiological parameters during sustained anesthesia in rats. *Lab. Anim. Sci.* 1978, **28**: 157–162.
17. Wixson SK, White WJ, Hughes Jr HC, Lang CM, Marshall WK. The effects of pentobarbital, fentanyl-droperidol, ketamine-xylazine and ketamine-diazepam on core and surface body temperature regulation in adult male rats. *Lab. Anim. Sci.* 1987, **37**: 743–749.
18. Hu C, Flecknell PA, Liles JH. Fentanyl and medetomidine anesthesia in the rat and its reversal using atipamazole and either nalbuphine or butorphanol. *Lab. Anim.* 1992, **26**: 15–22.
19. Brown JN, Thorne PR, Nuttall AL. Blood pressure and other physiological responses in awake and anesthetized guinea pigs. *Lab. Anim. Sci.* 1989, **39**: 142–148.
20. Field KJ, White WJ, Lang CM. Anaesthetic effects of chloral hydrate, pentobarbitone and urethane in adult male rats. *Lab. Anim.* 1993, **27**: 258–269.
21. Field KJ, Lang CM. Hazards of urethane (ethyl carbamate) a review of the literature. *Lab. Anim.* 1988, **22**: 255–262.
22. Zeller W, Meier G, Burki K, Panoussis B. Adverse effects of tribromoethanol as used in the production of transgenic mice. *Lab. Anim.* 1998, **32**: 407–413.
23. Alpert M, Goldstein D, Triner, L. Technique of endotracheal intubation in rats. *Lab. Anim. Sci.* 1982, **32**: 78–79.
24. Thet LA. A simple method of intubating rats under direct vision. *Lab. Anim. Sci.* 1983, **33**: 368–369.
25. Costa DL, Lehmann JR, Harold WM, Drew RT. Transoral tracheal intubation of rodents using a fiberoptic laryngoscope. *Lab. Anim. Sci.* 1986, **36**: 256–261.
26. Wood M, Wood AJ. Contrasting effects of halothane, isoflurane, and enflurane on in vivo drug metabolism in the rat. *Anesth. Analg.* 1984, **63**: 709–714.
27. Eisele PH, Woodle ES, Hunter GC, Talken L, Ward RE. Anesthetic, preoperative and postoperative considerations for liver transplantation in swine. *Lab. Anim. Sci.* 1986, **36**: 402–405.
28. Carruba MO, Bondiolotti G, Picotti GB, Catteruccia N, Da Prada M. Effects of diethyl ether, halothane, ketamine and urethane on sympathetic activity in the rat. *Eur. J. Pharmacol.* 1987, **134**: 15–24.
29. de Segura IAG. *Anaesthesia and Analgesia of Exotic Animals: Rodents and Rabbits.* Available online at http://www.vin.com/proceedings/Proceedings.plx?CID=WSAVA2002&PID=2567, 2004.
30. DeYoung DW. *Anesthesia, Surgery, Analgesia and Euthanasia.* Available online at http://www.ahsc.arizona.edu/uac/notes/classes/ANESTHESIA/anesthesia03.html, 2003.
31. UCSF. *Rodent Anesthesia and Surgical Management.* Available online at http://www.research.ucsf.edu/aw/Policies/awGlAnesSurg.asp, 2004.

32. Phifer CB, Terry LM. Use of hypothermia for general anesthesia in preweanling rodents. *Physiol. Behav.* 1986, **38**: 887–890.
33. Park CM, Clegg KE, Harvey-Clark CJ, Hollenberg MJ. Improved techniques for successful neonatal rat surgery. *Lab. Anim. Sci.* 1992, **42**: 508–513.
34. Sarajas HS, Oja SS. Effect of anesthesia and/or hypothermia on cerebral free amino acids in young rats. *Devel. Psychobiol.* 1973, **6**: 385–392.

6

Euthanasia in small animals

TURGUT TATLISUMAK

Only rarely does an animal experiment end in the natural death of the animal. In most cases, the animals must be killed following the completion of the experiment and certain tissue samples or organs must be collected. Even if the animal is fairly healthy after the experiment and even if it is not necessary to collect tissues, releasing laboratory animals into nature is strictly forbidden. Euthanasia is an important part of animal experimentation and every researcher who uses animals should be aware of the techniques and principles involved. There are a number of universally approved methods for euthanasia, but they may differ in different countries and different institutions even within the same country. This chapter will discuss the main methods of euthanasia. Every researcher must first consult the relevant authorities in their institution that provide permission for animal experiments, including the method of sacrifice. Only trained and competent personnel may carry out euthanasia within dedicated/suitable and approved facilities and only using methods approved by relevant authorities. Most animal facilities have veterinary physicians who are available for consultation and training purposes. The method for euthanasia should always be stated in detail in study plans and applications to the institutional body for animal care and use for scientific purposes. The method of euthanasia varies according to the animal species, number, nature of the experiment, and the intention of use of various organs for further research following death. Other animals and unnecessary personnel must not witness or hear the euthanasia procedures.

The term euthanasia comes from the Greek words for "easy death" (*eu*, good, *thanatos*, death).[1] The basic principle in euthanasia is to kill the animal with the least amount of distress and pain and to use a safe, reliable, rapid, and inexpensive method. Euthanasia methods should result in rapid loss of consciousness followed by cardiac or respiratory arrest and the ultimate, irreversible loss of brain function.[2] Usually, it is recommended to first anesthetize the animal before the final euthanasia procedure except in some rare situations. Proper and gentle handling before euthanasia is crucial to minimize discomfort to the animal and for safety of the personnel. Stress and pain inevitably

Handbook of Experimental Neurology, ed. Turgut Tatlisumak and Marc Fisher. Published by Cambridge University Press. © Cambridge University Press 2006.

cause several changes in physiologic parameters of the animal to be euthana-tized and may affect the results of the experiment.

There are a number of methods for euthanasia and they can be divided into two main groups as chemical and mechanical (physical).

6.1 Chemical methods

6.1.1 Inhalant anesthetics

Anesthesia and euthanasia with inhalant gas anesthetics require a transparent chamber with a pipe system that leads the gas in. The chamber must be intact and not allow leakage. Induction of anesthesia and loss of consciousness is more rapid if the inhalational agent concentration is high in the chamber. Some of these agents should be avoided for euthanasia purposes because of various risks. Halothane and isoflurane induce anesthesia rapidly and are very effective for euthanasia. Enflurane is less effective and may cause convulsions. Among the inhalants, halothane, isoflurane, and enflurane are generally acceptable for euthanasia especially in small animals.[3]

6.1.2 Carbon dioxide and carbon monoxide

Carbon dioxide is normally found in air in scarce amounts, is odorless, and heavier than air. The animal should be placed in a closed chamber and carbon dioxide with high concentration (preferably 100%) is allowed to flow in. Exposure to slowly increasing concentrations is preferred, because this lets the animal first fall into sleep (CO_2 narcosis) and later leads to death. Direct exposure to high concentrations may lead to suffocation. A glass or plastic system allows the researcher to observe the animal without opening the lid. At concentrations of 80–100% animals become unconscious within tens of sec-onds and respiratory arrest occurs in few minutes.[4] The animal should be left in the tank for several minutes to ascertain death. If the experiments necessi-tate use of large numbers of animals, this may be a good choice of method and a large euthanasia chamber can be built. Safety measures are important, as CO_2 is difficult to detect. Compressed CO_2 from cylinders is the only accep-table source because the inflow can be precisely regulated. Dry ice, fire extin-guishers, or chemicals are no longer permitted as sources of CO_2. An optimal flow rate of CO_2 should displace more than 20% of the chamber volume per minute.

Carbon monoxide (CO) is a colorless and odorless gas. It is neither explosive nor flammable, except at very high concentrations. CO binds rapidly and irreversibly to hemoglobin to form a carboxyhemoglobin complex. Consequently, erythrocytes cannot bind to oxygen and hypoxemia leads to death. CO euthanasia is also a quick and effective method, but the gas is difficult to detect, it is toxic, and therefore is risky for personnel. Furthermore, its use may be associated with agitation and convulsions in animals.[5] CO euthanasia should be avoided unless superb equipment, training, and safety measures are all arranged. In any case, it does not have any major advantage over the other measures of euthanasia.

6.1.3 Overanesthesia with non-inhalant agents

This is the simplest, easiest, and the most inexpensive method for killing animals. It is a commonly used method combined with or without exsanguination. The preferred drug is sodium pentobarbital at a dose of 120 mg/kg given either intravenously or intraperitoneally (intracardiac injection can only be used in heavily sedated or unconscious animals). Barbiturates depress the nervous system in a descending order, starting from the brain cortex with rapid loss of consciousness evolving into anesthesia, then deep anesthesia, and followed by respiratory depression, and later cardiac arrest within minutes. When the animal is apparently dead, it should still undergo cervical dislocation or decapitation to ensure death. This is the method of choice when cardiac perfusion-fixation is to follow. A combination of barbiturates with neuromuscular agents is not a suitable euthanasia method.

6.1.4 Intravenous or intracardiac potassium chloride injection

Potassium is strongly cardiotoxic and intracardiac/intravenous application results in cardiac arrest in seconds only. Potassium should never be given in conscious animals. However, if the animal is already anesthetized, this is a rapid and reliable method of euthanasia. Immediately following the injection muscle twitching and clonic spasms frequently occur.

6.2 Mechanical/physical methods

Mechanical methods of euthanasia are rapid and induce less fear and distress in animals. However, they require extensive training and as most of them involve trauma, they are potentially dangerous to personnel. Most physical methods seem brutal and displeasing, but when properly applied, they may be very humane.

6.2.1 Cervical dislocation

Cervical dislocation is appropriate for small animals in experienced hands. Especially mice and young rats can be killed with cervical dislocation. The animal should be held firmly with a rod-like instrument or a pencil located on its neck with one hand and hind limbs or the tail firmly held in the other hand. While the object is strongly pushed downwards to the junction of the head and the body, the animal is pulled down (backwards) leading to separation of the first cervical vertebra from skull base and massive damage to cervical tissues especially to cervical spinal cord (Fig. 6.1). Usually the body and all extremities contract one or more times (decerebration) and then relax. Electrical activity in

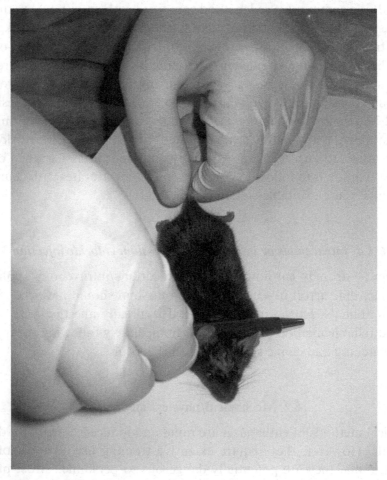

Figure 6.1. Cervical dislocation in a mouse. The procedure is performed under general anesthesia. A pen is used for pressing down on the neck.

brain cortex persists for 10 or more seconds following cervical dislocation,[6] therefore, although not strictly required, use of anesthesia or sedation prior to cervical dislocation is strongly encouraged.

6.2.2 Decapitation

Although it appears to be barbaric, this method is certain and quick and has some advantages. It allows for collection of blood and brain tissue, it is quick, certain, and inexpensive. The animal is placed under the guillotine and is decapitated with a quick full movement. A contraction in the body and extremities follows as in the above method. Some researchers use this method without prior anesthesia; we suggest that even decapitation should always be combined with prior anesthesia or sedation unless scientifically justified. Guillotines of various sizes for decapitation are available (Fig. 6.2). Sharp

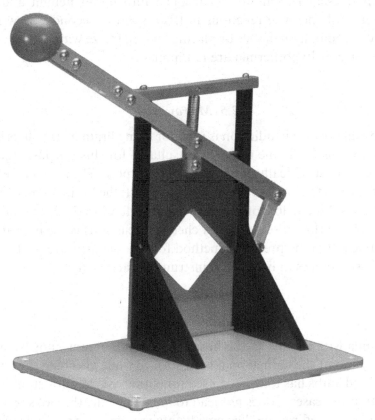

Figure 6.2. A commercially available guillotine for rodents. (Photograph courtesy of Dr Julian Williams, World Precision Instruments, Stevenage, UK.)

blades can also be used for very small-sized animals such as newborn mice. This technique carries a risk of injury to the personnel.

6.2.3 Exsanguination

Exsanguination can be performed with various methods, such as cardiac puncture through the thoracic wall, cutting a major artery open, cardiac perfusion, or by decapitation using a guillotine. Exsanguination gives an opportunity to collect large volumes of blood. Exsanguination is a suitable method in anesthetized animals.

6.2.4 Rapid freezing

Quick freezing by immersing into liquid nitrogen or liquid helium is rarely needed and has been largely abandoned. When used, it must be done under general anesthesia. The animal is dropped into liquid helium and freezes immediately. All chemical reactions in tissues end in seconds. Slow freezing by placing the animal on dry ice or placing in deep freeze with or without prior anesthesia or slow hypothermia are not humane.

6.2.5 Microwaving

Heating by microwave irradiation is used for fixing brain metabolites in vivo.[7] Microwave ovens for home use are not suitable for this purpose; there exist microwave ovens specifically designed for this purpose. The microwave irradiation is directed to the head of the mouse or the rat; the brain temperature rises to 80–90 °C resulting in loss of consciousness in a few hundreds of milliseconds and death in less than a second.[8] All chemical reactions cease in brain and it becomes fixed. It is the preferred method for reliable measurement of chemically labile substances in brain. The instruments are costly.

6.2.6 Head trauma

Brain trauma with a blow to the head (e.g., with a hammer) or by suddenly hitting the head of the animal on a hard surface while grabbing the animal by its tail or hind limbs has long been used for euthanasia and for stunning small animals. In many cases it does not lead to immediate death, looks brutal, may lead to external bleeding, and has no advantage over other methods of euthanasia. Furthermore, it cannot be applied to brain research if the brain must be collected for further examination. Even though this is an acceptable method in many countries other methods are preferable.

6.3 Euthanasia for fetuses and neonates

In the early phase of pregnancy (less than 2 weeks) neural development is minimal and pain perception is unlikely. Euthanasia of the mother or removal of the fetus will be sufficient. In the later phase of pregnancy (over 2 weeks) pain pathways are developed. In these fetuses, barbiturates are appropriate and can be followed by decapitation or cervical dislocation. Rapid freezing requires prior anesthesia.[9]

In neonates, anesthetics alone or combined with following mechanical measures (cervical dislocation or decapitation) is the method of choice. CO_2 narcosis is also an efficient method, but since mouse and rat fetuses and neonates are extremely resistant to CO_2 narcosis, it necessitates substantially longer exposure times (30 min or longer) to CO_2. If the animal is older than 2 weeks of age, they can be euthanatized in a way similar to adult rodents.[9]

6.4 Methods not suitable for euthanasia

Use of ether and chloroform has largely been abandoned because of safety reasons. Ether is extremely flammable and not acceptable unless used with adequate protection against the risk of explosion. Furthermore, it is an irritant to eyes and nose. Although it is not widely forbidden, there are several more appropriate methods. Nitrous oxide (N_2O) is not sufficient to induce anesthesia even at high concentrations and has a potential risk of abuse. Use of muscle relaxants without simultaneous application of anesthetics must be avoided since they lead to paralysis of respiratory muscles while consciousness preserves and the animal suffocates, and therefore are not a humane method of killing animals. Methods always unacceptable in an awake animal include potassium chloride injection, magnesium sulfate injection, strychnine, neuromuscular blocking agents, exsanguination, air embolism, and chloroform (hazardous to personnel). Electrocution is not a suitable method in small animals and should be avoided.[2]

Acknowledgments

This work is supported in part by the Helsinki University Central Hospital, the University of Helsinki, the Finnish Medical Foundation, the Sigrid

Juselius Foundation, and the Maire Taponen Foundation, all located in Helsinki, Finland.

References

1. *Merriam Webster's Collegiate Dictionary*, 10th edn. Springfield, MA: Merriam Webster, 1994.
2. American Veterinary Medical Association Panel on Euthanasia. 2000 Report of the AVMA Panel on Euthanasia. *J. Am. Vet. Med. Ass.* 2001, **218**: 669–696.
3. Booth NH. Inhalant anesthetics. In Booth NH, McDonald LE (eds.) *Veterinary Pharmacology and Therapeutics*, 6th edn. Ames, IA: Iowa State University Press, 1988, pp. 181–211.
4. Coenen AM, Drinkenberg WH, Hoenderken R, van Luijtelaar EL. Carbon dioxide euthanasia in rats: oxygen supplementation minimizes signs of agitation and asphyxia. *Lab. Anim.* 1995, **29**: 262–268.
5. Simonsen HB, Thordal-Christensen AA, Ockens N. Carbon monoxide and carbon dioxide euthanasia of cats: duration and animal behavior. *Br. Vet. J.* 1981, **137**: 274–278.
6. Vanderwolf CH, Buzsaki G, Cain DP, Cooley RK, Robertson B. Neocortical and hippocampal electrical activity following decapitation in the rat. *Brain Res.* 1988, **451**: 340–344.
7. Schneider DR, Felt BT, Rappaport MS, Goldman H. Development and use of a non-restraining waveguide chamber for rapid microwave radiation killing of the mouse and neonate rat. *J. Pharmacol. Meth.* 1982, **8**: 265–274.
8. Ikarashi Y, Maruyama Y, Stavinoha WB. Study of the use of the microwave magnetic field for the rapid inactivation of brain enzymes. *J. Pharmacol.* 1984, **35**: 371–387.
9. NIH Animal Research Advisory Committee. *Guidelines for the Euthanasia of Mouse and Rat Fetuses and Neonates*. Available online at http://oacu.od.nih.gov/ARAC/euthmous.htm, 2001.

7

Various surgical procedures in rodents

RENÉ REMIE

7.1 Principles of surgery

Surgery in laboratory animals, regardless of species and size, is governed by the same principles as those for surgery of human beings.

A basic principle in surgery is Halstead's contribution of not doing harm to the tissue. In fact this is only one of a set of interrelated principles composed of tissue handling and exposure, asepsis and hemostasis.

- Tissue handling. Remember that every time you pick up tissue with your instruments, you kill cells. Try to kill as few cells as possible. Be goal-oriented in your approach and remember that sharp dissection is generally less traumatic than blunt dissection.
- Exposure. Make sure your view is unobstructed, with proper illumination and physical access. This means that the wound you make should be sufficient in size and certainly not too small. Do not worry about the healing of the wound, as it is not primarily affected by its size, but rather by appropriate approximation of the wound edges.
- Asepsis. Conditions favorable to bacterial growth must be avoided. First of all a meticulous sterile technique must be followed. Second, but equally important, dead tissue and foreign materials should be removed together with blood or serum residues.
- Hemostasis. Especially in small laboratory animals blood loss can have serious consequences eventually resulting in the untimely death of your animal. Clamping or applying light pressure can stop almost all bleedings. Other ways are coagulation (mono-or bipolar), cauterization, ligation and chemical treatment with collagen and/or ADP-containing hemostatics.

7.1.1 The surgeon

In the beginning the study of surgical and especially microsurgical techniques makes many mental and physical demands. Attention to detail and a high

Handbook of Experimental Neurology, ed. Turgut Tatlisumak and Marc Fisher. Published by Cambridge University Press. © Cambridge University Press 2006.

concentration are very important when learning new techniques. When using a microscope, you do not have a direct eye-to-hand contact and you must develop an awareness of the fact that even simple movements in a significantly smaller world are more complex than when they are "life-size." Under the operating microscope not only are the objects enlarged, but at the same time your movements are magnified between 8 and 40 times. Also the physical ability required to co-ordinate one's movements decreases in proportion to the magnification used.

Individual preparation

Listed below are some suggestions to improve your performance.

- Make sure that the environment is quiet. A dedicated operating theatre is ideal.
- Try to avoid any mental stress.
- Make sure that your table is at the right height, giving adequate support to your arms. Sit upright to avoid strain injury to your shoulders, neck, and back.
- Plan your exercises. You need to be able to devote all your time to the exercise. Make sure that you have no appointments, and that you cannot be disturbed by telephone calls, etc. It is unrealistic to expect to perform well when your attention is divided or you act hastily.
- Try to avoid heavy physical exertion during the 24 hours preceding the surgical exercise, as this will interfere with your fine muscular control and probably will increase your tremor. Recently it was shown that experienced surgeons recover very quickly (within 4 hours) from heavy exercise.[1]
- Do not change any habits relating to your intake of coffee, as radical increase or decrease will increase your tremor.
- Do not become discouraged when something has gone wrong. If you encounter a difficulty, evaluate it and try to correct it before you continue. Do not let frustration become your greatest enemy.
- Do not work for too long at a stretch. Surgery is very fatiguing. If possible take a 10-minute break every hour, otherwise you will lose concentration and your co-ordination and learning ability will be reduced.

Planning

When a surgical procedure unfamiliar to the investigator is to be carried out, it is good practice for the work to be well planned. This will enable the investigator to feel and act calmly and confidently, while the animal gets the best possible treatment. So planning and preparation of an operation are important, and often underestimated. You should commence an operation preferably in the morning, in order to provide optimal postoperative care. The same is true for surgery at the end of the week, unless proper attention can be provided over the weekend.

Before you start an operation make sure that you have everything you need at your disposal. Preparation of a checklist of requirements before surgery is begun is helpful. It is most frustrating when you have to leave the operating theatre to search for things you urgently require, not to mention the break it causes in the aseptic technique.

For detailed instructions the reader is referred to Acland[2] and Remie *et al.*[3]

Anatomy

A thorough knowledge of the animal's anatomy is essential as it will reassure you whilst performing an operation. Do not start an operation until you are familiar with all the structures in the area of interest. Animals killed after being used in an experiment make ideal learning material. Use the operation microscope to look in detail at all kinds of tissue and learn how to handle the tissues with your instruments. For example, try dissecting some blood vessels to see how much tension they can withstand. As you will see, the majority of functions during microdissection are performed by slight pronation and supination movements of the fingers and forearm. Small spreading movements parallel to the blood vessel (or other structures) will prevent tearing of branches. Even while dissecting dead animals try to use atraumatic techniques, i.e., do not grab the whole thickness of the blood vessel between the jaws of your forceps. Pick it up only by its outer layer, the adventitia. The least damage you cause to the blood vessels and the surrounding tissues the better. For the study of rat and mouse anatomy the work of Greene,[4] Hebel and Stromberg,[5] and Iwaki and Hayakawa[6] are highly recommended.

Spatial relationships In anatomy, the basis defining all spatial relationships is the imaginary median plane, which runs from the head to the tail (Fig. 7.1). This plane divides the body into two equal (right and left) halves. Another imaginary plane is the sagittal plane, which runs parallel to the median plane. The sagittal plane also divides the animal into two, not necessary equal (left and right) sections. So there can be many sagittal planes but, by definition, only one median plane. The transverse plane lies perpendicular to the median plane; it divides the animal into a rostral, to define structures which are lying in the direction of the head, and a caudal part, which defines structures situated in the direction of the tail.

The transverse planes are traversed in turn by the coronal planes; these divide the body into a ventral and a dorsal component. The terms "proximal" and "distal" respectively relate to the anatomical definition of towards and away from the center, the median line, or point of attachment or origin.

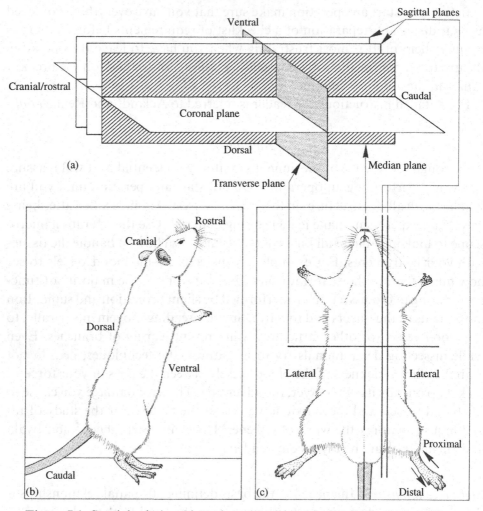

Figure 7.1. Spatial relationships, given (a) schematically, (b) in the standing animal, and (c) in the animal in supine position.

On the head itself we use the terms rostral and caudal, while in the rest of the body we use cranial and caudal. In the brain we use the term anterior instead of rostral and posterior instead of caudal.

7.2 Basic instrumentation

7.2.1 Surgical instruments

There are three main categories of surgical instruments: those that cut, grasp, or retract tissue. Always choose the instrument of proper size and strength to do the job. Try to get your own set of instruments. These should be of a good quality and must be well maintained. Do not begin with old, worn out, or obsolete equipment. Once you have acquired your set, do not lend it out.

Your set should consist of:

Macro instruments

- Anatomical or dissecting forceps (straight)
- Anatomical or dissecting forceps (90°-angled)
- A pair of fine-toothed forceps
- A pair of ring-handled scissors (straight, sharp/sharp, or sharp/blunt)
- A needle holder (Matthieu or Castroviejo)
- An artery forceps, baby-Mosquito, or micro-Halstead clamp
- Towel clips (Backhaus)
- Baby Dieffenbach Serrefines (bulldog hemostatic clamps)
- An instrument case

Micro instruments

- Two jeweler's forceps (No. 5, Dumont)
- One jeweler's forceps 45°-angled (Dumont)
- A micro needle holder (Barraquer-type), without a lock
- A pair of ring-handled dissecting scissors with gently curved blades
- A pair of fine 45°-angled iridectomy scissors (Wecker-type)
- Vessel clamps including a clamp applicator
  Two 12-mm single clamps (Acland, Biemer, or Heifetz)

Micro instruments should not be too long; 11–12 cm is suitable. An advantage of the Barraquer needle holder is that the round grips allow easy rotating movements.

Clamps can be divided into venous and arterial types, the latter having a higher shutting strength. One must be careful with clips that have a very high shutting strength, as they will damage the tissue.

Always clean your instruments immediately after surgery with tap water. Every now and then clean your instruments by placing them in an ultrasonicator. Before storing the instruments they must be dried and oiled using standard instrument oil. Some operations will require specialized instruments in addition.

7.2.2 The operating area

The physical environment in which surgery is to be performed can vary from a specially designed and sophisticated surgical suite to a small area on a laboratory bench. What is important is that the area is easily kept clean and uncluttered and is away from general human traffic. The liberal use of a disinfectant on all surfaces can be useful to reduce the room population of unwanted microorganisms and dust.

Operating table

Specially designed operating tables, or boards, made from metal, plastic, or silicon rubber are available and considerably aid surgery of small animals. Such tables may incorporate a heating facility which is very useful and is able to maintain the animals' temperature. Other most helpful accessories for surgery of small animals, such as small skin and tissue retractors, are available from commercial sources (Lone Star Medical Products, Inc.).

For simple operations on small animals a silicon plate (25×30 cm) may suffice. Silicon can be kept clean easily and may even be sterilized.

Lighting

A portable cold-illumination lighting system which can be regulated to give diffuse or pinpoint lighting is very effective. Proper lighting is of enormous help for surgery of all animals and the use of special surgical theater lights is highly recommended.

Other apparatus and accessories

The apparatus required for surgery will depend on the type of surgery being carried out, the species being used, and whether the surgery is an active part of an experiment. Similarly, surgical accessories such as gauze, drapes, cotton wool, etc., will be variously required. All apparatus should be clean and dust-free and preferably wiped down with a detergent or disinfectant. Some apparatus and accessories will be required to be sterile and this can be achieved by autoclaving or alternatively with suitable glass and metal apparatus, by dry heat in an oven at 160 °C for at least 1 hr. Plastic items can only satisfactorily be sterilized by irradiation but in many cases it is acceptable to use them after they have been disinfected in, for example, 0.5% aqueous chlorhexidine. Plastic cannulae disinfected in this way and rinsed with sterile saline have been kept in various parts of the body of both large and small animals for long periods of time without producing infection.

7.2.3 The animals

Animals should be allowed to acclimatize to their new environment for a period of 7 to 14 days. This is to make sure that metabolic and hormonal changes, as a result of a stressful transport, are eliminated. It is a good habit to keep records of body weight and of food and water consumption. A severe loss of body weight and a reduced intake of food and water are strong indications that the animal is in pain and adequate measures should be taken.

Given the fact that small rodents do not vomit during induction of anesthesia, it is not necessary to deprive them of food prior to the operation.

Preparation of the incision site

It is necessary to remove hair from the site of incision and from a sufficient area around it so that hair does not get into the wound. Apart from the possibility of causing infection by virtue of associated bacteria, hair can irritate the wound and delay healing. However, since short hair can be adequately disinfected, it is not always necessary to remove it for simple operations in rats and mice. Removal of hair should be carried out with clippers and a razor can then be used if required, though clipping suffices in most cases. The incision site must then be wiped liberally with an antiseptic such as 70% ethyl or isopropyl alcohol, or 0.5% chlorhexidine or 0.1% benzalconium chloride in 70% alcohol. Also very commonly used for larger animals in particular are tincture of iodine containing at least 1% free iodine and 10% povidone-iodine solution.

Do not use cream to remove the hair of the anesthetized animals, since it contains toxic components.

The incision

Making the incision is carried out with a scalpel and a sharp blade, though scissors are more frequently employed for the small animals. Some knowledge of anatomy is useful in determining where incisions into skin and muscle should be made, for example, when obtaining access to the trachea or associated structures such as the carotid arteries. These lie beneath the sternohyoid muscle, which is in two halves kept together by overlying connective tissue. Merely tearing the connective tissue will allow separation of the two muscle halves without damaging them and thus permit an approach to the underlying tissues.

Temperature

Animals undergoing surgery lose heat due to suppression of the thermoregulating center in the hypothalamus. The smaller the animal the faster the heat loss and for the mouse this can be alarming, with a 7-°C drop in body temperature within the first 10 min being quite possible (depending on the environmental temperature). Methods of monitoring body temperature vary from sophisticated automatic recording apparatus to the simple thermometer placed in the rectum. Any of these can be used for any of the common laboratory species.

Since a substantial drop in body temperature puts the animal at risk (anesthetics are more potent at lower temperatures) the temperature should be maintained near normal during the operation. This can be done using special (thermostatically controlled) heating pads on which the animal lies.

Fluid balance

Animals may lose substantial amounts of water and minerals during surgery, by evaporation of tissue fluid, loss of blood, and during respiration. Dehydration puts the animal at considerable risk, and if much fluid is lost it must be promptly replaced. Maintenance of fluid balance is a complex matter, but an interim measure is to give warm sterile saline. Any route of administration can be used and although the intravenous route is to be preferred, the fluid can be given intraperitoneally or subcutaneously as these routes are more accessible in the small animals.

Drying of tissues from prolonged exposure during surgery must be avoided and this can be prevented by applying warm saline or a saline-soaked gauze pad to the tissue.

Hemorrhage

Some bleeding during surgery is inevitable but blood loss at all times must be minimized and even mild loss can result in the animal showing signs of shock. Persistent bleeding must be stopped promptly. There are several methods to effect hemostasis, including clamping, ligation, electrocautery, and bipolar coagulation.

The bipolar coagulator is an indispensable surgical instrument that contributes to high-grade hemostasis and increases speed, leading to a higher efficiency of operation. Learn to use the coagulator properly with an appropriate pair of clean oiled bipolar forceps as this will reduce sticking of the forceps to the tissue.

If bleeding has occurred, excess blood must be removed before the wound is closed; otherwise it acts as an ideal medium for bacterial growth.

7.2.4 Suture materials

The primary function of suture is to hold tissue together. In the first week of wound healing in the rat, the strength of the wound is only 10–15% of the original strength of the unwounded tissue. This means that you have to adjust your choice of suture to the rate of tissue healing. Another important property is the tissue reaction caused by the suture. Generally absorbable sutures cause less reaction compared to the non-absorbable ones. Sutures should be removed after about 7 days.

Try to avoid excessively tight sutures as you allow bacteria to be protected in tissues made ischemic by pressure. Also avoid too many sutures making large ischemic portions, resulting in infection.

Today, both absorbable (polydioxanone, polyglycolic acid, and polylactic acid or a combination thereof) and non-absorbable materials are used. Most suture materials are of high quality; they pull easily through tissue and can be knotted securely. Mechanical performance of knotted sutures is generally measured by knot break load, minimum numbers of throws required for knot security, knot rundown force, first throw holding force, and tissue drag force.[7,8]

As a rule of thumb you should always use absorbable material. Only in case you want to fixate something (cannula or electrode) should you use non-absorbable sutures.

In rats the maximum suture size is 4–0 for closure of the abdominal cavity; in mice a 5–0 or 6–0 suture will do. Inside the animal, for ligation of small vessels etc., we only use 6–0 and 7–0 sutures.

Tying knots

In small animal surgery only instrument knots are tied. Knot tying starts with picking up the suture with the forceps. A loop (throw) is made on the tip of the needle holder which is placed just above the wound edges. Depending on the tension between the wound edges, single or double throws (to increase the friction in the first half of the knot) are made around the tip of the needle holder. Next the short end of the suture is grasped with the needle holder and the loop is pulled off, whilst moving each hand to the other side of the wound. Gently tightened to such extend that the wound edges are just approximated. This is the first half of the knot. Do not let go of the suture held with the forceps, but immediately make a second loop around the needle holder which again should be just above the wound edges in the middle of the V formed by the drawstrings of the suture. Pull off the loop and tighten the knot. You will see that the first half of the knot is progressively tightened during this procedure.

It is essential to maintain equal tension on the strands during knot tying. If you keep one strand under tension whilst the loop is pulled off, the knot will tumble and slip.

The configuration of a knot can be classified into two general types by the relation between the ears of the knot and the loop. When the right ear and loop of two throws exit on the same side of the knot (parallel to each other), the knot

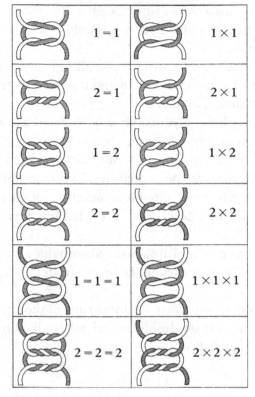

Figure 7.2. Different types of knots.

is judged to be square or reef. In case the right ear and loop exit on or cross different sides of the knot, it is called a granny knot. The above-described knot with two throws to overcome tension on the wound edges is called a friction or surgeon's knot. Tera and Åberg devised a simple description of a knot's configuration (Fig. 7.2).[9] The number of wraps for each throw is indicated by the appropriate arabic number. The relationship between each throw, being either cross or parallel, is given by the symbols $\times$ or $=$, respectively. In accordance with this code, the square knot is designated $1 = 1$, and the granny knot as 1×1, while the simple surgeon's knot is $2 = 1$ (this knot should not be used). A surgeon's knot with an extra half knot for security is represented by $2 = 1 = 1$. By following the above-mentioned sequence you will always tie $1 = 1$ or $2 = 1 = 1$ knots.

Wound closure and care

Gentle tissue handling combined with careful hemostasis, thorough debridement, and careful aseptic techniques decrease the risk of infections and promote healing.

7.2.5 Sterilization of instruments

Surgical asepsis

The opinion is widespread amongst scientists that rodents in particular are especially resistant to surgical infection, but evidence from work on intentional infection of these animals with pathogenic bacteria suggests that this may not be true. Considering the ubiquity of microorganisms, it is fortunate that only a small percentage is capable of causing diseases. It is against these pathogens that numerous methods of sanitization, disinfection, and sterilization have been developed. Although the rat has a remarkable resistance to the development of wound infection it is, however, frivolous to neglect aseptic technique for the surgical procedures. Surgery in the laboratory rat should therefore be governed by the same basic principles as those for surgery on human beings.

Surgical asepsis can be defined as the body of techniques that are designed to maintain an object or area in a condition as free of all microorganisms as possible. Unfortunately, the opinion amongst researchers that aseptic technique is a waste of time and money is still widespread.

Surgery on laboratory animals nowadays is often characterized by the use of so called "sanitary clean technique," meaning that the principles of aseptic surgery are completely neglected during procedures on small rodents. Most researchers varnish over these shortcomings by saying that a high percentage of animals remain alive after the operation. However, not the fact that the animals stay alive but rather the fact that they can be used as reliable models giving useful results should be the argument.

Asepsis during surgery seems far more important than is generally realized.[10] The literature about this specific topic is unfortunately limited.[11] This is probably due to the fact that the untimely death of an animal is seldom connected to the conditions during surgery. As a consequence more animals than strictly necessary are often being used. Furthermore, the consequences on the welfare aspects of the animals are unknown. The work of Baker on natural pathogens of laboratory animals and their effects on research gives additional arguments not to be reluctant with the application of aseptic technique.[12]

Another outcome of bad aseptic technique is the reduction of long-term patency rates of inserted catheters.[13] In our hands permanent jugular vein catheters can remain patent for up to 6 months (and sometimes even longer) when both catheters and surgical instruments are sterilized before use, in addition to some standard precautions (see below). When using non-sterile catheters and instruments, the patency is drastically reduced to between 1 and 2 weeks. But not only is patency affected, the recovery of the animal is also delayed and the time needed to return to the preoperative weight is extended.

A high level of aseptic technique can be achieved using the following procedures:

- Sterilization (generally achieved by autoclaving) of surgical instruments and all materials that are permanently implanted in the animal.
- Ask an assistant to help you during surgery.
- The use of proper scrub when washing hands, e.g., Betadine scrub (a polyvinylpyrrolidone–iodine solution), Hibiscrub (chlorhexidine solution).
- The use of rubber gloves: this was an important element in the transition from antiseptic surgery (killing microorganisms that are already present) to aseptic surgery (keeping the environment free from microorganisms from the outset).
- Subsequent disinfection with Sterillium® (isopropanol, n-propanol, and ethylhexadecyldimethyl ammonium ethylsulfate).
- The use of sterile suture materials, hypodermic needles and syringes, and sterile solutions (saline and heparin).
- A clean operating area, including a silicon rubber plate ($30 \times 25 \times 1$ cm) which can easily be sterilized or disinfected using 0.5% of an aqueous chlorhexidine solution or 70% ethanol.
- During surgery try to avoid talking, sneezing, and coughing, or making unnecessary body movements.

Furthermore you should know what is sterile and what is contaminated. Needless to say only sterile things may be touched by the surgeon. In case of doubt consider the object as contaminated.

For a wealth of information concerning good surgical practice (GSP) the reader is referred to the work of Tracy.[14]

In addition to the above-mentioned precautions animals could be administered an antibiotic in case a break of aseptic technique is likely to occur or when the total operating time exceeds 180 min. A single dosage of 150 mg/kg amoxycillin subcutaneously (s.c.) or ampicillin (150 mg/kg s.c.) given 10 min prior to the operation will give adequate protection against possible infections. Alternatively Baytril® (Enrofloxacin, Bayer) could be administered subcutaneous at a dose of 4 mg/kg body weight.

7.2.6 Anesthesia

Inhalation anesthesia is preferred above injectable anesthesia, as it allows for a better control of the anesthetic depth. We now routinely use isoflurane in combination with oxygen and nitrous oxide or air (50–50%). Concentration of isoflurane strongly depends on the strain and the concomitant use of nitrous oxide. Following induction it is most convenient to maintain anesthesia using a facemask. Make sure you remove waste and access anesthetic gases using a validated gas-scavenging system in order to protect you from unknown side effects.

When using stereotaxic equipment, special nose adapters for rats are available for the Kopf stereotaxic apparatus.

7.2.7 Solutions

All solutions used should be sterile and used at body temperature.

7.3 Catheterization of veins and arteries

7.3.1 Blood sampling

Blood samples are often needed in biomedical research. There are numerous ways in which blood can be sampled from the laboratory animals. Techniques can be divided into three categories, being acute without surgery, acute with surgery (anesthetized animals), and chronic models.

Acute techniques without surgery include:

- puncture of the ophthalmic venous plexus
- puncture of the heart
- cutting the tail vein
- decapitation.

In all these methods, the animal is anesthetized, handled, or restrained. This causes adverse reactions in the animal, such as a rise of glucose, prolactin, catecholamine, and corticosteroid levels. Needless to say that these changes may interfere with results of the experiment. Cutting of the tail vein can be done without anesthesia and seems to give reliable results.[15]

With surgery, while the animal remains anesthetized during the complete experiment:

- catheterization of the jugular vein
- catheterization of the carotid artery
- catheterization of the femoral vein
- catheterization of the femoral artery.

In these acute models the anesthetic has a marked influence on a number of physiological parameters.

These influences can be avoided by taking blood samples from surgically prepared animal models with permanent catheters. The techniques allow blood samples to be taken from freely moving animals without disturbing them. Several techniques have been put forward.

Techniques used with surgery (permanent catheters) include:

- catheterization of the jugular vein
- catheterization of the femoral vein
- catheterization of the carotid artery
- catheterization of the femoral artery.

Permanent catheterization of the jugular vein was described in the rat and the ground squirrel by Popovic *et al.* in 1963.[16] Catheterization of the jugular vein in combination with a head attachment apparatus allowing easy connection of catheters was first introduced by Steffens.[17] These techniques enable continuous blood sampling from the general circulation and even infusion of fluids in the freely moving rat. During sampling or infusion the animal remains undisturbed, which is of vital importance in experiments monitoring behavior or where stress factors are expected to influence results. Several modifications have been introduced amongst which are the ones by Brown and Hedge who introduced the L-shaped adapter,[18] Nicolaidis *et al.* who used an additional stainless steel head bolt,[19] and Dons and Havlik who used a multilayered catheter.[20] A good overview of methods for vascular access and collection of body fluids from the laboratory rat has been given by Cocchetto and Bjornsson.[21]

Catheters and their preparation

Catheters can be made of different materials, having different biocompatibility and thrombogenetic properties. For acute catheterization polyethylene, polyvinyl chloride, or polyurethane catheters are used. The catheters should be cut under 45° as the beveled end allows for easy insertion.

Permanent catheters used in rats and mice are preferably made of silicon rubber. Silicon tubing is rather flexible, causes hardly any immunity problems, and can be sterilized easily. As a routine we use Silastic® or Silclear™ medical-grade tubing from Dow Corning or Degania Silicone respectively. These tubings are available in various sizes. Alternatively you may use commercially available catheters such as those provided by Instech. Normally these catheters are cut rectangular ensuring minimal damage to intima.

To enhance biocompatibility and reduce thrombogenicity catheters might be coated (e.g. CBAS, or Hydromer).

7.3.2 *Acute catheterizations*

Catheterization of the femoral vessels (vein or artery)

Since this technique is almost the same for the artery and vein, it is described as one. A skin incision of approximately 1.5 cm is made starting at the point where the femoral vessels leave the abdominal cavity towards the hind leg. The underlying fat is carefully dissected using small forceps to expose the femoral vessels. Regular flushing with warm sterile saline is carried out throughout the procedure. At this point, you should separate the vein from the artery, leaving the saphenous nerve untouched. The vessels are manipulated by their adventitia using jeweler's forceps. Any residual fat and connective tissue is removed over a distance of approximately 12 mm. At this point it should be easy to raise the vessels by inserting the tip of the forceps beneath each one of them. Subsequently, two ligatures (6–0 silk) are placed around the vessel, a distal one that will tie off the vein or artery and a proximal one to tie the vessel around the catheter once it is inserted. Catheterization is facilitated by clamping the distal ligature close to the vessel to put it under slight tension, thus stabilizing and lifting the vessel. Before cutting a V-shaped hole in the vessel close to the distal ligature, using microvascular scissors, a clamp should be placed on the vessel just above the proximal ligature and the catheter, previously primed with sterile heparinized saline (50 IU/ml) is gently inserted into the vein using straight anatomical forceps. To secure the catheter the drawstring of the distal ligature should be tied around the catheter. Slightly open the clamp to check for leaking and patency.

As an alternative to cutting a hole in the vessel, a sterile 23-gauge needle fitted to a 1-ml syringe with the needle tip bent to a 90° angle can be used. This method works best for the artery. Using it on the vein may result in an uncontrolled longitudinal hole.

Catheterization of the jugular vein

A 1.5 cm incision should be made just above the right clavicle (Fig. 7.3). This place can be easily found by drawing imaginary lines between the animal's right ear and its left armpit, and between its right armpit and the chin.

Using two or three spreading movements with sharp scissors, connective and adipose tissue are pushed aside and the external jugular vein is exposed and mobilized over a distance of about 1 cm.

Small artery forceps (micro-Halstead or baby-Mosquito) are used to clamp the vessel as rostral as possible. The vein should then be ligated rostral to the clamp using 6–0 silk. A second ligature should be put loosely around the vessel.

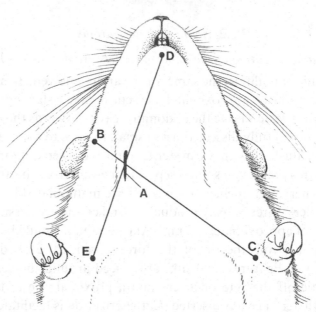

Figure 7.3. The correct place for an incision to catheterize the jugular vein. The imaginary lines between the animal's right ear and its left armpit (B–C), and between the chin and its right armpit (D–E) should be used to locate the exact place of incision (A).

Using iridectomy scissors, a V-shaped hole should be cut in the vein just proximal to the clamp. Prior to its insertion into the vessel, the catheter must be connected via a 23-gauge needle to a 1-ml syringe filled with a sterile heparinized saline solution (50 IU/ml). After insertion the second ligature must be tied, the artery forceps removed, and the first ligature tied to secure the catheter.

Catheterization of the carotid artery

The ventral neck area from the lower mandible to the sternum should be shaven. This area is then disinfected using chlorhexidine solution. A longitudinal incision should be made along the ventral midline. The membrane overlying the glands should be opened and the glands pushed aside with curved jeweler's forceps. The right carotid artery can be found lateral to the muscles overlying the trachea. The carotid artery should be mobilized for a distance of 12 mm in caudal direction. Make sure that the vagus nerve, which is lying next to the artery, is carefully dissected from the carotid artery without being damaged. The artery should then be ligated with 6–0 silk. This ligature should be tightened and put under minimal tension in rostral direction. A vessel clamp should be placed 10 mm caudal from the bifurcation. This will prevent extensive bleeding when the vessel is cut. A V-shaped hole should be cut 1 mm caudal from the bifurcation using micro-scissors. Prior to its insertion into the vessel, the catheter must be connected to a 1-ml syringe filled with sterile heparinized saline solution (50 IU/ml). As described before, a modified 23-gauge needle with its tip bent to a 90° angle can also be used to puncture and subsequently catheterize the vessel. The catheter should be pushed in until its tip reaches the vessel clamp.

The proximal ligature should be tied with the first half of a square knot. This will prevent the cannula being pushed out (blood pressure) when the vessel clamp is released, while it is still possible to advance the catheter into the artery. To be sure that the cannula is not pushed out, the inserted part of the cannula must be held in place with the jeweler's forceps while the cannula is pushed further using anatomical forceps. The second half of the square knot should now be tied and the distal ligature should be tied to secure the catheter.

7.3.3 Chronic catheterization

Catheterization of the jugular vein

The technique described below is one of the most simple and reliable, and it should be regarded as one of the basic techniques in catheterization of blood vessels.[22]

The operation can be divided into four parts:

(1) preparation of the crown of the head
(2) catheterization of the jugular vein
(3) subcutaneous tunneling of the catheter
(4) fixation of the catheter.

After the neck of the animal has been shaved on the right side, the skin should be disinfected with chlorhexidine solution. An incision should be made just above the right clavicle (Fig. 7.3). This place can be easily found by drawing imaginary lines between the animal's right ear and its left armpit, and between the chin and its right armpit.

Using two or three spreading movements with sharp scissors connective and adipose tissue are pushed aside and the jugular vein is exposed. The division of the external jugular into the maxillary vein and the linguofacial vein should be identified. This bifurcation is recognizable by the presence of a small lymph node. At this point one should choose the largest vessel for catheterization and mobilize it over a distance of about 5 mm.

Small artery forceps (micro-Halstead or baby-Mosquito) are used to clamp the vessel 3 mm rostral from the bifurcation. The vein should then be ligated

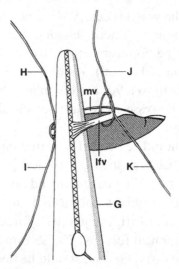

Figure 7.4. Placing a clamp and ligation of the vessel. Small artery forceps (G) (micro-Halstead or baby-Mosquito) are used to clamp the vessel. The cranial ligature (H/I) is tightened while the caudal ligature (J/K) is placed loosely around the vessel. mv, maxillary vein; lfv, linguofacial vein.

rostral to the clamp using 6–0 silk. A second ligature should be put loosely around the vessel (Fig. 7.4). Using iridectomy scissors, a V-shaped hole should be cut in the vein 2 mm rostral from the bifurcation. Prior to its insertion into the vessel, the sterile catheter must be connected via a 23-gauge needle to a 1-ml syringe filled with a heparinized saline solution (50 IU/ml). No air bubbles should be left in the catheter. Using sharp-pointed jeweler's forceps to dilate the vessel, the catheter should be slid between the legs of the forceps and gently pushed into the vessel until the silicon ring reaches the V-shaped hole. Sometimes whilst trying to push the catheter gently into the vessel, it bounces on release. The catheter will almost certainly have entered the subclavicular vein. This can be remedied by pulling the catheter back, whilst still leaving it inside the vessel, then pushing it back in gently while lifting the animal's chest by the skin. When the silicon ring has reached the vessel, the tip of the catheter should now be at the level of the right atrium. This can be checked by removing the needle and the syringe and looking at the fluid in the free end of the catheter. During inspiration the fluid should be sucked into the catheter, while during expiration the fluid should be pushed back (intrathoracic pressure). Moreover, the heart frequency should be superimposed on the respiratory-induced fluid movements. The catheter should be further checked by aspirating some blood, and the catheter should be flushed gently with heparinized saline solution. The artery forceps should now be removed, the caudal ligature gently tied, and the rostral ligature used to anchor the catheter to the vessel. Subsequently, the syringe should be removed and the catheter gently clamped using a small microvascular clamp. To ensure that the catheter cannot move, one drawstring of each ligature should be cross-tied.

Subcutaneous tunneling Small artery forceps are pushed in longitudinally under the skin in a caudal direction to a distance of about 3 cm. Subsequently, the forceps should be turned anticlockwise through an angle of 90 degrees, and pushed in the direction of the incision in the neck. The catheter should be grasped by the forceps and pulled back. Always make sure that the catheter makes a smooth curve ensuring that the animal can move freely without tearing the catheter. The forceps should then be removed and replaced by a small microvascular clamp. Subsequently the catheter is flushed with sterile saline, connected to an L-shaped adapter, and filled with a catheter lock solution. Finally the wound in the neck of the animal should be closed with two absorbable sutures (for details see Remie *et al.*[3]).

Fixation of catheters The head of the animal should be shaven and disinfected with a chlorhexidine solution. An incision of approximately 2 cm should be made in the crown of the head. This will provide enough space to mount three stainless steel screws (1.1 mm in diameter and 4.2 mm in length) in the crown of the skull which are used for additional anchoring. The membranous tissue should be removed, using curved jeweler's forceps, and the bregma (the point on the top of the skull where the coronal and sagittal sutures meet) is then exposed. With a 3/0-round dental drill, three holes should be made, two on the left and one on the right of the bregma. The stainless steel dental drill should be loosely held between the thumb and forefinger to allow rotating movements. To ensure that the underlying tissues such as the dura, the rostral sagittal sinus, or the transverse sinus are not punctured, the conical end of the drill is covered with a piece of polyethylene tubing leaving about 2 mm of the tip uncovered. If you have access to a mechanical drill, this procedure can be carried out very quickly. Make sure that you drill the holes with a sharp drill bit rotating at low speed, as high-speed drilling will dehydrate the bone structure leading to necrosis. The screws are fitted into the holes using specially prepared surgical forceps and a small screwdriver (see Fig. 7.5). They are tightened to such an extent that approximately 2 mm is left between the skull and the head of the screws. Prior to fixation, the catheter has to be slid over the short end of the L-shaped adaptor. To serve this purpose you may use some diethyl ether to make the silicon tubing even more supple and the catheter will slide smoothly over the stainless steel tubing. Catheters placed in blood vessels

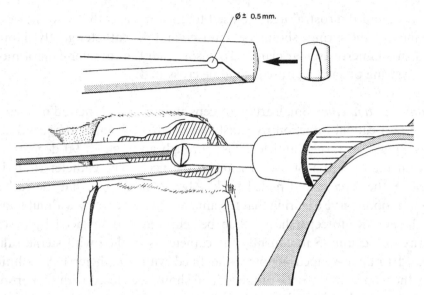

Figure 7.5. The specially prepared surgical forceps hold the stainless steel screw for easy insertion.

should now be flushed with saline (0.5 ml) and filled with a catheter lock solution. The long end of the L-shaped stainless steel adapter should be closed with a piece of heat-sealed polyethylene tubing. Next, the catheter together with the L-shaped adaptor should be fixed to the skull with suitable glue. Make sure the glue flows properly under the heads of the screws and that it is wrapped around the vertical part of the adaptor as this will prevent any movement.

Traditionally glues used to fixate catheters or electrodes on the crown of the head were taken from the dental praxis. Two-component acrylic glue was the standard during a long period of time. Due to the exothermic reaction during curing, the temperature of 1 g of glue could rise to 80 °C.[23] Other problems with this glue were the moderate binding to a wet surface and the relative long curing time (5 min). Today we prefer to use glasionomeric glue such as Fuji CG. This glue binds to moist surfaces and develops less exothermic heat. E. N. Spoelstra (personal communication) tested different pretreatments of the bony surface of the skull. Etching with diluted acid gel or mechanical roughening of the surface gave good binding. In case the glue has optimal binding it is not necessary to use additional anchoring screws.

On their website Alzet advocates the use of cyanoacrylate gel (CAG) (Loctite 454 Adhesive) instead of dental cement.[24] The results indicate that the use of CAG significantly reduced surgical time for the preparation of intracerebroventricular (ICV) implants in rats and had no adverse effects on the postoperative period when compared to the dental cement technique. Also, the advantage of the CAG technique was reduction of the number of screws used for the implant, resulting in less trauma to the skull, and reduction of the size of the headcap. In addition, the transparent nature of the gel may allow early visual detection of inflammation and infection under the headcap.

As an alternative to the head attachment a button can be used. There are a number of different types of implantable buttons available. Tethering buttons are generally attached by suturing in place under the skin or on top of the skin in the scapular area. The button allows the catheter to be externalized and attached to a spring tether. The button may also be held in place with a rodent jacket without suturing the button to the rat.

The type of button used depends on the needs of the research. Stainless steel buttons have been used for many years. They can be autoclaved and reused virtually without wear. Stainless steel buttons appear to be best suited for short-term studies, i.e., those lasting less than 7 days. Longer use of the stainless steel buttons can cause adverse tissue reaction.

Polysulfone buttons are rigid buttons that can be autoclaved and can be reused. Another type of button is the Dacron mesh button. This button has a Dacron mesh screen base and a soft plastic tip. The mesh base allows the tissue to infiltrate the material on longer studies. This produces an excellent attachment between the button and the animal. The flexible, soft, plastic tip creates a simple, yet effective, method to attach the button to the spring tether. Dacron mesh buttons are not reusable, but are relatively inexpensive.

Catheter lock solutions The patency life can be affected by many factors including flushing regimen, catheter material, and lock solutions used to fill the lumen of the catheter. Luo *et al.* studied several lock solutions with respect to their ability to maintain patency of unmanipulated, indwelling polyurethane vascular catheters in rats, as the use of a vascular flushing regimen would give unwanted variation:[25]

Heparinized saline Sodium heparin (10 000 IU/ml) was added to physiological saline (0.9%) to make a final concentration of 500 IU/ml.

Heparinized dextrose Sodium heparin (10 000 IU/ml) was added to 50% dextrose solution to make a final concentration of 500 IU/ml.

Heparinized polyvinyl pyrrolidone (PVP) Sodium heparin (10 000 IU/ml) and PVP (SIGMA PVP-40) was added to physiological saline (0.9%) to make a final concentration of 500 IU heparin/ml and 1 g PVP/ml in the final solution.

Heparinized glycerol Sodium heparin (10 000 IU/ml) was added to a glycerol solution (1.26 g/ml) to make a solution with a final concentration of 500 IU/ml of heparin.

Recovery after surgery Before you start using your animals, you should allow them to recover completely. In the past we used the return to preoperative weight as a sign that the animal had recovered completely. Today, however, using telemetric devices we know that it takes at least 7–9 days before the circadian rhythm has returned to normal. This is long after the animal has returned to its preoperative weight.

7.4 Craniectomy and craniotomy

7.4.1 Craniectomy

Craniectomy is defined as the removal of the brain. In most experimental work on the brain it is necessary to perfuse and remove the brain after the experiment(s). In this way one can see the exact location of, e.g., electrodes, lesions, infusion cannulae, or dialysis probes. Therefore we have to perfuse the brain with saline and formaldehyde fixative (10%) respectively. Perfusion can simply be performed using two reservoirs, one filled with saline and the other with 10% formaldehyde. Using a three-way stopcock both fluids may be perfused through the same needle (19-gauge).

Cardiac perfusion-fixation and removal of the brain

The animal should be deeply anesthetized using twice the amount of barbiturate needed for surgical anesthesia. Open the abdomen via a medial laparotomy, and open the thorax by cutting the ribs. Insert a perfusion needle into the left ventricle of the heart. Keep the needle in place by clamping it with a hemostatic forceps onto the point where the needle enters the heart. Next cut a hole in the right atrium to allow blood to be drained from the head. Keep on flushing with saline solution until the effluent is clear and subsequently switch to formaldehyde perfusion (250 ml). Next the brain can be removed.

Make an incision from behind the ears to the nose. Cut the skin from the skull down to the nose. Remove the temporal muscles from the skull and the first two vertebrae. Next remove the cranial bone using small bone cutters until the olfactory bulbs are visible. Cut the dura and lift the brain, starting with the anterior part. Cut the cranial nerves, lift the rest of the brain and cut the upper part of the spinal cord. Continue the fixation process by replacing the brain in formaldehyde (10%) during 3 days. Now you are ready for sectioning and staining.

7.4.2 Craniotomy

Craniotomy is defined as an operation on the skull or an incision into the skull. Surgery on the head is easier than surgery on other parts of the body, because there is little risk of excessive hemorrhage and the area is easily exposed.

Stereotaxic brain surgery is one of the techniques used to apply mono- or bipolar needle-shaped electrodes, infusion catheters, or sample catheters for the collection of cerebrospinal fluid.

In this section some basic principles in the use of stereotaxic equipment will be discussed. Furthermore some frequently use techniques will be described.

Anatomy

As with all surgery, a thorough knowledge of the anatomy of the area of interest is of vital importance. Fortunately there are a number of atlases available describing different aspects of the rat brain.[26]

If we look at the skull diagram of a 290-g Wistar rat in dorsal and lateral view, important landmarks are: bregma, lambda, and the interaural line (see Fig. 7.6).[27] Note that lambda is 0.3 mm anterior to the coronal plane passing through the interaural line.

The principle of stereotaxic surgery is based upon the constant relationship between these landmarks on the skull and parts of the brain. A system of three co-ordinates is used to determine a specific location in the brain relative to one of these landmarks:

Anterior–posterior (A–P)
Dorsal–ventral (D–V)
Lateral (Lat)

Stereotaxic brain surgery

Preparation of the animal Animals (adult Wistar rats of either sex) should preferable weigh between 250 and 350 g.[28,29] There may be some differences in craniometric and stereotaxic data for rats of different strain, sex, and weight; however, no substantial stereotaxic error will occur when rats of 290 g of a different strain and sex are used.[27] For the use of stereotaxis in newborn rats, the reader is referred to Cunningham and McKay.[30]

After the animal has been anesthetized, the head of the animal is shaved and disinfected. The rat is placed in a Kopf small-animal stereotaxic instrument.

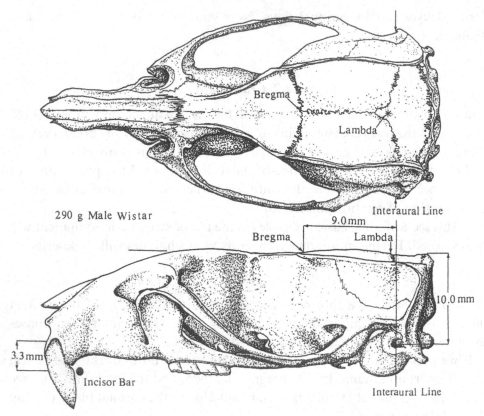

Figure 7.6. Dorsal and lateral view of the skull of a 290-g male Wistar rat, showing bregma, lambda, and the interaural line. (From Paxinos and Watson[27]).

The head will be fixed in three places, the two bony ear canals and the upper jaw. Start with inserting the ear bars into both ear canals. The head should pivot freely about the interaural axis and should have little lateral movement. Move the incisor bar under the upper incisors. Place the nose clamp over the nose, gently retract the incisor bar anteriorly and tighten it. Next the incisor bar should be adjusted vertically until the heights of lambda and bregma are equal (both in a coronal plane), resulting in a flat skull position. For the implantation procedure it is imperative that all the periosteum is removed from the crown of the head, ensuring that the glue will properly adhere to the skull. After positioning of the implantable device three additional holes may be drilled in the skull.

Positioning of implantable devices To determine the exact position of an implantable device (electrode, catheter, microdialysis probe, etc.) you have to use a stereotaxic atlas (Paxinos and Watson[27] is highly recommended). After the animal has been placed in the stereotaxic instrument, the implantable device is clamped into the electrode carrier. Make sure that the device is straight and has a 90° angle to the coronal plane. Next the tip of the device is adjusted directly above the bregma and the reading for the A–P and the Lat zero point are taken. Subsequently calculate the readings after the distances given in the stereotaxic atlas are added or subtracted from the A–P and Lat zero readings. The device should now be moved to the newly calculated A–P and Lat position. The device is lowered until it just touches the skull, giving the vertical zero reading. Calculate what the final reading must be in order for the tip of the device to penetrate the brain to the specific depth. When the device is in the newly calculated position, it should be slightly raised, and the place on the skull where the hole has to be drilled should be marked with a sharp pencil. Move the electrode aside and drill a hole of sufficient diameter in the skull at the pencil mark. Next the device should again be positioned in the A–P and Lat planes, according to the previous calculation. Now the device is lowered over the required distance to the reading of the calculated vertical placement (D–V value).

Lesion or stimulation using electrodes Monopolar electrodes can be used to damage or stimulate brain areas by passing an electrical current between the relative small surface area on the tip of the electrode, to a relative large amount of body tissue acting as a ground terminal. Electrodes are preferably made of platinum, and should be insulated. A two-component epoxy resin can be used for insulation. Simply dip the electrode in once or twice and let the resin cure. Next 0.5 mm of the tip is freed of the insulation using a scalpel blade.

Always connect the positive terminal (anode) of the current source to the electrode, thus preventing the formation of hydrogen and oxygen. The cathode should be clamped on a muscular layer on the head. After the lesion has been made, the electrode is removed and the hole in the skull is closed with bone wax. Next the skin is closed using interrupted suture technique.

Bipolar electrodes are very similar to the monopolar ones. They are commercially available but you can also build them yourself. Before implantation of the bipolar electrode, it should be soldered to a miniature connector (e.g., an IC foot).

Technically, the bipolar electrode is implanted in the same way as the monopolar electrode. After the electrode has been placed in a specific brain region, according to the calculated A–P, Lat, and D–V values, the electrode together with the small IC foot connector are glued to the skull using acrylic dental cement. Note that the electrode carrier is still holding the electrode during this process. After the dental cement has cured the skin should be closed around the connector using absorbable sutures (4–0).

Electroencephalography Electroencephalography (EEG) recording requires specialized equipment and technique. The signals picked up from the cortex are of very low voltage and should be derived as close to the source as possible. Electrode placement therefore is of vital importance.[31] We routinely use 1-mm stainless steel screws. The screws are equipped with 2 cm long small-diameter non-insulated stainless steel wires, which are point-welded to the top of the screw. The screws are placed on the crown of the head: the first one 2 mm posterior and 2 mm lateral to bregma and the second one 2 mm anterior and 2 mm lateral to lambda. A third screw is used for additional anchoring and can also be used as a ground electrode. The wires of all three screws are soldered (in situ) to a small connector.

Signals may be registered via a multi-channel electrical swivel while the animal is kept in a slowly rotating cage (to keep it awake) placed in a Faraday cage. More sophisticated is the use of a telemetric device that can be magnetically switched on and off, ensuring a long lifespan of the battery (approximately 1 year).

Central nervous system injections and infusions Several techniques have been described for placement of a catheter in one of the ventricles of the rat for injection, sampling, and infusion. Most techniques are rather simple and use a combination of an external guide cannula and an internal cannula. A very reliable and inexpensive cannula and injection system for local chemical brain stimulation with small volumes of fluids has been described by Strubbe.[32] This system, which will be described below, has several advantages over those mentioned in the literature. Its construction is very simple, it is inexpensive and therefore disposable, it allows bilateral infusions without disturbing the animal and it gives you a direct visual check of the rate at which the fluid enters the brain.

The system consists of a permanent guide (outer) cannula, made from a disposable hypodermic 23-gauge needle. The colored plastic is removed with the exception of the white fixed inner ring. The thin plastic layer above the ring is removed using a sharp knife. The needle is cut to a length depending on the depth of the brain area to be stimulated. After disinfection in chlorhexidine solution, the cannula tip is placed stereotaxically as described above. The plastic ring being just above the surface of the skull is now fixed using acrylic dental cement and three screws to anchor the cement to the skull. A poly-ethylene cap (inner diameter (ID) 0.58 mm, outer diameter (OD) 0.96 mm) is placed on the outer cannula. In case bilateral cannulas are wanted, they can be mounted in a brass bar with holes at the required distance and can be glued together with dental cement.

The inner cannula consists of a stainless steel tube (ID 0.1 mm, OD 0.29 mm) and should be exactly 3 mm longer than the guide cannula. Over these 3 mm a polyethylene tube is slipped (ID 0.29 mm, OD 0.61 mm). A silicon cuff (ID 0.5 mm, OD 1.0 mm) is slid over this connection.

On the other end of the polyethylene tube a silicon cuff (ID 0.5 mm, OD 1.0 mm) is placed. Over this cuff a second silicon tube (ID 1.0 mm, OD 3.0 mm) is slipped. A small nail with a head of suitable size (plunger) is pushed into the silicon tube and the injection system is ready.

The injection system is first filled completely with methylene blue (1% in saline). Subsequently the nail is pushed down and slightly pulled back again until an air bubble can just be perceived above the inner cannula. Now the tip of the inner cannula is placed in the fluid to be injected. The nail is pulled up so that the infusion tube is filled with that fluid. The inner cannula is then placed into the outer cannula. The silicon cuff on the lower end of the injection tube serves to attach it firmly to the guide cannula. The injection can now be made by pushing down the nail. The air bubble, separating methylene blue from the injection fluid, may serve as a marker for reading the volume administered. This volume can be calculated from the diameter of the polyethylene tubing.

Microdialysis

Chemical interplay between cells occurs in the extracellular fluid, a compartment usually overlooked due to the fact that it is hard to access experimentally. Many experimental approaches have been suggested to get information about the extracellular environment of the intact brain, for example ventricular perfusion, cortical cup perfusion and push–pull cannulas. The introduction of a dialysis membrane into the tissue has provided the first generally applicable way of interacting with the extracellular compartment. Brain dialysis is a good technique for the investigation of in vivo release of neurotransmitters and amino acids.[33–37] It has some advantages over other techniques such as push–pull perfusion, which has the risk of doing mechanical damage to the tissue, and in vivo voltammetry,[38,39] where it is often uncertain what the chemical identity of the detected material is.[37,40]

Today a range of different probes is used, e.g., the transstriatal, the U-shaped, the I-shaped, and the commercially available Carnegie cannulae.

Four different types of intracerebral microdialysis probes have been characterized.[41] Every type of dialysis probe causes a certain amount of damage when implanted into the brain. In acute experiments the best results were obtained using the I-shaped probe. In the chronic situation (24 hr after implantation) all probes performed well. During the second day after implantation, conditions were optimal to carry out dialysis experiments. After 48 hr certain restrictions are to be expected due to elevated K^+ levels in the neuronal tissue.

The transstriatal probe displayed a high output as it perfuses bilateral brain structures, but from an animal welfare point of view, much discomfort is produced due to damage done to the temporal muscles.

Details about perfusion fluids and other practical aspects can be found in reference 42.

7.5 Non-invasive and invasive measurement of blood pressure in rodents

Experiments with acutely prepared, anesthetized, or immobilized laboratory animals has been the standard for many years. The greater part of physiological and pharmacological knowledge on blood pressure, its regulation, and the influence of drugs on the cardiovascular system has been derived from these experiments. The site of measurement was either the carotid artery or the femoral artery.

Although valuable, this information is obscured by direct effects of anesthesia and surgical intervention. General anesthesia, for example, has a considerable impact on base-line blood flow, myocardial function (pressure) respiration, etc. Therefore, if subtle effects are to be measured, the need for refined methods becomes apparent.

The two most commonly used techniques for measuring blood pressure in small laboratory animals such as rats and mice are the indirect tail-cuff method and the direct measurement using an exteriorized catheter connected to a pressure transducer. Disadvantages of these methods are reviewed in references 43 and 44.

Radiotelemetry with an implantable transmitter, which minimizes exposure to stress, provides a way to obtain accurate and reliable measurements from awake and freely moving animals. Blood pressure measurements via radiotelemetry have been described for small laboratory animals from rabbits to mice.[45] From an animal welfare point of view radiotelemetry has another advantage, being the possibility of group housing the animals. This is very complicated in animals having an exteriorized catheter, as cage-mates will gnaw on the stoppers, closing the catheters and leading to the untimely death of the animal. In this section the surgical aspects of the radiotelemetry techniques currently used to monitor and measure blood pressure in awake animals will be described.

7.5.1 Tail cuff

A common technique currently employed for monitoring blood pressure in conscious rats and mice is the tail-cuff device. The tail-cuff method has the advantage of being non-invasive. The technique is dependent on maintaining a minimum amount of blood flow in the tail, and any physiological, pharmacological, or environmental factor that affects tail blood flow will affect the blood pressure measurement. In addition, mice are subject to the stress of handling, heating, and restraint, to which they do not seem to adapt, even after considerable training.

Considerable measurement errors however have been found using the tail-cuff technique in rats.[46] Systolic arterial pressure measurements with this method in conditioned Sprague-Dawley rats may deviate from measurements obtained by simultaneous aortic cannulation by as much as 37 mm Hg.[47] Such errors result in additional variability in data. In light of the fact that only a few momentary measurements are possible in rats that are subjected to stimuli such as handling, restraint, and heating, this high variability may interfere with the detection of small chronic changes in pressure.

7.5.2 Exteriorized catheters

Another common technique currently employed for monitoring blood pressure in conscious rats and mice is the use of an exteriorized catheter that refers pressure to a transducer located nearby. This technique involves placement of an open-lumen catheter in an artery and exteriorizing it at a site inaccessible to the animal, usually in the nape of the neck or at the crown of the head. Measurements of pulsatile arterial pressure and heart rate can thus be obtained. However, accurate measurements of systolic and diastolic pressure are difficult to obtain. There is often a poor dynamic response due to the small size of the catheters used for cannulation of mice arteries, significant catheter compliance, and a relatively long length of conduit from the point of cannulation to the transducer. The resulting damping renders measurements of systolic and diastolic pressure unreliable.

Probably the most significant drawback of this technique is that catheter patency is short. A carefully conducted study on measurement of blood pressure in mice using exteriorized catheters showed a failure rate of 50% by the end of the fourth week of implantation.[48]

There appear to be no documented scientific studies on whether the use of exteriorized catheters in mice results in stress artifacts. However, in rats, significantly higher levels of systolic and mean blood pressure (both +17 mm Hg) have been found when recorded by indwelling and exteriorized catheters vs. implanted radiotelemetry devices.[49] The authors hypothesized that the differences in blood pressure and heart rate were due to the stress associated with performing cardiovascular measurements through externalized catheters.

7.5.3 Radiotelemetry

The radiotelemetry technique can circumvent many of the problems associated with conventional methods (e.g., tail cuff, exteriorized catheters) of monitoring blood pressure in mice and rats. The implantable devices provide accurate and reliable measurements of systolic, diastolic and mean blood pressure as well as heart rate and locomotor activity from freely moving rats and mice single housed in their home cages.[49–52]

Data acquisition system

The commercially available radiotelemetry system for rats and mice (Data Sciences International (DSI), St. Paul, MN) used in all studies mentioned below, measured systolic, diastolic and mean blood pressure as well as heart rate and locomotor activity. An implantable blood pressure transmitter (rat: TA11PA-C40, DSI; mouse: TA11PA-C20, DSI) provides a direct measure of arterial pressure. The transmitter signals are coded in a pulse position modulated serial bit stream, which is received and monitored by the receiver (RPC-1, DSI) placed underneath the animal's cage.

The signals from the receiver are consolidated by the multiplexer (Data Exchange Matrix™, DSI) stored and analyzed on a PC with analyzing software (Dataquest™, A.R.T.™, DSI). In order to compensate for changes in atmospheric pressure, ambient barometric pressure is also measured (APR-1, DSI) and subtracted from the telemetered pressure by the data collection system (Dataquest™, A.R.T.™).

Systolic, diastolic, and mean blood pressure as well as heart rate and locomotor activity are monitored and stored every 5 min for 10 s. Systolic, diastolic, and mean blood pressure as well as heart rate data are extracted from the blood pressure waveform. Locomotor activity is obtained by the system through monitoring changes in the received signal strength occurring upon animal movement. Changes in signal strength of more than a predetermined threshold generate a digital pulse which is counted by the acquisition system. It is important to note that for detection of activity the transmitter has to move. Therefore, with the transmitter implanted intraperitoneally, slight head movements during grooming or eating are not registered as activity.

Blood pressure transmitters

For blood pressure measurements the fluid-filled catheter is placed into the appropriate blood vessel (usually the abdominal aorta, thoracic aorta, femoral artery, pulmonary artery, or carotid artery). The transmitter consists of a hermetically sealed thermoplastic cylinder housing (for rats: length 30 mm, diameter 14 mm; for mice: length 24 mm, diameter 10 mm), coated with silicone elastomer to provide the necessary biocompatibility. Total weight of the rat implant is 9.0 g and of the mouse implant 3.4 g; volume displacement is 4.5 ml and 1.9 ml, respectively.

A transmitter contains an amplifier, a battery, radio frequency electronics, a low-viscosity fluid-filled catheter (for rats: diameter 0.7 mm, length 8 cm; for mice: diameter 0.4 mm, length 5 cm) attached to the sensor located in the body of the transmitter and a magnetically activated switch that allows the device to be turned on and off in vivo. The lumen of the catheter is filled with a low-viscosity fluid, while the distal 2 mm of the thin-walled tip is filled with a blood-compatible gel which prevents blood from entering the catheter lumen. An antithrombogenic film is applied to the distal 1 cm of the catheter. A suture tab molded into the housing provides three sites for securing the device during implantation.

In rats and mice, blood pressure catheters are usually inserted into the abdominal aorta just caudal to the left renal artery, while the body of the transmitter is positioned in the peritoneal cavity. An alternative approach has been developed for measuring blood pressure in mice, whereby thoracic aorta implantation of the pressure-sensing catheter is combined with subcutaneous placement of the transmitter body along the right flank.[52] The carotid artery was used to insert the catheter, which was advanced till the tip was located in the aortic arch. The results of this study showed that the above-mentioned approach is a reliable method for measuring mean arterial pressure and heart rate for 50–60 days in mice weighing 22 g (minimum weight was 17 g). This placement also allowed mice to get pregnant.

However, although placing the blood pressure catheter in the carotid rather than in the abdominal aorta of the mouse can permit a less invasive operation procedure and does not interfere with peritoneal volume, one must be aware of the fact that the circle of Willis (circulus arteriosus cerebri) is not completely developed or shows large variation in some strains of mice and thus the carotid approach is not advised for these strains.[53,54]

Preoperative procedures The small telemetric transmitters are implanted either subcutaneously or in the peritoneal cavity of the animals through a midline laparotomy. Before implanting the transmitter body in the peritoneal cavity make sure that the transmitter is at least at room temperature or even better at body temperature. Open the sterile transmitter package, remove the implant device with sterile forceps, and immerse the device in warm sterile saline. Soak the implant for at least 15 min prior to implantation (the reason for this is the fact that the catheter is very hydrophilic and, if not hydrated, will absorb water from the bloodstream). This can cause the gel to recede slightly due to catheter expansion leaving a dead space at the tip of the catheter which could increase the risk of blood clot formation.

All animals are prepared for surgery in a room separate from the operating theater. After the abdominal area has been clipped the animal should be disinfected (iodine or chlorhexidine in alcohol), placed on a sterile silicon plate, covered with a sterile drape and placed under a binocular operation microscope on a thermostatically controlled heating pad that maintains body temperature at 36–37 °C during the operation.

Surgery (abdominal aorta) After median laparotomy the intestines are gently pushed in cranial direction using a roll of warm saline-soaked sterile gauze bent into a horseshoe shape. This allows easy access to the infrarenal abdominal aorta. Under the operation microscope, the lower abdominal aorta is carefully cleaned of adventitia at the place where the catheter will be inserted. If necessary, additional vasodilatation of the exposed part of the aorta can be achieved using 2% lidocaine solution. Without further dissection the vessels can be clamped with suitable microvascular clips (Biemer, Acland etc.).

Once clamped a small hole is made about 2 mm cranial to the iliac bifurcation using a 23-gauge hypodermic injection needle bent at a 90° angle. Using the hollow side of the needle as a guide, the catheter of the transmitter is inserted upstream into the aorta over a length of 5–6 mm with the aid of a vessel cannulation forceps. The tip should now be located about 2 mm caudal to the left renal artery.

Catheterization with the aid of a bent needle is a reliable technique for the insertion of rigid catheters. When introducing soft catheters such as silicon, it is advantageous to use Vannas scissors to cut a small hole in the blood vessel. In cases where the use of tissue glue is contraindicated, one could use a purse-string suture with the appropriate diameter (this, however, requires advanced microsurgical skills).

The area is then cleaned with a cotton wool stick and the catheter insertion site sealed with a small amount of tissue adhesive (15–20 μl). One could fill two (one spare for emergencies) small pipette-tips with the required volume.

The clamps can be removed while the catheter entry site is observed for leakage. The cannulated aorta may be again irrigated with 2% lidocaine to prevent vessel spasm. Subsequently the insertion site is covered with a 3×5 mm cellulose fiber patch. The patch is secured to the surrounding tissues with tissue glue, thus both anchoring the catheter and fostering connective tissue growth. Subsequently, the gauze is removed and the peritoneal cavity is flooded with warm sterile saline.

The transmitter body is positioned in the peritoneal cavity, and sutured to the abdominal wall. Next the abdominal cavity is closed with an absorbable suture using running technique with 5-mm bite size. Take care not to place the suture rib between the two muscular layers, as this will result in a hernia. Make sure that the muscles are properly approximated without putting too much tension on the suture and the knots. To complete the operation, the skin incision should be closed, again using absorbable suture material (4–0 for rats and 5–0 for mice).

Surgery (carotid artery) The animals are anesthetized and the neck is shaved and disinfected. Animals are placed on their backs on a heating pad with their forelimbs secured using adhesive tape. As described above, a ventral midline neck incision is made from the lower part of the mandible caudally to the sternum (2–3 cm), and the submandibular glands are gently separated using sharp dissection. The left common carotid artery (located just lateral from the sternohyoid muscle) is isolated using fine forceps, and retracted. During preparation of the carotid artery, take care not to touch or damage the vagus nerve which runs next to the artery as this could lead to the untimely death of the animal. Subsequently after placing two small vessel clamps, a tiny incision is made using the same technique as described for the aorta. The pressure-sensing catheter is carefully inserted into the left carotid artery by using a vessel cannulation forceps. In mice it should be advanced over a distance of 10 mm letting the tip just entered the aortic arch. In rats this distance is approximately 18 mm, but it is a good habit to check the distance in the strain of rats that you are using for your experiments. The catheter is secured by ligatures, and the transmitter body is inserted subcutaneously into a small pouch along the right ventral flank. The neck incision is closed and the animals are kept warm until they have fully recovered from anesthesia. Alternatively, the transmitter body can be placed on the back at the mid-scapular region of the mouse.[55] In short, the upper back is shaved, and a horizontal incision is made. The transmitter is placed in the opening and sutured to both the muscle and the skin (with the suture loop around the probe) via the suture rib on the transmitter body. A separate ventral neck incision is then made, the catheter is tunneled subcutaneously to the neck, and the catheterization procedure is carried out the same way.

Postoperative care After surgery, the animals are placed in an incubator (32 °C) for 1 hr. Together with their non-implanted cage-mates, they are then returned to a clean home cage partially placed on a heating pad, for at least 24 hr after surgery so that the animals can choose a comfortable temperature. To prevent harassment of the implanted animals by their cage-mates, the abdomen of each non-implanted animal should be gently rubbed with gauze moistened with 70% ethanol ensuring all animals carried a novel, strange odor for a short period of time. Besides normal food and water, Solid Drink® (Triple-A Trading, Otterloo, the Netherlands), moistened food pellets, and food 'porridge' made with 3% glucose solution may be provided additionally for 4 days. After implantation, animals are administered the non-steroidal anti-inflammatory drug rimadyl (Carprofen, Pfizer Animal Health) for 2 days after surgery.

7.6 Intracranial pressure measurement

One of the best ways of measuring intracranial pressure is by using radio-telemetry. The most elegant way is to place the tip of the pressure catheter in the cisterna magna.

7.6.1 Placement of the catheter tip

Following the same procedure as described above the skin is opened on the crown of the head and a 1-mm trepan drill is used to make a hole in the skull 2 mm from the occipital bone.[56] In rats varying in body weight from 150 to 300 g the catheter is placed in the cisterna magna over a distance of 9–11 mm measured from the top of the skull. The angle of insertion should approximately be 60° to the flat skull position, with the tip pointing in caudal direction. Once inserted the catheter is fixed using tissue glue to cover the hole and glasionomeric glue to further fixate the catheter in its 60° position. Subsequently the transmitter body is placed subcutaneously and sutured to the skin. Take care not to kink the catheter; and make sure the whole curve of the catheter is covered with glue. Next the skin is closed over the glue using absorbable sutures.

7.7 Recording of body, brain, and muscle temperature

Body temperature in the rat is usually recorded via the rectum. Today small electronic thermometers come with a variety of sizes of sensor probes (thermistors, thermocouples). However, handling the animal during measurement (even for 15 s) will inevitably lead to a rise in body temperature. Measuring more animals in a row will lead to stress-induced hyperthermia.[57]

Ideally, cerebral ischemia studies should measure brain temperature, as even slight hypothermia conveys protection against cerebral ischemia. It is well known that brain and body temperatures can dissociate under anesthesia and especially during ischemia.[58,59] Under normal circumstances, however, brain and body temperatures correlate reasonably well.

The preferred method of continual temperature measurement in rodents is via implanted telemetry probes. Telemetry probes have several advantages over conventional methods of measuring temperature (e.g., rectal probe):

- less stress to the animal
- rectal temperature measurements can result in a stress-induced fever (peak of ~1 °C, duration of ~1 hr)
- continual and automated data collection and storage
- better feedback regulation of temperature, resulting in better, more consistent and valid data
- use of fewer animals.

7.7.1 Implantation

Probes are available to measure core temperature (abdominal implant) or brain temperature. These probes are mounted on the skull. A core temperature probe (TA10TA-F40, DSI) is used.[60] It is sterilized and can be implanted into the abdominal cavity. For mice and gerbils smaller models are available. A brain temperature probe (model XMFH-BP) is manufactured by Mini-Mitter Co. (Bend, OR, USA). The probe with glued-on base assembly (cannula and nut) can be glued to the skull using glasionomeric glue. The probe tip is sterilized prior to use and the cannula is implanted under general anesthesia. Depending on the area of interest the tip of the probe can be implanted in different brain areas.

7.7.2 Muscular temperature

Muscular temperature can easily be measured by injection of a probe into the muscle of interest. The IPTT-200 programmable temperature transponder (dimensions 2.2 × 14 mm) is one of the leading transponders.[61] These precoded or programmable injectable transponders for electronic animal identification and body temperature monitoring can be programmed with 32 characters of choice. The temperature sensor has an accuracy of 0.1 °C. It is encapsulated in biocompatible glass and has an antimigration feature. It takes special equipment to read out these transponders.

References

1. Hsu PA, Cooley BC. Effect of exercise on microsurgical hand tremor. *Microsurgery* 2003, **23**: 323–327.
2. Acland, RD (ed.) *Microsurgery Practice Manual.* St. Louis, MO: C.V. Mosby, 1980.
3. Remie R, Rensema JW, van Wunnik GHJ, van Dongen JJ. General principles of microsurgery. In van Dongen JJ, Remie R, Rensema JW, van Wunnik GHJ, (eds.) *Manual of Microsurgery on the Laboratory Rat.* Amsterdam: Elsevier, 1990, pp. 11–15.
4. Greene EC. *Anatomy of the Rat.* New York: Hafner, 1963.
5. Hebel R, Stromberg MW. *Anatomy and Embryology of the Laboratory Rat.* Wörthsee, Germany: BioMed Verlag, 1986.
6. Iwaki T, Hayakawa T. *A Color Atlas of Sectional Anatomy of the Mouse.* Tokyo: Adthree, 2001.
7. Faulkner BC, Tribble CG, Thacker JG, Rodeheaver GT, Edlich RF. Knot performance of polypropylene sutures. *J. Biomed. Mat. Res.* 1996, **33**: 187–192.
8. Faulkner BC, Gear AJL, Hellewell TB, Watkins FH, Edlich RF. Biomechanical performance of a braided absorbable suture. *J. Long-Term Effects Med. Implants* 1996, **6**: 169–179.
9. Tera H, Aberg C. Tensile strengths of twelve types of knot employed in surgery, using different suture materials. *Acta Chir. Scand.* 1976, **142**: 1–7.
10. Bradfield JF, Schachtman TR, McLaughlin RM, Steffen EK. Behavioral and physiologic effects of inapparent wound infection in rats. *Lab. Anim. Sci.* 1992, **42**: 572–578.
11. Waynforth HB. Standards of surgery for rodents: do we need to change? *Scand. Lab. Anim. Sci.* 1993, **20**: 43–46.
12. Baker DG. *Natural Pathogens of Laboratory Animals: Their Effects on Research.* Washington, DC: American Society for Microbiology Press, 2003.
13. Popp MB, Brennan MF. Long-term vascular access in the rat: importance of asepsis. *Am. J. Physiol.* 1981, **241**: H606–H612.
14. Tracy DL (ed.) *Mosby's Fundamentals of Veterinary Technology: Small Animal Surgical Nursing.* St. Louis, MO: C.V. Mosby, 1994.
15. Fluttert M, Dalm S, Oitzl MS. A refined method for sequential blood sampling by tail incision in rats. *Lab. Anim.* 2000, **34**: 372–378.
16. Popovic V, Kent KM, Popovic P. Technique of permanent cannulation of the right ventricle in rats and ground squirrels (28437). *Proc. Soc. Exp. Biol. Med.* 1963, **113**: 599–602.
17. Steffens AB. A method for frequent sampling of blood and continuous infusion of fluids in the rat without disturbing the animal. *Physiol. Behav.* 1969, **4**: 833–836.
18. Brown MR, Hedge GA. Thyroid secretion in the unanesthetized, stress-free rat and its suppression by pentobarbital. *Neuroendocrinology* 1972, **9**: 158–174.

19. Nicolaidis S, Rowland N, Meile MJ, Jallat PM, Pesez A. Brief communication: A flexible technique for long term infusions in unrestrained rats. *Pharmacol. Biochem. Behav.* 1974, **2**: 131–136.

20. Dons RF, Havlik R. A multilayered cannula for long-term blood sampling of unrestrained rats. *Lab. Anim. Sci.* 1986, **36**: 544–547.

21. Cocchetto DM, Bjornsson TD. Methods for vascular access and collection of body fluids from the laboratory rat. *J. Pharmaceut. Sci.* 1983, **72**: 465–492.

22. Remie R, van Dongen JJ, Rensema JW. Permanent cannulation of the jugular vein (acc. to Steffens). In van Dongen JJ, Remie R, Rensema JW, van Wunnik GHJ, (eds.) *Manual of Microsurgery on the Laboratory Rat.* Amsterdam: Elsevier, 1990, pp. 159–170.

23. Agterberg MJH. Het rokende brein. *Biotechniek* 2001, **40**: 139–145.

24. Criado A. Use of cyanoacrylate gel as a substitute for dental cement in intracerebroventricular cannulations in rats. *Contemp. Topics* 2003, **42**: 13–16.

25. Luo YS, Luo YL, Ashford EB, *et al.* Comparison of catheter lock solutions in rats. Proceedings of the American Association for Laboratory Animal Science 2000, San Diego. Available online at http://www.criver.com/pdf/cath_lock_ solutions.pdf, 2000.

26. http://www.kopfinstruments.com/Atlas/Rat.htm.

27. Paxinos G, Watson C. *The Rat Brain in Stereotaxic Coordinates*, 4th edn. New York: Academic Press, 1998.

28. Paxinos G, Watson C, Pennisi M, Topple A. Bregma, lambda and the interaural midpoint in stereotaxic surgery with rats of different sex, strain and weight. *J. Neurosci. Methods* 1985, **13**: 139–143.

29. Kline J, Reid KH. Variability of bregma in 300 gram Long-Evans and Sprague-Dawley rats. *Physiol. Behav.* 1984, **33**: 301–303.

30. Cunningham MG, McKay RD. A hypothermic miniaturized stereotaxic instrument for surgery in newborn rats. *J. Neurosci. Methods* 1993, **47**: 105–114.

31. Rosenberg RS, Bergmann BM, Rechtschaffen A. Variations in slow wave activity during sleep in the rat. *Physiol. Behav.* 1976, **17**: 931–938.

32. Strubbe JH. Insulin, glucose and feeding behaviour in the rat: a reappraisal of the glucostatic theory. Ph.D. thesis, University of Groningen, the Netherlands, 1975.

33. Zetterstrom T, Sharp T, Marsden CA, Ungerstedt U. In vivo measurement of dopamine and its metabolites by intracerebral dialysis: changes after d-amphetamine. *J. Neurochem.* 1983, **41**: 1769–1773.

34. Ungerstedt U. Measurement of neurotransmitter release in vivo by intracranial dialysis. In Marsden CA (ed.) *Measurement of Neurotransmitter Release in Vivo.* New York: John Wiley, 1984, pp. 81–105.

35. Imperato A, Di Chiara G. Trans-striatal dialysis coupled to reverse phase high performance liquid chromatography with electrochemical detection: a new method for the study of the in vivo release of endogenous dopamine and metabolites. *J. Neurosci.* 1984, **4**: 966–977.

36. Westerink BH, De Vries JB. Characterization of in vivo dopamine release as determined by brain microdialysis after acute and subchronic implantations: methodological aspects. *J. Neurochem.* 1988, **51**: 683–687.

37. Ungerstedt U. Introduction to intracerebral microdialysis. In Robinson TE, Justice Jr JB (eds.) *Microdialysis in the Neurosciences.* Amsterdam: Elsevier, 1991, pp. 3–22.

38. Gonon F, Buda M, Cespuglio R, Jouvet M, Pujol JF. In vivo electrochemical detection of catechols in the neostriatum of anaesthetized rats: dopamine or DOPAC? *Nature* 1980, **286**: 902–904.
39. Ewing AG, Wightman RM, Dayton MA. In vivo voltammetry with electrodes that discriminate between dopamine and ascorbate. *Brain Res.* 1982, **249**: 361–370.
40. Westerink BHC, Justice Jr JB. Microdialysis compared with other in vivo release models. In Robinson TE, Justice Jr JB (eds.) *Microdialysis in the Neurosciences* Amsterdam: Elsevier, 1991, pp. 23–43.
41. Santiago M, Westerink BH. Characterization of the in vivo release of dopamine as recorded by different types of intracerebral microdialysis probes. *Naunyn Schmiedebergs Arch. Pharmacol.* 1990, **342**: 407–414.
42. Robinson TE, Justice Jr JB (eds.) *Microdialysis in the Neurosciences*. Amsterdam: Elsevier, 1991.
43. Brockway BP, Hassler CR. Application of radio telemetry to cardiovascular measurement and recording of blood pressure, heart rate, and activity in rat via radiotelemetry. *Clin. Exp. Hyper.* 1991, **3**: 885–895.
44. Kramer K, Kinter LB. Evaluation and applications of radio-telemetry in small laboratory animals. *Physiol. Genom.* 2003, **13**: 197–205.
45. Kramer K. Applications and evaluation of radio-telemetry in small laboratory animals. Ph.D. thesis, University of Utrecht, the Netherlands, 2000.
46. Bunag RD. Facts and fallacies about measuring blood pressure in rats. *Clin. Exper. Hyper. Theory and Practice A5* 1983, **5**: 1659–1681.
47. Bunag RD, McCubbin JW, Page IH. Lack of correlation between direct and indirect measurements of arterial pressure in unanaesthetized rats. *Cardiovasc. Res.* 1971, **5**: 24–31.
48. Mattson DL. Long-term measurement of arterial blood pressure in conscious mice. *Am. J. Physiol.* 1998, **271**: R564–R570.
49. Bazil MK, Krulan C, Webb RL. Telemetric monitoring of cardiovascular parameters in conscious spontaneously hypertensive rats. *J. Cardiovasc. Pharmacol.* 1993, **22**: 897–905.
50. Brockway BP, Mills PA, Azar SH. A new method for continuous chronic measurement and recording of blood pressure, heart rate and activity in the rat via radio-telemetry. *Clin. Exper. Hyper. Theory and Practice A13* 1991, **5**: 885–895.
51. Mills PA, Huetteman DA, Brockway BP, *et al.* A new method for measurement of blood pressure, heart rate, and activity in the mouse by radio-telemetry. *J. Appl. Physiol.* 2000, **88**: 1537–1544.
52. Butz GM, Davisson RL. Long-term telemetric measurement of cardiovascular parameters in awake mice: a physiological genomics tool. *Physiol. Genom.* 2001, **5**: 89–97.
53. Barone FC, Knudsen DJ, Nelson AH, Feuerstein GZ, Willette RN. Mouse strain differences in susceptibility to cerebral ischemia are related to cerebral vascular anatomy. *J. Cereb. Blood Flow Metab.* 1993, **13**: 683–692.
54. Ward HB, Baker TG, McLaren A. A histological study of the gonads of T16H/XSxr hermaphrodite mice. *J. Anat.* 1988, **158**: 65–75.
55. Carlson SH, Wyss MJ. Long-term telemetric recording of arterial pressure and heart rate in mice fed basal and high NaCl diets. *Hypertension* 2000, **35**: e1–e5.

56. Bouman HJ, Wimersma Greidanus TB. A rapid and simple cannulation technique for repeated sampling of cerebrospinal fluid in freely moving rats. *Brain Res. Bull.* 1979, **4**: 575–577.

57. Van der Heyden JAM, Zethof TJJ, Tolboom JTBM, Olivier B. Stress-induced hyperthermia in singly housed mice. *Physiol. Behav.* 1997, **62**: 463–470.

58. Colbourne F, Sutherland G, Auer RN. An automated system for regulating brain temperature in awake and freely-moving rodents. *J. Neurosci. Methods* 1996, **67**: 185–190.

59. DeBow S, Colbourne F. Brain temperature measurement and regulation in awake and freely moving rodents. *Methods* 2003, **30**: 167–171.

60. Clement JG, Mills P, Brockway B. Use of telemetry to record body temperature and activity in mice. *J. Pharmacol. Methods* 1989, **21**: 129–140.

61. http://www.plexx.nl/UK/index.htm.

8

Genetically engineered animals

CAROLINA M. MAIER, LILLY HSIEH, AND PAK H. CHAN

8.1 Introduction

Animal models that recreate specific pathogenic events and their corresponding behavioral outcomes are indispensable tools for exploring the underlying
pathophysiologic mechanisms of disease and for investigating therapeutic
strategies prior to testing them in human patients. Although rodents have a
long tradition as models for human neurological diseases, they have received
increasing attention in light of genetic engineering methods that have made
it possible to create precisely defined genetic changes. The development of
transgenic technology, a tool that allows sophisticated manipulation of the
genome, has provided an unprecedented opportunity to expand our understanding of many aspects of neuronal development, function, and disease.

Transgenic animals are specific variants of species following the introduction
and/or integration of a new gene or genes into the genome of the host animal.
Transgenic technology is now routinely used to increase the level of (overexpress) particular proteins or enzymes in animals or to mutate or inactivate a
particular gene using a "knockout" approach. One of the most commonly used
animals in transgenic techniques is the mouse, a species in which transgene
microinjections into the pronuclei of fertilized oocytes and the subsequent
expression of the transgene in the animal have been carefully worked out.

Since their development in the 1980s, the transgenic and knockout technologies have allowed us to examine the regulation of gene expression and the
pathophysiology of its alterations. The ability to cause overexpression of
genes, to insert reporter genes controlled by specific gene promoters, and to
ablate single genes has also allowed us to ascertain the factors involved in cell
differentiation,[1–3] to manipulate oncogenesis,[4–6] to identify new molecules and
specify substrates,[7,8] to elucidate signal transduction pathways,[9–11] and to
examine novel therapeutic strategies for the management of patients with
neurological disorders.[12–15]

Handbook of Experimental Neurology, ed. Turgut Tatlisumak and Marc Fisher. Published by Cambridge
University Press. © Cambridge University Press 2006.

Although the rapid advancement of genetic engineering has made it possible to create extremely elegant experiments involving transgenic and knockout rodents, many of these animals develop not only impressive but sometimes unexpected phenotypes, making their interpretation a major challenge to researchers.

In this chapter, we will give a short overview of the methods used to generate genetically modified animals and the possible ways to analyze them. We will also review some of the challenges that are encountered when using genetically engineered rodents to model human neurological disorders, the strategies used to overcome them, the success stories that have ensued, and the lessons learned. The vast array and complexity of genetic animal models precludes us from discussing all, or even most, of the neurological diseases that have benefited from this technology. Instead, we will focus mainly on oxidative stress-related disorders, with particular emphasis on stroke, to provide insights into the benefits and limitations of using genetically manipulated animals as research study tools.

8.2 Beyond the link between gene and disorder

Alterations in the information encoded by genes that regulate critical steps of brain development and function can disrupt the normal course of development, and have profound consequences on neuronal processes. Genetically modified animal models have helped to elucidate the contribution of specific gene alterations and gene–environment interactions to the phenotype of several forms of neurological disorders, including Huntington's disease,[16] familial forms of Alzheimer's disease,[17] and Parkinson's disease,[18,19] amyotrophic lateral sclerosis (ALS),[20,21] spinocerebellar ataxias,[22] Down and Rett syndromes,[23,24] and X-linked forms of mental retardation.[25]

A handful of genetic models that have made substantial contributions to the study of some of the above-mentioned disorders (in addition to those discussed in the text) are listed in Table 8.1.

Although the list of genetically altered animals is very limited, it serves to illustrate the impact of transgenic technology. The ability to manipulate specific genes has been useful in establishing the gene–disorder link and has also provided researchers with a powerful tool to explore the mechanisms involved in a particular diseased state. For example, genetically engineered animals have elucidated the necessary elements required for the tissue-specific and cell-specific expression of hormones; they have identified novel molecules; they have confirmed the role of precursor cells in cell differentiation; and they have allowed the exploration of quantitative relationships between abnormal

Table 8.1. *Genetically modified animal models that have contributed to the study of human diseases*

Disease	Transgene (TG)/knockout (KO)	Objective/purpose	Reference
Alzheimer's disease	PDAPP	Used to understand the process of amyloid plaque formation and test candidate therapies	26
	TG2576	Used to replicate human-like tau pathologies	27
	FTPD-17 (various mutations)	Used to study possible tau kinases that play a	28
	P25	role in tau pathology	29
	P301L X APP TG	Used to study beta-amyloid and tau interactions	30
	APP/presenilin TG	Used to study role of presinilin mutation in amyloid plaque formation	31
	APP/ApoE	Used to study the effect of ApoE in plaque formation	32
	APP/ACT	ACT is expressed in astrocytes and is found in amyloid plaques; used to study the role of inflammation in Alzheimer's disease	33
Parkinson's disease	Alpha-synuclein TG A53T	Used to study alpha-synuclein-induced neurodegeneration (fibrillar and nonfibrillar)	34
	Alpha-synuclein KO	Shows necessity of alpha-synuclein for DA neuron death with MPTP treatment	35
Huntington's disease	hdh KO	Complete deletion is lethal; Huntington's disease not caused by loss of function	36
	huntingtin TG	Show gene dosage effect	37
	R6/2 line	Show functional loss preceding cell loss	38
		Evidence of protein aggregates	39
	Conditional TG huntingtin model	Show reversal of neuropathology and motor dysfunction when expression stopped	40
Amyotrophic lateral sclerosis (ALS-PDC)	APO E TG	Explore the interaction of cycad toxin and possible genetic cofactors	41

	mSOD1 TG	Ubiquitous expression leads to formation of ALS-like disease in mice	42
Stroke	NR2 A KO	Used to study role of excitotoxicity in ischemia	43
	GluR2 TG		44
	GLT-1 HT KO		45
	Three isoforms of superoxide dismutase (SOD)	Oxidative stress	46
	TG and KO		47, 48
	nNOS KO		49
	eNOS KO		50
	BAK KO		51
	XIAP TG		52
	IL-α/IL-ß KO	Inflammation	53
	mICE TG		54
	MAC-1 KO		55
	Intercellular adhesion molecule (ICAM) KO		56
	tPA KO	Extracellular enzymes	57
	MMP9 KO		58
Muscular dystrophy	ALP KO	Used to determine whether it participates in muscle development	59
	Utrophin TG	Test whether it can replace dystrophin to ameliorate symptoms of MS	60
	Mbnl1	Sequestration of MBNL proteins contributes to pathogenesis of muscular dystrophy	61

gene products and the disease state. Furthermore, transgenic and knockout animals have enabled us to investigate specific molecular and cellular mechanisms associated with cell dysfunction and death. Thus, the development of this revolutionary technology has not only advanced the discovery and characterization of pathogenic mutations associated with major human neurodegenerative diseases, it has also advanced the study of multifaceted disease states such as stroke, traumatic brain injury, neuroinflammation, neuroimmune conditions, and tumorigenesis.[62–67]

Mice are the preferred species for the above studies for two main reasons. First, mice are quite similar to humans in terms of genetic and physiological aspects, which makes them suitable for modeling human neurological disorders. Second, the murine genome has been extensively mapped and lends itself well to embryonic cell technology.[66]

8.3 Methods for the production of transgenic mice

The most commonly used method for creating transgenic mice is the microinjection of the DNA of interest (transgene) into the pronuclei of fertilized mouse oocytes.[68] This technique is used to introduce a linear DNA fragment (genomic or cDNA with the proper promoter), which contains sequences required for directing correct transcriptional initiation, and for encoding a gene product (protein, enzyme) that can be readily identified using various biochemical and immunocytochemical assays. Pronuclear microinjection of DNA leads to random integration of various copies of the injected DNA into a single site on a mouse chromosome. The injected DNA is present in the germline and is transmitted to the next generation. In some instances, the injected DNA can integrate into multiple sites of the genome, giving rise to a mosaic founder mouse. Another way to produce transgenic mice is by using pluripotent embryonic stem (ES) cells,[69] which are initially obtained from the inner cell mass of a mouse blastocyst and established in culture.[70] ES cells can be produced with a foreign gene and subsequently screened for the integration of transgenes. These ES cells with the transgene can be microinjected into the blastocyst of a mouse embryo, resulting in a chimeric mouse. The mating of chimeric mice with wild-type mice will produce heterozygous offspring that contain the transgene.

It is critical to verify that the animals generated have only the desired genetic alteration, given that apparently normal transgenic animals may have very subtle abnormalities in gene expression.[71] Various molecular biological and biochemical techniques, including Southern blot (DNA), polymerase chain reaction (PCR), Northern blot (RNA), reverse transcriptase (RT) PCR, and

Western blot (protein immunoreactivity) and enzymatic assays can be used to identify the gene or the gene products.

8.3.1 Making the human SOD1 transgenic mouse

An example of a successful transgenic animal that has rendered numerous findings in the study of cerebral ischemia is the human copper/zinc (Cu/Zn)-superoxide dismutase (SOD1) transgenic mouse. The making of this transgenic animal was done by cloning SOD1 cDNA from mRNA and by cloning SOD1 genomic DNA from lambda phage.

Cloning SOD1 cDNA from mRNA was accomplished by isolating total poly(A)-containing RNA from simian virus 40 (SV40)-transformed human fibroblasts and fractionating the RNA through a linear sucrose gradient. The fractions were then tested by in vitro translation and immunoprecipitation, which identified the 11s fraction as having the desired mRNA. From that fraction, double-stranded (ds) DNA was synthesized by the use of RT, DNA polymerase, and nuclease S1. The dsDNA encoding SOD1 was then inserted into the Pst I site of pBR322, and the plasmid constructs were used to transform *Escherichia coli* HB101. Finally, the plasmid DNA containing the SOD1 cDNA was isolated from *E. coli*.

For cloning SOD1 genomic DNA from lambda phage, the human genomic library Ch4 was screened by fishing out the bacterial phage plaque that hybridized with ^{32}P-labeled SOD1 cDNA. Lambda phage clones having the nucleotide sequences of the SOD1 functional gene were identified and the SOD1 gene fragment was excised with *Eco*R1. The fragment was then inserted into EcoRa site of pHG165, the plasmid digested with *Bam* H1 and a *Bam* H1 fragment containing a neoresistant marker, which was ligated to the pGSOD to make a pGSOD-SV neoconstruct.[72] The 14.5 kb *Eco*R1-*Bam* H1 fragment of the human Cu/Zn-SOD gene was cloned in the same sites in pBluescript II(+) K/S and maintained in the *E. coli* DH5 alpha strain. For in vitro injection, the human Cu/Zn-SOD gene in the *Eco*R1-*Bam* H1 fragment could be separated from the bacterial sequence. That clone was used successfully to generate transgenic mice with increased SOD1 activity.[73]

The next step in this process was to microinject the DNA fragments into the embryos. Mice of strain B6SJL were used due to their high success rate in incorporating transgenes. Following hormonal stimulation to enhance egg production, females were mated with B6SJL males and euthanized within 6–9 hr to ensure that the fertilized eggs were still at the 1-cell pronuclear stage. The embryos were then flushed out of the oviduct and maintained in a special medium where the injection process took place immediately. The embryos were held with suction in the microinjection apparatus, with a vibration-free injection stage, while the DNA microinjection was carried out. The surviving injected embryos were then reimplanted into the oviducts of pseudo-pregnant CD-1 or CD-57 female mice (previously mated with vasectomized males) with a 15–20% birth rate.

8.3.2 Identifying the gene and gene products

Screening, identification, and characterization of the *Sod1* gene and SOD1 protein/enzyme were systematically performed. First, Southern blot analysis was carried out using DNA purified from the tails of the pups. The founder mice were mated with non-transgenic mice, producing true transgenic progeny (i.e., carrying the *Sod1* gene in all their cells). Northern blot analysis was carried out to examine SOD1 mRNA, while tissue expression of Cu/Zn-SOD was analyzed by non-denaturing polyacrylamide gel electrophoresis. The transgenic mice were also identified by a PCR screening method.[74] The method, based on rapid preparation of a small amount of genomic DNA, used two specific PCR primers to amplify a small DNA fragment that was specific for the transgene. The PCR primers specific for the human Cu/Zn-SOD gene were designed according to the known DNA sequences, tested, and applied to the screening of transgenic mice.

Expression of SOD1 transgenes was confirmed by RT-PCR amplification, while mapping of the chromosome localization of Cu/Zn-SOD and determination of the copy number was done by fluorescence in situ hybridization (FISH). As a final step, expression of Cu/Zn-SOD in mouse neurons and astrocytes was identified in the primary culture of cortical neurons and astrocytes.

8.4 Methods for the production of knockout mice

Another approach for studying gene function is to mutate the particular gene of interest using homologous recombination-mediated gene targeting in ES cells that subsequently generate mice carrying null mutation through germline transmission.[75] This molecular genetic approach was used to target the inducible, mitochondria-specific manganese (Mn)-SOD. To investigate the role of Mn-SOD in the complex network of cellular antioxidative defense systems and to distinguish its actions from those of the constitutively expressed cytoplasmic Cu/Zn-SOD, the mouse MnSOD gene (*Sod2*) was inactivated by homologous recombination. This lead to the development of knockout mice with reduced or no MnSOD activity.

The replacement-type targeting vector was constructed from a genomic clone containing *Sod2* isolated from a C57BL/6 genomic DNA library. Exons 2 and 3 of the 16 kb *Sod2* sequence, and their corresponding exon–intron junction region, were sequenced. The remainder was mapped with restriction enzyme digestion and Southern blot analysis using human cDNA as the probe. The neomycin cassette containing the DNA polymerase II promoter (PolII) and bovine growth hormone polyadenylation signal was flanked by *Sod2* genomic sequences, a 1.7 kb *Bal*I (in exon 2) to *Bal*I (in intron 2) fragment at the 5′ side and a 7.3 kb *Xba*I (in intron 3) to *Eco*RI fragment at the 3′ side. A HSV-*tk* driven by a phosphoglycerate kinase-1 (*pgk*) promoter was placed 5′ upstream of the 1.7 kb fragment. pBluescript was used as the cloning vector.

CB-1 ES cells were derived from a blastocyst harvested from a C57BL/6 J female bred to a F_1 Robertsonian hybrid. The ES cells were grown on mitomycin C-treated, neomycin-resistant embryo fibroblasts to 90% confluence. At passage 7, 1×10^7 ES cells were transfected with 10 µg linearized targeting vector by electroporation. Transfected ES cells were selected with G418 and FIAU (1 (2-deoxy, 2 fluoro-B-D arabinofuranosyl)-5-iodouracil) for 7 days. Thirteen doubly resistant colonies were identified as properly targeted (out of 173 transfected colonies). Five knockout colonies were obtained, with approximately 50% reduction in MnSOD enzymatic activity. RT-PCR analysis demonstrated the knockout mutant colonies that produced both normal and truncated MnSOD mRNAs. To produce the mutant mice, ES cells in groups of 5–10 were injected into CD1 zygotes. The injected zygotes that developed to healthy blastocysts were transferred to pseudopregnant B6D2 females. Homozygous and heterozygous MnSOD knockout mice were identified and characterized.[76,77]

8.5 The production of transgenic rats

The successful development of SOD1 and SOD2 mutant mice has allowed researchers to study the mechanisms underlying the complex neuronal responses to ischemic insults by subjecting these animals to various models of stroke, brain trauma, and spinal cord injury. Yet despite the ability to model neurodegenerative conditions in those animals, the need for using a larger animal such as the rat was still prevalent. First, stroke models (focal, global, or thrombotic in nature) were well established in rats. Second, the physiological parameters, brain anatomy, cerebrovascular structures and stroke risk factors had been characterized in rats to much greater depth and detail than in mice. The rat would also allow studies that were difficult, if not impossible, in mice

due to their small size (e.g., electrophysiology, microdialysis, systemic variables, regional cerebral blood flow and metabolism, multi-organ physiology)
or due to poorly defined neurologic responses and behavioral deficits in mice.

Thus, a substantial amount of effort was placed in developing an SOD1
transgenic rat. To generate transgenic rats, a 14 kb *Bam*HI-*Eco*RI genomic
fragment of the *Sod1* gene (with five exons) was used, along with its own
promoter. The SOD1 genomic DNA was purified and diluted prior to injection into fertilized eggs obtained from female Sprague-Dawley rats. Injected
zygotes were transfected into pseudopregnant female Sprague-Dawley rats
and pups were born 24 days from the day of transfer. The site of transgene
integration was determined by FISH. Transgenic animals were identified by
expression of the human SOD1 enzyme from red blood cell lysates using
isoelectric focusing gel electrophoresis and staining for SOD1 activity with
nitroblue tetrazolium. Determination of total enzyme activity of Cu/Zn-SOD
and evaluation of the cerebral vasculature were also carried out.[78]

8.6 Challenges of gene targeting and emerging strategies

One of the frequently encountered difficulties when using the classic gene targeting strategy (ES cells and homologous recombination) is that, since it uses the
germline mutation, mutations in developmentally essential genes can induce
serious defects or embryonic lethality.[79] For example, inactivation of the *Sod2*
gene as described above resulted in a lethal phenotype of the homozygous $(-/-)$
mutant. While there was no prenatal loss of homozygous mutant mice by PCR
screening and they were of normal size and without structural defects at birth,
the $-/-$ neonates were hypotonic, hypothermic, and paler than their wild-type
litter-mates.[76] This was not surprising, given that defects in embryonic development are observed frequently in knockout mice. However, the homozygous
animals fatigued rapidly after any type of exertion and by post-partum days
4–5, nearly 38% of the $-/-$ animals were dead, with the remaining ones severely
growth-retarded. Mortality rates approached 100% by day 10. The precise cause
of death remained unknown, but cardiac abnormalities (resulting from high
levels of oxidative stress) were the suspected culprits.

Of note, when mid-gestation lethality occurs following targeted gene disruption, a careful examination of extraembryonic tissues should be carried
out, followed by a chimeric analysis using tetraploid embryos.[80] In the case of
SOD2 knockout mice, heterozygous animals proved to be more than adequate
for examining the role of Mn-SOD. *Sod2* $-/+$ mice had no discernable
abnormal phenotype at 9 months of age, and this lack of phenotype could
not be attributed to the induction of MnSOD in those animals since MnSOD

activity was reduced by 49–55% of +/+ activity in brain, heart, liver, and kidney. Furthermore, Cu/Zn-SOD activity was unaltered in heterozygous SOD2-deficient mice.

Aside from embryonic lethality and anatomical and physiological defects, another problem with classic gene targeting is that it can only be used to study the function of a particular gene in the context of the specificity of the cell lineage and developmental progression. It is also important to keep in mind that introducing a specific mutation into the mouse genome does not really model a phenotype that was acquired by a somatic mutation in a human, as is the case with most forms of cancer.[79] Other common problems with simple gene targeting include compensatory mechanisms and functional redundancies, as well as the creation of multifarious phenotypes.[80] That is, a genetic alteration can have effects on multiple different cell and tissue types, resulting in a complex phenotype in which it is difficult to distinguish between direct gene function in a particular tissue versus secondary effects ensuing from altered gene function in other tissues.

To overcome the above limitations, scientists have developed very elegant strategies. These include the use of organ-, tissue-, or cell-specific gene targeting, also known as conditional gene targeting[79,81,82] and transgene rescues.[80] This is possible by the availability of well-characterized promoters. The specific targeting of transgene expression can be modulated not only by tissue-specific promoters, but also by employing inducible strategies. Examples of such strategies are the tetracycline-inducible method[83] and site-specific recombination systems such as Cre/loxP[84] and Flp/Frt.[85] The Cre/loxP system consists of a mouse strain harboring a "floxed" targeted gene (i.e., a gene flanked by loxP sites) that can be crossed to various strains of mice expressing Cre recombinase in a specific tissue or cell type (or even in a developmentally regulated manner).[84,86] The Cre recombinase catalyzes DNA recombination between loxP sites, resulting in either deletion of the intervening DNA segment and one loxP site or inversion (flipping) of the intervening DNA segment and two loxP sites. The Cre- and loxP-containing strains of mice are usually developed independently, and then crossed to generate offspring. The result is that the targeted gene is inactivated only in tissues expressing Cre and remains inactive in all other tissues. The Cre/loxP system has recently been used to examine the role of synGAP, a brain-specific Ras/Rap GTPase-activating protein, in apoptotic neuronal death,[87] and to show that brain-specific deletion of neuropathy target esterase results in neurodegeneration.[88] The Flp/Frt works in a similar manner. Flp (named for its ability to or "flip" a DNA segment in *Saccharomyces cerevisiae*), is able to recombine specific sequences of DNA with high fidelity without the need for cofactors. Flp recombines DNA at the *FRT* site (Flp recombinase recognition target) in both actively dividing and postmitotic cells, as well as in most tissue types.[89]

8.7 The impact of transgenic technology

The generation of rats and mice with specific SOD mutations has proved invaluable for studying the role of oxygen radicals in the pathogenesis of neuronal death, as well as other neurodegenerative disorders.[90] For example, a landmark study identified mutations in the gene encoding SOD1 that account for approximately 2% of all ALS and 20% of familial ALS cases.[90] More than 70 different mutations of the SOD protein have been identified.[92] Because all SOD1 mutations result in an autosomal dominant phenotype of ALS with similar pathological features, the general consensus in the field is that they all must work through the same mechanism, but exactly how this happens is not fully understood. The research on ALS serves as an example of the success and challenges of using genetically engineered animals. The initial description of SOD1 gene alterations in ALS lead researchers to hypothesize that the disease was caused by an excess of superoxide anion due to loss of SOD1 function.[93] However, studies on knockout mice null for SOD1 have shown that these animals do not develop motor neuron degeneration. The same is true for mice overexpressing human wild-type SOD1, indicating that alterations in SOD activity are not sufficient or necessary for the ALS phenotype in these mice. On the other hand, overexpression of mutant SOD1 in mice causes motor neuron disease despite the presence of elevated SOD1 activity.[94] A pathological hallmark of ALS is the accumulation of neurofilaments, which are part of the slow axonal transport system in motor neurons. Transgenic mice expressing two human SOD1 mutations linked to familial ALS show a slowing of axonal transport at least 6 months before the onset of clinical features or pathological changes.[95] However, intact neurofilament structure is not required for mutant SOD1-mediated motor neuron death, as evidenced by studies on NFL-KO mice.[96]

In Alzheimer's dementia, peptides derived from proteolytic processing of the β-amyloid precursor protein (APP), including the amyloid-β peptide, play an important role in the pathogenesis of this disease. Transgenic mice overexpressing APP have a profound and selective impairment in endothelium-dependent regulation of the neocortical microcirculation. This dysfunction is not observed in transgenic mice expressing both APP and SOD1 or in APP transgenics that undergo topical application of SOD to the cerebral cortex.[97]

SOD1 transgenic mice have also provided evidence for a role of SOD in Parkinson's disease, where the most prominent pathological feature is selective degeneration of dopaminergic neurons in the substantia nigra pars compacta of the midbrain, resulting in decreased dopamine levels in the striatum. Midbrain dopaminergic neurons from SOD1 transgenic mice show better survival in vitro than those from non-transgenic litter-mates, and when transplanted into Parkinsonian model rats, they show better survival as well as better functional recovery.[98]

Work in our laboratory has shown that ischemic infarction is significantly reduced at 3 or 24 hr in mice overexpressing SOD1 compared with wild-type litter-mates after transient focal cerebral ischemia.[46] However, these animals are not protected against permanent middle cerebral artery occlusion, lending further support to the notion that oxidative stress plays a role in reperfusion injury. Following focal cerebral ischemia, SOD1 knockout[99] and SOD2 knockout[47] animals are more susceptible to ischemic injury compared with wild-type animals.

Traumatic brain injury has also been studied using SOD transgenic and SOD knockout mice. Levels of CuZn are significantly correlated with inhibition of cerebral edema formation 4 hr following trauma, and lesion size 2 weeks after contusion injury is significantly smaller in SOD1 overexpressors compared with their wild-type litter-mates. At 15 days post injury, transgenic animals also have improved neurologic function, suggesting an SOD1-mediated neuroprotective effect. Neuroprotection is also evident in SOD1 and in extracellular SOD overexpressing mice following cold injury-induced brain edema.[100] The importance of extracellular SOD on neurologic outcome after both severe and moderate closed head injury has also been shown in extracellular SOD overexpressors tested in the Morris water maze.[101]

It is important to highlight the fact that many human diseases have a polygenic component. A stroke-related example includes the genetic susceptibility to two major risk factors, namely atherosclerosis and hypertension. Both of these disease states have genetic equivalents in mice. Creating genetic animal models with combinations of various susceptible genes may help to develop more realistic animal models of neurological disorders.

8.8 Summary

Identifying the role of specific genes in neuropathologies provides a framework in which to understand key stages of human brain development and function. Genetic linkage analysis, which has allowed us to identify the genes responsible for neurological conditions such as Huntington's disease, familial forms of Alzheimer's disease and Parkinson's disease, and ALS, has been a powerful research tool. Another giant step in experimental neurology has come from genetically engineered animals, particularly mice, which have allowed us to further our understanding of the molecular and cellular pathogenesis of neurological diseases. A DNA fragment, microinjected into pronuclei, can reprogram the genome, thereby inducing the transformation of the mouse through transmission of a new mutation. These transgenic mice often produce the protein product of the introduced gene, providing us with powerful animal models of human disease states. Similarly, site-directed mutagenesis that leads to ablation or knockout of a specific gene has yielded invaluable information to the study of mechanisms underlying neurological conditions. The field of genetic engineering is quickly advancing toward the development of temporal and cell type-specific control of gene expression. Such advances will help to further elucidate the role of specific genes on a vast array of neurological disorders and will provide a basis for testing novel therapeutic strategies.

References

1. Garcia AD, Doan NB, Imura T, *et al.* GFAP-expressing progenitors are the principal source of constitutive neurogenesis in adult mouse forebrain. *Nature Neurosci.* 2004, **7**: 1233–1241.
2. De Marchis S, Temoney F, Erdelvi F, *et al.* GABAergic phenotypic differentiation of a subpopulation of subventricular derived migrating progenitors. *Eur. J. Neurosci.* 2004, **20**: 1307–1317.
3. Wen PH, Shao X, Shao Z, *et al.* Overexpression of wild type but not an FAD mutant presenilin-1 promotes neurogenesis in the hippocampus of adult mice. *Neurobiol. Dis.* 2002, **10**: 8–19.
4. Le Menuet D, Viengchareun S, Penfornis P, *et al.* Targeted oncogenesis reveals a distinct tissue-specific utilization of alternative promoters of the human mineralocorticoid receptor gene in transgenic mice. *J. Biol. Chem.* 2000, **275**: 7878–7886.
5. Steinbach JP, Kozmik Z, Pfeffer P, *et al.* Overexpression of Pax5 is not sufficient for neoplastic transformation of mouse neuroectoderm. *Int. J. Cancer* 2001, **93**: 459–467.
6. Tong WM, Ohgaki H, Huang H, *et al.* Null mutation of DNA strand break-binding molecule poly(ADP-ribose) polymerase causes medulloblastomas in p53($-/-$) mice. *Am. J. Pathol.* 2003, **162**: 343–352.
7. Moy LY, Tsai LH. Cyclin-dependent kinase 5 phosphorylates serine 31 of tyrosine hydroxylase and regulates its stability. *J. Biol. Chem.* 2004, **279**: 54487–54493.
8. Hyun DH, Lee M, Hattori N, *et al.* Effect of wild-type or mutant Parkin on oxidative damage, nitric oxide, antioxidant defenses, and the proteasome. *J. Biol. Chem.* 2002, **277**: 28572–28577.
9. Saito A, Hayashi T, Okuno S, *et al.* Modulation of the Omi/HtrA2 signaling pathway after transient focal cerebral ischemia in mouse brains that overexpress SOD1. *Brain Res. Mol. Brain Res.* 2004, **127**: 89–95.
10. Pizoli CE, Jinnah HA, Billingsley ML, *et al.* Abnormal cerebellar signaling induces dystonia in mice. *J. Neurosci.* 2002, **22**: 7825–7833.

11. Winder DG, Mansuy IM, Osman M, *et al*. Genetic and pharmacological evidence for a novel, intermediate phase of long-term potentiation suppressed by calcineurin. *Cell* 1998, **92**: 25–37.

12. Casas C, Sergeant N, Itier JM, *et al*. Massive CA1/2 neuronal loss with intraneuronal and N-terminal truncated Abeta42 accumulation in a novel Alzheimer transgenic model. *Am. J. Pathol.* 2004, **165**: 1289–1300.

13. Manley GT, Binder DK, Papadopoulos MC, *et al*. New insights into water transport and edema in the central nervous system from phenotype analysis of aquaporin-4 null mice. *Neuroscience* 2004, **129**: 983–991.

14. Okamura N, Suemotu T, Shiomitsu T, *et al*. A novel imaging probe for in vivo detection of neuritic and diffuse amyloid plaques in the brain. *J. Mol. Neurosci.* 2004, **24**: 247–255.

15. Richards JG, Higgins GA, Ouagazzal AM, *et al*. PS2APP transgenic mice, coexpressing hPS2mut and hAPPswe, show age-related cognitive deficits associated with discrete brain amyloid deposition and inflammation. *J. Neurosci.* 2003, **23**: 8989–9003.

16. Menalled LB, Chesselet MF. Mouse models of Huntington's disease. *Trends Pharmacol. Sci.* 2002, **23**: 32–39.

17. Janus C, Chishti MA, Westaway D. Transgenic mouse models of Alzheimer's disease. *Biochim. Biophys. Acta* 2000, **1502**: 63–75.

18. Dawson TM, Dawson VL. Neuroprotective and neurorestorative strategies for Parkinson's disease. *Nature Neurosci.* 2002, **5** (Suppl.): 1058–1061.

19. Lim KL, Dawson VL, Dawson TM. The genetics of Parkinson's disease. *Curr. Neurol. Neurosci. Rep.* 2002, **2**: 439–446.

20. Bruijn LI, Houseweart MK, Kato S, *et al*. Aggregation and motor neuron toxicity of an ALS-linked SOD1 mutant independent from wild-type SOD1. *Science* 1998, **281**: 1851–1854.

21. Rakhit R, Cunningham P, Furtos-Matei A, *et al*. Oxidation-induced misfolding and aggregation of superoxide dismutase and its implications for amyotrophic lateral sclerosis. *J. Biol. Chem.* 2002, **277**: 47551–47556.

22. Burright EN, Orr HT, Clark HB. Mouse models of human CAG repeat disorders. *Brain Pathol.* 1997, **7**: 965–977.

23. Glaze DG. Rett syndrome: of girls and mice – lessons for regression in autism. *Ment. Retard. Devel. Disabil. Res. Rev.* 2004, **10**: 154–158.

24. Reeves RH, Irving NG, Moran TH, *et al*. A mouse model for Down syndrome exhibits learning and behaviour deficits. *Nature Genet.* 1995, **11**: 177–184.

25. Heinzer AK, McGuinness MC, Lu JF, *et al*. Mouse models and genetic modifiers in X-linked adrenoleukodystrophy. *Adv. Exp. Med. Biol.* 2003, **544**: 75–93.

26. Games D. Adams R, Alessandrini R, *et al*. Alzheimer-type neuropathology in transgenic mice overexpressing V717 F beta-amyloid precursor protein. *Nature* 1995, **373**: 523–527.

27. Hsiao K, Chapman P, Nilsen S, *et al*. Correlative memory deficits, Abeta elevation, and amyloid plaques in transgenic mice. *Science* 1996, **274**: 99–102.

28. Phinney AL, Horne P, Yang J, *et al*. Mouse models of Alzheimer's disease: the long and filamentous road. *Neurol. Res.* 2003, **25**: 590–600.

29. Ahlijanian MK, Barrezueta NX, Williams RD, *et al*. Hyperphosphorylated tau and neurofilament and cytoskeletal disruptions in mice overexpressing human p25, an activator of cdk5. *Proc. Natl Acad. Sci. USA* 2000, **97**: 2910–2915.

30. Lewis J, Dickson DW, Lin WL, *et al*. Enhanced neurofibrillary degeneration in transgenic mice expressing mutant tau and APP. *Science* 2001, **293**: 1487–1491.

31. Holcomb L, Gordon MN, McGowan E, *et al.* Accelerated Alzheimer-type phenotype in transgenic mice carrying both mutant amyloid precursor protein and presenilin 1 transgenes. *Nature Med.* 1998, **4**: 97–100.

32. Holtzman DM, Bales KR, Wu S, *et al.* Expression of human apolipoprotein E reduces amyloid-beta deposition in a mouse model of Alzheimer's disease. *J. Clin. Invest.* 1999, **103**: R15–R21.

33. Mucke L, Masliah E, Yu GQ, *et al.* High-level neuronal expression of abeta 1–42 in wild-type human amyloid protein precursor transgenic mice: synaptotoxicity without plaque formation. *J. Neurosci.* 2000, **20**: 4050–4058.

34. Lee MK, Stirling W, Xu Y, *et al.* Human alpha-synuclein-harboring familial Parkinson's disease-linked Ala-53 → Thr mutation causes neurodegenerative disease with alpha-synuclein aggregation in transgenic mice. *Proc. Natl Acad. Sci. USA* 2002, **99**: 8968–8973.

35. Dauer W, Kholodilov N, Vila M, *et al.* Resistance of alpha-synuclein null mice to the parkinsonian neurotoxin MPTP. *Proc. Natl Acad. Sci. USA* 2002, **99**: 14524–14529.

36. Barnes GT, Duyao MP, Ambrose CM, *et al.* Mouse Huntington's disease gene homolog (Hdh). *Somat. Cell Mol. Genet.* 1994, **20**: 87–97.

37. Lin CH, Tallaksen-Greene S, Chien WM, *et al.* Neurological abnormalities in a knock-in mouse model of Huntington's disease. *Hum. Mol. Genet.* 2001, **10**: 137–144.

38. Lione LA, Carten RJ, Hunt MJ, *et al.* Selective discrimination learning impairments in mice expressing the human Huntington's disease mutation. *J. Neurosci.* 1999, **19**: 10428–10437.

39. Morton AJ, Lagan MA, Skepper JN, *et al.* Progressive formation of inclusions in the striatum and hippocampus of mice transgenic for the human Huntington's disease mutation. *J. Neurocytol.* 2000, **29**: 679–702.

40. Yamamoto A, Lucas JJ, Hen R. Reversal of neuropathology and motor dysfunction in a conditional model of Huntington's disease. *Cell* 2000, **101**: 57–66.

41. Wilson JM, Khabazian I, Pow DV, *et al.* Decrease in glial glutamate transporter variants and excitatory amino acid receptor down-regulation in a murine model of ALS-PDC. *Neuromol. Med.* 2003, **3**: 105–118.

42. Dal Canto MC, Gurney ME. Neuropathological changes in two lines of mice carrying a transgene for mutant human Cu, Zn SOD, and in mice overexpressing wild type human SOD: a model of familial amyotrophic lateral sclerosis (FALS). *Brain Res.* 1995, **676**: 25–40.

43. Morikawa E, Mori H, Kiyama Y, *et al.* Attenuation of focal ischemic brain injury in mice deficient in the epsilon1 (NR2A) subunit of NMDA receptor. *J. Neurosci.* 1998, **18**: 9727–9732.

44. Sans N, Vissel B, Petralia RS, *et al.* Aberrant formation of glutamate receptor complexes in hippocampal neurons of mice lacking the GluR2 AMPA receptor subunit. *J. Neurosci.* 2003, **23**: 9367–9373.

45. Namura S, Maeno H, Takami S, *et al.* Inhibition of glial glutamate transporter GLT-1 augments brain edema after transient focal cerebral ischemia in mice. *Neurosci. Lett.* 2002, **324**: 117–120.

46. Yang G, Chan PH, Chen J, *et al.* Human copper-zinc superoxide dismutase transgenic mice are highly resistant to reperfusion injury after focal cerebral ischemia. *Stroke* 1994, **25**: 165–170.

47. Murakami K, Kondo T, Kawase M, *et al.* Mitochondrial susceptibility to oxidative stress exacerbates cerebral infarction that follows permanent focal

cerebral ischemia in mutant mice with manganese superoxide dismutase deficiency. *J. Neurosci.* 1998, **18**: 205–213.

48. Sheng H, Bart RD, Oury TD, *et al.* Mice overexpressing extracellular superoxide dismutase have increased resistance to focal cerebral ischemia. *Neuroscience* 1999, **88**: 185–191.

49. Samdani AF, Dawson TM, Dawson VL. Nitric oxide synthase in models of focal ischemia. *Stroke* 1997, **28**: 1283–1288.

50. Huang Z, Huang PL, Ma J, *et al.* Enlarged infarcts in endothelial nitric oxide synthase knockout mice are attenuated by nitro-L-arginine. *J. Cereb. Blood Flow Metab.* 1996, **16**: 981–987.

51. Fannjiang Y, Kim CH, Huganir RL, *et al.* BAK alters neuronal excitability and can switch from anti- to pro-death function during postnatal development. *Devel. Cell* 2003, **4**: 575–585.

52. Trapp T, Korhonen L, Besselmann M, *et al.* Transgenic mice overexpressing XIAP in neurons show better outcome after transient cerebral ischemia. *Mol. Cell Neurosci.* 2003, **23**: 302–313.

53. Boutin H, LeFeuvre RA, Horai R, *et al.* Role of IL-1alpha and IL-1beta in ischemic brain damage. *J. Neurosci.* 2001, **21**: 5528–5534.

54. Friedlander RM, Gagliardini V, Hara H, *et al.* Expression of a dominant negative mutant of interleukin-1 beta converting enzyme in transgenic mice prevents neuronal cell death induced by trophic factor withdrawal and ischemic brain injury. *J. Exp. Med.* 1997, **185**: 933–940.

55. Soriano SG, Coxon A, Wang YF, *et al.* Mice deficient in Mac-1 (CD11b/CD18) are less susceptible to cerebral ischemia/reperfusion injury. *Stroke* 1999, **30**: 134–139.

56. Ishikawa M, Cooper D, Russell J, *et al.* Molecular determinants of the prothrombogenic and inflammatory phenotype assumed by the postischemic cerebral microcirculation. *Stroke* 2003, **34**: 1777–1782.

57. Wang YF, Tsirka SE, Strickland S, *et al.* Tissue plasminogen activator (tPA) increases neuronal damage after focal cerebral ischemia in wild-type and tPA-deficient mice. *Nature Med.* 1998, **4**: 228–231.

58. Asahi M, Sumii T, Fini ME, *et al.* Matrix metalloproteinase 2 gene knockout has no effect on acute brain injury after focal ischemia. *NeuroReport* 2001, **12**: 3003–3007.

59. Jo K, Rutten B, Bunn RC, *et al.* Actinin-associated LIM protein-deficient mice maintain normal development and structure of skeletal muscle. *Mol. Cell Biol.* 2001, **21**: 1682–1687.

60. Dennis CL, Tinsley JM, Deconinck AE, *et al.* Molecular and functional analysis of the utrophin promoter. *Nucleic Acids Res.* 1996, **24**: 1646–1652.

61. Kanadia RN, Johnstone KA, Mankodi A, *et al.* A muscleblind knockout model for myotonic dystrophy. *Science* 2003, **302**: 1978–1980.

62. Chan PH. Reactive oxygen radicals in signaling and damage in the ischemic brain. *J. Cereb. Blood Flow Metab.* 2001, **21**: 2–14.

63. Chan PH. Epstein CJ, Li Y, *et al.* Transgenic mice and knockout mutants in the study of oxidative stress in brain injury. *J. Neurotrauma* 1995, **12**: 815–824.

64. Hesselager G, Holland EC. Using mice to decipher the molecular genetics of brain tumors. *Neurosurgery* 2003, **53**: 685–694; discussion 695.

65. Kalaria RN, Viitanen M, Kalimo H, *et al.* The pathogenesis of CADASIL: an update. *J. Neurol. Sci.* 2004, **226**: 35–39.

66. Longhi L, Saatman KE, Raghupathi R, *et al.* A review and rationale for the use of genetically engineered animals in the study of traumatic brain injury. *J. Cereb. Blood Flow Metab.* 2001, **21**: 1241–1258.

67. McCullough L, Wu L, Haughey N, *et al*. Neuroprotective function of the PGE2 EP2 receptor in cerebral ischemia. *J. Neurosci.* 2004, **24**: 257–268.
68. Gordon JW, Scangos GA, Plotkin DJ, *et al*. Genetic transformation of mouse embryos by microinjection of purified DNA. *Proc. Natl Acad. Sci. USA* 1980, **77**: 7380–7384.
69. Wagner EF. EMBO medal review: On transferring genes into stem cells and mice. *EMBO J.* 1990, **9**: 3024–3032.
70. Evans MJ, Kaufman MH. Establishment in culture of pluripotential cells from mouse embryos. *Nature* 1981, **292**: 154–156.
71. Humpherys D, Eggan K, Akutsu H, *et al*. Epigenetic instability in ES cells and cloned mice. *Science* 2001, **293**: 95–97.
72. Elroy-Stein O, Bernstein Y, Groner Y. Overproduction of human Cu/Zn-superoxide dismutase in transfected cells: extenuation of paraquat-mediated cytotoxicity and enhancement of lipid peroxidation. *EMBO J.* 1986, **5**: 615–622.
73. Epstein CJ, Avraham KB, Lovett M, *et al*. Transgenic mice with increased Cu/Zn-superoxide dismutase activity: animal model of dosage effects in Down syndrome. *Proc. Natl Acad. Sci. USA* 1987, **84**: 8044–8048.
74. White BA. *PCR Protocols: Current Methods and Applications*. Totowa, NJ: Humana Press, 1993.
75. Thomas KR, Capecchi MR. Site-directed mutagenesis by gene targeting in mouse embryo-derived stem cells. *Cell* 1987, **51**: 503–512.
76. Li Y, Huang TT, Carlson EJ, *et al*. Dilated cardiomyopathy and neonatal lethality in mutant mice lacking manganese superoxide dismutase. *Nature Genet.* 1995, **11**: 376–381.
77. Li Y, Carlson EJ, Murakami K, *et al*. Targeted expression of human CuZn superoxide dismutase gene in mouse central nervous system. *J. Neurosci. Methods* 1999, **89**: 49–55.
78. Chan PH, Kawase M, Murakami K, *et al*. Overexpression of SOD1 in transgenic rats protects vulnerable neurons against ischemic damage after global cerebral ischemia and reperfusion. *J. Neurosci.* 1998, **18**: 8292–8299.
79. Sung YH, Song J, Lee HW. Functional genomics approach using mice. *J. Biochem. Mol. Biol.* 2004, **37**: 122–132.
80. Lee D, Threadgill DW. Investigating gene function using mouse models. *Curr. Opin. Genet. Devel.* 2004, **14**: 246–252.
81. Kwan KM. Conditional alleles in mice: practical considerations for tissue-specific knockouts. *Genesis* 2002, **32**: 49–62.
82. Schnutgen F, Doerflinger N, Calleja C, *et al*. A directional strategy for monitoring Cre-mediated recombination at the cellular level in the mouse. *Nature Biotechnol.* 2003, **21**: 562–565.
83. Gossen M, Freundlieb S, Bender G, *et al*. Transcriptional activation by tetra-cyclines in mammalian cells. *Science* 1995, **268**: 1766–1769.
84. Orban PC, Chui D, Marth JD. Tissue- and site-specific DNA recombination in transgenic mice. *Proc. Natl Acad. Sci. USA* 1992, **89**: 6861–6865.
85. Dymecki SM. Flp recombinase promotes site-specific DNA recombination in embryonic stem cells and transgenic mice. *Proc. Natl Acad. Sci. USA* 1996, **93**: 6191–6196.
86. Rajewsky K, Gu H, Kuhn R, *et al*. Conditional gene targeting. *J. Clin. Invest.* 1996, **98**: 600–603.
87. Knuesel I, Elliott A, Chen HJ, *et al*. A role for synGAP in regulating neuronal apoptosis. *Eur. J. Neurosci.* 2005, **21**: 611–621.

88. Akassoglou K, Malester B, Xu J, *et al.* Brain-specific deletion of neuropathy target esterase/swisscheese results in neurodegeneration. *Proc. Natl Acad. Sci. USA* 2004, **101**: 5075–5080.

89. Branda CS, Dymecki SM. Talking about a revolution: the impact of site-specific recombinases on genetic analyses in mice. *Devel. Cell* 2004, **6**: 7–28.

90. Maier CM, Chan PH. Role of superoxide dismutases in oxidative damage and neurodegenerative disorders. *Neuroscientist* 2002, **8**: 323–334.

91. Rosen DR, Siddique T, Patterson D, *et al.* Mutations in Cu/Zn superoxide dismutase gene are associated with familial amyotrophic lateral sclerosis. *Nature* 1993, **362**: 59–62.

92. Brown Jr RH. Superoxide dismutase and familial amyotrophic lateral sclerosis: new insights into mechanisms and treatments. *Ann. Neurol.* 1996, **39**: 145–146.

93. Rosen DR. Mutations in Cu/Zn superoxide dismutase gene are associated with familial amyotrophic lateral sclerosis. *Nature* 1993, **364**: 362.

94. Gurney ME, Pu H, Chiu AY, *et al.* Motor neuron degeneration in mice that express a human Cu, Zn superoxide dismutase mutation. *Science* 1994, **264**: 1772–1775.

95. Williamson TL, Cleveland DW. Slowing of axonal transport is a very early event in the toxicity of ALS-linked SOD1 mutants to motor neurons. *Nature Neurosci.* 1999, **2**: 50–56.

96. Al-Chalabi A, Leigh PN. Recent advances in amyotrophic lateral sclerosis. *Curr. Opin. Neurol.* 2000, **13**: 397–405.

97. Iadecola C, Zhang F, Niwa K, *et al.* SOD1 rescues cerebral endothelial dysfunction in mice overexpressing amyloid precursor protein. *Nature Neurosci.* 1999, **2**: 157–161.

98. Nakao N, Frodl EM, Widner H, *et al.* Overexpressing Cu/Zn superoxide dismutase enhances survival of transplanted neurons in a rat model of Parkinson's disease. *Nature Med.* 1995, **1**: 226–231.

99. Kondo T, Reaume AG, Huang TT, *et al.* Reduction of CuZn-superoxide dismutase activity exacerbates neuronal cell injury and edema formation after transient focal cerebral ischemia. *J. Neurosci.* 1997, **17**: 4180–4189.

100. Lewen A, Matz P, Chan PH. Free radical pathways in CNS injury. *J. Neurotrauma* 2000, **17**: 871–890.

101. Pineda JA, Aono M, Sheng H, *et al.* Extracellular superoxide dismutase overexpression improves behavioral outcome from closed head injury in the mouse. *J. Neurotrauma* 2001, **18**: 625–634.

9

Imaging in experimental neurology

MARC FISHER, ENG H. LO, AND MICHAEL LEV

9.1 Introduction

The availability of advanced imaging techniques has revolutionized the evaluation of many clinical neurological disorders. Similarly, the availability of
advanced imaging techniques has enhanced the utility of animal models
related to the study of these disorders. Currently, the most available and useful
imaging techniques in animal models of neurological disorders are those
related to magnetic resonance imaging (MRI) applications, computerized
tomography (CT), and positron emission tomography (PET). This chapter
will introduce the basic concepts related to these various imaging modalities
and then discuss their application to neurological disorders with a focus on
acute ischemic brain injury.

9.2 Magnetic resonance imaging

A wide variety of MRI techniques are currently available for use in animals
and patients. The range of MRI modalities and their main uses are provided in
Table 9.1. The initial MRI modalities employed were T1- and T2-weighted
imaging that evaluated the density of water proton spins.[1] Water protons in
relatively unrestricted fluid spaces have higher T1 and T2 values, while these
protons in more restricted environments such as brain edema, hemorrhages, or
tumors have lower values. These two MRI modalities are associated with an
increase in interstitial water content of the brain, as seen with the development
of vasogenic edema.[2] Conventional T1 and T2 MRI have been used widely in
clinical imaging for two decades and have also been used extensively in animal
models of brain ischemia, tumors, traumatic injury, and multiple sclerosis
(MS). The predominant utility of T1 and T2 MRI is to define the anatomical
localization and extent of tissue injury. T1 MRI with the injection of a paramagnetic contrast agent such as dimegluminegadopentate (Gd_DTPA) can
provide information about the integrity of the blood–brain barrier.[3] In

Handbook of Experimental Neurology, ed. Turgut Tatlisumak and Marc Fisher. Published by Cambridge
University Press. © Cambridge University Press 2006.

Table 9.1. *Magnetic resonance imaging (MRI) methods and their utility*

Method	Utility
T2-weighted MRI	Detect vasogenic edema
Contrast-enhanced T1-weighted MRI	Evaluate blood–brain barrier injury
Diffusion-weighted MRI	Marker of cytotoxic edema that can detect regions of ischemic injury very early onset
Perfusion-weighted MRI	Evaluate perfusion in the microvasculature and detect regions of hypoperfusion
Blood oxygenation level-dependent (BOLD) MRI	Evaluate subtle flow changes and demonstrate regions of brain activation
Susceptibility-weighted MRI	Detect intracerebral hemorrhage
Magnetic resonance angiography	Evaluate the status of the vasculature

conditions associated with disruption of the blood–brain barrier, the intravenously administered contrast agent leaks out into the brain parenchyma, leading to enhancement on T1 MRI. In brain tumors, contrast-enhanced T1 MRI can be used to delineate characteristics of the tumor and responses to therapy.[4] Contrast-enhanced T1 MRI has also been used in stroke models to assess blood–brain barrier permeability and potentially to evaluate the risk for hemorrhagic transformation.[5] Disruption of the blood–brain barrier with contrast-enhanced T1 MRI has been studied in models of experimental allergic encephalomyelitis, a model with similarities to MS. The presence of blood–brain barrier disruption can help to distinguish acute and chronic lesions in this disorder.[6] Contrast-enhanced T1 MRI is commonly used clinically to evaluate disease activity in MS patients and responses to immunomodulatory therapy.

Diffusion-weighted MRI (DWI) exploits the ability of MRI to measure the apparent diffusion coefficient (ADC) of water molecule protons in brain tissue.[7] ADC is acquired by adding strong pulse gradients to standard MRI sequences to determine the random movement of these protons in brain tissue. ADC values are higher in areas of relatively unrestricted diffusion such as the cerebral spinal fluid and vary also between white and gray matter within the brain parenchyma. With acute ischemic brain injury, ADC values decline rapidly, leading to an obvious region of hyperintensity on DWI.[8] The precise mechanism for the ADC decline after focal ischemic brain injury remains to be clarified. One leading hypothesis is that the ADC decline in ischemic tissue is related to the abrupt shift of water from the extracellular space to the intracellular space as a consequence of ischemia-induced failure of high-energy metabolism, i.e., the development of cytotoxic brain edema.[9] Other potential explanations for the rapid ADC decline seen in focal brain ischemia include an increase in tortuosity and changes of intracellular organelles. Rapid ADC declines are not limited to focal ischemic brain injury and are also observed after global brain ischemia, hypoglycemia, and seizures. DWI has been used extensively in animal stroke models to evaluate the temporal and spatial evolution of ischemic brain injury.[10] Additionally, DWI can provide an in vivo assessment tool for the evaluation of acute stroke therapies in animals. Information can be gathered in animal models concerning the time period required for maximal therapeutic effects and the precise location where the therapy is most effective.[11,12] This information is potentially invaluable for determining how best to proceed with further development of purported neuroprotective and thrombolytic interventions for acute ischemic stroke because the presumed target of such therapies is to reduce the extent of ischemic injury. DWI provides a unique in vivo assessment tool that can then be translated from animal stroke models to clinical trials. DWI has also been used in brain tumor modeling to evaluate therapeutic responses. In a glioma model, reduction of tumor burden was associated with an increase in ADC values.[13]

Another important application for DWI in experimental ischemia is its ability to detect the presence of secondary injury. Brain regions with initially reduced ADC values, detected shortly after stroke onset, are potentially reversible with early reperfusion or the use of neuroprotective agents.[14] In rats, reperfusion after 30 min of temporary focal ischemia is associated with complete or near-complete reversal of ADC abnormalities within 60–90 min. However, it was observed by many investigators that a portion of the ADC reversal can have a secondary decline in ADC values beginning hours later.[15,16] Secondary ADC declines are more likely to occur where initial ADC values are lower and where initial brain perfusion is most affected. These secondary ADC declines after reperfusion may represent the consequences of reperfusion injury and are an area of interest for future investigations. In stroke patients, similar secondary ADC declines after successful reperfusion have also been described, but the clinical consequences of these late ADC changes remain uncertain.[17]

Perfusion-weighted MRI (PWI) can be used to evaluate perfusion in the brain microvasculature in both animals and humans. PWI is currently performed by two techniques. The more commonly performed PWI technique is bolus-tracking that employs the injection of a contrast agent such as Gd_DPTA with a paramagnetic effect that impairs the acquisition of a $T2^*$-signal.[18] Multiple, repetitive $T2^*$ images are obtained beginning shortly before the injection of the contrast agent and then they are repeated every second for 30 s or longer to generate a signal intensity curve. The signal intensity curve can be utilized to generate perfusion-related parameters such as the mean transit time (MTT), cerebral blood volume, and an index of cerebral blood flow (CBF). Determining of the arterial input function and appropriate deconvolution leads to enhanced precision of CBF measurements with bolus tracking PWI.[18] Perfusion MRI maps are most commonly generated using MTT values of time to peak of the signal intensity curve. In addition to the generally qualitative CBF data determined by bolus-tracking PWI, another disadvantage is the technique cannot be performed repetitively over a short time period because of recirculation of the contrast agent and potential toxicity with multiple injections of the contrast agent. The other PWI technique is arterial spin labeling PWI (ASL), which involves the non-invasive labeling of water protons in the blood. With ASL, selective inversion of the water protons in the blood is done by disturbing their spins with a radiofrequency pulse just before they enter the brain, i.e., in the neck.[19] The tagged spins are then detected in the brain and compared to control images and CBF can be determined. With the continuous ASL approach using a two-coil system, quantitative CBF measurements across the entire rat brain can be obtained.

Both bolus-tracking and ASL perfusion imaging have been applied to animal stroke models and stroke patients. A number of investigators have used bolus-tracking PWI to evaluate perfusion changes in a variety of stroke models. Combining DWI and bolus-tracking PWI in stroke patients led to the development of the diffusion/perfusion mismatch concept as an approximation for the detection of ischemic but not irreversibly injured brain tissue, i.e., the ischemic penumbra.[20] The presence of the diffusion/perfusion mismatch is now being utilized in stroke trials to try to extend the therapeutic time window beyond the current 3 hr of proven benefit with t-pa. The diffusion/perfusion mismatch has not been extensively evaluated in animal stroke models until recently. In a rat model of permanent focal ischemia, using ASL to generate quantitative CBF values and DWI to generate absolute ADC values, it was observed that no significant volume of mismatch between the diffusion and perfusion lesions (Fig. 9.1) was detectable beyond 60 min after the onset of ischemia.[21] An elegant evaluation of individual pixels in this model demonstrated that almost all of the pixels in the mismatch zone shortly after stroke onset migrated to the irreversibly injured or ischemic core region over the initial 3 hr after the induction of ischemia. The same type of analysis was performed in rats subjected to 60 min of temporary focal ischemia.[22] Initially, a diffusion/perfusion mismatch similar to that observed in permanent ischemia was observed. After mechanical reperfusion the volume of the

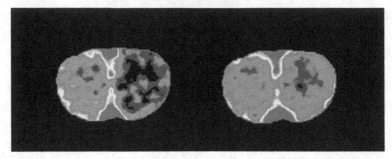

Figure 9.1. Images from a rat 1 hr after middle cerebral artery occlusion demonstrating a larger perfusion lesion on the right-sided image compared to the diffusion lesion on the left-sided image, a diffusion/perfusion mismatch.

diffusion abnormality decreased dramatically and the histologically defined infarct volume was approximately 40% smaller in the 60-min reperfusion group than in the permanent ischemia group. Using the individual pixel assessment approach, it was observed that 28% of the pixels in the ischemic core region just prior to the 60-min time point were salvaged and 90% of the pixels in the mismatch region were salvaged. These experiments demonstrate the level of sophisticated data available with the application of currently available DWI and PWI to animal stroke models. The data also exemplify that the current simplistic approach to the identification of the ischemic penumbra in animals and humans by the diffusion/perfusion mismatch approach will have to be modified. It is now abundantly clear that a portion of the ischemic region identified by DWI in animal stroke models and stroke patients is reversible early after stroke onset.[23] Additionally, the more mildly affected part of the PWI lesion represents oligemic tissue not destined for infarction. Future iterations of predictive models using DWI- and PWI-derived data will have to more precisely characterize injured tissue early after stroke onset to guide therapeutic decisions and evaluate therapeutic responses. Such sophisticated data analysis for determining the potential for tissue salvage could also be applied to animal models of global ischemia and traumatic injury. The addition of other MRI data such as anisotropy and magnetization transfer values might enhance the predictive modeling. Incorporating automated, unsupervised segmentation techniques such as K mean or Fuzzy-c clustering and the iterative self-organizing data analysis algorithm (ISODATA) will likely provide much additional useful information about tissue characteristics in a variety of brain disorders that use MRI in preclinical modeling.

The detection of intracerebral hemorrhage with MRI was considered problematic, but recent clinical studies suggest that both DWI and susceptibility-weighted imaging with T2* sequences can reliably determine the presence of acute bleeding.[24] Such MRI approaches have also been applied in animal models.[25] The paramagnetic effect of deoxyghemoglobin in the cerebral hemorrhage leads to signal loss on T2* and an obvious region of hypointensity. Therefore, DWI and susceptibility-weighted MRI can be used in animal stroke models to evaluate the expansion of intracerebral hemorrhages and to determine if hemorrhagic conversion has occurred.

Functional MRI (fMRI) is being widely used in a variety of models of neurological disorders to evaluate brain activation and function. The blood oxygenation level-dependent (BOLD) technique is most commonly used to perform fMRI. BOLD imaging also takes advantage of the paramagnetic effects of deoxyhemoglobin and the diamagnetic effects of oxyhemoglobin.[26] The paramagnetic effect of deoxyhemoglobin interferes with the acquisition of T2* signal similar to but to a lesser extent than exogenous contrast agents such as Gd_DPTA. With local brain activation, an increase in metabolic demand leads to an increase in CBF. The increase in CBF increases local oxygen supply that is greater than the increase in oxygen demand and an increase in BOLD MRI signal. This imbalance forms the basis of fMRI that can map regions of brain activation to a variety of stimuli both temporally and spatially. Preactivation maps are compared with postactivation maps to determine where the increase in blood flow has occurred in response to the activation paradigm. Brain activation paradigms have been applied in models of cardiac arrest, stroke, and Parkinson's disease to assess functional activity in specific brain regions.[27,28] After recovery from stroke, fMRI has been used to evaluate the functional reorganization pattern in the ipsilateral and contralateral hemispheres.[29] In a seizure model, fMRI was used to locate the origin and propagation of seizure foci.[30] BOLD imaging has been used in tumor modeling to evaluate the status of the microvasculature in the tumor and to distinguish between viable and necrotic regions within tumors.[31]

Magnetic resonance angiography (MRA) is a widely used MRI modality in clinical practice that is less commonly utilized in animal models because of difficulties with relatively low in-plane resolution. With technical advances, MRA should become more applicable to the smaller vasculature of most animal models. MRA acquisition is dependent upon flow-related enhancement of unsaturated, fully magnetized spins in the blood that flow into the imaging plane.[32] This enhancement is maximized by emphasizing flow-related signal and minimizing intraluminal dephasing. Applying repetitive radiofrequency pulses to saturate stationary tissue in the imaging slice suppresses stationary signal and enhances the signal from flowing blood. High-resolution MRA studies have been performed in rats and mice.[33] In stroke models, MRA can be used to document vascular occlusion and the response to t-pa. MRA can thus be used along with diffusion/perfusion MRI in stroke models to provide a comprehensive battery of MRI-based assessments that can be extrapolated to human studies.

A relatively new MRI technique with exciting capabilities for future applications is molecular imaging that can be used to detect and evaluate processes at a cellular or molecular level. With molecular imaging, targeted molecular probes such as monoclonal antibodies labeled with a label detectable by MRI are used.[34] Gene activation or enzymatic activity can be directly evaluated and localized within the brain. The function of brain tumor cells and endothelial cells have been initial targets of molecular imaging and more widespread applications will emerge.[35] Another new MRI application is the capability to track labeled cells in the brain. Labeled stem cells injected into the brain can be traced over time to determine their migration pattern. In a stroke model, it was observed that stem cells injected into the contralateral hemisphere migrated across the corpus callosum and appeared in great quantities in the infarct region.[36] The ability to evaluate molecular events and to map the migration of injected stem cells will find applications in other areas of experimental neurology soon.

9.3 Computed X-ray tomography

Initial studies with conventional CT in animal models of stroke suffered from the same caveats that somewhat limited early clinical utility. The basic CT signal is derived from changes in X-ray beam attenuation, which is in turn dependent on tissue electron density. Thus, standard CT is sensitive only to changes in brain density, such as that which occurs after edema or outright infarction. Such changes may be on the order of only a few Hounsfield units (the standard CT measure of tissue density), often barely detectable by the human eye. Non-contrast enhanced CT may additionally reveal dense vessels or sulcal effacement in early ischemic strokes. Cerebral infarction would be easily visible in delayed times after stroke onset. These findings were confirmed in experimental models of cerebral ischemia in non-human primates, and final infarct volumes correlated well with histological results.[37] The efficacy of reperfusion therapies have also been demonstrated using CT. Urokinase successfully resolved vascular occlusions and reductions in the expected progression of CT-defined infarcts correlated well with improved neurological outcomes.[38] Currently, unenhanced CT is clinically used to primarily exclude hemorrhage prior to thrombolytic therapy.

Contrast-enhanced CT is valuable in the diagnostic evaluation of patients with acute stroke both for its vascular angiographic and its parenchymal perfusion components. CT angiography is highly accurate in the detection of large vessel occlusions.[39] With newer 4-, 8-, or 16-slice multidetector helical scanners, a complete neurovascular workup may be accomplished, from the great vessels of the aortic arch, through the circle of Willis, up to the skull vertex, in well under a minute, with an additional 5–10 min for advanced three-dimensional reconstruction of vascular anatomy. Although diffusion-weighted MRI is clearly the more sensitive technique for small brainstem or lacunar infarcts, CT angiography has the advantage of speed, low cost, and perhaps most importantly, availability. The CT angiogram source images may also provide convenient whole brain blood volume weighted visualization of the brain parenchyma (see discussion on dynamic first-pass perfusion CT below). With the use of contrast enhancement, came also the promise that blood–brain barrier leakage would be detectable. However, initial tests in cats subjected to focal cerebral ischemia revealed that robust changes in Hounsfield units was not reliably correlated with Evans blue dye assays of blood–brain barrier leakage.[40] This limitation may speak to both the relative sizes of the contrast agent versus the magnitude of disruption of the blood–brain barrier, as well as the nature of its kinetics, which can be multiphasic (i.e., opening and closing of the barrier over time). Indeed, comparisons of serum protein leakage immunohistochemistry versus MR imaging of gadolinium leakage in a rabbit model of focal stroke showed that similar mismatches were present,[41] thus suggesting that this limitation is not CT-specific.

With the advent of xenon-enhanced CT, changes in cerebral perfusion could be detected.[42] This in vivo imaging method showed that regions of perfusion deficits were quantitatively detectable within ischemic zones in animal models of focal cerebral ischemia[43] as well as in models of global cerebral ischemia following cardiac arrest.[44] Profiles of ischemic blood flow dynamics and autoregulation have all been investigated using this technique.

More recently, dynamic CT perfusion imaging has come to the forefront. The fundamental approach is similar to that used in dynamic gadolinium-enhanced MRI. A bolus injection of a typically iodinated contrast agent is performed, and fast-repeated CT scanning is used to measure the first-pass transit curves of the agent through the brain. Standard calculations can then be used to map transit times, peak times, areas under curve, etc., to derive indirect measures of cerebral blood flow and volume. Indeed, it has even been suggested that due to the more linear characteristics of the iodine X-ray attenuation curves, this method may be more reliable compared to the gadolinium bolus used in MRI.[45] By calculating correlation coefficients that represent the integrity of hemodynamics relative to normal brain, one can map the hemodynamic perturbations that arise after cerebral ischemia. Changes in

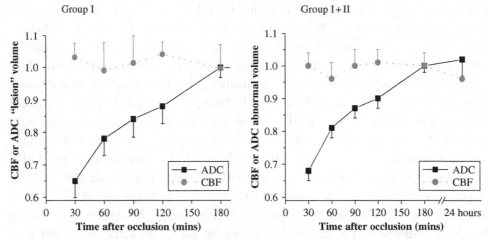

Figure 9.2. Dynamic first-pass CT imaging yields perfusion images in a rat model of focal cerebral ischemia. Left image shows the extensive ischemia induced by placement of a homologous blood clot in the middle cerebral artery. At 2 hrs, the rat was treated with 10 mg/kg of tPA intravenously. One hour later, right image shows that perfusion is mostly restored.

hemodynamic decay that mirror the collapse of the ischemic penumbra have been mapped using dynamic CT in rabbit models of focal ischemia.[46,47] In rats treated with antagonists of the amino-3-hydroxy-5-methyl-4-isoxazol proprionic acid (AMPA) type glutamate receptor, collapse of the ischemic penumbra was prevented.[48] This method has also been applied to test the hypothesis that hemodynamic support in the ischemic penumbra is sustained by nitric oxide derived from endothelial nitric oxide synthase (eNOS). In eNOS-deficient knockout mice, penumbra was significantly reduced compared to wild-type mice.[49] This combination of functional imaging and transgenic mouse technology promises to be highly valuable for dissecting the molecular mechanisms of stroke and to follow the effects of thrombolytic therapy (Fig. 9.2).

Changes in dynamic CT can also be calculated as absolute quantitative levels of cerebral blood flow and volume.[50] In a non-human primate model of stroke, this approach was found to be highly predictive of tissue infarction.[51] Recently, this approach has been successfully applied to clinical stroke as well.[52–55] In MRI, the diffusion/perfusion mismatch is considered by many as an indirect way to begin to assess the ischemic penumbra. While one cannot measure "diffusion" in CT, there are at least some data suggesting that blood volume/blood flow "mismatches" may also provide a somewhat analogous index of penumbra-like regions after focal ischemia. With the advent of many research CT facilities with increased spatial resolution, animal models can be used to test these hypotheses. Although some limitations may apply in terms of limited brain volume coverage, the rapid and widespread availability of dynamic perfusion CT compared to MRI may offer this method as a feasible alternative in some situations. One possible solution to limited coverage might be the use of two distinct cine acquisitions with two contrast bolus injections, resulting in twice the coverage volume. In the near future, the next generation of helical CT scanners with longer detector matrices may significantly increase the volume of brain that can be imaged.

9.4 Positron emission tomography

Positron emission tomography (PET) is an imaging modality that can provide sensitive, quantitative information about energy metabolism and cerebral perfusion. With the use of ^{15}O-labeled tracers such as oxygen, water of carbon dioxide CBF, cerebral blood volume (CBV), cerebral metabolic rate of oxygen (CMRO$_2$), and oxygen extraction fraction (OEF) can be quantified in different brain regions and temporally assessed.[56] With the use of fluorine-18 (^{18}F)-fluoro-2-deoxy-D-glucose in PET studies, brain glucose utilization can be quantitatively evaluated.[57] Radiolabeled ligands which bind to receptors such as the benzodiazepine or the dopamine receptor are used in PET studies that evaluate neuronal integrity, as well as receptor kinetics and integrity.[58]

PET studies with ^{15}O-labeled tracers have been used extensively in animal studies to evaluate the basic pathophysiology of ischemic brain injury and to determine tissue fate over time. PET provides quantitative data about CBF, CBV, OEF, and CMRO$_2$. This information has been used to determine varying levels of ischemic compromise.[59] Regions with very low CBF, collapsed CBV, and markedly reduced CMRO$_2$ represent irreversible injury, i.e., necrosis. Regions with moderately reduced CBF and increased CBV and OEF represent ischemic penumbra. The penumbra is the ischemic tissue that is potentially salvageable with timely reperfusion where the vasculature and brain parenchyma is trying to compensate for the reduction in CBF. Lastly, an oligemic zone with a modest reduction in CBF and increase in CBV and OEF can also be identified. This oligemic zone typically does not evolve into infarction.

PET has been used in cat and primate stroke models to evaluate tissue evolution over time and the responses to timely reperfusion. Early after stroke onset, substantial amounts of the ischemic zone has PET characteristics reflecting penumbral and oligemic properties.[60] Over time, the penumbral zone evolves into the ischemic core or necrotic zone without intervention. The time course for this evolution in primates is typically many hours, implying a prolonged time window for potential intervention with reperfusion therapy or neuroprotection. Studies have demonstrated that early reperfusion is capable of salvaging part of the ischemic penumbra.[61] A recent study in primates reperfused after 20 hr of middle cerebral artery occlusion demonstrated that part of the penumbral zone identified early after occlusion as a region with high OEF and reduced CBF could be salvaged even with this relatively late time of reperfusion.[62] Similar types of PET studies have been performed in humans, but human application of PET has been limited by lack of general availability, cost, and the complexity of data analysis. Receptor binding PET studies have also been performed in animal stroke models to evaluate tissue characteristics.[63] The radioligands used in these studies can identify irreversibly injured ischemic tissue and ischemic tissue that is hypoxic, but not yet necrotic. PET studies of reperfusion stroke models have confirmed the presence of postreperfusion hyperperfusion.[64] In cats, postreperfusion hyperperfusion improved outcome and lessened the probability of histologically confirmed tissue injury. This phenomenon also occurs in stroke patients and is associated with improved outcome.

PET studies with ^{18}F-DOPA have been performed in primate models of Parkinson's disease to evaluate striatal levels of dopamine and the concentration of dopamenergic neurons in the substantia nigra.[65] PET studies in Parkinson's disease models have also been performed with radiolabeled ligands to the dopamine transporter.[66] These studies provide information on the density of dopaminergic axon terminals. The effect of treatment on dopaminergic function can also be assessed with these PET techniques.

References

1. Beaulieu C, Moseley ME. Diffusion-weighted and perfusion-weighted magnetic resonance imaging in clinical stroke. In Fisher M, Bogousslavsky J (eds.) *Current Review of Cerebrovascular Disease*, 4th edn. Philadelphia, PA: Current Medicine, 2001, pp. 59–68.
2. van Bruggen N, Roberts TP, Cremer JE. The application of magnetic resonance imaging to the study of experimental cerebral ischemia. *Cerebrovasc. Brain Metab. Rev.* 1994, **6**: 180–210.
3. Runge VM, Price AC, Wehr CJ, Atkinson JB. Contrast enhanced MRI: evaluation of a canine model of osmotic blood–brain barrier disruption. *Invest. Radiol.* 1985, **20**: 830–844.
4. Schmiedl UP, Kenney J, Maravilla KR. Kinetics of pathologic blood–brain-barrier permeability in an astrocytic glioma using contrast-enhanced MR. *Am. J. Neuroradiol.* 1992, **13**: 5–14.
5. Knight RA, Barker PB, Fagan SC, *et al.* Prediction of impending hemorrhagic transformation in ischemic stroke using magnetic resonance imaging in rats. *Stroke* 1998, **29**: 144–151.

6. Silver NC, Good CD, Barker GJ, *et al*. Sensitivity of contrast enhanced MRI in multiple sclerosis: effects of gadolinium dose, magnetization transfer contrast and delayed imaging. *Brain* 1997, **120**: 1149–1161.

7. Neumann-Haefelin T, Moseley ME, Albers GW. New magnetic resonance imaging methods for cerebrovascular disease: emerging clinical applications. *Ann. Neurol.* 2000, **31**: 559–570.

8. Fisher M, Albers GW. Application of diffusion-perfusion magnetic resonance imaging in acute ischemic stroke. *Neurology* 1999, **52**: 1750–1756.

9. van der Toorn A, Skyova E, Dijkhuizen RM, *et al*. Dynamic changes in water ADC, energy metabolism, extracellular space volume and tortuosity in neonatal rat brain during global ischemia. *Mag. Res. Med.* 1996, **36**: 52–60.

10. Dijkhuizen RM, Nicolay K. Magnetic resonance imaging in experimental models of brain disorders. *J. Cereb. Blood Flow Metab.* 2003, **23**: 1383–1402.

11. Reith W, Hasegawa Y, Latour LL, *et al*. Multislice diffusion mapping for 3-D evolution of cerebral ischemia in a rat stroke model. *Neurology* 1995, **45**: 172–177.

12. Li F, Carano RAD, Irie K, *et al*. Neuroprotective effects of a novel broad spectrum cation channel blocker LOE 908MS on experimental focal ischemia. *J. Magn. Res. Imaging* 1999, **10**: 138–145.

13. Chenevert TL, Mckeever PE, Ross BD. Monitoring early response of experiemental brain tumors to therapy using diffusion magnetic resonance imaging. *Clin. Cancer Res.* 1997, **3**: 1457–1466.

14. Fiehler J, Foth M, Kucinski T, *et al*. Severe ADC decreases do not predict irreversible tissue damage in humans. *Stroke* 2002, **33**: 79–86.

15. Li F, Liu KF, Silva A, *et al*. Secondary decline in apparent diffusion coefficient and neurological outcome after a short period of focal brain ischemia in rats. *Ann. Neurol.* 2000, **48**: 236–244.

16. Ringer TM, Neumann-Haefelin T, Sobel RA, Moseley ME, Yenari MA. Reversal of early diffusion-weighted magnetic resonance abnormalities does not necessarily reflect tissue salvage in experimental cerebral ischemia. *Stroke* 2001, **32**: 2362–2369.

17. Kidwell CS, Saver JL, Mattiello J, *et al*. Thrombolytic reversal of acute human cerebral ischemic injury shown by diffusion/perfusion magnetic resonance imaging. *Ann. Neurol.* 2000, **47**: 462–469.

18. Calamante F, Thomas DL, Pell GS, Wiersma J, Turner R. Measuring cerebral blood flow using magnetic resonance imaging techniques. *J. Cereb. Blood Flow Metab.* 1999, **19**: 701–735.

19. Williams DS, Detre JA, Leigh JS, Koretsky AP. Magnetic resonance imaging of perfusion using spin inversion of arterial water. *Proc. Natl Acad. Sci. USA* 1992, **89**: 212–216.

20. Meng X, Shen Q, Fisher M, Sotak CH, Duong TQ. Characterizing the diffusion/ perfusion mismatch evolution in permanent and temporary experimental ischemic stroke models. *Ann. Neurol.* 2004, **55**: 207–212.

21. Shen Q, Meng X, Fisher M, Sotak CH, Duong TQ. Pixel-by-pixel spatiotemporal progression of focal ischemia derived using quantitative perfusion and diffusion imaging. *J. Cereb. Blood Flow Metab.* 2003, **23**: 1479–1488.

22. Shen Q, Fisher M, Sotak CH, Duong TQ. Effect of reperfusion on ADC and CBF pixel-by-pixel dynamics in stroke: characterizing tissue fates using quantitative diffusion and perfusion imaging. *J. Cereb. Blood Flow Metab.* 2004, **24**: 280–290.

23. Kidwell CS, Alger JR, Saver JL. Beyond mismatch: evolving paradigms in imaging the ischemic penumbra with multimodal magnetic resonance imaging. *Stroke* 2003, **34**: 2729–2735.

24. Fiebach JB, Schellinger PD, Gass A, *et al.* Stroke magnetic resonance imaging is accurate in hyperacute intracerebral hemorrhage: a multicenter study on the validity of stroke imaging. *Stroke* 2004, **35**: 502–506.

25. Gustafsson O, Rossitti S, Ericsson A, Raininko R. MR imaging of experimentally induced intracranial hemorrhage. *Acta Radiol.* 1999, **40**: 360–368.

26. Ogawa S, Tank DW, Menon R, *et al.* Intrinsic signal changes accompanying sensory stimulation: functional brain mapping with magnetic resonance imaging. *Proc. Natl Acad. Sci. USA* 1992, **89**: 5951–5955.

27. Ono Y, Morikawa S, Inubishi T, Shimizu H, Yoshimoto T. T2*-weighted magnetic resonance imaging of cerebrovascular reactivity in rat reversible cerebral ischemia. *Brain Res.* 1997, **744**: 207–215.

28. Pelled G, Bergman H, Goelman G. Bilateral overactivation of the sensorimotor cortex in the unilateral rodent model of Parkinson's disease: a functional magnetic resonance imaging study. *Eur. J. Neurosci.* 2002, **15**: 389–394.

29. Cramer SC, Nelles G, Benson RR, *et al.* A functional MRI study of subjects recovered from hemispheric stroke. *Stroke* 1997, **28**: 2518–2527.

30. Opdam HI, Federico P, Jackson GD, *et al.* A sheep model for the study of focal epilepsy with concurrent intracranial EEG and functional MRI. *Epilepsia* 2002, **43**: 779–787.

31. Mazurchuk R, Zhou R, Straubinger RM, Chau RI, Grossman Z. Functional magnetic resonance (fMR) imaging of rat brain tumor model: implications for evaluation of tumor microvasculature and therapeutic response. *Magn. Res. Imaging* 1999, **17**: 537–548.

32. Weber J, Forsting M. Magnetic resonance angiography. In Fisher M, Bogousslavsky J (eds.) *Current Review of Cerebrovascular Disease*, 4th edn. Philadelphia, PA: Current Medicine, 2001, pp. 85–92.

33. Hilger T, Niessen F, Diedenhofen M, Hossmann K, Hoehn-Berlage M. Magnetic resonance angiography of thromboembolic stroke in rats. *J. Cereb. Blood Flow Metab.* 2002, **22**: 652–662.

34. Blasberg R. Imaging gene expression and endogenous molecular processes: molecular imaging. *J. Cereb. Blood Flow Metab.* 2002, **22**: 1157–1164.

35. Sipkins DA, Giijbels K, Tropper FD, *et al.* ICAM-1 expression in autoimmune encephalitis visualized using magnetic resonance imaging. *J. Neuroimmun.* 2001, **104**: 1–9.

36. Hoehn-Berlage M, Kustermann E, Blunk J, *et al.* Monitoring of implanted stem cell migration in vivo. *Proc. Natl Acad. Sci. USA* 2002, **99**: 16267–16272.

37. Pevsner PH. Computed tomography in a primate stroke model using selective balloon catheter arterial occlusion. *J. Comput. Asst. Tomogr.* 1997, **3**: 105–108.

38. Del Zoppo GJ, Copeland BR, Waltz TP, *et al.* The beneficial effect of intracarotid urokinase on acute stroke in a baboon model. *Stroke* 1986, **17**: 638–643.

39. Kuroiwa T, Seida M, Tomida S, *et al.* Discrepancies among CT, histological and BBB findings in early cerebral ischemia. *J. Neurosurg.* 1986, **65**: 517–524.

40. Lev MH, Farkas J, Rodriguez VR, *et al.* CT angiography in the rapid triage of patients with hyperacute stroke: accuracy in the detection of large vessel thrombus. *J. Comput. Asst. Tomogr.* 2001, **25**: 520–528.

41. Lo EH, Pan Y, Matsumoto K, Kowall NW. Blood–brain barrier disruption in experimental focal ischemia: comparison between in vivo MRI and immunocyto-chemistry. *Magn. Res. Imaging* 1994, **12**: 403–411.
42. Gur D, Yonas H, Herbert D, *et al.* Xenon enhanced dynamic computed tomography: multilevel cerebral blood flow studies. *J. Comput. Asst. Tomogr.* 1981, **5**: 334–340.
43. Yonas H, Gur D, Claassen D, Wolfson Jr SK, Moossy J. Stable xenon enhanced computed tomography in the study of clinical and pathologic correlates of focal ischemia in baboons. *Stroke* 1988, **19**: 228–238.
44. Yonas H, Gur D, Classen D, Wolfson SK, Moossy J. Stable xenon enhanced CT measurement of cerebral blood flow in reversible focal ischemia in baboons. *J. Neurosurg.* 1990, **73**: 266–273.
45. Wolfson SK, Safar P, Reich H, *et al.* Dynamic heterogeneity of cerebral perfusion after prolonged cardiac arrest in dogs measured by stable xenon CT technique. *Resuscitation* 1992, **23**: 1–20.
46. Lo EH, Rogowska J, Batchelder KF, Wolf GL. Hemodynamic alterations in focal cerebral ischemia: temporal correlation analysis for functional imaging. *Neurol. Res.* 1996, **18**: 150–156.
47. Lo EH, Rogowska J, Bogorodzki P, *et al.* Temporal correlation analysis of penumbral dynamics in focal cerebral ischemia. *J. Cereb. Blood Flow Metab.* 1996, **16**: 60–68.
48. Shimizu-Sasamata M, Kano T, Rogowska J, *et al.* YM872, a highly water-soluble AMPA antagonist, reduces brain damage in the hemodynamic penumbra after permanent focal ischemia in rats. *Stroke* 1998, **29**: 2141–2148.
49. Lo EH, Hara H, Rogowska J, *et al.* Temporal correlation mapping analysis of the hemodynamic penumbra in mutant mice deficient in endothelial nitric oxide synthase gene expression. *Stroke* 1994, **27**: 1381–1386.
50. Hamberg LM, Hunter GJ, Kierstead D, *et al.* Measurement of quantitative cerebral blood volume with subtraction 3D-fCT. *Am. J. Neuroradiol.* 1996, **17**: 1861–1869.
51. Hamberg LM, Hunter GJ, Maynard KI, *et al.* Functional CT perfusion imaging in predicting the extent of cerebral infarction from a 3 hr middle cerebral artery occlusion in a primate model of stroke. *Am. J. Neuroradiol.* 2002, **23**: 1013–1021.
52. Hunter GJ, Hamberg LM, Ponzo JA, *et al.* Assessment of cerebral perfusion and arterial anatomy in hyperacute stroke with three-dimensional functional CT: early clinical results. *Am. J. Neuroradiol.* 1998, **19**: 29–37.
53. Lev MH, Segal AZ, Farkas J, *et al.* Utility of perfusion-weighted CT imaging in acute middle cerebral artery stroke treated with intra-arterial thrombolysis: prediction of final infarct volume and clinical outcome. *Stroke* 2001, **32**: 2021–2028.
54. Wintermark M, Reichhart M, Thiran JP, *et al.* Prognostic accuracy of cerebral blood flow measurement by perfusion computed tomography, at the time of emergency room admission, in acute stroke patients. *Ann. Neurol.* 2002, **51**: 417–432.
55. Eastwood JD, Lev MH, Provenzale JM. Perfusion CT with iodinated contrast material. *Am. J. Roentgenol.* 2003, **180**: 3–12.
56. Baron JC. Clinical use of positron emission computed tomography in cerebrovascular disease. *Neurosurg. Clin America.* 1996, **7**: 653–664.
57. Baron JC, Frackowiak RSJ, Herholz K, *et al.* Use of positron emission tomography in the investigation of cerebral hemodynamics and energy metabolism in cerebrovascular disease. *J. Cereb. Blood Flow Metab.* 1989, **9**: 723–742.

58. Lee CS, Samii A, Sossi V, *et al.* In vivo positron emission tomographic evidence for compensatory changes in post synaptic dopaminergic nerve terminals in Parkinson's disease. *Ann. Neurol.* 2000, **47**: 493–500.
59. Marchal G, Serrati C, Rioux P, *et al.* PET imaging of cerebral perfusion and oxygen consumption in acute ischaemic stroke, relationship to outcome. *Lancet* 1993, **341**: 925.
60. Yong AR, Sette G, Touzani O, *et al.* Relationship between high oxygen extraction fraction in the acute stage and final infarction in reversible middle cerebral artery occlusion. *J. Cereb. Blood Flow Metab.* 1996, **16**: 1176–1188.
61. Young AR, Touzani O, Derlon JM, *et al.* Early reperfusion in the anesthetized baboon reduces brain damage following middle cerebral artery occlusion. *Stroke* 1997, **28**: 632–638.
62. Giffard C, Young AR, Kerouche N, Derlon JM, Baron JC. Outcome of acutely ischemic brain tissue in prolonged middle cerebral artery occlusion. *J. Cereb. Blood Flow Metab.* 2004, **24**: 495–508.
63. Wantanbe N, Young AR, Garcia JH, *et al.* Focal cerebral ischemia and chronic stage reduced flumazeril uptake in anesthetized baboons. *J. Cereb. Blood Flow Metab.* 1999, **19**: S16.
64. Heiss WD, Graff R, Lottgen J, *et al.* Repeat positron emission tomographic studies in transient middle cerebral artery occlusion in cats: residual perfusion and efficacy of postischemic reperfusion. *J. Cereb. Blood Flow Metab.* 1997, **17**: 388–400.
65. Pate BD, Kawamata T, Yamada T, *et al.* Correlation of striatal fluorodopa uptake in the MPTP monkey with dopaminergic indices. *Ann. Neurol.* 1993, **34**: 331–338.
66. Poyot T, Couda F, Gregoire M–C, *et al.* Anatomic and biochemical correlates of the dopamine transporter ligand[11] C-PE21 in normal and parkinsonian primates. *J. Cereb. Blood Flow Metab.* 2001, **21**: 782–792.

10

Safety in animal facilities

TARJA KOHILA

10.1 Introduction

The research animal facility is perhaps the most highly regulated area of interaction between humans and animals. Informing staff members and researchers of the risks posed by research animals is one of many expectations that must be met by institutions. Research animal facilities often house several different animal species. Each animal has a unique physiological, anatomical, and microbiological profile that affects its potential to harm personnel. The institutions are responsible for conveying information regarding research animal risks to large numbers of personnel and researchers with diverse backgrounds. The challenge of animal risk assessment is to select essential and easily understood information to help people who work with animals. Providing too little information to the researchers is unacceptable, but overwhelming detail is equally likely to miss the scientific target of experiments.

Laboratory animal facilities are simply a special type of laboratory. As a general principle, the biosafety level (facilities, practices, and operational requirements) recommended for working with infectious agents in vivo and in vitro are comparable with a microbiological laboratory where hazardous conditions are caused by personnel, and by the equipment. In the animal room, the activities of the animals themselves can present new hazards. Animals may generate aerosols, they may bite and scratch, and they may be infected with a zoonotic disease transferable from animals to humans.

10.2 General hazards

Since 1967 rodent breeding units have been recommended to be built behind a "barrier," a so-called specific-pathogen-free (SPF) space separated from the main laboratory. It is based on the need to standardize the microbiological conditions for the animals and for the quality of the research. Nowadays it is

Handbook of Experimental Neurology, ed. Turgut Tatlisumak and Marc Fisher. Published by Cambridge University Press. © Cambridge University Press 2006.

common to maintain a safe working practice in a healthy environment for both animals and personnel and this determines the design, fabric, contents, and work routines of the laboratory animal facility.

Hazards associated with the housekeeping of animals can be avoided by common-sense precautions. One example of physical hazards is probably water. Floors should be made of an impermeable, non-slip material that can be easily cleaned, and are suitable for non-slip footwear. Waste materials should be classified according to their constituents and their particular hazards. Empty aerosol cans, organic solvents and scintillation fluid, quantities of paper, and dense forms of plastic must be excluded from general or clinical waste and any sharps, scalpel blades, or needles should be in robust containers. Disposal of chemical and radioactive waste will not be dealt with in this chapter. The bags of waste should not be too heavy if manual handling is necessary. Workplace injury records highlight the frequency of injuries caused by lifting, moving, or pulling heavy refuse bags and equipment. This is particularly relevant in laboratory animal facilities. Animal rooms, laboratories, equipment, and procedures should be designed, selected, and developed to provide for ergonomically sound operations that reduce the potential of physical injury to personnel. Safety equipment should be properly maintained and routinely calibrated.

10.3 Personal hygiene and protective clothing

It is essential that all personnel maintain a high standard of personal cleanliness. The importance of personal hygiene cannot be overemphasized and requires sufficient hand washbasins and bactericidal soap dispensers that should be available for staff and researchers. Rest rooms and a canteen space should be separate from the animal areas, and washing and showering facilities should also be available. Disposable gloves, masks, head covers, coats, coveralls, and shoe covers might be desirable in all circumstances. Also protective clothing should be changed when moving from one area to another inside the animal facility. Clean protective clothing should be provided as often as necessary. Personnel working in areas where they might be exposed to contaminated airborne particulate material or vapors should be provided with suitable respiratory protection. Personnel should not be permitted to eat, drink, use tobacco products, or apply cosmetics inside animal rooms. Because of their isolated nature some areas like barrier animal facilities, individual ventilated cage areas, isolators, and biohazard areas are at risk if staff and researchers do not comply with requirements and local safety rules on entry to the animal facility.

10.4 Infectious hazards and zoonoses

In laboratory animal facilities, workplace exposure to zoonotic pathogens, agents transmitted to humans from vertebrate animals or their tissues, might be an occupational hazard. The risks to animal facility users posed by infectious agents can be divided into two distinct areas: experimental infections and zoonotic infections.

Zoonosis surveillance should be a part of an occupational health program. Anyway, there is no known risk of zoonotic disease development from typical exposure to microbial flora of laboratory mice and rats. Commercially raised laboratory rodents have non-pathogenic, well-defined microbial flora. Mice obtained through facility-approved sources will be free of lymphocytic choriomeningitis virus and other zoonotic agents. Rats obtained through facility-approved sources will be free of hantavirus, *Leptospira* spp., *Salmonella* spp., and *Ornithonyssus bacoti* mites. There is minor risk when importing and exporting animals between research institutes which do not follow any health monitoring programs or test animals regularly. There is also a minor risk of scratch wounds or bites associated with handling laboratory rodents. There is also a moderate risk of injury or infection due to rodent bites, especially rat bites, which may produce deep puncture wounds. Risk of rat-bite fever is minimal due to the eradication of the causative agents from commercial rat colonies. Appropriate methods for rodent restraint and wearing protective clothing reduce the risk of scratch and bite wounds. Most organisms are harmless and can be matched by those carried by personnel working with animals.

In the UK the Advisory Committee on Dangerous Pathogens has categorized biological agents into four groups:[1]

Group 1 A biological agent unlikely to cause human disease

Group 2 A biological agent that can cause human disease and may be a hazard to employees; it is unlikely to spread to the community and effective treatment is usually available

Group 3 A biological agent that can cause severe human disease and is a hazard to employees

Group 4 A biological agent that causes severe human disease and is a serious hazard to employees; it is likely to spread to the community and there is usually no effective treatment available.

In principle, laboratory animals pose a minor risk not only from the microorganism under study but also from any potentially zoonoses that they may be carrying. Thus all areas containing animals should be considered as posing some degree of risk even when being used simply to house and breeding laboratory animals from commercial sources.

The expansion and improvement of high-containment animal facilities has been driven by the threat of terrorism, economics, the emergence of new pathogens, and the re-emergence of other pathogens in new areas. Working with highly infectious viral agents requires a team of trained scientists, laboratory technicians, veterinarians, animal care staff, biological safety officers, engineers, and physical plant staff to ensure safety, biocontainment, and the well-being of animals, while providing essential scientific data. The challenges of working with infectious disease agents in high levels of containment, and some solutions to these challenges.[2]

10.5 Chemical and radiation hazards

The main natural chemical hazards associated with animal work are allergens in animal products. Sterilizing agents, disinfectants, detergents, corrosive cleaning chemicals, drugs, and chemicals in experiments are also encountered. Exposure to hazardous chemicals may arise from contact with metabolites in animal excretions and secretions through the skin and in exhaled gases.

Chemical safety is an essential element of an effective occupational health and safety program. Controlling exposure to chemical agents requires a careful process of hazard recognition, risk assessment, development of control measures, communication of the risks and control measures, and training to ensure that the indicated controls will be utilized. Managing chemical safety in animal care and use presents a unique challenge, in part because research is frequently conducted in two very different environments, the research laboratory and the animal care facility. The chemical agents specific to each of these environments are typically well understood by the employees working there; however, the extent of understanding may not be adequate when these individuals, or chemicals, cross over into the other environment or are used by not so well-trained researchers. In addition, many chemicals utilized in animal research are not typically used in the research laboratory, and therefore the level of employee knowledge and proficiency may be less compared with more routinely used materials. Finally, the research protocol may involve the exposure of laboratory animals to either toxic chemicals or chemicals with unknown hazards. Such animal protocols require careful review to minimize the potential for unanticipated exposures of the research staff or animal care personnel. Numerous guidelines and regulations are cited, which define the standard of practice for the safe use of chemicals.[3]

Certain chemicals are known to be sensitizers and that is a chronic health problem that affects only some individuals in an exposed population following repeated exposures. The hazardous chemicals must be evaluated by suppliers and information given to users in the form of certificates and adequate labeling which includes an indication of danger.

Techniques involving the administration of radioactive materials or exposure of laboratory animals to ionizing radiation sources are now widely used in biomedical research. Nowadays non-ionizing radiation from ultrasound, microwaves, and magnetic fields have found increasing applications in biology and medicine and applications of these techniques also involve the use of laboratory animals. The basics of radiation protection are to minimize or prevent injury to personnel and to the general population. In order to achieve this objective it is necessary to ensure that all work involving radiation sources or radioactive materials is carried out carefully and with strict observance of the local and national principles and legislation. Especially the disposal of radioactive waste is now strictly controlled in an increasing number of countries because of public concern. Because all sources of ionizing and non-ionizing radiations are a potential risk to human health both the employing organization and the individual worker must adopt a thoroughly responsible attitude to radiation work. It is essential that before starting to work with radioactive materials all personnel are fully trained and understand the nature of the risks and the reasons underlying the safety procedures and instructions.

10.6 Laboratory animal allergies

Certain animal-derived materials contain sensitizing chemicals. Examples include urine and dander. In an animal facility, without proper precautions, some personnel will succumb to developing a sensitization to these materials. This occupational illness is known as laboratory animal allergy (LAA). It is not possible to predict which individuals will be susceptible and once developed laboratory animal allergy may limit the ability to continue working with the sensitizing species of animals.

Laboratory animal allergy is an important threat to the occupational health of those who work with rats and mice and it may affect up to 56% of all personnel exposed to laboratory animals. Animal allergens include small proteins that can be found in dander, hair, saliva, urine, feces, and serum. Several specific allergens have been isolated from mice, rats, guinea pigs, rabbits, cats, and dogs. Recent studies indicate that the majority of clinically important aeroallergens are biochemically active.[4] The most common laboratory animal allergies are to rat and mouse antigens. In 1977 the urine of rats and mice was identified as an important source of allergens.[5] The low molecular weight of the urine of adult male animals was particularly potent at causing bronchoconstriction and a positive skin test response in sensitive subjects. The composition of rat urine is dependent on the age and sex of the animal, but there is no significant difference in the urinary allergens from different strains of rat.[6] The most common sources of rat or mouse allergens are urine, pelt, fur, and serum. Exposure to these may occur through the direct handling of animals or via dirty bedding and other materials which have had contact with animals.

The fact is that most laboratory animal species produce allergenic proteins and that is why laboratory animal allergy and its prevention have recently received increased attention within the biomedical research field. There is a moderate to significant risk of development of laboratory animal allergy and approximately 50% of people who work regularly with rats will become allergic and about 10% of the workforce will develop asthma.[7] Early diagnosis should be confirmed and where possible the patient is removed from the exposure area. Wearing personal protective equipment (mask, gloves, laboratory coat) and using appropriate equipment (laminar airflow hoods, individual ventilated cages, isolators, etc.) can minimize a risk to sensitization. In summary, the incidence of laboratory animal allergy can be reduced by effective, integrated health risk management, with the conscientious use of engineering, procedural and personal control measures. Engineering controls are the first line of defense and include room and building ventilation and humidity control systems, local ventilation systems including safety hoods, isolators or individually ventilated cages and racks for animals, and vacuum systems for experimental working. Building designs that enclose and separate animal use space from public space will lead to the correct standard and such engineering and architectural features help to control allergens within the animal facility and minimize contamination of office or other public areas.

10.7 Risk assessment

An effective occupational health and safety program ensures that the risks associated with the experimental use of animals are reduced to acceptable levels. Professional personnel who conduct and support research programs that involve hazardous biologic, chemical, or physical and radiation agents should be qualified to assess dangers associated with the programs and to select safeguards appropriate to the risks. Potential hazards that are involved in experimental animal use should be identified and evaluated. Safety specialists with knowledge in appropriate disciplines should be involved in the assessment of risks associated with hazardous activities and in the development of procedures to manage such risk.[8]

References

1. Wood M, Smith MW. *Health and Safety in Laboratory Animal Facilities.* London: Laboratory Animals Ltd, 1999.
2. Copps J. Issues related to the use of animals in biocontainment research facilities. *Inst. Lab. Anim. Res. J.* 2005, **46**: 34–43.
3. Thomann WR. Chemical safety in animal care, use, and research. *Inst. Lab. Anim. Res. J.* 2003, **44**: 13–19.
4. Stewart GA, Thompson PJ. The biochemistry of common aeroallergens. *Clin. Exp. Allergy* 1996, **26**: 1020–1044.
5. Newman-Taylor AJ. Laboratory animal allergy. *Eur. J. Respir. Dis. Suppl.* 1982, **123**: 60–64.
6. Lutsky I, Fink JN, Kidd J, Dahlberg MJ, Yunginger JW. Allergenic properties of rat urine and pelt extracts. *J. Allergy Clin. Immunol.* 1985, **75**: 279–284.
7. Preece RM, Renström A. Laboratory animal allergy. In Hau J, Van Hoosier GL Jr (eds.) *Handbook of Laboratory Animal Science*, 2nd edn. Boca Raton, FL: CRC Press, 2002, pp. 107–126.
8. Clark JM. Planning for safety: biological and chemical hazards. *Lab. Anim.* 2005, **22**: 33–38.

11

Behavioral testing in small-animal models: ischemic stroke

LARRY B. GOLDSTEIN

The ultimate validation of any animal model of human disease is the extent to which it simulates the parameter of interest. Depending on its purpose, the model may attempt to mimic the pathology and/or pathophysiology of a disease process, or predict the impact of putative therapeutic interventions. In the case of neurological disease, the ultimate outcome is behavioral. For example, in humans, the outcome of interest for patients with movement disorders is the preservation or return of normal motoric function, for persons afflicted with Alzheimer's disease it is the maintenance or restoration of normal cognition and for those with stroke or traumatic brain injury it is the return to their premorbid functional status. Although the fundamental features of simple stimulus–response relationships and even more complex environmental–behavioral interactions are remarkably preserved across species, the complete repertoire of human behaviors and their response to neurological disease are uniquely complex. Therefore, animal models will always be found to be wanting. Despite this fundamental limitation, animal behavior can provide critical insights into the functional consequences of human neurological disease and the potential benefit and toxicity of therapeutic interventions. They are particularly important as functional outcomes may be dissociated from the extent of neurological injury due to differences in the post-injury recovery process.[1,2]

11.1 Limitations and principles

The limitations of small-animal behavioral models become apparent when considering the differences in even seemingly simple functional abilities as compared to humans. Olfaction and sensory data obtained through whisker stimulation are of much greater importance to the "activities of daily living" of rodents than humans. Rodents are quadrapedal and humans bipedal, representing a fundamental difference in the neurobiological processes underlying gait. Humans have an opposable thumb that is essential for digital manipulation and grasping, also quite different than in rodents. Although mammals

Handbook of Experimental Neurology, ed. Turgut Tatlisumak and Marc Fisher. Published by Cambridge University Press. © Cambridge University Press 2006.

such as non-human primates, whales, and porpoises may communicate through complex vocalizations in many ways analogous to human speech, there is no evidence of such capabilities in rodents. Testing of human abstract thinking cannot be readily simulated in other animals. Therefore, animal models can provide data that may be relevant to some of the deficits resulting from neurological disease or injury in humans, but generally cannot simulate the entire range of impairments found in humans.

The role of behavioral compensation or substitution is an important principle to consider when evaluating an animal's functional response to neurological injury. Just as a human with a paralyzed arm can perform activities such as driving an automobile, dressing, or bathing using the uninvolved limb, laboratory animals can accomplish involved tasks using alternative strategies.[3] Even if the impaired limb is used to complete a task, it may be used differently than before the neurological injury occurred. It is also important to recognize that post-injury behavioral experience has a direct effect on anatomical changes that occur in the brain after injury.[3] Lesion-induced neuronal degeneration can also lead to an enhanced responsiveness to post-injury behavioral experience.[3]

In considering the use of different behavioral tests and paradigms, it needs to be understood that it is often difficult to isolate the specific impairment(s) underlying a performance deficit. For example, sensory, motor, perceptual and cognitive limitations can all contribute to a rat's difficulty negotiating a maze. Although frequently critical for behavioral psychologists interested in understanding the functional importance of a specific central structure, it is difficult (and from the standpoint of animal models of human disease often not important) to isolate individual components of an overall behavioral abnormality. However, it can be useful when attempting to extrapolate the results of behavioral studies to humans.

11.2 General experimental considerations

A series of other factors need to be considered when evaluating the behavioral outcomes of small-animal models of ischemic stroke. These studies have traditionally employed young, male rats housed individually or in small groups in cages devoid of any complex environmental stimuli. This would be analogous to modeling strokes occurring only in young men held in solitary confinement before and after the event.

The difference in the capacity for behavioral recovery following brain injury between young and aged animals is well known.[4] For motor function, differences in recovery may in part be due to an increase in age-related impairments in balance and co-ordination[5] that correlate with loss of cerebellar noradrenergic function.[6]

However, even differences in age of a few months can affect recovery after focal brain injury.[7,8] Gender-specific differences in the response to brain injury and resultant behavioral impairments are also being increasingly recognized.[9–11]

Numerous studies in laboratory animals show that environmental complexity can have a direct impact on anatomical brain plasticity.[3,12] Housing in complex environments is associated with overall and regionally specific increases in brain weight, cortical depth, hippocampal thickness, callosal size, and cortical glial density[12] and have effects on both neuronal morphology[12,13] and connectivity.[14] It has also long been recognized that even housing animals in complex environments as compared to a standard cage either before or after brain injury can lead to less severe functional deficits and more favorable outcomes,[15–18] although some debate remains as to whether this represents true recovery or enhancement of compensatory behavioral strategies.[12,19]

In addition to general environmental factors, a large number of laboratory studies show the important impact of post-brain injury training on functional motor recovery.[13,20,21] As summarized in these detailed reviews, exercise can increase levels of neurotrophic factors such as brain-derived neurotrophic factor (BDNF), enhance neurogenesis, and improve learning. Rehabilitative training is associated with specific improvements in motor function after cortex injury in several behavioral paradigms,[22–28] particularly when this training is coupled with housing in complex environments.[25,26] Experimental studies in squirrel monkeys suggest that repetitive use of the impaired hand is required for maintenance of the spared portion of the hand representation after motor cortex infarction.[29] However, overuse of the affected limb during vulnerable periods after experimental brain injury is associated with both exacerbation of the underlying brain damage, and in some cases, poorer sensorimotor performance.[3,30–35] In ischemia models, despite exacerbation of injury with exercise begun immediately after the injury, functional outcome is still improved.[34,36] Intensive training after the first 3–5 days after focal brain injury does not exacerbate lesion size or negatively affect outcome.[24,28] Further, delaying training for longer periods can diminish this effect.[26]

11.3 Individual behavioral tests

The individual behavioral tests described below were chosen as being representative of those commonly employed in studies evaluating post-stroke and brain injury deficits and recovery (Table 11.1). The list is far from comprehensive as there are a myriad of behavioral testing paradigms that can be used for specific purposes. General descriptions are given and their relationship to focal ischemic injuries discussed in the sections that follow.

Table 11.1. *Examples of tests that can be used in the behavioral assessment of rats after focal ischemia*

Forelimb posture
Tactile placing (forelimb and hindlimb)
Proprioceptive placing (forelimb and hindlimb)
Visual placing
Open field behavior
Resistance to lateral pressure
Vertical screen test
Foot-fault test
Running wheel
Beam-walking
Head-movement dependent orientation
Rotarod
Somatosensory asymmetry test
Limb-use asymmetry (cylinder) test
Corner test
Staircase test
Water maze

11.3.1 Forelimb posture

Rats are suspended gently by the tail 1 m above the floor. Normal rats extend both forelimbs. Rats with recent cortical infarction consistently flex the forelimb contralateral to the injured hemisphere.[37]

11.3.2 Tactile placing (forelimb and hindlimb)

The examiner supports the animal's trunk with its limbs hanging freely. The dorsum of the limb being tested is gently touched against the edge of a platform.[38] A placing response is present when the appropriate limb is lifted and the foot is placed on the platform. Forelimb placing can also be assessed by brushing the rat's vibrissae on the edge of a platform.[39] Intact animals place the forelimbs of both sides quickly onto the top of the platform. Animals with unilateral cortical injury have varying degrees of impaired placing of the contralateral forelimb (measured as a percentage of 10 trials).

Early studies in several species dating to the 1930s show that the corticospinal tract is important for placing responses.[38] In rats, tactile forelimb placing responses appear around postnatal day 7 with hindlimb responses appearing around postnatal day 13.[38] The development of placing responses temporally correlates with the postnatal growth of corticospinal axons into the gray matter of the spinal cord.[38] Hindlimb proprioceptive responses decline with age. In one study, the response was present in 90% of rats 6–12 months of age, but in only 24% older than 24 months.[40]

11.3.3 Proprioceptive placing (forelimb and hindlimb)

The examiner supports the animal's trunk displacing the limb (i.e., hip and knee extension and ankle plantar flexion) after the dorsum of the paw touches the edge of a platform.[38] A placing response is present when the appropriate limb is lifted and the foot is placed on the platform. In rats, proprioceptive forelimb placing responses appear around postnatal day 4 with hindlimb responses appearing around postnatal day 9.[38]

11.3.4 Visual placing

The examiner supports the animal with its forelimbs free, and it is then slowly lowered towards the edge of a platform. The response is present if the animal extends its forelimbs toward the platform before physical contact.[40]

11.3.5 Open field behavior

The animals are placed on a flat surface ($\sim$80 $\times$ 100 cm) marked off into evenly spaced rectangles. The observer records the number of squares entered over a specified period of time (e.g., 2 min).[40] The number of upward rears, grooming behaviors, and stereotypic behaviors can also be recorded. Similar types of data can be obtained with the use of automated devices (e.g., infrared beam crossings) or using different sizes of open fields.[41] Between the ages of 6 and 30 months, there are not significant differences in the number of squares entered, upward rears or in the proportions of rats exhibiting grooming behaviors.[40] However, if an elevated platform is used for assessing open field behavior, rats older than 2 years have a greater tendency to fall that is thought to be related to vestibular or proprioceptive sensory impairments.[40] Latency to begin movement when placed on the open field and the tendency for circling locomotion can also be assessed.

11.3.6 Resistance to lateral pressure

Rats are placed on a sheet of soft, plastic-coated paper that can be firmly gripped by their claws. The examiner holds the animal's tail and applies gentle lateral pressure behind the rat's shoulder until the forelimbs slide several centimeters.[37] Normal rats resist sliding whereas rats with hemispheric lesions have reduced resistance to lateral push toward the paretic side.

11.3.7 Vertical screen test

This is designed to assess forelimb and hindlimb strength. Rats are placed on a screen ($\sim$50 × 20 cm with 15 mm^2 grid openings) in the horizontal position.[42] The screen is then rotated over 2 s to the vertical position. A score of 0 is given if the rat maintains its grip for 5 s, 0.5 if the rat slips, but does not fall, 1 if the rat falls within 5 s and 2 if it falls immediately.[42]

11.3.8 Foot-fault test

The test is intended to assess limb use and placing deficits during locomotion.[43] Rats are placed on an elevated grid floor (e.g., $\sim$30 × 30 cm with grid openings $\sim$3 cm^2) for 2 min.[42,43] Rats place their paws on the wire frame while ambulating with a 'foot-fault' occurring when a foot falls through a grid opening. When they occur, foot-faults are usually symmetric in intact animals.[43] The total number of limb steps and the numbers of forelimb and hindlimb foot-faults are recorded. A "foot-fault index" can then be calculated (number of contralateral forelimb or hindlimb foot-faults minus the number of ipsilateral forelimb or hindlimb foot-faults as a percentage of the total number of forelimb steps).[43]

Lesions of the caudal forelimb cortex in rats cause a deficit manifest as an increase in contralateral forelimb foot-faults on the first postoperative day that spontaneously declines to control levels over the first 2 weeks.[44] Damage in the rostral forelimb, anteromedial, or hindlimb corticies does not result in consistent forelimb deficits with this test. An increase in hindlimb foot-faults does not occur consistently after lesions affecting any of these areas.[44]

11.3.9 Running wheel

This can be considered as a variation of the foot-fault test. Rats are placed in a closed running wheel with 2-cm spaced rungs and videotaped.[45] A given number (e.g., 100) of steps are recorded and the numbers of footslips between the rungs are counted for the forepaw contralateral and ipsilateral to a cortex injury. The number of errors is then obtained by subtracting the ipsilateral from the contralateral footslips.

11.3.10 Beam-walking

The test is intended to assess the impact of a hindlimb sensorimotor cortex lesion on a rat's locomotor abilities. The behavioral testing apparatus consists of a goal box located at one end of a 2.5 × 122 cm elevated wooden beam.[46,47]

A switch-activated source of bright light and white noise were located at the start end of the beam and served as avoidance/activating stimuli. For each training or testing trial, the rat is placed at the start end of the beam opposite to the goal box. If the rat does not begin to traverse the beam after 10 s, the light and noise stimuli are activated and continued until the rat's nose entered the goal box or for a total of 80 s at which time the trial was terminated. On the first day of training, each rat is given a series of three approximate trials. Motor performance is rated on a 7-point scale (1, the rat is unable to place the affected hindpaw on the horizontal surface of the beam; 2, the rat places the affected hindpaw on the horizontal surface of the beam and maintains balance for at least 5 s; 3, the rat traverses the beam while dragging the affected hindpaw; 4, the rat traverses the beam and at least once places the affected hindpaw on the horizontal surface of the beam; 5, the rat crosses the beam and places the affected hindlimb on the horizontal surface of the beam to aid less than half its steps; 6, the rat uses the affected hindpaw to aid more than half its steps; and 7, the rat traverses the beam with no more than two footslips). Other systems for scoring the deficit using this type of apparatus have also been devised[48] and the test can also be successfully used for assessing locomotor performance in mice.[49] Time to run the beam can also be measured.[50] Another variation is to place a "ladder" consisting of a series of spaced dowels or wires over the length of the beam.[45]

Using the 7-point rating scale, rats generally recover to pre-lesion levels of performance over approximately 2 weeks after unilateral sensorimotor cortex ablation.[47] This permits studies aimed at assessing factors that may accelerate, delay, or block spontaneous recovery.

11.3.11 Rotarod

The rotarod test can be used to assess co-ordinated walking.[51] Rats are placed on a rotating cylinder with the speed of rotation slowly increasing at a predefined rate. The mean duration that a rat can stay on the device without falling or griping is recorded.

11.3.12 Somatosensory asymmetry test

The assessment includes two tests. The first determines the presence or absence of an asymmetry and the second measures its magnitude.[39,43,44] An animal is removed from its home cage and an adhesive label (113 mm^2) is attached to the distal radial region of each forelimb. The animal is then returned to its home cage and the latency and order of stimulus contact/removal are recorded for each of four trials. After unilateral cortical lesions, rats preferentially remove the adhesive tape ipsilateral to the side of the injury. If an ipsilateral bias is present (the ipsilateral stimulus is contacted first on greater 70% of the trials), the size of the contralateral stimulus is progressively increased and the size of the ipsilateral stimulus is simultaneously decreased by an equal amount (14.1 mm^2) until the ipsilateral bias is no longer present. The degree of bias is proportional to the amount of brain injury and decreases over time as the animal recovers.[43]

Lesions of the rat rostral forelimb cortex, caudal forelimb cortex, and anteromedial cortex slow latencies to contact and remove the patch contralateral to the lesion on the first day after surgery.[44] There is no effect of a lesion in the hindlimb cortex. The effect from lesions of the caudal forelimb and anteromedial cortex resolves by day 14, but the effect of lesions of the rostral forelimb cortex persists as long as 56 days after surgery. Rats with rostral forelimb cortex lesions also have a greater initial magnitude of asymmetry as compared with those with lesions that affect the caudal forelimb or anteromedial cortices.[44] Asymmetries remain in rats with rostral forelimb cortex lesions for as long as 4 weeks with the asymmetries in rats with caudal forelimb or anteromedial cortex injuries returning to pre-lesion levels before that time.[44]

11.3.13 Limb-use asymmetry (cylinder) test

This test is designed to measure the level of preference for using the non-impaired forelimb for weight-shifting movements during spontaneous vertical exploration.[39] Rats are placed in a transparent cylinder (~20 cm diameter and ~30 cm high) and videotaped for 3–10 min. A mirror is placed behind the cylinder to permit recording of forelimb movements when the animal is turned away from the camera. Several behaviors can be scored using slow-motion videotapes. These include: (a) the independent use of the forelimbs for contacting the wall during a full rear, to initiate weight-shifting movements, or to regain the center of gravity while moving laterally in the vertical position; (b) independent use of the right or left forelimbs to land after a rear; (c) simultaneous use of both forelimbs for contacting the walls of the cylinder during full rears and for lateral movements along the wall; and (d) simultaneous use of both forelimbs for landing following a rear.[39] Each behavior can then be expressed as a percentage use of the non-impaired forelimb relative to the total number of limb use observations, the percent use of the impaired forelimb relative to the total number of limb use observations for wall movements, etc., and a variety of calculations can be performed.

11.3.14 Corner test

The corner test was devised to assess vibrissae-induced sensory responses in mice.[52] In its home cage, a mouse is placed between two $30 \times 20 \times 1$ cm boards attached at a 30° angle. The mouse is placed between the two boards facing the corner. Vibrissae on both sides are stimulated as the animal moves towards the corner. It then rears and turns to face the open end. The turns in each direction over a series of 10 trials are recorded.

11.3.15 Staircase test

The staircase test evaluates lateralized forepaw dexterity.[53] The apparatus consists of a test box from which extends a corridor with a series of steps. Rats are required to reach into the corridor with either their left or right forepaws to retrieve small food pellets. The farther pellets are progressively more difficult to reach. The number of pellets retrieved over a given period by the forepaw ipsilateral and contralateral to a sensorimotor cortex injury is measured for each testing session. In addition, the rats can be videotaped to analyze the patterns of reaching and grasping movements.

11.3.16 Water maze

Mazes are used to test an animal's learning capacity and memory. A variety of different types of mazes have been developed for different purposes, but the Morris water maze has proven particularly useful.[54] Rats placed in a circular pool of opaque water rapidly learn to escape by finding and climbing on to a small platform hidden just beneath the surface based on visuospatial cues. Comparing the latency for escape for a visible versus a submerged platform provides a control for sensory, motor, or perceptually related deficits. For example, a comparison of performance with a submerged as compared with a visible platform identifies rats with hippocampal (impaired) vs. cortical (unimpaired) lesions.[54] Detailed analysis of the pathways hippocampal-lesioned rats use to attempt to find the hidden platform also differs from unlesioned animals that use a random searching pattern. A variety of sophisticated analyses can be performed depending on the individual experiment.

11.4 Use in focal ischemia models

In reviewing the use of the various behavioral tests previously described in rodent models of focal ischemia, it should be noted that there can be significant differences in their utility depending on strain differences and occlusion site.[55] Laboratory procedures may differ in any of several important ways that can have a profound impact on the results of behavioral-based outcomes. As a result, the section that follows should be viewed as providing a general discussion. It is imperative that appropriate controls be utilized to reduce the likelihood of spurious results. These potential differences also underscore the need to use several different types of assessments and models based on experiments carried out in multiple laboratories when assessing behavioral results. Tests used in several studies of permanent or transient middle cerebral artery occlusion are given in Table 11.2.

11.4.1 Forelimb posture

As indicated above, rats with recent cortical infarction consistently flex the forelimb contralateral to the injured hemisphere.[37] This can be used to determine whether an animal has had an ischemic injury and can serve as an inclusion/exclusion criterion as sham-operates show no deficit.[56] Contralateral forelimb flexion is present in most rat strains after middle cerebral artery (MCA) occlusion.[57] The duration of transient MCA occlusion correlates with the duration of forelimb flexion over a 10-s trial.[45] Forelimb flexion may persist as long as 2 weeks after MCA occlusion[42,56,57] but was no longer evident after about 20 days in one study[42] and 37 days in another.[57]

11.4.2 Tactile placing (forelimb and hindlimb)

There is a severe deficit of vibrissae-associated forelimb placing over the first 2 weeks after permanent MCA occlusion in rats.[39] This improved to pre-stroke levels by 23 days in one study.[42] A second study also noted spontaneous improvement over time, but not to pre-stroke levels by 21–30 days.[39]

11.4.3 Visual placing

Rats with MCA occlusions can have a severe visual placing deficit 2 days after infarction; however, a difference between rats with MCA occlusion and sham-operated controls is no longer evident by 16 days.[57]

11.4.4 Open field behavior

Rats with hemispheric infarction tend to circle towards the paretic side when walking in an open field.[37,57] This behavior tends to decrease over time and in

Table 11.2. *Examples of studies using behavioral assessments of rats after focal ischemic injury*

Study	Animal	Model[a]	Follow-up[b]	Forelimb posture	Tactile placing	Proprioceptive placing	Visual placing	Open field	Lateral pressure
Bederson et al.[37]	Rat	P-MCAO	24 hr	✓				✓	✓
Yamamoto et al.[58]	Rat	P-MCAO	16 w					✓	
Andersen et al.[59]	Rat	P-MCAO	27 d					✓	
Markgraf et al.[42]	Rat	P-MCAO	5 w	✓	✓	✓	✓		
van der Staay et al.[57]	Rat	P-MCAO	37 d	✓	✓		✓	✓	
Aronowski et al.[45]	Rat	T-MCAO	21 d	✓					
Schallert et al.[39]	Rat	P-MCAO	30 d		✓				
Modo et al.[56]	Rat	T-MCAO	12 w	✓	✓		✓	✓	
Chen et al.[61]	Rat	T-MCAO	5 w	✓	✓		✓	✓	
Zhang et al.[52]	Mouse	P-MCAO	90 d						
Maguire et al.[2]	Rat	P-MCAO	28 d	✓	✓				✓
Li et al.[62]	Rat	T-MCAO	6 w	✓				✓	

one study was no longer apparent by 37 days.[57] The amount of spontaneous movement may not differ between rats with MCA occlusion as compared to sham-operated animals over 8 weeks of observation.[58] This may differ according to rat strain, with some (e.g., F344, SHR-SP, and WISW) having at least an initial increase in latency for the initiation of movement.[57]

11.4.5 *Resistance to lateral pressure*

Resistance to lateral pressure is one component of a composite neurological scoring system.[37] As part of that scoring system, there is a general relationship between the extent of histologically defined injury and impairments.

Assessment									
Vertical screen	Foot-fault	Run wheel	Beam-walk	Rotarod	Somatosensory asymmetry	Cylinder	Corner	Water maze	Other
									✓
			✓		✓				✓
✓	✓				✓			✓	
✓									✓
		✓	✓		✓				✓
					✓	✓			
	✓			✓	✓			✓	✓
			✓	✓					✓
	✓						✓		✓
						✓	✓		✓

Notes:
[a] P-MCAO, permanent middle cerebral artery occlusion; T-MCAO, transient middle cerebral artery occlusion.
[b] hr, hours; d, days; w, weeks.

11.4.6 *Vertical screen test*

The test is relatively insensitive for the detection of neurological impairments after permanent MCA occlusion with at least one study finding no difference between rats with ischemic injury and sham-operated controls.[42]

11.4.7 *Foot-fault test*

Rats with an MCA occlusion have significantly greater numbers of contra-lateral foot-faults for as long as 8 weeks and return to control levels by 11 weeks.[56] The foot-fault test has also been used to assess the effects of MCA occlusion in mice.[52] Deficits are apparent as soon as the animals can be tested and return to control levels by 90 days.

11.4.8 Running wheel

The number of errors of a rat on the running wheel differ as a function of the duration of ischemia after transient MCA occlusion with the number of foot-faults remaining stable over 21 days.[45] In one study, 45 min of transient ischemia resulted in a behavioral deficit that was 46% of maximum.[45]

11.4.9 Beam-walking

Rats tend to slip more frequently with the forepaw contralateral to the side of a transient MCA occlusion[45,59] with the degree of deficit correlating with the duration of the ischemia.[45] The test has also been adapted for use in mice.[49]

11.4.10 Somatosensory asymmetry test

Rats with transient MCA occlusion preferentially remove the piece of tape applied to the ipsilateral forelimb.[42,45,56,59] One study found slow improvement over time with MCA-occluded rats reaching control levels of performance by 20 days after stroke.[42] Another study, also in rats with permanent MCA occlusion, reported minimal recovery by 21–30 days.[39] The degree of asymmetry (assessed by increasing the size of the contralateral stimulus while decreasing the size of the ipsilateral stimulus until the bias is neutralized) correlates with the duration of ischemia.[45] The deficit can recover within days, with recovery to base-line also correlating with the duration of ischemia.[45,59] However, other studies find that although some improvements occur, deficits are still detectable as long as 18 weeks after infarction.[56]

11.4.11 Limb-use asymmetry (cylinder) test

Rats have a moderate limb use asymmetry for wall exploration during the acute period (1–14 days) after permanent MCA occlusion.[39]

11.4.12 Corner test

The corner test has also be used to assess mice after MCA occlusion.[52] The deficits in mice recover, but not back to base-line levels over the first 90 days after infarction.[52]

Table 11.3. *Examples of studies using composite neurological scores*

Study	Animal	Model[a]	Follow-up (days)	Composite score test components												Scale points
				Forelimb posture	Tactile placing	Visual placing	Open field	Lateral pressure	Run wheel	Beam walk	Somato-sensory asymm.	Other reflexes	Righting	Tilting	Grasp	
Bederson et al.[37]	Rat	P-MCAO	1	✓			✓	✓								3
Longa et al.[63]	Rat	T-MCAO	3	✓			✓									4
Aronowski et al.[45]	Rat	T-MCAO	21	✓					✓		✓					20
Modo et al.[56]	Rat	T-MCAO	5	✓	✓	✓	✓						✓	✓	✓	7
Hunter et al.[64]	Mouse	P-MCAO	7	✓	✓		✓						✓	✓	✓	21
Chen et al.[61]	Rat	T-MCAO	35	✓	✓	✓	✓			✓		✓				18
Li et al.[62]	Mouse	T-MCAO	7	✓			✓									4

Note:
[a] P-MCAO, permanent middle cerebral artery occlusion; T-MCAO, transient middle cerebral artery occlusion.

11.4.13 Water maze

Abnormalities of visuospatial learning as reflected in Morris water maze testing are evident several weeks after hemispheric infarction in rats.[41,42,56] As with non-lesioned rats, performance improves over time indicating visuospatial learning.[42,56] There is no difference in latencies to reach a visible platform indicating an absence of a primary motor deficit.[42] The test is also sensitive to the effects of transient global ischemia that can selectively affect vulnerable neuronal populations, including those in the hippocampus.[60]

11.5 Graded neurological evaluations

Several graded neurological evaluations have been devised to provide a composite score reflecting an animal's overall level of neurological impairment (Table 11.3). These may be composed of several of the individual tests listed in Table 11.2, or involve assessments in addition to those listed in Table 11.1. There is no general agreement regarding the individual components of these scales, nor the duration of testing that may be required.

11.6 Ongoing issues

The critical test of a therapeutic intervention is whether it affects clinically relevant outcomes. In human stroke studies, several widely used scales assessing impairments, disabilities, social handicaps, and quality of life have been adopted. As is apparent from reviewing Tables 11.2 and 11.3, unlike the situation in human trials, a specific group of behavioral tests for the measurement of functional deficits after focal ischemia in rodents have not be embraced. This situation is likely to continue until the predictive value of a specific group of behavioral tests can be established.

References

1. Irle E. Lesion size and recovery of function: some new perspectives. *Brain Res. Rev.* 1987, **12**: 307–320.
2. Maguire S, Strittmatter R, Chandra S, Barone FC. Stroke-prone rats exhibit prolonged behavioral deficits without increased brain injury: an indication of disrupted post-stroke brain recovery of function. *Neurosci. Lett.* 2004, **354**: 229–233.
3. Jones TA, Bury SD, Adkins-Muir DL, *et al.* Importance of behavioral manipulations and measures in rat models of brain damage and brain repair. *Inst. Lab. Anim. Res. J.* 2003, **44**: 144–152.

4. Brailowsky S, Knight RT. Recovery from GABA-mediated hemiplegia in young and aged rats: effects of catecholaminergic manipulations. *Neurobiol. Aging* 1987, **8**: 441–447.
5. Wallace JE, Krauter E, Campbell BA. Motor and reflexive behavior in the aging rat. *J. Gerontol.* 1980, **35**: 364–370.
6. Bickford P. Motor learning deficits in aged rats are correlated with loss of cerebellar noradrenergic function. *Brain Res.* 1993, **620**: 133–138.
7. Goldstein LB, Bullman S. Age but not sex affects motor recovery after unilateral sensorimotor cortex suction-ablation in the rat. *Restor. Neurol. Neurosci.* 1999, **15**: 39–43.
8. Hoane MR, Lasley LA, Akstulewicz SL. Middle age increases tissue vulnerability and impairs sensorimotor and cognitive recovery following traumatic brain injury in the rat. *Behav. Brain Res.* 2004, **153**: 189–197.
9. Roof RL, Zhang Q, Glasier MM, Stein DG. Gender-specific impairment on Morris water maze task after entorhinal cortex lesion. *Behav. Brain Res.* 1993, **57**: 47–51.
10. Roof RL, Duvdevani R, Stein DG. Gender influences outcome of brain injury: progesterone plays a protective role. *Brain Res.* 1993, **607**: 333–336.
11. Li K, Futrell N, Tovar S, *et al.* Gender influences the magnitude of the inflammatory response within embolic cerebral infarcts in young rats. *Stroke* 1966, **27**: 498–503.
12. Rose FD, Al-Khamees K, Davey MJ, Attree EA. Environmental enrichment following brain damage: an aid to recovery or compensation? *Behav. Brain Res.* 1993, **5**: 93–100.
13. Kolb B, Forgie M, Gibb R, Gorny G, Rowntree S. Age, experience and the changing brain. *Neurosci. Biobehav. Rev.* 1998, **22**: 143–159.
14. Beaulieu C, Colonnier M. Richness of environment affects the numbers of contacts formed by boutons containing flat vesicles but does not alter the number of these boutons per neuron. *J. Comp. Neurol.* 1988, **274**: 347–356.
15. Johansson BB. Functional outcome in rats transferred to an enriched environment 15 days after focal brain ischemia. *Stroke* 1996, **27**: 324–326.
16. Will B, Kelche C. Environmental approaches to recovery of function from brain damage: a review of animal studies (1981 to 1991). *Adv. Exp. Med. Biol.* 1992, **325**: 79–103.
17. Hamm RJ, Temple MD, O'Dell DM, Pike BR, Lyeth BG. Exposure to environmental complexity promotes recovery of cognitive function after traumatic brain injury. *J. Neurotrauma* 1996, **13**: 41–47.
18. Schallert T, Woodlee MT, Fleming SM. Experimental focal ischemic injury: behavior–brain interactions and issues of animal handling and housing. *Inst. Lab. Anim. Res. J.* 2003, **44**: 130–143.
19. Rose FD, Davey MJ, Attree EA. How does environmental enrichment aid performance following cortical injury in the rat? *NeuroReport* 1993, **4**: 163–166.
20. Cotman CW, Berchtold NC. Exercise: a behavioral intervention to enhance brain health and plasticity. *Trends Neurosci.* 2002, **25**: 295–301.
21. Kleim JA, Jones TA, Schallert T. Motor enrichment and the induction of plasticity before or after brain injury. *Neurochem. Res.* 2003, **28**: 1757–1769.
22. Goldstein LB, Davis JN. Beam-walking in rats: studies towards developing an animal model of functional recovery after brain injury. *J. Neurosci. Methods* 1990, **31**: 101–107.
23. Goldstein LB, Davis JN. Post-lesion practice and amphetamine-facilitated recovery of beam-walking in the rat. *Restor. Neurol. Neurosci.* 1990, **1**: 311–314.

24. Nudo RJ, Wise BM, SiFuentes F, Milliken GW. Neural substrates for the effects of rehabilitative training on motor recovery after ischemic infarct. *Science* 1996, **272**: 1791–1794.

25. Biernaskie J, Corbett D. Enriched rehabilitative training promotes improved forelimb motor function and enhanced dendritic growth after focal ischemic injury. *J. Neurosci.* 2001, **21**: 5272–5280.

26. Biernaskie J, Chernenko G, Corbett D. Efficacy of rehabilitative experience declines with time after focal ischemic brain injury. *J. Neurosci.* 2004, **24**: 1245–1254.

27. Delay ER, Rudolph TL. Crossmodal training reduces behavioral deficits in rats after either auditory or visual cortex lesions. *Physiol. Behav.* 1994, **55**: 293–300.

28. Jones TA, Chu CJ, Grande LA, Gregory AD. Motor skills training enhances lesion-induced structural plasticity in the motor cortex of adult rats. *J. Neurosci.* 1999, **19**: 10153–10163.

29. Friel KM, Heddings AA, Nudo RJ. Effects of postlesion experience on behavioral recovery and neurophysiologic reorganization after cortical injury in primates. *Neurorehab. Neur. Repair* 2000, **14**: 187–198.

30. Humm JL, Kozlowski DA, Bland ST, James DC, Schallert T. Use-dependent exaggeration of brain injury: is glutamate involved? *Exp. Neurol.* 1999, **157**: 349–358.

31. Bland ST, Schallert T, Strong R, Aronowski J, Grotta JC. Early exclusive use of the affected forelimb after moderate transient focal ischemia in rats: functional and anatomic outcome. *Stroke* 2000, **31**: 1144–1151.

32. Kozlowski DA, James DC, Schallert T. Use-dependent exaggeration of neuronal injury after unilateral sensorimotor cortex lesions. *J. Neurosci.* 1996, **16**: 4776–4786.

33. Humm JL, Kozlowski DA, James DC, Gotts JE, Schallert T. Use-dependent exacerbation of brain damage occurs during an early post-lesion vulnerable period. *Brain Res.* 1998, **783**: 286–292.

34. Risedal A, Zeng J, Johansson BB. Early training may exacerbate brain damage after focal brain ischemia in the rat. *J. Cereb. Blood Flow Metab.* 1999, **19**: 997–1003.

35. Leasure JL, Schallert T. Consequences of forced disuse of the impaired forelimb after unilateral cortical injury. *Behav. Brain Res.* 2004, **150**: 83–91.

36. Farrell R, Evans S, Corbett D. Environmental enrichment enhances recovery of function but exacerbates ischemic cell death. *Neuroscience* 2001, **107**: 585–592.

37. Bederson JB, Pitts LH, Tsuji M, *et al.* Rat middle cerebral artery occlusion: evaluation of the model and development of a neurological examination. *Stroke* 1986, **17**: 472–476.

38. Donatelle JM. Growth of the corticospinal tract and the development of placing reactions in the postnatal rat. *J. Comp. Neurol.* 1977, **175**: 207–232.

39. Schallert T, Fleming SM, Leasure JL, Tillerson JL, Bland ST. CNS plasticity and assessment of forelimb sensorimotor outcome in unilateral rat models of stroke, cortical ablation, parkinsonism and spinal cord injury. *Neuropharmacology* 2000, **39**: 777–787.

40. Marshall JF. Sensorimotor disturbances in the aging rodent. *J. Gerontol.* 1982, **37**: 548–554.

41. Lyden PD, Lonzo LM, Nunez SY, *et al.* Effect of ischemic cerebral volume changes on behavior. *Behav. Brain Res.* 1997, **87**: 59–67.

42. Markgraf CG, Green EJ, Hurwitz BE, *et al.* Sensorimotor and cognitive consequences of middle cerebral artery occlusion in rats. *Brain Res.* 1992, **575**: 238–246.
43. Hernandez TD, Schallert T. Seizures and recovery from experimental brain damage. *Exp. Neurol.* 1988, **102**: 318–324.
44. Barth TM, Jones TA, Schallert T. Functional subdivisions of the rat somatic sensorimotor cortex. *Behav. Brain Res.* 1990, **39**: 73–95.
45. Aronowski J, Samways E, Strong R, Rhoades HM, Grotta JC. An alternative method for the quantitation of neuronal damage after experimental middle cerebral artery occlusion in rats: analysis of behavioral deficit. *J. Cereb. Blood Flow Metab.* 1996, **16**: 705–713.
46. Feeney DM, Gonzalez A, Law WA. Amphetamine, haloperidol, and experience interact to affect the rate of recovery after motor cortex injury. *Science* 1982, **217**: 855–857.
47. Goldstein LB. Beam-walking in rats: the measurement of motor recovery after injury to the cerebral cortex. *Neurosci. Protocols* 1993, **10**: 1–13.
48. Brailowsky S, Knight RT, Blood K. G-aminobutyric acid-induced potentiation of cortical hemiplegia. *Brain Res.* 1986, **362**: 322–330.
49. Goldstein LB, Vitek MP, Dawson H, Bullman S. Expression of the apolipoproteine gene does not affect motor recovery after sensorimotor cortex injury in the mouse. *Neuroscience* 2000, **99**: 705–710.
50. Dixon CA, Clifton GL, Lighthall JW, Yaghami AA, Hayes RL. A controlled cortical impact model of traumatic brain injury in the rat. *J. Neurosci. Methods* 1991, **39**: 253–262.
51. Hamm RJ, Pike BR, O'Dell DM, Lyeth BG, Jenkins LW. The rotarod test: an evaluation of its effectiveness in assessing motor deficits following traumatic brain injury. *J. Neurotrauma* 1994, **11**: 187–196.
52. Zhang L, Schallert T, Zhang ZG, *et al.* A test for detecting long-term sensorimotor dysfunction in the mouse after focal cerebral ischemia. *J. Neurosci. Methods* 2002, **117**: 207–214.
53. Montoya CP, Campbell-Hope LJ, Pemberton KD, Dunnett SB. The "staircase test": a measure of independent forelimb reaching and grasping abilities in rats. *J. Neurosci. Methods* 1991, **36**: 219–228.
54. Morris RG, Garrud P, Rawlins JN, O'Keefe J. Place navigation impaired in rats with hippocampal lesions. *Nature* 1982, **297**: 681–683.
55. van der Staay FJ, Augstein K-H, Horváth E. Sensorimotor impairments in rats with cerebral infarction, induced by unilateral occlusion of the left middle cerebral artery: strain differences and effects of the occlusion site. *Brain Res.* 1996, **735**: 271–284.
56. Modo M, Stroemer RP, Tang E, *et al.* Neurological sequelae and long-term behavioural assessment of rats with transient middle cerebral artery occlusion. *J. Neurosci. Methods* 2000, **104**: 99–109.
57. van der Staay FJ, Augstein K-H, Horváth E. Sensorimotor impairments in Wistar Kyoto rats with cerebral infarction, induced by unilateral occlusion of the middle cerebral artery: recovery of function. *Brain Res.* 1996, **715**: 180–188.
58. Yamamoto M, Tamura A, Kirino T, Shimizu M, Sano K. Behavioral changes after focal cerebral ischemia by left middle cerebral artery occlusion in rats. *Brain Res.* 1988, **452**: 323–328.
59. Andersen CS, Andersen AB, Finger S. Neurological correlates of unilateral and bilateral "strokes" of the middle cerebral artery in the rat. *Physiol. Behavi.* 1991, **50**: 263–269.

60. Nunn J, Hodges H. Cognitive deficits induced by global cerebral ischaemia: relationship to brain damage and reversal by transplants. *Behav. Brain Res.* 1994, **65**: 1–31.
61. Chen J, Sanberg PR, Li Y, *et al.* Intravenous administration of human umbilical cord blood reduces behavioral deficits after stroke in rats. *Stroke* 2001, **32**: 2682–2688.
62. Li XL, Blizzard KK, Zeng ZY, *et al.* Chronic behavioral testing after focal ischemia in the mouse: functional recovery and the effects of gender. *Exp. Neurol.* 2004, **187**: 94–104.
63. Longa EZ, Weinstein PR, Carlson S, Cummins R. Reversible middle cerebral artery occlusion without craniectomy in rats. *Stroke* 1989, **20**: 84–91.
64. Hunter AJ, Hatcher J, Virley D, *et al.* Functional assessments in mice and rats after focal stroke. *Neuropharmacology* 2000, **39**: 806–816.

12

Methods for analyzing brain tissue

PÄIVI LIESI

12.1 Introduction

Analysis of the brain tissue depends on the experimental setup and question, and needs to be decided by each investigator. However, one should bear in mind that the health of animals as well as the diet they eat will inevitably affect the results obtained. Even though it is commonly thought to be so, the experiment does not start from the day the brains are dissected out and subjected to analysis but from the way animals are handled, fed, and cared for.

12.2 Fixation of brain tissue

Fixation is needed to stop degradation of the tissue and to preserve both structure and tissue antigens for analysis. Chemicals used for fixation are compounds that form cross-linking bonds between the components of the tissue and thereby literally fix/preserve them in the state they existed during life. The more cross-linking in the fixative, the more it can preserve the structural morphology of the tissue. The most commonly used fixatives in the order of their cross-linking properties are: glutaraldehyde, formaldehyde, paraformaldehyde, and p-benzoquinone. In addition, different alcohols (acetone, methanol) can be used as fixatives, but they dissolve lipids and therefore do not preserve structure as well.

For electron microscopic analysis of the brain, 1–2% glutaraldehyde is the preferred fixative. For immunocytochemical demonstration of tissue antigens at light microscopic level, 2–4% paraformaldehyde or 0.4% p-benzoquinone are the best alternatives. The length of time and temperature of fixation need to be determined in each situation, but as a general rule, fixation at +4 °C for 15 min for 10–20 μm cryostat sections or immersion fixation at +4 °C for 24 hr for pieces of brain tissue works well. The general logic behind fixation is to fix tissue sufficiently to preserve the structure, but not too much to mask the antigenic sites of the tissue.

Handbook of Experimental Neurology, ed. Turgut Tatlisumak and Marc Fisher. Published by Cambridge University Press. © Cambridge University Press 2006.

12.3 Storage and handling of the brain tissue

Fixed brain tissue can be frozen and stored at $-70\,°C$. The fixed tissue can also be stored in a buffer solution (phosphate buffer or phosphate buffered saline pH 7–8) at $+4\,°C$ for prolonged periods of time (months) provided that sodium azide (NaN_3) is added to 0.01% final concentration to prevent growth of bacteria. However, one must remember that fixation is a reversible procedure and some of the fixative will be washed away during long-term storage. Thus, it is recommended to store the tissue in a buffer solution for just the necessary time and to preserve the tissue permanently by mounting it in paraffin wax for light microscopy and staining or in plastic mounting media for cutting of ultrathin sections for electron microscopy. Paraffin sections are cut with a microtome and are generally 1–4 μm thick. For electron microscopy one uses a microtome with specialized diamond knives and sections are about 0.1–0.01 μm thick. If frozen tissue is to be stored, the only proper method of storage is to maintain tissue in ultra freezers at -70–$80\,°C$.

12.4 Brain for analysis: what one cannot do

(1) One should never store frozen brain tissues at $-20\,°C$. The only safe way of storage is at $-70\,°C$ or below.
(2) One should not store cut cryostat sections at $-20\,°C$ and not even at $-70\,°C$ for longer periods of time.
(3) Never store frozen brain inside the cryostat chamber (the cryostat defrosts itself once a day).
(4) Never leave fixed pieces of tissue or cut sections intended for immunocytochemistry in buffer solutions for longer than necessary. Washing for immunocytochemistry is to rinse away any unbound antibodies and not to recover an enzyme after fixation like in conventional histochemistry. This difference in principles is often forgotten and surface antigens are therefore lost with extensive washing.

12.5 Staining methods for brain: analysis of different cellular components

A number of staining methods to visualize different cellular components of the brain are available. The most commonly used ones, such as hematoxylin–eosin (H–E) staining, demonstrate basophilic components (such as DNA and RNA) as blue and acidophilic components (in the cytoplasm) as pinkish color. Thus, H–E allows detection of nuclei, nucleoli, and Nissl bodies (large accumulations of rough endoplasmic reticulum) in neurons and glial cells, but does not reveal intracytoplasmic details. Silver staining methods are difficult to master but they allow random demonstration of neuronal and glial fibers with their smallest details. Myelin can be detected by specific stains (such as Luxol fast blue), and amyloid depositions in the brain in Alzheimer's disease with stains such as Congo red. At present, identification of different central nervous system (CNS) cell types (neurons vs. astrocytes, oligodendrocytes vs. microglial cells) is largely based on immunocytochemical demonstration of cell type specific proteins. For example, neurofilaments are expressed by neurons, glial fibrillary acidic protein by astrocytes, and myelin basic protein by oligodendrocytes. Thus, antibodies against those proteins allow reliable demonstration of cell types expressing such proteins.

12.6 Brain for cells in tissue culture

Embryonic rodent brain, early postnatal rodent cerebellum (P0–P10) and embryonic rodent hippocampus (E18–P5) are the best sources of viable neurons in culture. Pure cultures of glial cells (astrocytes) can be obtained from early postnatal rat brain (P0–P5) while mouse astrocytes are more difficult to isolate and cultures are often contaminated with meningeal fibroblasts. Note that different plastics may have very different properties. For example, rat astrocytes refuse to attach onto Nunc plastic dishes, but they attach well on Corning and Falcon dishes. If one wishes to obtain highly pure neuronal cultures, one needs to use serum-free media (such as Neurobasal from Gibco) and substrates such as poly-D-lysine (the D-form is not eaten up by cells) or laminin-1 that support attachment and viability of neurons over the glial elements. Several manuals give detailed descriptions of different culture methods.[1,2]

12.7 Brain for immunocytochemical analysis

Immunocytochemistry is based on detection of tissue antigens by their specific antibodies (i.e., primary antibodies) followed by detection of the primary antibody by a secondary antibody coupled to a fluorochrome/enzyme that allows visualization of the antigen–antibody reaction (Fig. 12.1). The secondary antibody is usually commercially available and from a different species than the primary one. If one wishes to do double immunolabeling using two primary antibodies from two different species (for example, rabbit anti-X and mouse anti-Y), the secondary antibodies, e.g., anti-rabbit-fluorescein isothiocyanate (FITC) and anti-mouse-tetramethyl rhodamine isothiocyanate (TRITC), must be from the same third species (such as goat, donkey). The most commonly used methods of immunocytochemistry are as

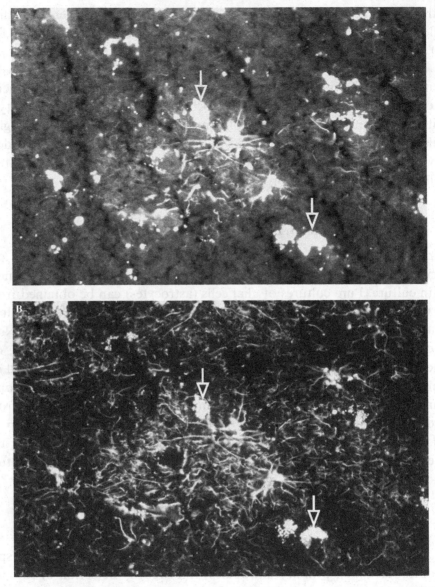

Figure 12.1. Immunocytochemistry for (A) alpha 1 laminin and (B) glial fibrillary acidic protein (GFAP) in brain tissue in Alzheimer's disease. In (A), astrocytes around a senile plaque express immunoreactivity for alpha 1 laminin. Immunoreactivity is apparent in both cell bodies and fibers while lipofuscin granules (open arrows), easily recognized under the microscope by their yellow autofluorescence, show granular autofluorescence. In (B), double immunocytochemistry for GFAP verifies that the cell bodies and fibers in (A) belong to reactive astrocytes. Open arrows point to the lipofuscin granules also seen in (A).

follows: indirect immunofluorescence or peroxidase method, peroxidase/anti-peroxidase (PAP) method, biotin–avidin method, and direct immunodetection by labeled primary antibody. The sensitivity of the direct method is considerably less than that of indirect methods. The PAP method is considered more sensitive than the indirect method but less sensitive than biotin–avidin detection. The exact principles and procedures are explained in references 3 and 4.

Success in immunocytochemical analysis of brain tissue is based on appropriate fixation, processing/cutting, and microscopic analysis of the sections. The best method must be experimentally determined for each antigen/antibody combination, and depends on a number of factors, such as the distribution of antigen (e.g., cell surface vs. cytoplasm), quality of antibodies (monoclonal vs. polyclonal), and microscopes available (fluorescence vs. light microscopy vs. electron microscopy). However, certain basic principles do exist and can be followed to systematically search for the optimal results.

Most antigens and antibodies are fixation sensitive. As a general rule, one has to balance between preservation of antigenicity and/or tissue. The more cross-linking fixatives that are good at preserving the tissue and most suitable for electron microscopy (such as glutaraldehyde) are usually less suitable for immunocytochemistry, because their cross-linking capability often masks the antigenic sites. They also cause a lot of non-specific background that will even further mask the antigens one might want to detect. The most commonly used fixatives for light and fluorescence microscopic analysis of brain tissue include 2–4% paraformaldehyde, 100% cold ($-20\,^\circ$C) methanol (sometimes acetone), and 0.4% *p*-benzoquinone. The latter is less cross-linking than paraformaldehyde, and has been specifically developed for detection of neuroactive peptides, such as vasoactive intestinal polypeptide (VIP), substance P, etc.

There are several alternatives for the method of fixation. One can fix by transcardial perfusion, immersion or applying a post-fixation method. The latter is best applicable for frozen brain tissue that one can section first in 10–20-µm cryostat sections, let them dry for 1–2 hr at room temperature and then fix them by immersion for a short period of time (10–15 min). Alternatively, one can fix the brain and also flush the blood out by transcardial perfusion with the fixative, and freeze the brain immediately or after 12-hr immersion in the fixative at $+4\,^\circ$C. Perfusion is the preferred method if one wants to process the brains into paraffin and cut semithin paraffin sections for in situ hybridization or immunocytochemistry or just for plain morphology.

For most polyclonal and monoclonal antibodies, a brief fixation (10–15 min) of cryostat sections is quite beneficial. If one needs to cut down the background of tissue (such as lipids in adult rat brain), one should use cold freshly prepared 0.4% *p*-benzoquinone for 15 min at $+4\,^\circ$C in the dark. The fixation (either with

Table 12.1. *Methodology for detecting most brain antigens in cryostat sections using indirect immunofluorescence*

1. Cut 10–20-µm cryostat sections of CNS tissue.
2. Leave to dry at room temperature for 1–3 hr.
3. Fix in staining jars for 15 min at +4 °C either in freshly prepared ice-cold 0.4% *p*-benzoquinone/PBS pH 7.4 or in 2% paraformaldehyde/PBS. (Note that the *p*-benzoquinone fixative must be protected from light and that fresh fixative has to be prepared each time. The right color is light yellow – if it turns brownish, it should not be used.)
4. After fixation rinse with PBS three times without incubation.
5. Dehydrate the sections by using a rising series of ethanol as follows: 50% ETOH/ distilled water(DW) – 70% ETOH/DW – 96% ETOH/DW – 100% ETOH – xylene. (Note that each step of ETOH incubation is for 15 min at room temperature and incubation in xylene is for 10 min.)
6. Rehydrate the sections by using a reverse order of alcohols with the same incubation times: 100% – 96% – 70% – 50% – PBS. (Note that all solutions should be freshly prepared, and that after the xylene step, we usually wash in 100% ETOH three times to get rid of the solvent.)
7. Once in PBS, the sections are rinsed three times without incubation and then incubated in PBS for 30 min at room temperature. Then the sections are rinsed in PBS again and incubated in PBS for 15 min at room temperature. (Note that the second incubation in PBS is done in a manner such that only six slides are in one jar. This is to make sure that all the sections are properly rehydrated.)
8. The sections are incubated overnight at +4 °C with a blocking serum. One should use the normal serum of the same animal as is used for the second antibody step. For example, most of our second antibodies are made in goat, and therefore we use normal goat serum diluted 1 : 30 in PBS.
9. The first (primary) antibody is applied at pre-tested dilutions on sections after tapping the excess normal goat serum on a tissue (no washing at this point). We normally also dilute the primary antibodies in the normal serum of the second antibody animal (e.g., goat). This prevents purified immunoglobulin G (IgG) molecules sticking onto the walls of Eppendorf tubes. (Note that all diluted primary antibodies are stored at +4 °C, and not frozen. Again this is to avoid aggregation of the antibodies. Note also that the primary antibodies are allowed to bind to their specific sites for 24 hr at +4 °C. An antiserum is usually used at 1 : 2000 to 1 : 10 000 and a purified IgG at 1–10 µg/ml.)
10. The first antibody step is followed by a brief wash in PBS. The sections are not incubated in PBS but rinsed vigorously to detach unbound antibodies from the sections.
11. In the secondary antibody step, one incubates sections at room temperature with a secondary antibody coupled to a fluorochrome (either FITC or TRITC). The dilution of the secondary antibody depends on the strength of the antibody. We generally use antibodies from Cappel Laboratories or from Jackson Laboratories, and they can be diluted at 1 : 500 to 1 : 1000.
12. After a brief wash, the sections are mounted in PBS : glycerol (1 : 1). We use a special glycerol for microscopy (Merck, Germany). (Note that PBS: glycerol allows one to recover the sections and re-incubate the slides with some other antibodies, etc. This is useful for many different purposes and allows flexibility depending on the results.)

paraformaldehyde or *p*-benzoquinone) should be followed by dehydration/ rehydration steps through xylene. This is to reduce background even further and also to dissolve the lipids that may help to make the antigens more accessible by the antibodies. We have successfully used *p*-benzoquinone for most antigens and tissues using the protocol described in detail in Table 12.1 and in our selected publications.[5,6]

12.8 Brain for biochemical analysis

For biochemical analysis of brain tissue, one may want to freeze the tissue first and then grind it into fine powder in liquid nitrogen using a pestle and mortar. Once the tissue is a fine powder, it can be transferred into a 50-ml Falcon tube (or some other sterile tube) using liquid nitrogen. Once liquid nitrogen is evaporated one pours into the 50 ml Falcon tube a suitable buffer for dissolving the proteins. For example, we have used the NET buffer (in mM: 400 NaCl, 50 Tris-HCl pH8, 5 EDTA pH8, 1% NP40) containing protease inhibitors, such as phenylmethanesulfonyl fluoride (PMSF) at 1–2 mM. The powdered tissue is then kept on ice ($+4\,°C$), and passed through a 21-gauge needle in a 10-ml syringe five to ten times to augment the dissolution of the proteins. Then the tissue is incubated on a shaker for 30–60 min at $+4\,°C$ to allow the proteins to dissolve into the buffer. Finally, undissolved material is pelleted using low-speed centrifugation at 1000 rpm for 10 min. The dissolved material is transferred into a new tube and used for analysis of proteins by gel electrophoresis followed by Western blotting.

Alternatively, one can use an Ultraturrax homogenizer, mesh, or Pasteur pipette to break the fresh tissue into small pieces and then follow the same protocol as described for frozen tissues to dissolve the proteins for analysis.

12.9 Brain for molecular biological analysis

For molecular analysis of RNA or DNA one can freeze down the brain tissue and use the same method of homogenization as for proteins. Alternatively, one can homogenize the freshly prepared brain tissue using an Ultraturrax homogenizer to isolate RNA. Genomic DNA is large and degrades easily, which prevents use of the Ultraturrax method. Nowadays, several companies (Ambion, for example), specialized in the preparation of high-quality RNA and DNA, will provide excellent kits and detailed instructions for isolation of RNA and DNA. Such methods work well on brain tissues at all ages. The RNA or DNA isolated can be subjected to analysis using Northern (RNA) or Southern (DNA) blotting or polymerase chain reaction (PCR). For in situ hybridization, e.g., in situ detection of intracytoplasmic mRNA coding for a specific protein, one should have the brain as paraffin sections or frozen sections.[6,7,8] The former provides better preservation of tissue during the harsh treatments of the protocol. As probes, one can use either ^{35}S-antisense RNA probes[6,7] or short (100–1000 bp) complementary DNA probes labeled using oligolabeling and digoxygenin-coupled deoxyuridine triphosphate (dUTP).[8] The in situ method is based on binding of antisense RNA probe or complementary DNA to the specific mRNA present in tissue. In the radioactive method, the slides are processed for autoradiography that detects the mRNA/labeled antisense RNA complexes as grainy precipitation. In the digoxygenin method, the mRNA/digoxygenin-labeled complementary DNA complexes are detected by anti-digoxygenin antibodies coupled either to alkaline phosphatase or a fluorochrome.

References

1. Fedoroff S, Hertz L (eds.) *Cell, Tissue and Organ Cultures in Neurobiology*. San Diego, CA: Academic Press, 1977.
2. Banker G, Goslin G (eds.) *Culturing Nerve Cells*. Cambridge, MA: MIT Press, 1991.
3. Sternberger, LA. *Immunocytochemistry*. New York: John Wiley, 1979.
4. Bullock GR, Petrusz P. *Techniques in Immunocytochemistry*, vols. 1–3. San Diego, CA: Academic Press, 1985.
5. Liesi P, Silver J. Is glial laminin involved in axon guidance in the mammalian CNS? *Devel. Biol.* 1988, **130**: 774–785.
6. Wiksten M, Liebkind R, Laatikainen T, Liesi P. γ1 laminin and its biologically active KDI-domain may guide axons in the floor plate of the embryonic human spinal cord. *J. Neurosci. Res.* 2003, **71**: 338–352.
7. Wilkinson DG, Bailes JA, Champion JE, McMahon AP. A molecular analysis of mouse development from 8 to 10 days post coitum detects changes only in embryonic globin expression. *Development* 1987, **99**: 493–500.
8. Wilkinson DG, Nieto MA. Detection of messenger RNA by in situ hybridization to tissue sections and whole mounts. *Methods Enzymol.* 1993, **225**: 361–373.

13

Targeting molecular constructs of cellular function and injury through in vitro and in vivo experimental models

ZHAO ZHONG CHONG, FAQI LI, AND KENNETH MAIESE

13.1 Introduction

At present, over 23 million people in the United States suffer from central nervous system disorders. Globally, this number reaches a level of 368 million people. Yet, no effective therapy for the prevention or treatment of acute or chronic neuronal injury exists. As a result, identification of novel cellular pathways that determine neuronal survival and regulate programmed cell death or apoptosis in the nervous system become essential for the effective development of therapeutic strategies against neuronal injury. To achieve this goal, use of both in vitro and in vivo models of cell injury become essential to elucidate the mechanisms that determine intrinsic cell destruction and inflammatory cell demise.

In this chapter, we provide detailed methods for the preparation and analysis of experimental cell injury in several different cell and tissue animal models employed in the Maiese laboratory. The cell cultures from the central nervous system can provide a unique tool for the investigation of the cellular and molecular mechanisms that are involved in acute and chronic neurodegenerative disease. The utilization of a cell culture system avoids the complex environment of tissue or animal models that require multiple cell types to function in concert. By using isolated living cells, studies can focus upon specific signal transduction pathways that determine cellular function and cellular response to injury. Ultimately, knowledge gained at the cellular level must be transferred into experimental animal models in order to fully comprehend the physiological and pathological function of the brain. Animal models not only provide a window into the intimate relationship of multiple cell types and systems during injury, but also allow some predication of clinical impairment through models of behavior assessment.

Handbook of Experimental Neurology, ed. Turgut Tatlisumak and Marc Fisher. Published by Cambridge University Press. © Cambridge University Press 2006.

13.2 Cell culture methods

13.2.1 Primary hippocampal neuronal cultures

The high vulnerability of hippocampus to injury has led to the frequent application of hippocampus as research target to study neurodegeneration.[1,2] During acute and chronic neurodegenerative diseases such as cerebral ischemia and Alzheimer's disease, the neuronal loss occurs in selective regions in which the neuronal population is vulnerable to the injury insult. Consequently, the culture of rodent hippocampal neurons has been extensively employed in neuroscience. We employ a modified method from Furshpan and Potter[3] for the culture of rat or mouse hippocampal neurons.[4,5]

Materials

Animals Pregnant Sprague-Dawley rats (gestation day 19).

Equipment
    35 mm dish; 60 mm dishes; 150 mm dishes
    Dissection microscope; phase-contrast microscope
    Forceps (large and small sizes); microdissection forceps and microscissor.

Solutions
    Modified 112 (120 ml)
        70 ml 2.5 M glucose
        25 ml 0.2 M L-glutamine
        25 ml penicillin/streptomycin solution (contains 10 000 units penicillin and 10 mg
            streptomycin per ml)
        Filter with 0.2 μm 150 ml filter
        Store at $-20\,°C$ in 4.8 ml aliquots
    Modified Stable Vitamin Mix (SVM)
        198 ml distilled water in beaker, add
        0.6 g L-proline
        0.6 g L-cysteine
        0.2 g *para*-aminobenzoic acid
        80 mg vitamin B_{12}
        0.4 g chloline chloride
        1.0 g fumaric acid
        16 mg coenzyme A
        Stir at low temperature
        Add 0.4 g d-biotin and 100 mg dl-6, 8-thiocytic acid to 10 ml distilled water and
            shake to suspend. Then quickly pipette out 2.0 ml and add to the beaker.

Stir for 2 hr (may not dissolve completely)
Store at $-20\,^{\circ}$C in 10 ml aliquots
Transferrin solution
  100 mg transferrin
  20 ml phosphate buffered saline solution
  Filter with 0.2 μm filter
  Store at $-20\,^{\circ}$C in 1.0 ml aliquot
Putrescine solution
  40 mg putrescine
  25 ml PBS
  Filter with 0.2 μm filter
  Store at $-20\,^{\circ}$C in 1.0 ml aliquot
Insulin/transferrin/selenite (ITS)
  ITS 1 vial (Sigma, I-1884, contains 5 mg insulin from bovine pancreas, 25 mg
    human transferrin, and 25 μg sodium selenite)
  45 ml sterile water
  Store at $-20\,^{\circ}$C in 1.0 ml aliquot
Progesterone
  1 mg progesterone
  50 ml water
  Filter with 0.2 μm filter
  Store at $-20\,^{\circ}$C in 402 μl aliquot
0.15 M $NaHCO_3$
  6.3 g $NaHCO_3$
  500 ml water
  Filter with 0.2 μm filter
  Store at 4 $^{\circ}$C
100 μg/ml polylysine stock solution
  5 mg polylysine
  50 ml sterile water
  Store at $-20\,^{\circ}$C in 12 ml aliquots
Leibovitz's L-15 medium
L-17 Growth medium
  500 ml L-15 medium
  105 ml 0.15 M $NaHCO_3$
  2.75 ml SVM
  Store at 4 $^{\circ}$C
L-17 medium with additives (ready for culture)
  178.30 ml L-17 growth medium
  0.9 ml SVM
  4.8 ml modified 112
  13.0 ml rat serum

402 µl progesterone

10 ml ITS

10 ml putrescine

10 ml transferrin

(Note: mix ITS, putrescine, and transferrin separately)

Hank's balanced salt solution with Ca^{2+} and Mg^{2+} (HBSS+)

Hank's balanced salt solution without Ca^{2+} and Mg^{2+} (HBSS−)

1M HEPES stock solution

6.508 g HEPES

25 ml distilled water

Filters with 0.2 µm filter

HEPES buffer (500 ml)

5 ml 1M HEPES stock solution (final concentration 10 mM)

0.5 g $NaHCO_3$ (final concentration 11.9 mM)

4.09 NaCl (final concentration 140 mM)

0.37 g KCl (final concentration 10 mM)

Water to 500 ml, pH 7.4

Filter with 0.2 µm filter.

Procedure

(1) Preparation of dishes

    (a) Place five 35 mm dishes in each 150 mm dish

    (b) Thaw laminin (1 mg/ml) under the hood and vortex

    (c) Mix 500 µl laminin in 25.5 ml sterile water

    (d) Vortex

    (e) Thaw 12 ml 100 µg/ml polylysine aliquot at 37 °C water bath

    (f) Mix 12 ml polylysine in 18 ml sterile water

    (g) Vortex

    (h) Add 500 µl laminin into each 35 mm dish

    (i) Add 500 µl polylysine into each 35 mm dish

    (j) Rotate 150 mm dish to make sure that each 35 mm dish is covered by coating fluid

    (k) Wrap the 150 mm dish in foil and place it in 37 °C 5% CO_2 incubator

(2) Incubate overnight

(3) Removal of excess laminin/polylysine

    (a) Remove excess laminin/polylysine with sterile Pasteur pipette by touching along the side of the dish

    (b) Add 1 ml sterile water into the dish

    (c) Remove the water

    (d) Repeat (b) and (c) one more time

    (e) Add 0.5 ml growth medium

    (f) Store at 37 °C 5% CO_2 incubator

(4) Separation of hippocampi
  (a) Make 30 ml HBSS+ solution
      30 ml HBSS+
      300 µl 100 mm sodium pyruvate (final concentration 1 mM)
      300 µl 1 M HEPES (final concentration 10 mM)
      Incubate at 37 °C water bath
  (b) Make 30 ml HBSS− solution
      30 ml HBSS−
      300 µl 100 mm sodium pyruvate (final concentration 1 mM)
      300 µl 1 M HEPES (final concentration is 10 mM)
      Incubate at 37 °C in water bath
  (c) Place autoclaved surgical instruments on gauze
  (d) Euthanize the 19-day pregnant rat with CO_2; remove pups from the mother and put them on gauze
  (e) Dip pup in 70% alcohol for a while and then pin the pup through with 22-gauge needles
  (f) Make a T-type incision; clip skin over the head longitudinally down the middle and then to each side; cut skull to expose forebrain
  (g) Cut the olfactory bulbs and the cerebellum; put hemispheres into a 60 mm dish containing HBSS− solution
  (h) Separate hemispheres with scissor and hippocampus from each hemisphere
  (i) Put all hippocampi into another 60 mm dish with 12 ml HBSS− solution
  (j) Transfer the hippocampi to a 50 ml polypropylene centrifuge tube
(5) Culture of hippocampal neurons
  (a) Triturate 10 times using 10 ml pipette with a 1 ml tip and then add 24 ml HBSS+ solution
  (b) Allow non-dispersed tissues to settle for 3 min and then transfer the supernatant to a 30 ml centrifuge tube
  (c) Centrifuge at $200 \times g$ for 2–3 min; remove the supernatant and add 1 ml growth medium to disperse the cells; take an aliquot for counting
  (d) Add proper volume of growth medium to yield final concentration of 6×10^5 to 1.0×10^6 cells/ml
  (e) Add 1 ml cell suspension into each 35 mm dish and incubate at 37 °C in 5% CO_2 incubator.

(Note: The slow trituration of cells is advised to avoid injury of the neurons.)

13.2.2 *Rat cerebral microvascular endothelial cells*

The cerebral microvascular endothelial cells that line microvessels play a crucial role in maintaining the normal function of the central nervous system. Endothelial cell damage during cerebral ischemia may exacerbate brain injury through the loss of integrity of the blood–brain barrier and the production of vasogenic brain edema.[6] The in vitro study of cerebral microvascular endothelial cells is critical for understanding the mechanisms underlying normal function of the central nervous system and the pathophysiological process of neurodegeneration. The culture method of rat cerebral microvascular endothelial cells is developed based on a collagenase/dispase digestion protocol.[7–9]

Materials

Animals Three Sprague-Dawley adult rats

Equipment
    35 mm dishes; 60 mm dishes; 150 mm dishes; 30 ml centrifuge tubes
    Forceps (large and small sizes); microdissection forceps and microscissor
    Scalpel and needle-nosed tweezers
    Underpad; sterile gauze
    5 ml glass tissue grinder
    High-speed centrifuge

Solutions
    10 × PBS
        8.4 g KH_2PO_4
        25.5 g $NaH_2PO_4 \cdot 6H_2O$
        42.5 g NaCl
        1.0 g KCl
        500 ml distilled water, pH 7.4
    15% dextran
        15 g dextran (MW 100 000 to 200 000)
        100 ml HEPES buffer
    Dissociation medium
        500 ml medium 199
        500 mg collagenase/dispase
        2.5 ml antibiotic–antimycotic solution
        Store at −20 °C in 20 ml aliquots
    Percoll (colloidal silica gradient) solution
        43 ml Percoll
        5 ml 10 × PBS
        1.5 ml 1M HEPES
        0.5 ml antibiotic–antimycotic solution
    40 ml dissociation medium
    10 ml heat-inactivated fetal bovine serum
        Aliquot 30 ml into 30 ml centrifuge tubes
        Centrifuge at 14 500 rpm (10 °C) for 70 min and store at 4 °C

200 mm L-glutamine
    1.461 g L-glutamine
    50 ml distilled water
    Store at −20 °C in 1 ml aliquots
1% gelatin
    250 mg gelatin
    25 ml sterilized water
    Incubate in 37 °C water bath for 1 hr
    20 mg/ml endothelial cell growth supplement
    25 mg endothelial cell growth supplement
    1.25 ml M199
    Store at −20 °C in 100 μl aliquots
90 mg/ml heparin
    180 mg heparin
    2 ml Medium 199
    Store at −20 °C in 100 μl aliquots
Growth medium
    79 ml Medium 199
    20 ml heat-inactivated fetal bovine serum
    1 ml L-glutamine
    500 μl antibiotic–antimycotic solution
    100 μl 90 mg/ml heparin
    100 μl 20 mg/ml endothelial cell growth supplement
    Store at 4 °C.

Procedure

(1) Coat the dishes
    (a) Add 1 ml 1% gelatin to each 35 mm dish and total four to six dishes in a 150 mm dish
    (b) Incubate dish in 37 °C 5% CO_2 incubator for 1 hr
    (c) Wash dishes with HEPES buffer twice and then leave 1 ml HEPES buffer in dish. Incubate at 37 °C until use.
(2) Harvest the brains
    (a) Euthanize the rats by CO_2 and then bilateral pneumothorax
    (b) Pinch skin on the top of the head and cut off with large scissors
    (c) Cut off the skull along the middle line
    (d) Open the skull to expose brain
    (e) Remove the brain and place it in alcohol for 3 min
    (f) Transfer brains to HEPES buffer
    (g) Place the brain on a piece of sterile gauze soaked by HEPES buffer
    (h) Peel off meninges and then carefully remove white matter
    (i) Place the reminder of the brain in a 60 mm dish and then chop into small pieces

(3) Form cell slurry
  (a) Incubate brain chunks in 15 ml dissociation medium for 1–2 hrs at 37 °C; shake gently every 30 min
  (b) Take tissue grinder, sterile in alcohol for 2 hrs or overnight, rinse with HEPES buffer
  (c) Pour 5 ml tissue solution every time into the grinder and homogenize three times
  (d) Pour homogenized tissue into a 30 ml sterilized centrifuge tube
  (e) Wash the grinder with HEPES buffer to fill the remainder of the centrifuge tube

(4) Separate from myelin and neuronal component
  (a) Centrifuge at 1800 rpm for 6 min at room temperature.
  (b) Remove supernatant carefully and refill the tube with HEPES buffer, repeat twice more
  (c) Remove the supernatant for last time, add 15% dextran to centrifuge tube, and then mix
  (d) Centrifuge at 5800 rpm ($4000 \times g$) for 20 min at 4 °C
  (e) Pour upper myelin layer and supernatant into another 30 ml centrifuge tube; keep the first tube upside down over cap to prevent myelin residues from sliding down into cells
  (f) Add dextran to the supernatant repeat steps (d) and (e)
  (g) Remove the myelin residues from the tube using cotton swabs
  (h) Add 1 ml HEPES buffer to the cells and transfer to a 1.5 ml centrifuge tube; flick tube to break cell pellet
  (i) Centrifuge at 2500 rpm for 15 s, remove the supernatant, and repeat twice more
  (j) Remove supernatant, disperse in 5 ml dissociation medium, and then incubate at 37 °C for 1–2 hr

(5) Separate vascular elements and red blood cells
  (a) Centrifuge at 1800 rpm for 6 min to spin down the cells; remove supernatant
  (b) Add 500 µl HEPES buffer to resuspend the pellet and add to a 30 ml centrifuge tube containing Percoll solution (Note: do not disturb the gradient layer of Percoll solution – add cell suspension one drop followed another with the tip near the surface of solution)
  (c) Centrifuge at 13 000 rpm ($20\,000 \times g$) for 20 min at 10 °C. Transfer the middle layer (endothelial cells) to a new 30 ml centrifuge tube
  (d) Centrifuge at 4500 rpm for 6 min and then remove the supernatant
  (e) Add HEPES buffer to resuspend the cells and then centrifuge at 1800 rpm for 6 min; repeat one more time; remove supernatant for last time
  (f) Add 4.5–6 ml growth medium to resuspend the cells and then add 1.5 ml to each 35 mm dish; incubate at 37 °C in 5% CO_2 incubator
  (g) After 3–5 days, endothelial cells can be observed under the microscope

(6) The passage of endothelial cells
   (a) Remove growth medium from dishes
   (b) Add 0.5 ml 0.25% trypsin to wash the dish and then remove trypsin
   (c) Add 1 ml 0.25% trypsin (37 °C) to each dish; incubate at 37 °C for 3 min
   (d) Triturate three to eight times with 1000 ml pipette tip; check cells under phase-contrast microscope; if some cells still attached, repeat trituration
   (e) Add 1 ml growth medium containing serum to inactivate trypsin and transfer cell suspension to 30 ml centrifuge tube; wash dish with medium one time and fill the remainder of the tube with medium
   (f) Centrifuge at 1800 rpm for 6 min at 20 °C and then remove supernatant
   (g) Add desired volume of growth medium and triturate three times to disperse cells
   (h) Add cell suspension to dishes and incubate at 37 °C in 5% CO_2 incubator
   (i) The subculturing ratio is 1 : 2 or 1 : 3.

13.2.3 Primary microglia cultures

Microglia are monocyte-derived immunocompetent cells that enter the central nervous system during embryonic development and function in a similar way to peripheral macrophages. During an insult to the brain, microglia are the cells that are initially responsible for host defense. Microglial activation and the phagocytic removal of apoptotic cells within the central nervous system play an important role during development, tissue homeostasis, and host defense. Culture of microglial cells is performed by the modified method[10,11] of Giulian and Baker.[12] Microglial cells are identified by α-naphthyl acetate esterase, OX-42, and isolectin B4 from *griffonia*. The cells do not stain for glial fibrillary acidic protein (GFAP).

Materials

Animals Pregnant Sprague-Dawley rats (gestation day 19)

Equipment
   60 mm dishes; 72 cm^3 flasks
   Dissection microscope; phase-contrast microscope
   Forceps (large and small sizes); microdissection forceps and microscissor

Solutions
   Dulbecco's modified Eagle F-12 medium (DMEM/F-12)
   Heat-inactivated fetal bovine serum (FBS)
   Penicillin (10 000 IU/ml) /streptomycin (10 mg/ml) solution

Growth medium
    89 ml DMEM/F-12
    10 ml FBS
    1 ml penicillin/streptomycin solution
    100 µg/ml polylysine stock solution
      5 mg polylysine
      50 ml sterile water
      Store at $-20\,°C$ in 10 ml aliquots
    Hank's balanced salt solution with Ca^{2+} and Mg^{2+} (HBSS+)
    Hank's balanced salt solution without Ca^{2+} and Mg^{2+} (HBSS−).

Procedure

(1) Add 10 ml distilled water in 10 ml polylysine stock solution
(2) Add 4 ml polylysine solution to each $75\,cm^3$ flask; place flask in hood overnight
(3) Wash three times with sterilized water before use
(4) Make 30 ml HBSS+ solution
    30 ml HBSS+
    300 µl 100 mm sodium pyruvate (final concentration 1 mM)
    300 µl 1 M HEPES (final concentration 10 mM)
    Incubate at $37\,°C$ in water bath
(5) Make 30 ml HBSS− solution
    30 ml HBSS−
    300 µl 100 mm sodium pyruvate (final concentration 1 mM)
    300 µl 1 M HEPES (final concentration 10 mM)
    Incubate at $37\,°C$ in water bath
(6) Placed autoclaved surgical instruments on gauze
(7) Euthanize the 19-day pregnant rat with CO_2; remove pups from the mother and put them on gauze
(8) Dip pups in 70% alcohol and then pin pups through with 22-gauge needles
(9) Clip skin over the head longitudinally and then to each side; cut skull to expose forebrain
(10) Cut the olfactory bulbs and the cerebellum; put hemispheres into a 60 mm dish containing HBSS+ solution
(11) Separate hemispheres with scissors and cortices from each hemisphere and put into another 60 mm dish with 12 ml HBSS+ solution
(12) Transfer the cortices to a 50 ml polypropylene centrifuge tube; triturate 10 times using 10 ml pipette with a 1 ml tip; add 24 ml HBSS+ solution
(13) Allow non-dispersed tissues to settle for 3 min; transfer the supernatant to a 30 ml centrifuge tube
(14) Centrifuge at 2500 rpm for 5 min; remove the supernatant and add 1 ml growth medium to disperse the cells; take an aliquot for counting

(15) Add proper volume of growth medium (10–15 ml per flask) to yield final density of $0.8–1 \times 10^7$ cells per flask

(16) Renew growth media every 3–5 days. After 10–14 days in culture, purify microglia by shaking (180 rpm) on reciprocal shaker for 15 hr at 37 °C

(17) Put microglia suspension into 25 cm³ flasks for adhesion; following 3 hr of adhesion, remove medium, resuspend microglia with growth media, and reseed them according to experiment.

13.2.4 Assessment of microglial activation

In our culture systems, microglia activation is achieved by conditioning for 3–5 hr with media from neurons or endothelial cells 24 hr following an injury. In this process, the externalization of membrane phosphatidylserine (PS) residues in neurons or endothelial cells induced by the injury is sufficient for the induction of microglial activation. Microglial activation is determined by detection of proliferating cell nuclear antigen (PCNA) expression[13] and bromo-deoxyuridine (BrdU) uptake.[14]

Materials

Fluorescence microscope
Shaker
PBS, ice cold
  4% paraformaldehyde
  83 ml 2.26% NaH_2PO_4
  17 ml 2.52% NaOH
  Heat to 60~80 °C in a covered container
  Add 4 g paraformaldehyde and stir until dissolved and filter
BrdU
0.2% triton
Primary mouse anti-PCNA or anti-BrdU antibody
Biotinylated anti-mouse immunoglobulin G (IgG)
Fluorescein avidin
Fluorodexyuridine.

Procedure

(a) Prepare several 35 mm dishes of microglia for staining
(b) Wash the dish with PBS one time
(c) Add 4% paraformaldehyde to each dish to fix the cell for 30 min at room temperature or overnight at 4 °C
(d) Wash with 1 ml PBS for 10 min, repeat twice more

(e) Remove the PBS; add 1 ml 0.2% triton and incubate at room temperature for 15 min

(f) Add 1 ml primary mouse anti-PCNA antibody (1 : 100) solution; incubate at 4 °C for 24 hr after gently shaking for 5–10 min at room temperature (to avoid drying of the dish, put 35 mm dishes into a 150 mm dish and cover with parafilm)

(g) For detection of BrdU uptake, apply BrdU (10 µM) and fluorodexyuridine (1 µM) to the cultures 1 hr prior to the time of fixation; following fixation, incubate with primary mouse anti-BrdU antibody (1 : 100) solution at 4 °C for 24 hr

(h) Wash with PBS for 5 min and repeat twice more

(i) Add 1 ml biotinylated anti-mouse antibody (1 : 50) and incubate at room temperature for 2 hr

(j) Wash three times with PBS for 3 min each

(k) Add fluorescein avidin solution (1 : 50), cover with foil, and incubate at room temperature for 2 hr

(l) Wash with PBS three times for 3 min each

(m) Carry out detection under fluorescence microscope using fluorescent excitation light at 490 nm and detecting emission at 585 nm.

13.2.5 Human neuroblastoma SH-SY5Y cell line

SH-SY5Y cells exhibit morphological features of primary cultured neurons after differentiation. In contrast to primary neuronal cultures, cell lines such as SH-SY5Y cells offer an ideal research tool for the generation of stable clones during the assessment of gene expression or silencing.[10,11]

Solutions

Eagle's Minimum Essential alpha-Medium (EMEM)
  100 mm sodium pyruvate
  75 g/l sodium bicarbonate
  7.5 g sodium bicarbonate
  Distilled water to 100 ml
  Store in 2 ml aliquots
Heat-inactivated fetal bovine serum (FBS)
Penicillin (10 000 IU/ml) /streptomycin (10 mg/ml) solution
Growth medium 100 ml
  86 ml EMEM
  10 ml FBS
  2 ml 75 g/l sodium bicarbonate (final concentration 1.5 g/l)
  1 ml 100 mm sodium pyruvate
  1 ml penicillin/streptomycin solution
  pH is less than or equal to 7.3.

Procedure

(a) The cells are stored in liquid nitrogen; thaw the cells at 37 °C water bath within 2 min

(b) Transfer the cells to a 50 ml centrifuge tube containing desired volume of growth medium

(c) Triturate three times gently and then culture in flasks or dishes; incubate at 37 °C in 5% CO_2 incubator; change medium every 3–5 days

(d) When subculturing the cells, remove medium carefully as the cells loosely adhere to dish or flask; add 0.25% pre-warmed trypsin solution; keep the dishes at room temperature for 3 min; triturate cells several times and transfer to a 30 ml centrifuge tube; wash the dishes one time using growth medium; fill the remaining volume of the tube with medium

(e) Centrifuge at 1800 rpm for 3 min at room temperature; remove the supernatant and add desired volume of growth medium (subculture ratio is 1:10 to 1:20)

(f) Add cell suspension to dishes and incubate in 5% CO_2 incubator

(g) The third to sixth passage of SH-SY5Y is used for experiments when cells reach 60–70% confluence.

13.2.6 SH-SY5Y cell line differentiation

When the cells reach 60% confluence, remove the medium and add fresh EMEM containing retinoic acid (RA). The stock solution of RA (10 mM) in dimethylsulfoxide (DMSO) is directly applied to cultures yielding a final concentration of 10 µM. The cultures are continuously incubated in a humidified atmosphere of 5% CO_2/95% room air at 37 °C for 48 hr until the cells are ready for experiments.[10,11]

13.3 Assessment of cellular injury in cell culture models

13.3.1 Trypan blue exclusion method for the assessment of cell viability

The disruption of cell membrane occurs during both necrosis and during the late phase of apoptosis. The integrity of cell membrane can be detected by cellular uptake of the dye trypan blue. Non-injured cells with intact membranes actively exclude the dye while cells with disrupted membrane accept the dye and stain blue in color. This method has been commonly used to detect cell viability.[7–9]

Materials

0.85% saline
0.4% (w/v) trypan blue (in 0.85% saline)

Light microscope
37 °C water bath.

Procedure

(1) Pre-warm sufficient volume of 0.4% trypan blue solution in 37 °C water bath
(2) Take several dishes (35 mm) of cells from CO_2 incubator
(3) Add 200 µl 0.4% trypan blue solution into each dish
(4) Incubate 10 min at 37 °C in water bath
(5) Remove the medium containing trypan blue and add 1 ml pre-warmed growth medium
(6) Observe cells under microscope; select eight different fields from each dish and count the number of stained and unstained cells
(7) Calculate the average number of surviving cells per dish
(8) Calculate the average of percentage survival of cells in each group.

13.3.2 Assessment of apoptotic injury (two independent pathways)

Cellular self-destruction known as programmed cell death (PCD) or apoptosis plays a significant role during neuronal degeneration. The biochemical and physiologic features of PCD include the loss of plasma membrane asymmetry, nuclear chromatin condensation, and DNA fragmentation. In most scenarios, PCD is considered to be a significant contributor of cellular injury during neurodegenerative disease.

Two independent pathways have been demonstrated to lead to cellular PCD that involve the externalization of membrane PS residues[15,16] and genomic DNA degradation. Membrane phospholipids are asymmetrically distributed across the cellular membrane bilayer with the membrane PS residues positioned in the inner leaflet of cells under normal conditions. Exposure of PS residues is believed to occur prior to genomic DNA degradation and serves to "tag" injured cells for phagocytosis.[5,17,18] An additional role for membrane PS externalization in the vascular cell system is the activation of coagulation cascades. The externalization of PS in platelets or endothelial cells can promote the formation of a procoagulant surface.[19,20] In contrast, the cleavage of genomic DNA into fragments is a delayed event that occurs late during PCD. The degradation of genomic DNA through the activity of endogenous neuronal endonucleases is considered to be a committed event that results in neuronal demise.[21,22] Since DNA fragmentation and PS externalization can each lead to cellular injury, the two parameters are commonly used in the research of apoptosis in the central nervous system.

13.3.3 DNA fragmentation with terminal deoxytransferase

Materials

4% paraformaldehyde solution (25 ml)
  1.0 g paraformaldehyde
  50 mg picric acid
  12.5 µl glutaraldehyde
  pH 7.4
1% bovine serum albumin (50 ml)
  0.5 g bovine serum albumin
  50 ml PBS
0.1% triton X-100 (20 ml)
  20 µl triton X-100
  20 ml PBS
Standard saline citrate buffer (20 ml)
  350 mg sodium chloride
  176 mg sodium citrate
  Distilled water to 20 ml
TdT (terminal deoxytransferase) buffer (50 ml)
  181.7 mg trizma base
  1.5 g sodium cacodylate
  11.9 mg cobalt chloride
  Distilled water to 50 ml
0.3% H_2O_2
  60 µl H_2O_2
  20 ml methanol
  Make immediately before using
TdT solution (15 ml)
  3 µl 11-bio-deoxyuridive triphosphate (dUTP)
  157 µl TdT (25 U/µl)
  15 ml TdT buffer
  Make before using
Peroxidase complex (20 ml)
  100 µl streptavidin peroxidase (0.1 µg)
  20 ml 1% bovine serum albumin
Peroxidase substrate kit (Vector Laboratory, Inc.)
  3,3′-diaminobenzidine (DAB)
  Buffer stock solution
  H_2O_2 solution
DAB substrate solution (20 ml)
  8 drops buffer stock solution
  16 drops DAB solution

8 drops H$_2$O$_2$ solution
20 ml tap water.

Procedure

(a) Prepare several dishes of cell cultures (e.g., 35 mm dishes)
(b) Remove the medium and wash dishes with 1 ml PBS
(c) Add 1 ml 4% paraformaldehyde solution and fix the cells for 30 min at room temperature or overnight at 4 °C
(d) Wash dishes with PBS three times for 2 min each
(e) Remove the PBS after final wash and add 1 ml 0.1% triton X-100
(f) Incubate at room temperature for 20 min
(g) Remove 0.1% triton X-100 solution and add 1 ml 0.3% H$_2$O$_2$ solution
(h) Incubate at room temperature for 30 min
(i) Wash dishes with PBS three times for 2 min each
(j) Add 0.5 ml TdT buffer at room temperature for 15 min
(k) Add 750 µl TdT solution containing 11-bio-dUTP and TdT
(l) Incubate for 60 min in a 37 °C humidified incubator
(m) Remove the TdT solution and add standard saline citrate buffer
(n) Incubate for 15 min at room temperature to stop reaction
(o) Wash dishes with PBS three times for 2 min each
(p) Add 1 ml 1% bovine serum albumin and incubate for 30–60 min at room temperature for blocking
(q) Add 1 ml peroxidase complex for 2 hr at room temperature
(r) Wash dishes with PBS three times for 2 min each
(s) Incubate in DAB substrate solution for 10 min at room temperature
(t) Wash with tap water
(u) Counterstain with hematoxylin for 5 min at room temperature
(v) Wash with tap water, observe, or store at 4 °C.

13.3.4 *Annexin V labeling for phosphatidylserine exposure*

The externalization of PS is detected through labeling by annexin V conjugated to phycoerythrin (PE). PS is revealed by green fluorescence. We have developed the ability to follow living cells over time with this system and have illustrated that, under some conditions, membrane PS exposure is reversible and does not directly impact upon cell injury unless it is allowed to progress to late stages of apoptotic injury with DNA degradation.[5,18,23,24]

Materials

Annexin V conjugated to phycoerythrin (R&D Systems, Minneapolis, MN)
Binding buffer
   10 mm HEPES
   150 mm NaCl

5 mm KCl
1 mm MgCl$_2$
1.8 mm CaCl$_2$
Dissociation buffer
10 mm HEPES
150 mm NaCl
5 mm KCl
1 mm MgCl$_2$
Fluorescence microscope (Leica, McHenry, IL).

Procedure

The procedure is performed in primary hippocampal neurons as an example.

(a) Prepare two dishes (35 mm) at one time; pre-warm the binding and dissociation buffer in a 37 °C water bath
(b) Remove the medium and add 1 ml binding buffer to wash the dishes
(c) Wash one more time
(d) Turn off the light; make the application solution of annexin V (the original concentration is 30 μg/ml); in 100 μl annexin V stock solution, add 900 μl binding buffer, yielding the final concentration 3 μg/ml
(e) Remove the binding buffer in dishes after final wash
(f) Add 500 μl application solution of annexin V to each dish
(g) Cover the dish with foil and put dishes in 5% CO$_2$ incubator
(h) Incubate the dishes for 10 min
(i) Remove the annexin V solution
(j) Add binding buffer to wash the cells three times and remove the buffer after the last time
(k) Add 1 ml growth medium to the dishes
(l) Cover with foil and transfer the cells to dark room to observe the cells under fluorescence microscope; images are acquired using both transmitted light as well as fluorescent single-excitation light at 490 nm and detected emission at 585 nm; by drawing a grid on the bottom of the culture dishes, we can relocate the same field of cells for sequential imaging; the percentage of labeled neurons is counted in three to seven discrete fields
(m) After examination, the annexin V labeling can be detached by washing three times with dissociation buffer; add growth medium and put dishes back into incubator; incubate cells for a further specified period and redetect the PS exposure again using the same method.

13.4 In vitro models of injury

13.4.1 Anoxia

The primary insult of cerebral ischemia is the oxygen deficiency resulting from the interruption of supply of cerebral blood flow. In cell cultures, anoxic injury can be easily induced by keeping the cultures in an anoxic chamber. The model has been used to investigate signaling pathways leading to apoptosis of the central nervous system cells.[8,9,25] The model can also be used to evaluate neuroprotective agents.

Materials

Cell cultures
Anoxic chamber system (Sheldon Manufacturing, Cornelius, OR).

Procedure

(a) Prepare cell cultures that are required for experiment
(b) Transfer the cultures to the anoxic chamber (37 °C) filled with 90% N_2, 5% H_2, and 5% CO_2
(c) Keep the cultures in the chamber for 4 hr (neuron) and 12 hr (endothelial cells)
(d) Transfer the cultures to CO_2 incubator and incubate for a period according to experimental paradigms
(e) In our culture systems, anoxia yields about 30–40% survival revealed by the trypan blue staining 24 hr following 4 hr period of anoxia in neurons and 12 hr period of anoxia in endothelial cells.

13.4.2 Oxygen–glucose deprivation

Oxygen–glucose deprivation (OGD), which represents the combined deficiency of oxygen and glucose that occurs during cerebral ischemia, is one of the described in vitro injury models that can mimic the animal model of cerebral ischemia as well as oxidative stress. The model has been extensively applied in the research of cerebral ischemia.

Materials

Anoxic chamber system (Sheldon Manufacturing, Cornelius, OR)
Glucose-free Hank's balanced salt solution (HBSS)
   116 mm NaCl
   5.4 mm KCl
   0.8 mm $MgSO_4$
   1 mM NaH_2PO_4
   0.9 mm $CaCl_2$
   10 mg/l phenol red
   pH 7.4.

Procedure

(a) Remove culture medium and add pre-warmed HBSS
(b) Transfer the cultures to the anoxic chamber (37 °C) filled with 90% N_2, 5% H_2, and 5% CO_2

(c) After 3 hr (for neurons or differentiated SY5Y cells) or 8 hr (for endothelial cells), take the cultures out of the chamber

(d) Remove the HBSS.

(e) Add normal growth medium and incubate at 37 °C in CO_2 incubator for period by specific experimental paradigm

(f) In our culture systems, OGD insult yields about 30–40% survival revealed by trypan blue staining 24 hr following 3 hr period of OGD in neurons and 8 hr period of OGD in endothelial cells.

13.4.3 Nitric oxide toxicity

Generation of nitric oxide (NO) is considered to be one of the triggers for the subsequent induction of cell injury in cerebral microvascular endothelial cells and neurons. Enhanced expression of the enzyme responsible for NO production, nitric oxide synthase (NOS), has been associated with both chronic neuronal and vascular degeneration. Generally, two or three NO donors are applied for the experimental paradigms and the results from different NO donors are combined. More than one NO generator is employed to ensure that the biological effects observed are a result of NO generation rather than through by-products of the NO generators.[8,24,26–28]

Materials

NO donors
    6-(2-hydroxy-1-methyl-2-nitrosohydrazino)-*N*-Methyl-1-hexanamine (NOC-9)
    3-Morpholinosydnonimine (SIN-1)
    Sodium nitroprusside (SNP)
Neuronal or endothelial cell cultures.

Procedure

(a) Observe the cultures to ensure that the cells are growing

(b) Warm sufficient volume of growth medium in 50 ml tube in 37 °C water bath

(c) Calculate NO donors for neurons
    300 μM NOC-9: NOC-9 (mg) = [solution volume (ml) × 300 (μM) × 204.3 (MW)]/1 000 000
    300 μM SIN-1: SIN-1 (mg) = [solution volume (ml) × 300 (μM) × 170.2 (MW)]/ 1 000 000
    300 μM SNP: SNP (mg) = [solution volume (ml) × 300 (μM) × 298.0 (MW)]/ 1 000 000

(d) Weigh NO donors carefully in dark (turn off the light)

(e) Place the entire weight boat with NO donor into foil-covered 50 ml vial

(f) Quickly remove the media from culture dishes (35 mm dish for example) by suction under hood (turn off light)

(g) Add desired volume of warmed growth medium with (1.5 ml for each 35 mm dish) into a NO donor-containing vial

(h) Add 1.5 ml of NO donor-containing medium into dishes quickly and place the dishes into incubator for 5 min

(i) Remove the medium with NO by suction and place normal 1.5 ml growth medium into the dishes and incubate for period by specific experimental paradigm

(j) In our culture system of hippocampal neurons, NO insult yields about 30–40% survival revealed by the trypan blue staining 24 hr following NO treatment

(k) For cerebral microvascular endothelial cells, the concentration of 1000 µM of NO donors without removal is used to yield similar results to neurons.

13.5 In vivo models of injury

13.5.1 Permanent middle cerebral artery occlusion

Although applicable to rodent models of rats or mice, the following description applies to the rat model. Rodent models are extremely useful since they are less expensive to use than primates, cats, and dogs and possess a cranial circulation similar to humans. In regards to mouse models, they have provided excellent tools for gene manipulation experiments. The middle cerebral artery (MCA) occlusion model was initially introduced in rats.[29] The model is performed using a subtemporal craniotomy to expose the origin of the MCA.[30] Permanent focal ischemia is achieved by coagulation of the MCA. The reproducible infarct volume of the model is beneficial to evaluate neuroprotective agents, but this model is invasive and may alter the intracranial pressure which is affected when the dura is opened.

Materials

Male Sprague-Dawley rat, 250–300 g
Isofluorane
30% oxygen/70% nitrogen
Anesthetic vaporizer and flowmeter
Polysporin topical ointment
Cefazolin
Rat anesthesia mask
Homeothermic blanket system with rectal probe
Elastikon porous tape
Surgical instruments: dissecting microscope; microdissecting tweezers, scissors, and
    forceps; bone-cutting forceps; retractors; hand-held drill
Bipolar electric coagulation unit
Surgical 3–0 nylon suture
pH/blood gas analyzer
PE50 tube.

Procedure

(a) Anesthetize rat with 3% (v/v) isofluorane in 30% oxygen/70% nitrogen using an anesthetic vaporizer, flowmeter, and rat anesthesia mask

(b) Cannulate a femoral artery for arterial blood sampling of blood gases

(c) Place rat in the left lateral position and hold the anterior portion; maintain anesthesia with 1–2% (v/v) isofluorane; maintain body temperature at 37 °C using a rectal probe and a small homeothermic blanket system

(d) Place artificial tears in the rat's eyes and cover them with a small piece of porous tape to protect the eyes during surgery

(e) Shave the surgery area and smear with 70% ethanol

(f) Make a vertical skin incision at the midpoint between the left orbit and the external auditory canal (the length is about 2 cm)

(g) Make an incision around the superior and posterior margins of the temporalis muscle, scrape the muscle from the lateral aspect of the skull, and reflect it forwards

(h) Under a dissecting microscope, remove the zygomatic arch and make a hole using a hand-held drill with a diameter of 1.0–1.5 mm to expose the origin of MCA

(i) Remove pieces of skull to expose the MCA

(j) Remove the dura that covers the proximal MCA; occlude the MCA between the olfactory tract and the inferior cerebral vein by micropolar coagulation of bipolar coagulation unit

(k) Transect the MCA with microscissors and close the incision with nylon suture

(l) Apply polysporin topical ointment to the incision site

(m) Give 40 mg/kg cefazolin intraperitoneally to prevent infection.

13.5.2 Reversible middle cerebral artery occlusion

This model occludes the origin of the MCA by insertion of an intraluminal suture into the external carotid artery and then into the internal carotid artery to pass along the origin of MCA.[31] The model is non-invasive and can be used for either permanent or transient cerebral ischemia. The reliability of occlusion is determined by the degree of which the diameter of the monofilament matches the diameter of the internal carotid artery. Alternatively, this model is also performed in mice with a silicon-coated 8–0 monofilament suture.

Materials

Male Sprague-Dawley rat, 280–300 g
Isofluorane
30% oxygen/70% nitrogen
Chloral hydrate
10% buffered formalin (see recipe)

Wound clips
Anesthetic vaporizer and flowmeter
Dissecting microscope
Homeothermic temperature system
Animal clippers
Microdissecting tweezers, microdissecting scissors, microdissecting forceps, straight iris scissors, retractors,
5–0 silk suture, intraluminal monofilament occluder
3–0 nylon monofilament (the nylon monofilament should be silicon-coated and rounded at the tip to avoid vascular injury during the insertion).

Procedures

(a) Anesthetize rat with 3% isofluorane in 30% oxygen/70% nitrogen using an anesthetic vaporizer and flowmeter; fix the animal on its back; maintain body temperature at 37 °C with a homeothermic temperature system
(b) Make a 2 cm midline incision in the neck to expose the left common carotid, external carotid, and internal carotid arteries; dissect the arteries free from surrounding nerves and tissues; isolate and coagulate branches of the external carotid artery, such as the occipital artery, terminal lingual, and maxillary artery
(c) Separate the internal carotid artery from the adjacent vagus nerve; dissect its only extracranial branch pterygopalatine artery and ligate with 5–0 silk suture
(d) Loosely tie two 5–0 silk sutures around the external carotid artery stump, and apply a microaneurysm clip to the external carotid artery near its origin
(e) Tighten the silk suture at the terminal of external carotid artery and make a small opening close to the ligation; insert the monofilament through the opening and tighten the silk sutures around the lumen containing the filament
(f) Apply a microclip to common carotid artery; remove the microaneurysm clip from the external carotid artery
(g) Insert the monofilament into the lumen of internal carotid artery and advance the monofilament into the internal carotid artery for 20–22 mm (from the bifurcation of the common carotid artery); tighten the suture around the external carotid artery to prevent bleeding; remove the microclip from common carotid artery
(h) Close the neck incision with 3–0 suture
(i) Reperfusion is performed by withdrawal of monofilament suture and closure of the external carotid artery.

13.5.3 *Embolic model of focal cerebral ischemia*

In this model, induction of focal cerebral ischemia is performed through the injection of a pre-formed clot into middle cerebral artery.[32] The advantage of this model is its close pathophysiological similarity to clinical thromboembolic disease. In addition, since the clot is pre-formed and is confirmed prior to injection, the surgery period is reduced and the result becomes more reliable and reproducible.

Materials

Male Wistar rats, 300–350 g
PE50 tube
100 µl Hamilton syringe
Surgical tweezers, scissors, microdissecting forceps, straight iris scissors, retractors, animal clippers
Homeothermic blanket with rectal temperature probe
Chloride hydrate
30% oxygen/70% nitrous oxide
Halothane
Facemask
Thrombin.

Procedure

(a) Preparation of emboli: anesthetize a rat with 360 mg/kg chloride hydrate; withdraw 0.1 ml of blood through cardiac puncture using a 1.0 mm disposable syringe with a 23-gauge needle; Quickly (within 20 s) mix the blood with 25 µl 10 NIH U/l thrombin in a 1.5 ml Eppendorf tube; transfer the blood into a PE50 tube and store at 4 °C overnight; check the clot-rich portion of the tube and cut out for embolization.

(b) Anesthetize rat with 3.0% halothane and maintain with 1.5% halothane in a mixture of 30% oxygen/70% nitrous oxide with a facemask during surgery; keep the rectal temperature at about 37 °C

(c) Make a 1.5 cm incision in the midline of the ventral cervical skin; separate the right common carotid artery, right internal carotid artery, and right external carotid artery

(d) Ligate the distal portion of the external carotid artery; tie loosely with a 4–0 silk suture around the origin of the external carotid artery

(e) Apply microvascular clips to common carotid artery and internal carotid artery

(f) Modify the pre-clot-forming PE50 tube to make the tip be 0.3 mm in outside diameter; attach the tube to a 100-µl Hamilton syringe

(g) Make an opening on the external carotid artery by using microdissecting scissors; insert the clot-containing tube into external carotid artery; tighten the suture around the origin of the external carotid artery

(h) Remove the clip on internal carotid artery; advance the tube to a length of 17 mm in the internal carotid artery until its tip is 1–2 mm away from the origin of the middle cerebral artery

(i) Inject 5 µl clot into the middle cerebral artery; keep the tube unmoved for 5 min

(j) Withdraw the tube gently and ligate the external carotid artery

(k) Remove the clip on common carotid artery and close the incision

(l) After it has recovered, place the rat in its cage

(m) The infarct volume is about 40% at 48 hr following the injection.

13.5.4 Global cerebral ischemia with a four-vessel occlusion model

The model induces global cerebral ischemia by combined occlusion of the bilateral common carotid arteries and both vertebral arteries.[33] The four-vessel occlusion (4-VO) rat model has been widely used to study mechanisms of ischemia-induced neuronal death, especially delayed neuronal cell death in the hippocampus. It also has been extensively used to evaluate the effects of neuroprotective drugs.

Materials

Male Wistar rats, 280–300 g
Isofluorane
Chloral hydrate
Stereotaxic apparatus
Rat anesthesia mask
Electric hair clippers
Surgical instruments: scissors, scalpel, forceps
Dissecting microscope
Wound clips
Rectal thermometer
Heat lamp
Monopolar electric coagulation unit.

Procedure

(a) Anesthetize rat with 3% isofluorane in 30% oxygen/70% nitrogen

(b) Place rat in stereotaxic apparatus, tighten earbars and adjust facemask to keep animal anesthetized

(c) Shave middle area of dorsal neck and swab area with 70% alcohol

(d) Make a 1 cm midline incision behind the occipital bone directly over the first two cervical vertebrae

(e) Under the dissecting microscope, expose the right and left alar foramina of the first cervical vertebra; the vertebral arteries pass beneath the alar foramen

(f) Insert the monopolar needle of monopolar coagulation unit into each alar foramen and electrocauterize both vertebral arteries to permanently occlude them

(g) Remove rat from stereotaxic apparatus; let the rat recover from anesthesia

(h) The following day, anesthesize and fix the rat on its back; shave ventral surface of the neck and swab the skin with 70% alcohol

(i) Make a midline ventral incision; dissect both common carotid arteries free from connective tissue and associated nerves

(j) Place the atraumatic arterial clasps to block blood flow of both common carotid arteries; remove the clasps 10–30 min later
(k) Rat should have no response to stimuli and should lose the ability to ambulate
(l) The delayed neuronal cell death occurs 3–7 days following a 10–30 min period of ischemia; ischemia for 20–30 min also causes neuronal cell death in cerebral cortex and striatum.

13.5.5 Ischemic preconditioning

Ischemic preconditioning is a phenomenon in which a brief administration of sublethal ischemia produces resistance to a subsequent detrimental ischemic insult.[34] Ischemic conditioning has been observed in global cerebral ischemia, focal cerebral ischemia, and ischemic injury in cell culture systems. The pre-conditioning model can be used to investigate the underlying mechanisms of endogenous protection and may function to find new therapeutic approaches for neurodegenerative disease. Methods for focal and global ischemic precon-ditioning are described below.

Focal cerebral in vivo ischemic preconditioning

This model is made through the rat model of a short-term period of reversible middle cerebral artery occlusion.[35]

Materials

Male Wistar rats, 230–250 g
30% oxygen/70% nitrogen
Halothane
Rat anesthesia mask
Electric hair clippers
Surgical instruments: scissors, scalpel, forceps
Wound clips
Rectal thermometer
Heat lamp
Surgical 3–0 nylon suture
pH/blood gas analyzer
PE50 tube
Blood pressure monitor
4–0 nylon monofilament thread.

Procedure

Following the induction of reversible MCA occlusion, a 30 min period of occlusion is induced. After the short-term occlusion, the animal is allowed free access to food and water. Four days later, the animal is anesthetized again. The physiological parameters are monitored through the cannulation of a femoral artery. MCA occlusion is then performed for a 3 hr period.

Global cerebral in vivo ischemic preconditioning

For global ischemic preconditioning in the rat, ischemia and ischemic preconditioning are produced by bilateral carotid occlusions and systemic hypotension (50 mm Hg) for various time periods. In some cases, brief periods of ischemic preconditioning, such as for 2 min prior to 10 min of global ischemia, can protect vulnerable ischemic tissue.[36]

Materials

Male Wistar rats, 250–300 g
30% oxygen/70% nitrogen
Halothane
Rat anesthesia mask
Electric hair clippers
Surgical instruments: scissors, scalpel, forceps
Wound clips
Rectal thermometer
Heat lamp
Surgical 3–0 nylon suture
pH/blood gas analyzer
PE50 tube
Blood pressure monitor.

Procedure

(a) Anesthetize rat with 3% (v/v) halothane in 30% oxygen/70% nitrogen using an anesthetic vaporizer, flowmeter, and rat anesthesia mask
(b) Cannulate femoral arteries with PE50 tube for arterial blood sampling of blood gases and blood pressure monitoring
(c) Maintain anesthesia with 1–2% (v/v) halothane; maintain body temperature at 37 °C using a rectal probe and a small homeothermic blanket system
(d) Shave the ventral area of the neck and smear with 70% ethanol
(e) Make a vertical 2 cm skin incision in the midpoint
(f) Dissect both common carotid arteries free from connective tissue and associated nerves
(g) Withdraw blood from femoral vein into a heparinized syringe to reduce blood pressure to 50 mm Hg
(h) Place the atraumatic arterial clasps for 2 min to block blood flow of both common carotid arteries

(i) Reject the shed blood into femoral vein and then close the incision; place the animal back into cage

(j) 24 hr later, repeat the procedure and block both common carotid arteries with hypotension for a 10 min period.

13.6 Behavior evaluation in the animal model

In the early studies, the evaluation of therapeutic agents in animal ischemic stroke was simply performed by histological method to count the neuronal loss or calculate infarct volume in a relatively short-term period following ischemia. Although histological assessment of neuronal or vascular injury following an experimental paradigm is important, assessment of functional recovery following an injury or therapeutic intervention is equally critical and may provide some insight toward clinical disability and recovery. Therefore, we briefly describe some common assessments of functional outcome in the animal model.

13.6.1 Neurological deficit score

Twenty-four hours following cortical injury and recovery from anesthesia, the animal is placed on a flat surface and raised by the tail. Animals following successful ischemic occlusion will exhibit specific features such as twisting and retraction of contralateral forepaw. The neurological deficits are determined by a modified Bederson's scoring system as follows:[38]

0 No observable deficit
1 Forelimb flexion
2 Forelimb flexion plus decreased resistance to lateral push
3 Unidirectional circling
4 Unidirectional circling plus decreased level of consciousness.

13.6.2 Cylinder test

The cylinder task for ischemic animals has been established to observe the forelimb-use bias following focal cerebral ischemia.[39] The cylinder should have sufficient width to allow movement and should be narrow enough to encourage the animal to rear or explore a wall. The top edge of the cylinder should be beyond the reach of the animal. The movement of the animal is observed through a camera and a mirror is placed behind the cylinder to observe and record forelimb movements with the animal at the opposite side of the camera. The animal is scored for 3–5 min for a series of movements with a scoring method as follows.

Forelimb placing scores Score when the animal rears, with one or both forelimbs placed on the wall

Simultaneous limb-use scores Score when the animal explores the wall by alternating right and left limb placement

Independent limb-use scores Score when the animal moves along the wall using one limb

Percentage use scores
  (a) Movements of the ipsilateral limb/the total number of movements
  (b) Movements of the contralateral limb/the total number of movements
  (c) Limb-bias use score = (a)–(b).

13.6.3 Elevated body swing test

The elevated body swing test was designed to evaluate asymmetric motor behavior.[40] Focal cerebral ischemia in animals impairs the movement of the contralateral limb, which can be detected by biased swing. It also can be used to evaluate the functional recovery following intervention with neuroprotective agents. Hold the rat by the base of the tail and elevate it 2.5 cm from the tabletop. Record the number and direction of times that the animal turns its body more than 10 degrees to either left or right side in 30 s. During recording, each animal has to return to the vertical position before the next swing is counted. Calculate the percentage of turns to the side contralateral to the injured cerebral hemisphere. For example, animals following focal cerebral ischemia demonstrate a strong tendency to turn toward the ipsilateral side.

13.6.4 Morris water maze test

The Morris water maze test was originally designed to evaluate the memory of rats.[41] Either focal or global cerebral ischemia often results in cognitive impairment. This test is performed in a water tank to evaluate the ability of rats to find the platform in the water and determine the retention of rat's reference memory.

The Morris maze consists of a circular black tank with a vertical wall or a sloping wall 153 cm in diameter at the top, 143 cm in diameter at the bottom, and 63 cm in depth. The tank is filled with water of 43.5 cm in height and the temperature is kept at approximately 22 °C. An escape platform (a black polyethylene cylinder) with a diameter of 11–13 cm is submerged 1.5 or 2 cm below the surface of the water and placed at one end of tank. The animal is released at the opposite end of the tank. A computer-interfaced camera tracking system is used to record the swim paths of the rats.

13.6.5 Passive avoidance test

Cognitive deficits following a cerebral insult can also be evaluated via the passive avoidance test.[42] The test is performed by using a step-down apparatus that consists of two compartments. The grid compartment (10×30 cm) is equipped with a grid floor for the delivery of an electric shock. The safe compartment has a plexiglass floor. The two compartments are separated by a guillotine door.

In the habitual trial, animals are placed in the safe compartment to get habituated to the apparatus. The door between the two compartments is opened for free entrance into the grid compartment. The acquisition trial is performed by placing the animal in the safe compartment and a 2 s 0.2–0.6 mA foot shock is delivered as soon as the animal enters into the grid compartment. The animal is taken back to its cage after 30 s. The retention trial is performed 24 hr later. The trial is performed in the same manner as the habitual trial, but without foot shock. During the trials, the latency to enter the grid compartment is recorded and is usually observed to be shorter with cerebral cortex injury.

References

1. Rami A, Ausmeir F, Winckler J, Krieglstein J. Differential effects of scopolamine on neuronal survival in ischemia and glutamate neurotoxicity: relationships to the excessive vulnerability of the dorsoseptal hippocampus. *J. Chem. Neuroanat.* 1997, **13**: 201–208.
2. Maiese K, Chong ZZ, Kang J. Transformation into treatment: novel therapeutics that begin within the cell. In Maiese K (ed.) *Neuronal and Vascular Plasticity: Elucidating Basic Cellular Mechanisms for Future Therapeutic Discovery.* Norwell, MA: Kluwer, 2003, pp. 1–26.
3. Furshpan EJ, Potter DD. Seizure-like activity and cellular damage in rat hippocampal neurons in cell culture. *Neuron* 1989, **3**: 199–207.
4. Chong ZZ, Lin SH, Kang JQ, Maiese K. The tyrosine phosphatase SHP2 modulates MAP kinase p38 and caspase 1 and 3 to foster neuronal survival. *Cell Mol. Neurobiol.* 2003, **23**: 561–578.
5. Maiese K, Vincent AM. Membrane asymmetry and DNA degradation: functionally distinct determinants of neuronal programmed cell death. *J. Neurosci. Res.* 2000, **59**: 568–580.
6. Faraci FM. Regulation of the cerebral circulation by endothelium. *Pharmacol. Ther.* 1992, **56**: 1–22.
7. Rupnick MA, Carey A, Williams SK. Phenotypic diversity in cultured cerebral microvascular endothelial cells. *In Vitro Cell Devel. Biol.* 1988, **24**: 435–444.
8. Lin SH, Maiese K. The metabotropic glutamate receptor system protects against ischemic free radical programmed cell death in rat brain endothelial cells. *J. Cereb. Blood Flow Metab.* 2001, **21**: 262–275.

9. Chong ZZ, Kang JQ, Maiese K. Erythropoietin is a novel vascular protectant through activation of Akt1 and mitochondrial modulation of cysteine proteases. *Circulation* 2002, **106**: 2973–2979.

10. Kang JQ, Chong ZZ, Maiese K. Critical role for Akt1 in the modulation of apoptotic phosphatidylserine exposure and microglial activation. *Mol. Pharmacol.* 2003, **64**: 557–569.

11. Kang JQ, Chong ZZ, Maiese K. Akt1 protects against inflammatory microglial activation through maintenance of membrane asymmetry and modulation of cysteine protease activity. *J. Neurosci. Res.* 2003, **74**: 37–51.

12. Giulian D, Baker TJ. Characterization of ameboid microglia isolated from developing mammalian brain. *J. Neurosci.* 1986, **6**: 2163–2178.

13. Williams K, Schwartz A, Corey S, *et al.* Proliferating cellular nuclear antigen expression as a marker of perivascular macrophages in simian immunodeficiency virus encephalitis. *Am. J. Pathol.* 2002, **161**: 575–585.

14. Martinez-Contreras A, Huerta M, Lopez-Perez S, *et al.* Astrocytic and microglia cells reactivity induced by neonatal administration of glutamate in cerebral cortex of the adult rats. *J. Neurosci. Res.* 2002, **67**: 200–210.

15. Chong ZZ, Kang JQ, Maiese K. Hematopoietic factor erythropoietin fosters neuroprotection through novel signal transduction cascades. *J. Cereb. Blood Flow Metab.* 2002, **22**: 503–514.

16. Chang GH, Barbaro NM, Pieper RO. Phosphatidylserine-dependent phago-cytosis of apoptotic glioma cells by normal human microglia, astrocytes, and glioma cells. *Neuro-oncol.* 2000, **2**: 174–183.

17. Jessel R, Haertel S, Socaciu C, Tykhonova S, Diehl HA. Kinetics of apoptotic markers in exogeneously induced apoptosis of EL4 cells. *J. Cell Mol. Med.* 2002, **6**: 82–92.

18. Chong ZZ, Kang JQ, Maiese K. Essential cellular regulatory elements of oxidative stress in early and late phases of apoptosis in the central nervous system. *Antioxid. Redox Signal.* 2004, **6**: 277–287.

19. Dombroski D, Balasubramanian K, Schroit AJ. Phosphatidylserine expression on cell surfaces promotes antibody- dependent aggregation and thrombosis in beta2-glycoprotein I-immune mice. *J. Autoimmun.* 2000, **14**: 221–229.

20. Bombeli T, Karsan A, Tait JF, Harlan JM. Apoptotic vascular endothelial cells become procoagulant. *Blood* 1997, **89**: 2429–2442.

21. Okamoto M, Matsumoto M, Ohtsuki T, *et al.* Internucleosomal DNA cleavage involved in ischemia-induced neuronal death. *Biochem. Biophys. Res. Commun.* 1993, **196**: 1356–1362.

22. Vincent AM, Maiese K. Nitric oxide induction of neuronal endonuclease activity in programmed cell death. *Exp. Cell Res.* 1999, **246**: 290–300.

23. Vincent AM, Maiese K. Direct temporal analysis of apoptosis induction in living adherent neurons. *J. Histochem. Cytochem.* 1999, **47**: 661–672.

24. Chong ZZ, Lin SH, Kang JQ, Maiese K. Erythropoietin prevents early and late neuronal demise through modulation of Akt1 and induction of caspase 1, 3, and 8. *J. Neurosci. Res.* 2003, **71**: 659–669.

25. Chong ZZ, Kang JQ, Maiese K. Apaf-1, Bcl-xL, cytochrome c, and caspase-9 form the critical elements for cerebral vascular protection by erythropoietin. *J. Cereb. Blood Flow Metab.* 2003, **23**: 320–330.

26. Maiese K, Chong ZZ. Nicotinamide: necessary nutrient emerges as a novel cytoprotectant for the brain. *Trends Pharmacol. Sci.* 2003, **24**: 228–232.

27. Chong ZZ, Kang JQ, Maiese K. Metabotropic glutamate receptors promote neuronal and vascular plasticity through novel intracellular pathways. *Histol. Histopathol.* 2003, **18**: 173–189.

28. Chong ZZ, Kang J, Maiese K. G-protein mediated metabotropic receptors offer novel avenues in neuronal and vascular cells for cytoprotective strategies. In Maiese K (ed.) *Neuronal and Vascular Plasticity: Elucidating Basic Cellular Mechanisms for Future Therapeutic Discovery.* Norwell, MA: Kluwer, 2003, pp. 257–298.

29. Tamura A, Graham DI, McCulloch J, Teasdale GM. Focal cerebral ischaemia in the rat: 1. Description of technique and early neuropathological consequences following middle cerebral artery occlusion. *J. Cereb. Blood Flow Metab.* 1981, **1**: 53–60.

30. Maiese K, Pek L, Berger SB, Reis DJ. Reduction in focal cerebral ischemia by agents acting at imidazole receptors. *J. Cereb. Blood Flow Metab.* 1992, **12**: 53–63.

31. Longa EZ, Weinstein PR, Carlson S, Cummins R. Reversible middle cerebral artery occlusion without craniectomy in rats. *Stroke* 1989, **20**: 84–91.

32. Wang CX, Yang T, Shuaib A. An improved version of embolic model of brain ischemic injury in the rat. *J. Neurosci. Methods* 2001, **109**: 147–151.

33. Pulsinelli WA, Brierley JB, Plum F. Temporal profile of neuronal damage in a model of transient forebrain ischemia. *Ann. Neurol.* 1982, **11**: 491–498.

34. Kitagawa K, Matsumoto M, Mabuchi T, *et al.* Ischemic tolerance in hippocampal CA1 neurons studied using contralateral controls. *Neuroscience* 1997, **81**: 989–998.

35. Matsushima K, Hakim AM. Transient forebrain ischemia protects against subsequent focal cerebral ischemia without changing cerebral perfusion. *Stroke* 1995, **26**: 1047–1052.

36. Alsbo CW, Wrang ML, Nielsen M, Diemer NH. Ischemic tolerance affects the adenylation state of GluR2 mRNA. *Neuroreport* 2000, **11**: 3279–3282.

37. Liu J, Ginis I, Spatz M, Hallenbeck JM. Hypoxic preconditioning protects cultured neurons against hypoxic stress via TNF-alpha and ceramide. *Am. J. Physiol. Cell Physiol.* 2000, **278**: C144–C153.

38. Bederson JB, Pitts LH, Tsuji M, *et al.* Rat middle cerebral artery occlusion: evaluation of the model and development of a neurologic examination. *Stroke* 1986, **17**: 472–476.

39. Schallert T, Hernandez TD, Barth TM. Recovery of function after brain damage: severe and chronic disruption by diazepam. *Brain Res.* 1986, **379**: 104–111.

40. Borlongan CV, Cahill DW, Sanberg PR. Locomotor and passive avoidance deficits following occlusion of the middle cerebral artery. *Physiol. Behav.* 1995, **58**: 909–917.

41. Morris RG, Garrud P, Rawlins JN, O'Keefe J. Place navigation impaired in rats with hippocampal lesions. *Nature* 1982, **297**: 681–683.

42. Kiprianova I, Sandkuhler J, Schwab S, Hoyer S, Spranger M. Brain-derived neurotrophic factor improves long-term potentiation and cognitive functions after transient forebrain ischemia in the rat. *Exp. Neurol.* 1999, **159**: 511–519.

14

Neuroimmunology and immune-related neuropathologies

BAO-GUO XIAO AND HANS LINK

14.1 Basic immunology

14.1.1 Systemic immunology

Immunology is a relatively new and rapidly developing field that is involved in most clinical diseases. In 1796, Edward Jenner discovered that cowpox or vaccinia induced protection against human smallpox, but he knew nothing of the infectious agents that cause disease. Late in the nineteenth century, Robert Koch proved that infectious diseases are caused by microorganisms. We now recognize four broad categories of disease-causing microorganisms or pathogens: viruses, bacteria, fungi, and parasites. In 1890, Emil von Behring and Shibasaburo Kitasato discovered that the serum of vaccinated individuals contained antibodies that specifically bound to the relevant pathogen. Both innate and adaptive immune responses depend on the activities of leukocytes.

The immune system is a complex network of specialized cells and organs that defend the body against foreign pathogens and maintain the balance between immunity and tolerance. The peripheral lymphoid organs (lymph node and spleen) are specialized to trap antigen and allow the initiation of adaptive immune responses. Once lymphocytes are mature, they leave the central lymphoid organs (thymus and bone marrow), and are capable of responding to foreign pathogens. Peripheral mature immune cells include lymphocytes (T cells and B cells), antigen presenting cells (macrophages and dendritic cells, DC) and nature killer (NK) cells. Armed effector T cells play a critical role in almost all adaptive immune responses. Both major histocompatibility complex (MHC) and co-stimulatory signals provided by professional antigen-presenting cells (APC) are required for the activation and expansion of T cells. Adhesion molecules and soluble factors influence immune cell migration, activation, and interaction. Increasing evidence demonstrates that cancer, autoimmune diseases, and certain other disorders

Handbook of Experimental Neurology, ed. Turgut Tatlisumak and Marc Fisher. Published by Cambridge University Press. © Cambridge University Press 2006.

are mediated by dysfunction of the immune system. One of the great future challenges of immunology is the control of the immune responses, so that unwanted immune responses can be suppressed and desirable responses elicited. To do this, we need to understand more about special microenvironments and the generation of immune responses within the central nervous system (CNS), and to control tissue damage mediated by immune responses in human disease.

14.1.2 Autoimmunity

Autoimmune disease occurs when a specific adaptive immune response is mounted against self-antigen(s). However, it is not clear what triggers the autoimmune responses, but both genetic and environmental factors are important. Theoretically speaking, autoimmune responses are common, but they attract medical attention only when they cause lasting tissue damage and clinical symptoms. Autoimmunity is initiated by a response involving T cells, cytotoxic T cell responses, and inappropriate activation of macrophages or DC that can cause extensive tissue damage, while inappropriate T cell help can initiate a harmful antibody response to self-antigens. To define a disease as autoimmune, the tissue damage must be caused by an immune response to self-antigens. Autoimmune diseases can be caused by autoantibodies or autoreactive T cells, and tissue damage may result from direct attack on the cells bearing the antigen, from immune complex formation, or from local inflammation. The most convincing form of proof that the immune response may cause autoimmunity is transfer of disease by transferring the active component of immune response (antibodies or immune cells) to an appropriate recipient. The current challenge is to identify the autoantigens recognized by T cells in autoimmunity, and to control the activity of these cells and the production of pathogenic autoantibodies.

14.2 Neuroimmunology

14.2.1 Special structure of the central nervous system

Blood–brain barrier

The blood–brain barrier (BBB) is responsible for the selective transport of molecules and cells from the systemic compartment into the CNS. The BBB is composed of a specialized microvascular endothelium and glial cell elements (astrocytes and microglia) that are in physical proximity to the endothelium. All the elements contribute to the so-called "immunological privilege" status of the CNS. However, this immune privilege of the CNS is not complete. There is likely a certain degree of ongoing trafficking of immune cells and molecules through the BBB. One thus considers that the CNS also needs a physiological immune surveillance by neuroimmune network, rather than only depending on BBB.

The specialized endothelial cells (EC) are a central component of the BBB that restricts immune cell infiltration and soluble molecule diffusion from the systemic compartment into the CNS. The functional events that define the BBB occur at the level of capillaries. Brain capillaries are composed of a fine network of tightly adherent EC, surrounded by a very narrow basal lamina. At the microscopic level, these EC show a typical continuous cobblestone appearance and have a high mitochondria content, which is thought to provide the energy required to develop high-resistance tight junctions. These tight junctions consist of strongly anastomosed plasma membranes of one or several EC which fuse and form a complex surface of ridges and grooves.

Astrocytes cast large processes or end feet which unsheath EC and cover the basement membrane of brain capillaries. Pericytes and perivascular microglia are widely distributed at the level of the BBB. Brain microvascular EC need constant input from the neuroglia in order to maintain BBB-related properties. A direct contact between EC and astrocytes has been deemed necessary to generate an optimal barrier. Activated glia can produce an array of chemokines and cytokines that increase the permeability of the EC barrier and act directly on immune cells or via EC to enhance the process of lymphocyte migration. The dynamic properties of the BBB construct a promising site for direct immunomodulatory therapies. A number of systemic therapies directed at specific molecules such as adhesion molecules and chemokine receptors of the BBB are under study in experimental models, and even in initial clinical trials.[1]

Resident cells of the central nervous system

Endothelial cells Besides the formation of the BBB, brain EC have been considered as potential APC because of their large cumulative surface and unique anatomical location between circulating T cells and the extravascular site of antigen exposure. Murine brain EC failed to induce T cell proliferation, although they can be induced to express MHC class II and co-stimulatory molecules in the presence of inflammatory cytokines, such as interferon gamma (IFN-γ). Human brain EC, despite expressing human leukocyte antigen (HLA) DR and co-stimulatory molecules, also downregulated the proliferation of $CD4^+$ T cells. These results reveal the possibility that although EC of BBB contribute to brain inflammation by cytokine and adhesion molecule production, they may also inhibit antigen-specific immune responses within the CNS.

Microglia The glial cells of the CNS, especially for microglia/CNS macrophages, have emerged as much more active players in neuroimmune interactions than was previously assumed. Microglia and astrocytes constitute the two main classes of immune cells within the CNS, where they actively participate in CNS immune reactions, including T cell reactivation and inflammatory molecule production. Microglia have an initial hematopoietic origin, likely explaining their multiple shared properties with circulating monocytes and tissue macrophages. Based on histological and immunophenotypic criteria, microglia can be subdivided into two major classes: (1) the ramified resting microglia residing in the parenchyma display a downregulated phenotype characterized by lack of endocytic and phagocytic activity, low expression of CD45, low or undetectable membrane ligands, and receptors that are essential for inducing typical macrophage functions; (2) activated or reactive microglia (i.e., perivascular cells) acquire macrophage differentiation markers and effector properties which induce inflammatory stimuli and overt inflammation. In addition, in the presence of granulocyte–macrophage colony-stimulating factor (GM-CSF), transforming growth factor beta 1 (TGF-β1) can trigger microglia to differentiate into dendriform cells. These morphologic features are similar to those of DC derived from bone marrow and spleen (Fig. 14.1).[2]

Microglia are very sensitive to several pathogens in the CNS microenvironment and rapidly become activated in inflammatory conditions. The activation pattern of microglia involves both morphological changes with hypertrophy and proliferation as well as functional differentiation with upregulated expression of MHC antigens. Upon activation, microglia are capable of secreting a range of immune regulating molecules, such as cytokines and chemokines in addition to non-specific inflammatory mediators, e.g., reactive oxygen species and nitric oxide (NO). At the end stage of activation, microglia become outright phagocytic, thus representing scavenger cells of the CNS. The activity of microglia can be both cytotoxic and protective and is profoundly affected by the nature of the tissue and the presence or absence of other immune cells.[3]

Under CNS inflammation, microglia can also differentiate into brain DC that might contribute to the chronicity of intracerebral T helper 1 (Th1) responses.[4] Microglia-derived interleukin-12 (IL-12) may contribute to Th1 skewing within the CNS and hence to the pathogenesis of Th1-mediated CNS disorders. Interestingly, Th1 cells, and to a lesser extent Th2 cells, also stimulate microglia to produce prostaglandin E_2 (PGE$_2$),[5] suggesting that negative

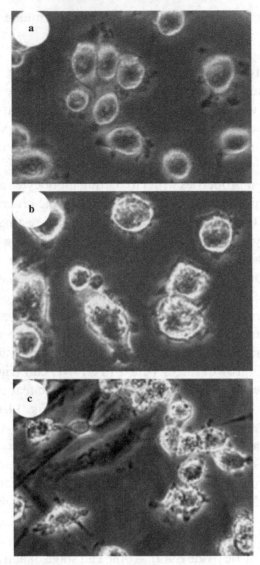

Figure 14.1. Morphologic comparison of (a) splenic dendritic cells (DC) and (b) bone marrow DC, and (c) glial cell-derived DC. Cells from spleen, bone marrow, and newborn rat brain were cultured in medium supplemented with granulocyte–macrophage colony-stimulating factor (GM-CSF) and interleukin-4 (IL-4). After 7 days, the photographs were obtained by phase-contrast microscopy. Morphologic features with irregular shaped veils by phase-contrast microscopy are similar among DC from spleen, bone marrow, and brain.

feedback mechanisms are induced which may prevent the Th1 development of newly recruited Th1 cells and stop inflammation. Besides Th1 response, microglia also promote Th2 responses within the CNS. During the course of tissue specific inflammation, activation of counter-regulatory mechanisms is essential to avoid escalation of inflammatory processes and allow recovery.

Astrocytes Astrocytes are the major glial cells within the CNS and have a number of important physiological properties to balance CNS suppressive environment. Besides contributing to structural and functional integrity of the BBB, astrocytes have at least three categories of functions: (1) astrocytes associated with synapses integrate neuronal inputs and release transmitters that modulate synaptic sensitivity, and regulate extracellular pH and K^+ levels; (2) astrocytes undergo a process of proliferation, morphological changes, and enhancement of glial fibrillary acidic protein (GFAP) expression, termed astrogliosis, a common hallmark of many neurodegenerative diseases; and (3) astrocytes function as immune effector cells to influence aspects of inflammation and immune reactivity, emphasizing the involvement of astrocytes in promoting Th2 responses.[6]

Numerous studies have confirmed the role of microglia as important APC within the CNS, while the role of astrocytes remains controversial. Astrocytes are the first CNS cell type shown to express MHC class II molecules upon IFN-γ stimulation in vitro. However, there are discrepancies in the literature regarding the ability of astrocytes to express MHC class II and co-stimulatory molecules (B7-1, B7-2, and CD40) both in vivo and in vitro. If astrocytes lack the capacity to deliver co-stimulatory signals to T cells and can not function as fully competent APC, these cells may induce T cell apoptosis or anergy. Astrocytes function as non-professional APC by promoting mainly Th2 responses and/or apoptosis of T cells, which may be important for recovery from Th1-mediated CNS inflammation. Several studies have shown that MHC class II positive astrocytes are not capable of stimulating T cell proliferation and, instead, actively induce suppression or apoptosis of $CD4^+$ T cells, presumably due to the lack of B7 expression. Astrocytes respond vigorously to any brain injury (e.g., tumor, stroke, Alzheimer's disease, and multiple sclerosis) and are postulated to play an important role in the fine tuning of brain inflammation by using death receptors to modulate pro- and anti-inflammatory effects.[7]

Neurons Neurons have long been known to signal to each other by various kinds of transmitter substances. Recent data have revealed that immune responses of microglia in the CNS are tightly controlled by neuronal signals and that glial cells also affect neurons and modulate synaptic activity. There are two principal pathways for the way in which neurons could regulate immune function of neighboring glial cells. First, normal physiologically active neurons have a general suppressive potential that prevents and limits the development of inflammatory responses, as well as possible concomitant bystander damage. For instance, microglia are kept in a quiescent state in the intact CNS by local interactions between the microglia receptor CD200 and its ligand, which is expressed on neurons.[8] In addition, neurons can suppress MHC expression in surrounding glial cells, in particular microglia and astrocytes. Neurons expressing Fas ligand (FasL) also induce T cell death. Antibodies blocking neuronal FasL were shown to have a protective effect on T cell survival.[9] Second, injury to neurons might rapidly trigger gene transcription of inflammation in neurons which, in turn, would stimulate nearby microglia and astrocytes. For example, death of neurons leads to the transformation of microglia into phagocytotic cells that remove cellular debris. Significant amounts of tumor necrosis factor alpha (TNF-α) and IL-1β are detectable at day 14 after facial nerve axotomy. These cytokines within the CNS are bidirectional, because they not only damage oligodendrocytes and neurons, but also cause T cell apoptosis. The balance between pro-inflammatory cytokines and local CNS-derived suppressive elements determines the outcome of inflammatory reactions in the CNS tissues.

Oligodendrocytes Oligodendrocytes, myelin-forming glial cells of the CNS, are vulnerable to damage in a variety of neurologic diseases.[10] Oligodendrocytes provide CNS axons with myelin sheaths through processes of various lengths. The lipid-rich myelin insulates axons, which increases conduction velocity. In addition, oligodendrocytes have trophic effects on axons. During development, immature oligodendrocytes undergo controlled migration, proliferation, and differentiation, influenced by various growth factors and axons. A number of genetically manipulated animal models have provided insights regarding myelination and the function of myelin components. Current research on myelin-related diseases, e.g., multiple sclerosis, focus on novel strategies for remyelination through transplantation of myelinating cells or stimulation of endogenous oligodendrocytes.

A growing literature suggests that oligodendrocytes can provide trophic support for neuronal survival and function. In particular, oligodendrocytes produce a number of growth factors, and influence the survival and/or function of neighboring neurons. Conversely, neural signals also influence oligodendrocyte function as trophic factor providers. In addition, oligodendrocytes may influence their own development and survival. In a number of cases, growth factors produced by oligodendrocytes have potent developmental and survival effects on the oligodendrocytes themselves. Like neurons, oligodendrocytes are highly sensitive to injury by oxidative stress, excitatory amino acids, and activation of apoptotic pathways. Understanding the mechanism of oligodendrocyte death could contribute to new therapeutic strategies to preserve or restore white matter function and structure after brain injury.

Taken together, oligodendrocytes and neurons are rather inert cells that can not be activated to induce strong immune responses and produce any wide variety of inflammatory mediators. In contrast, they are important target cells within the CNS, and easily damaged through cytotoxic molecules. Microglia and astrocytes are the most effective immune effector cells within the CNS. The sensitivity of microglia to microenvironmental changes enables them to function as sentinels, while astrocytes deactivate the microglia functions and suppress immune responses within the CNS, thereby contributing to the maintenance of the CNS immune privilege (Fig. 14.2).

Immune response of the CNS

Unlike most peripheral tissue, the CNS functions through a network of post-mitotic cells that are believed to be incapable of regeneration and hence cannot be replaced when aging or impaired. Being simultaneously essential for survival and unable to recover fully from injury, the CNS is in special need of protection from pathogens and damage. Immune surveillance and immune function of the CNS are conditional. They are minimal under healthy conditions but can be induced, whenever required. Several features are unique for this regulated type of immune responsiveness within the CNS.

Under healthy conditions Under normal conditions, the BBB prevents inflow of leukocytes, antibodies, complement factors, and cytokines into the brain parenchyma. Only a small number of T cells, which were triggered by an antigen-specific stimulus in peripheral immune organs, have the ability to pass through the BBB, but they cannot encounter the cells of the intact CNS. Although microglia of the healthy brain can have occasional contact with cellular components of the immune system and their release products, and also successfully present antigen and seems to be rather efficient in restimulating lymphocytes, these processes are under strict control.

First, the intact CNS lacks professional APC, like DC, macrophages, and B cells. The absence of functional APC within the CNS prevents the initiation and propagation of antigen-specific immune responses. Second, there is low level of MHC expression in the CNS. In particular, healthy brain is almost devoid of MHC class II, which would seem to disallow induction of CD4$^+$

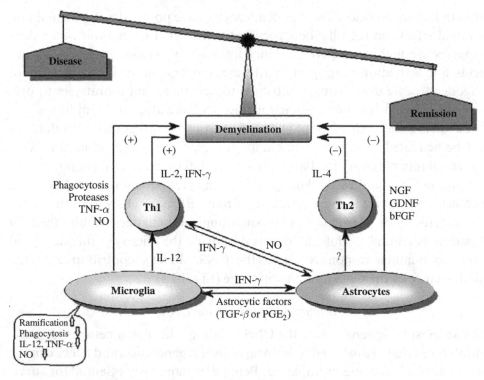

Figure 14.2. The balance between microglia and astrocytes in regulating Th1/Th2 cell responses and demyelinating processes. The left panel represents positive regulation of microglia by promotion of Th1 cell responses and production of proteases, tumor necrosis factor alpha (TNF-α), and nitric oxide (NO). The right panel demonstrates negative regulation of astrocytes by induction of Th2 cell responses and secretion of nerve growth factor (NGF), glial-cell-line-derived neurotrophic factor (GDNF), and basic fibroblast growth factor (bFGF). The lower panel indicates that astrocytes can deactivate microglia by astrocytic factors transforming growth factor beta (TGF-β) and prostaglandin E_2 (PGE$_2$). The production of PGE$_2$ by microglia presents a negative feedback mechanism, limiting the propagation of Th1 responses. Interferon gamma (IFN-γ) secreted by activated microglia and Th1 cells could induce PGE$_2$ and NO production by astrocytes and contribute to the downregulation of microglia and Th1 cell responses.

T cell responses. Third, CNS parenchymal tissue that contributes to relative immune privilege of the CNS may represent an immunosuppressive environment. Constitutive expression of FasL within the CNS can induce Fas-expressing leukocytes to apoptosis, thus conferring protection to the tissue.[11] Astrocytes seem to induce apoptosis of transformed T cells in vitro by FasL expression on astrocytes.[11] Fourth, normal physiologically active neurons have a general suppressive potential that prevents and limits the development of inflammation. Fifth, several soluble factors such as TGF-β,

IL-10, and TNF-related apoptosis-inducing ligand (TRAIL), also constitute an immunosuppressive environment within the CNS. Astrocytes have been identified as a major source of these immunomodulatory cytokines.

Under inflammatory/pathologic conditions The past few years have seen significant progress towards understanding the mechanisms of glial cells and inflammation within the CNS. Interestingly, almost all degenerative CNS diseases are associated with signs of CNS inflammation.[8] The spectrum of inflammatory diseases of the CNS has been steadily expanding from disorders such as multiple sclerosis (MS) with a proposed autoimmune background, to more diverse diseases, like Alzheimer's disease and stroke. However, the grade of the CNS inflammation in degenerative diseases strongly depends on immune responses of the diseases. In MS, "full-blown" immune activation is observed.[12] Microglia and astrocytes are induced to express MHC class I and II. Further, microglia express the co-stimulatory molecules B7-1 and B7-2, which allow primary initiation of antigen-specific immune responses. Recently, dendritic cells expressing CD11c have been observed in the perivascular area in mice with experimental allergic encephalomyelitis (EAE).[4] Inflammation is a key component of host defence responses to pathogens and injury, but it is now also recognized as a major contributor to diverse acute and chronic CNS disorders. During the development and persistence of inflammation, complement, adhesion molecules, cyclo-oxygenase enzymes and their products as well as cytokines are increased, as seen both in experimental and human CNS diseases. Interventional studies in experimental animals suggest that several of these factors contribute directly to neuronal injury. Some specific cytokines, such as IL-1 and TNF-α, have been strongly implicated in acute neurodegeneration such as stroke and traumatic brain injury. Glial cells and neurons produce or express all of the activation and regulatory proteins and the C3a/C5a receptors.

Inflammation may have beneficial as well as detrimental actions in the CNS. Activated microglia secrete pro-inflammatory cytokines such as TNF-α and IL-1β, activate complement factors, and promote release of free radicals,[13] which are toxic for neurons. Secretion of NO by stimulated microglia may underlie a more general pathway of T cell death in the CNS, thereby inducing apoptosis of infiltrating T cells and preventing the differentiation of microglia to become effective APC. DC within the CNS may also play a key role for maintaining immune privilege within the inflamed CNS.[14] Nevertheless, several anti-inflammatory principles have been suggested as putative treatments for CNS disorders that include both acute disease states and chronic neurodegenerative conditions. For example, the inflammatory and immune components of syndromes such as Alzheimer's disease and stroke may be amenable to treatment by anti-inflammatory and immunotherapeutic approaches.[15]

14.2.2 Special structure of the peripheral nervous system

Blood–nerve barrier

The blood–nerve barrier (BNB) is a cylindrical structure formed partly by membranes composed of tightly joined perineurial cell layers. In addition, there is a cylindrical structure made up of endoneural endothelial cells also united by specialized junctures.[16] These tend to keep blood away from axons and to impede the passage of circulating substances into the endoneural environment. Fluorescence label indicates that it was observed in the external nerve sheath and slightly in the endoneurium of these nerves, but was not observed within nerve fibers, suggesting that the vascular barrier in human peripheral nerves is incomplete.[17] Based on the present reports, the co-culture of peripheral nerve microvascular endothelial cells (PnMECs) and pericytes appears to be useful in constructing BNB model in vitro.

The BNB in peripheral nerves is important for maintaining the environment for axons. Breakdown of the barrier by nerve injury causes various pathologies, which are associated with changes in the expression of intercellular junctional proteins, including claudins, occludin, VE-cadherin, and connexin 43.[18]

Resident cells of the peripheral nervous system

Previous studies demonstrate that Schwann cells constitute the satellite cell of the peripheral nervous system (PNS), and they surround axons and motor nerve terminals. Besides maintaining insulation of axons and correct localization of ion channels, the relationships among Schwann cells, axons, and the perineurial barrier emphasize that Schwann cells play a key role in normal functions of the nerve. Schwann cells are responsible for action potential velocity through insulation of axons, maintenance of axonal caliber, immunological and functional integrity of the nerve through the perineurial BNB, and effective nerve regeneration. Schwann cells signal not only to themselves but also to the other cellular components within the nerve to act as major regulators of nerve development. In addition, Schwann cells utilize short focal tight junctions to provide morphological stabilization of the contact with the elongating axon, as well as small-scale gap junctions to facilitate traffic of substances between them. Nerve regeneration is not a simple phenomenon of axonal elongation on the part of the Schwann cell membrane, but is based on direct and dynamic communication between the axon and the neighboring Schwann cell, which may be partly associated with the mechanisms of neural regeneration.

Immune response of the peripheral nervous system

The PNS displays structural barriers and a lack of lymphatic drainage that strongly limit the access of molecules and cells from the immune system. In addition, the PNS has the ability to set up some specific mechanisms of immune protection to limit the pathogenicity of inflammatory processes following insults by pathogens. Schwann cells are among the most prominent cells that can display immune capabilities in the PNS. Numerous in vitro studies have shown that Schwann cells are indeed able to display properties of immune responses, ranging from the participation in antigen presentation, to secretion of pro- and anti-inflammatory cytokines, chemokines and neurotrophic factors. This could exacerbate a BNB breakdown that has been increasingly implicated in inflammatory demyelinating neuropathies. Schwann cells can reactivate P_0 and P_2 peptide-specific $CD4^+$ T cell lines. Activated T cells cause focal breakdown of the BNB, allowing circulating anti-myelin antibody to enter the endoneurium with consequent focal demyelination. Activated $CD4^+$ T cells may help B cells to produce antibodies against peripheral nerve components, thereby inducing activation of either complement or antibody-dependent cytolytic cells, or they may operate by recruiting macrophages to exert damage on peripheral nerve tissue. Using a T cell proliferation assay, it was observed that the expression of MHC class II by Schwann cells indicates a potential facultative role of Schwann cells in the presentation of antigen to neuritogenic T cells during inflammatory demyelinating neuropathies.[19] Human Schwann cells also express MHC class I antigens in vivo and thus may serve as cytotoxic targets for $CD8^+$ autoreactive T lymphocytes. Activated $CD8^+$ T cells or their soluble products have a direct cytotoxic effect on myelin and Schwann cells or, alternatively, can play a role as suppressor cells in recovery of patients with Guillain–Barré syndrome (GBS).

The BNB disruption may permit large molecules like immunoglobulins to enter the endoneurial space, contributing to development of autoimmune demyelinative neuropathy. Anti-GM1 antibody, frequently detected in sera from patients with inflammatory neuropathies, may contribute to BNB dysfunction and development of neuropathy. Intraneural injection of sera or purified immunoglobulin G (IgG) from patients with chronic inflammatory demyelinating polyradiculoneuropathy (CIDP) produced marked conduction block and demyelination, supporting an important role for anti-myelin/Schwann cell autoantibodies in the pathogenesis of CIDP at least in some patients. Accumulation of immunoglobulin was maximal during the worsening of neurological deficit, and declined rapidly before the onset of neurological recovery.[20] Ligation of the chemokine receptor CXCR4 on Schwann cells by HIV gp120 resulted in the release of RANTES ("regulated upon activation normally T cell expressed and secreted"), which induced dorsal root ganglion neurons to produce TNF-α and subsequent TNF receptor-1 (TNFR1) mediated neurotoxicity in an autocrine fashion, revealing that inter-action between Schwann cells and neurons may be pathogenically relevant in other peripheral neuropathies.[21]

14.3 Animal models of immune-mediated neuropathologies

While insight into human diseases is mainly based on biopsy material and in vitro analysis, a better understanding of the pathogenic mechanisms of these complex and heterogeneous disorders can be obtained from studies on animal models, offering the possibility to explore the complex interaction of genetic and immunological factors. Animal models for CNS autoimmune diseases provide a rational basis for studying mechanisms of pathogenesis and new immunother-apeutic strategies. However, no single animal model exists that mimics all the features of human diseases but the available models reflect specific facets.

14.3.1 Experimental autoimmune encephalomyelitis

Acute experimental autoimmune encephalomyelitis (EAE) can be reliably elicited in Lewis rats by immunization with myelin basic protein (MBP). The advantage of this model is high incidence (almost 100%) and low variation of clinical score, making it especially suitable for studies of new therapies. Sensitized T cells can generate adoptive EAE, giving conclusive proof of the pivotal pathogenic role of T cells. The value of the Lewis rat EAE model for the elucidation of the pathogenesis of MS is limited by the lack of spontaneous relapses, and also by the absence of demyelinating lesions. A significant amount of demyelination can be observed by co-transfer of anti-myelin oligo-dendrocyte glycoprotein (MOG) antibodies and encephalitogenic T cells or recombinant human MOG, when performed in Lewis rats or Lewis AV1 strains. EAE in mice shares many features with MS in humans because it has a chronic-relapsing course and also shows histopathological evidence of demyelination. Both actively induced EAE and adoptive transfer EAE can be investigated in different mice strains. The main advantage of mouse EAE is that genetically engineered mutants can be bred.

Theiler's murine encephalomyelitis viruses (TMEV) belong to the Picornaviridae and are natural pathogens of mice. In susceptible strains, such as SJL or DBA/1, persistent infection of the CNS with TMEV leads to chronic progressive and immune-mediated demyelination. Although TMEV-induced demyelinating disease is initiated by virus-specific CD4$^+$ T cells targeting virus persisting in the CNS, CD4$^+$ T cell responses against self myelin epitopes are also activated via epitope spreading, thereby contributing to development of chronic disease.[22] Histological features of the pathological lesion in TMEV infection and MS are very similar.

Cellular immunity in EAE

During the past two decades, emphasis has been placed on investigating the role of T lymphocytes in the pathological process of EAE since EAE can be passively transferred by myelin-reactive T cells that contain high levels of the pro-inflammatory cytokines IFN-γ and lymphotoxin/TNF-α, indicating that CD4$^+$ T cells of the Th1 subset are responsible for transfer of EAE. It is generally accepted that the encephalitogenic T cells cross the BBB and secrete pro-inflammatory cytokines and chemokines that attract other leukocytes to the local environment. The inflammatory lesions contain T cells and macrophages and/or microglia, as well as some B cells. In addition, myelin antigen-specific CD8$^+$ T cells are encephalitogenic and produce severe EAE in C57BL/6 mice.

Besides T cells, microglia and perivascular macrophages are believed to act as APC during the effector phase of EAE. If CNS-reactive T cells survive in the CNS, they have the potential to attack the CNS, through either their products or the recruitment of other inflammatory cells. Under inflammation, microglia express MHC class II molecules, and can present antigenic peptides to CD4$^+$ T cells. If microglia express co-stimulatory molecules such as B7-1 or B7-2, it may provide a co-stimulatory signal to T cells through CD28, thereby inducing the reactivation of infiltrating T cells within the CNS. By contrast, if microglia express CD95L it may ligate T cell CD95 and induce apoptosis of T cells. Microglia produce other proapoptotic signals such as NO, which can induce T cell apoptosis. Microglia also participate in the phagocytosis of apoptotic lymphocytes in the CNS. Phagocytosis of apoptotic cells is a general mechanism for clearing these cells from tissues. The interactions of T cells with microglia can lead to either proliferation or apoptosis of T cells. A possible role for astrocytes in EAE is that astrocytes present CNS antigens to T cells but fail to provide co-stimulatory signals, thereby leading to activation-induced T cell anergy. Astrocyte-derived soluble factor(s), rather than direct cell–cell interactions, seem to be responsible for the inhibitory effect of T and B cell

functions. Compared to microglia, supernatants from IFN-γ-stimulated astrocytes inhibit MBP-reactive T and B cell functions, indicating the role for
astrocytes in the inactivation of MBP-reactive T and B cells.[23]

CNS inflammation in EAE is associated with the proliferation of CD11b$^+$
brain cells that exhibit DC marker CD11c. CD11c$^+$ cells from inflamed brain
proved to be distinct from other microglia, but strikingly resembled bone
marrow-derived DC and thus were identified as DC. DC are more potent
stimulators of naive or allogeneic T cell proliferation. Consistently, a functional maturation of brain DC was observed to occur following the onset of
encephalitis.[4] These findings indicate that in addition to inflammatory macro-
phage-like brain cells, intraparenchymatical DC exist in autoimmune and
infectious encephalitis, and might contribute to the chronicity of intracerebral
Th1 responses. However, DC isolated from mice with EAE were unable to
prime naive T cells, and inhibited T cell proliferation, indicating that CNS DC
may play a key responsible role for maintaining immune privilege within the
inflamed CNS.[14] Results from our laboratory show that TGF-β1 contributes
to DC differentiation from glial cells in vitro,[2] and that TGF-β1-induced glial
cell-derived DC effectively inhibited the expansion of MBP-reactive T cells.[24]

Humoral immunity in EAE

Some of the controversy surrounding the role of antibodies in MS pathogenesis arises from the data obtained using models of EAE. On the one hand, EAE
is induced in susceptible animals following active immunization with various
myelin proteins or passive transfer of T cells specific for these myelin proteins.
B cells and antibodies are unable to induce EAE in susceptible animal strains.
No direct correlation has been found between antibody titers and disease
severity. Induction of EAE in B cell-deficient mice revealed that B cells and/
or antibodies are necessary in the generation of EAE immunized with peptides
of MBP and MOG.

On the other hand, evidence derived from recent studies of the MS lesion,
and of the EAE model has led to a renewed interest in a role for B cells and the
humoral immune system in the pathogenesis of MS and EAE. The demyelinating pathology is probably a consequence of synergy between autoimmune
T and B cells as extensive demyelinating lesions are observed in the rat
following adoptively transferred MBP-reactive T cells when subsequently
injected with anti-MOG antibodies. B cell-deficient mice were resistant to
EAE induced with MOG, whereas wild-type mice were susceptible to MOG-
induced EAE. Histological examination of spinal cord demonstrated a general
lack of inflammation and demyelinating pathology in the B cell-deficient mice.
These data suggest that B cells and antibodies are important to the disease

process. Anti-MOG antibodies also are critical to EAE induction in a primate (marmoset) model, and potentiate MBP-induced EAE in Lewis rats. In mice genetically engineered to produce high levels of MOG-specific antibodies, EAE was accelerated and disease severity exacerbated, even when EAE was induced by myelin antigens other than MOG.[25]

The variability in the pathogenicity of myelin antibodies is probably comparable to the heterogeneity of myelin-reactive T cells for the induction of EAE and is likely to be dependent on the isotype and epitope specificity of the antibodies or the ability to interact with fragment crystallizable (Fc) receptors or fix complement. The presence of C5a, a proteolytic fragment generated during complement activation cascade, has been documented during all stages (preclinical, early acute, peak, and remission phases) of EAE induced in rats by active immunization with spinal cord homogenate. It has been reported that demyelination and axonal damage occur in the presence of antibodies and require activation of the entire complement cascade, including the membrane attack complex (MAC) deposition.[26] In contrast, it has also been demonstrated that C3, a key component in complememt activation, is not essential in MOG-induced EAE in mice.[27] Absence of C5 resulted in fiber loss and extensive scarring, whereas presence of C5 favored axonal survival and more efficient remyelination.[28] The cellular source of CNS expression of C5aR has been shown to be mainly microglia, activated astrocytes, and infiltrating mononuclear cells.

14.3.2 Experimental autoimmune myasthenia gravis

In the 1970s, it was found that a syndrome similar to the human myasthenia gravis (MG) can be induced in experimental animals by immunization with electrophorus acetylcholine receptor (AChR). Experimental autoimmune myasthenia gravis (EAMG) has been induced in the monkey, dog, rabbit, guinea pig, rat, and mouse. Characteristics shared by human MG and animal EAMG include: muscular weakness and flaccid paralysis which is aggravated by exercise and relieved by cholinesterase inhibitors, hypersensitivity to curare, low-amplitude miniature endplate potentials, decrementing compound muscle action potentials, simplification of the postsynaptic membrane at neuromuscular junction, and the presence of circulating autoantibodies reactive with autologous AChR. Passive transfer EAMG can be induced by transfer of polyclonal or monoclonal anti-AChR antibodies. In inbred rat strains, the susceptibility for EAMG is Wistar Munich > Fischer > Lewis > Buffalo > Brown Norway > ACI > Wistar Kyoto > Kopenhagen > Wistar Furth. In mice, the strains with H-2^b haplotype are highly susceptible to EAMG, while those with H-2^q are intermediate in susceptibility, and strains with H-2^k and H-2^p haplotypes are relatively resistant.

Cellular immunity in EAMG

EAMG is a typical antibody-mediated disease, but the production of pathogenic antibodies by B cells may depend on T helper cells. When antibodies reach the endplates, the local debris of AChR antibody complexes is removed to the draining lymph nodes where the autoimmune response is maintained. The passive transfer of anti-AChR antibodies resulted in increased expression of AChR subunit genes, mainly at synaptic regions, and this may ensure a continuous supply of self-antigen. Depletion of $CD8^+$ T cells effectively suppressed clinical EAMG and anti-AChR antibody levels.[29] When $CD4^-8^-$ mutant mice were immunized with AChR, clinical EAMG was nearly completely prevented, accompanied with strongly reduced AChR-specific T and B cell responses.[30] $CD4^+$ T cells have a pathogenic role, by permitting and facilitating the synthesis of high-affinity anti-AChR antibodies. Th1 $CD4^+$ cells are especially important because they drive the synthesis of anti-AChR complement-fixing IgG subclasses. Binding of those antibodies to the muscle AChR at the neuromuscular junction will trigger the complement-mediated destruction of the postsynaptic membrane. Th2 cells secrete different cytokines, with different effects on the pathogenesis of EAMG. Among them, IL-10, which is a potent growth and differentiation factor for B cells, facilitates the development of EAMG.[31] In rat EAMG, both Th1 and Th2 cells are able to induce pathogenic anti-AChR antibodies. Manipulation of the Th1 and Th2 balance does not affect the severity of disease.[32] Unlike mouse IgG subclasses, both Th1- and Th2-associated rat IgG subclasses are capable of binding complement. In human, both Th1 and Th2 cells are able to induce the production of complement-binding antibodies. It can be concluded from these studies that rat EAMG models are more relevant for the study of human MG.

Humoral immunity in EAMG

Evidence for antibody-mediated damage of AChR is that EAMG can be induced by passive transfer of IgG or sera from patients with MG to mice, or from rats with EAMG to healthy rats. A majority of anti-AChR antibodies in EAMG are directed to the main immunogenic region (MIR) in the α subunit. Sequence analysis of monoclonal antibodies immortalized from B cells of EAMG animals reveals a high number of somatic mutations, indicating that the immune response is antigen-driven. The immunological attack of anti-AChR antibodies is directed at the postsynaptic membrane of the neuromuscular junction, where three regulatory mechanisms aim to limit or restore the damage:

(1) B cell-activating factor (BAFF)-derived B cell activation. EAMG is an antibody-mediated autoimmune disease. Blocking BAFF in vivo confirms that it is required for production of antigen-specific antibodies and development of germinal centers in the spleen. An increased BAFF is sufficient to cause antibody-mediated autoimmune diseases.[33] Increased levels of BAFF have been detected in serum from patients with systemic lupus erythematosus and rheumatoid arthritis, and the level of BAFF correlates with the level of autoantibodies.[34] AChR-pulsed DC induce peripheral tolerance to EAMG by possibly inhibiting the expression of BAFF and production of anti-AChR antibodies.[35]

(2) The role for complement and complement regulatory proteins. Muscle cells are able to upregulate the synthesis of complete regulatory proteins (CD55, CD59, and vitronectin) as a defensive mechanism against complement-mediated damage. When anti-AChR antibodies bind to the tip of the postsynaptic folds, the classical complement pathway is activated. This results in the formation of MAC, thereby affecting focal lysis of the postsynaptic membrane. Mice that lack CD55 are markedly more susceptible to AChR antibody-induced EAMG.[36] CD55 inhibits C3 production, and CD59 inhibits the formation of MAC.[36] Antibody blocking of CD55 in the presence of sensitizing antibody results in increased C3b deposition and significantly increased exosome lysis. Blockade of CD59 also results in significant lysis, while blocking both CD55 and CD59 exhibits additional lysis.[37] These molecules could be used as therapeutic agents to rapidly reverse a myasthenia crisis.

(3) The role of AChR anchor protein. Clustering of AChR is a critical step in neuromuscular synaptogenesis, and is induced by agrin and laminin which are thought to act through different signaling mechanisms. MG patients without detectable anti-AChR antibodies (about 15%) clearly have a humorally mediated disorder since they improve clinically with plasma exchange, and injection of their IgG or Ig fractions into mice results in defects in neuromuscular transmission. In these patients, IgG antibodies against the muscle-specific kinase (MuSK) have been described, which reduced agrin-induced AChR clustering in vitro.[38] These antibodies are not found in AChR antibody-positive MG and are predominantly IgG4.[39] MuSK, a surface membrane receptor essential for the development of the neuromuscular junction, is involved in maintaining AChR at high density at the synapse.

14.3.3 Experimental autoimmune neuritis

Since Waksman and Adams first described experimental autoimmune neuritis (EAN) in 1955 by inoculating rabbits with homogenized PNS tissue, investigators have studied EAN in various species. In susceptible rat strains, EAN can be actively induced by immunization with purified PNS myelin or peptides. Mice of strain SJL developed a mild neurological deficit and histological lesions characteristic of EAN, whereas BALB/c and C57BL/6 mice were relatively resistant to disease induction. Recently, EAN in C57BL/6 mice has been induced by active immunization with P_0 peptides 56–71 and 180–199 in combination with pertussis toxin. Acute EAN mirrors many of the morphological and electrophysiological aspects of GBS, and thus serves as an animal model for GBS. Chronic EAN has been developed as a model of the human CIDP. Chronic EAN was induced by immunization of rabbits with galactocerebroside. This model underscores the pathogenic contribution of circulating autoantibodies for the induction of demyelinating lesions. Adoptive transfer EAN of differing disease severity was induced by peripheral nervous myelin-specific T cells. Progressive nerve conduction changes consistent with demyelination in the sciatic nerve and lumbar nerve roots were observed during the disease. The electrophysiological changes in EAN induced by myelin-specific T cells are very similar to those seen clinically during GBS dominated by demyelination, whereas it has less resemblance to axonal forms of GBS.

Cellular immunity in EAN

Activated autoreactive T cells, which recognize peripheral nerve autoantigens in the presence of resident macrophages or Schwann cells, cross the BNB and generate an immune response within the PNS that orchestrates the invasion of T cells and macrophages/monocytes. Using $CD4^-8^-$, and B cell knockout mice, it was observed that CD4 and CD8T cells, but not B cells, play a critical role in the development of murine EAN. The importance of T cells is further supported by the prevention of EAN by treatment with antibodies directed at the α/β T cell receptor. Invasion of the PNS by T cells has been documented immunocytochemically, and the degree of cellular infiltration subsequently correlates well with the degree of nerve function deficit. T cell infiltration is the first pathological sign in EAN, accompanied by a rapid increase in permeability of the BNB. Before onset of clinical signs, most T cells express the $CD4^+$ phenotype, whereas $CD8^+$ T cells prevail after the peak of the disease and during recovery. Although macrophages greatly outnumber lymphocytes in affected peripheral nervous tissue, there is increasing evidence that a small population of target-specific T cells can control a vast majority of non-specific inflammatory cells and regulate their behavior. Resident macrophages constitutively express the MHC class II antigen and complement receptor 3 (CR3). The location of these cells adjacent to blood vessels presumably facilitates their interaction with trafficking T cells, thus serving as major APC in acute EAN. The activation and differentiation of autoreactive T cells within the PNS in turn results in recruitment of macrophages and B cells. This augments the damage in the PNS in an antibody-mediated and complement-dependent manner.

Humoral immunity in EAN

The importance of humoral factors in demyelinating diseases of the PNS is underlined by the therapeutic effect of plasma exchange and immunoabsorption in GBS. Although systemic injection of EAN serum alone cannot transfer the disease, specific demyelination occurs when antisera to galactocerebroside and to a much lesser degree to P_0 are injected intraneurally. Systemic administration of antibodies to galactocerebroside also enhances the demyelination produced by adoptive transfer of neurotogenic T cells. In galactocerebroside-induced EAN, circulating IgG antibodies to galactocerebroside in the serum and deposits of IgG in the spinal roots were detectable weeks before definite clinical, morphological, and electrophysiological alterations occurred. This model underscores the pathogenetic contribution of circulating autoantibodies for the induction of demyelinating lesions. High titers of circulating antibodies against galactocerebroside could be detected, whereas T cell infiltration was absent, and only moderate numbers of macrophages were observed. There are several mechanisms by which antibodies might mediate demyelination. First, upon binding to macrophages via the Fc receptor, they could direct these cells to autoantigenic structures and mediate antibody-dependent cytotoxicity. Second, antibodies may activate the classic complement pathway with subsequent formation of the terminal complement complex. Finally, antibodies may serve as a tool to opsonize target structures and promote their internalization by macrophages.

14.3.4 Immunotherapeutic strategies in CNS and PNS autoimmune diseases

Animal models have been crucial for understanding the major mechanisms of immune-mediated damage in human disorders and exploring therapeutic strategies, although they do not always mimic all the features of the human diseases. Only through animal models can we experimentally delineate the sequence of events in immune-mediated attacks, and design immunotherapeutic strategy. Immunosuppressive drugs have been introduced for the treatment of CNS and PNS autoimmune diseases in the early 1960s and are widely used. Long-term use of immunosuppressive drugs has been associated with a risk of development of malignant diseases or infection. In principle, all the different stages of cellular activation, transmigration, pro-inflammatory mediators, and effector mechanisms of the immune responses can be manipulated by immunotherapeutic strategies. The study of modern immunotherapies is moving rapidly in animal models, including EAE, EAMG, and EAN.

Therapeutic targets directed at the trimolecular complex

Because $CD4^+$ T cells are important mediators in the pathogenesis of autoimmune disease, they are ideal candidates for immunotherapy. Peripheral tolerance represents an attractive strategy to downregulate previously activated T cells and to suppress ongoing disease. Mucosal tolerance is a state of immune hyporesponsiveness induced by the oral or nasal exposure to antigens, depending on the dose of the oral or nasal antigen administered or combination with cytokines such as IL-4 and IL-10. Low dose of antigen stimulates regulatory T cell development, and leads to active immune suppression that is transferable via T cells. The active mechanism appears to be a cytokine-mediated immune deviation with predominant Th2 and Th3 (TGF-β) responses. In contrast, a high dose of oral antigen leads to clonal deletion and anergy. The active suppression by low dose oral tolerance can also suppress an unrelated immune response (bystander suppression), paving the way for therapy of autoimmune diseases.

Many therapeutic principles have been directed against the trimolecular complex, but this has proved to be very difficult to target. In most diseases, the target antigens have been poorly understood or cannot be identified at an individual level. Oral tolerance to antigens was successfully employed in a variety of experimental models for autoimmune diseases. The results obtained in experimental animal models led to the conduction of several clinical trials of oral tolerance in patients with autoimmune background. Conflicting but mostly negative results were obtained, and although some improvement was noted in some of the patients, broad-ranging clinical improvement has not yet been observed. Because of the large numbers of autoantigens involved in human autoimmune diseases, it might be difficult to identify individual patients who might respond to the administered antigen (homologous versus heterologous).

Therapeutic targets directed at co-stimulatory signals

A co-stimulatory second signal plays an important role for complete T cell activation. Therapeutic manipulation of these molecules is being investigated. The B7 family of cell surface molecules expressed on APC is capable of providing this second signal to T cells via two receptors, CD28 and CTLA-4. It appears that the co-stimulation provided by B7-1 is important in disease development, while B7-2 may play an important regulatory role. Similarly, anti-B7-1 administration was protective, while anti-B7-2 administration exacerbated EAE. Recent evidence suggests that peripheral tolerance of antigen-specific T cells induced in vivo may require CTLA-4 engagement of the tolerized T cells. Selective upregulation of CTLA-4 or blocking the B7–CD28 pathway may mediate peripheral tolerance. In the adoptive transfer model of EAE, CTLA-4 Ig inhibited the proliferation and IL-2 production of MBP-specific lymph node cells during activation in vitro, resulting in reduced clinical disease upon subsequent transfer.[40] In actively induced EAE, a single injection of CTLA-4 Ig inhibited the development of disease.

Therapeutic agents directed at intracellular signals, adhesion molecules, and cytokines

Approaches such as modulation of intracellular signaling pathways seem currently to hold more promise. Leflunomide, an inhibitor of tyrosine kinase signaling, has been successfully used in EAN, and may be a promising alternative for human autoimmune neuropathies. Another approach is to block cellular adhesion to the vessel wall and regression of inflammatory cells from the bloodstream to the target tissues. The integrin very late antigen 4 (VLA-4) has been shown to play a key role in the entry of antigen-specific T cells into the CNS during autoimmune demyelination. A synthetic antagonist of VLA-4 (TBC 3486) delayed disease onset and suppressed clinical severity and demyelination in chronic relapsing EAE.[41] Oral or subcutaneous administration of anti-inflammatory cytokines, such as IL-4, IL-10, and TGF-β, can effectively suppress severity of clinical signs in rat and mice EAE.

Therapeutic targets directed at gene delivery

Gene therapy protocols aimed to deliver therapeutic molecules into the CNS and PNS may represent an alternative therapeutic strategy in patients affected by inflammatory demyelinating diseases of the CNS and PNS where systemic therapies have shown limited therapeutic efficacy possibly due to the BBB or BNB. Primary T cells and hybridomas rapidly and preferentially home to the sites of inflammation in organ-specific autoimmune disease. These cells if transduced with retroviral vectors to drive expression of various "regulatory proteins," such as IL-4, IL-10, and IL-12p40, deliver these immunoregulatory proteins to the inflamed lesions by "peripheral" or intrathecal gene delivery, providing therapy for experimental models of autoimmune disease. The peripheral gene therapy approach shows some disadvantages, while the intrathecal gene delivery shows some major advantages: (1) availability of high levels of the "therapeutic molecule" in all areas of the CNS, (2) persistent therapeutic effect after a single vector administration, and (3) lack of interference with the peripheral immune system.

Therapeutic targets directed at dendritic cells

There is increasing evidence that DC could be used as a tool to induce peripheral tolerance. Immature DC, plasmacytoid DC and IL-10-modified DC can mediate immune tolerance by several different mechanisms. Several possibilities exist for rational modulation of DC to achieve therapeutic tolerance against autoimmune diseases. Lewis rats receiving TGF-β1-modified DC developed very mild symptoms of EAMG without loss of body weight.[42] IFN-γ-exposed DC also effectively treated acute and chronic-relapsing EAE in rats and mice. (Fig. 14.3)[43] These results demonstrate that different types of DC mediate peripheral tolerance possibly through different pathways. One approach for DC-based immunotherapy could be creation of optimal prerequisites to use autologous DC that are prepared from the individual patient with autoimmune disease, to render such DC tolerogenic by exposure in vitro to factors that promote tolerogenicity, and to reinfuse these pretreated DC to the patient in order to treat the ongoing autoimmune disease and prevent its future exacerbation.

Several immunotherapeutic strategies have frequently given favorable results in the experimental models, but have been shown not to be clinically effective. This could be due to several reasons. First, the homogeneity among animals used in the experimental models is non-existent in humans, in whom a given pathological condition instead may show a high variability. Second, the procedure of the experimental model itself does not correspond to the clinical situation seen in humans. Third, there may exist pathophysiological differences between experimental animals and humans. Fourth, the substances tested have different pathophysiological or pharmacological properties in the different species. Identifying the reasons for divergences between experimental and clinical situations can help to optimize experimental models so that they actually become comparable with the human diseases.

14.4 Concluding remarks

Taken together, recent advances have demonstrated a vast network of communication pathways between the nerve and immune systems. Lymphoid organs are innervated by branches of the autonomic nervous system. Accessory immune cells and lymphocytes have membrane receptors for most neurotransmitters and neuropeptides. These receptors are functional, and their activation leads to changes in immune functions, including cell proliferation and specific immune responses. Brain lesion can induce a number of changes in the function of the immune responses. The communication

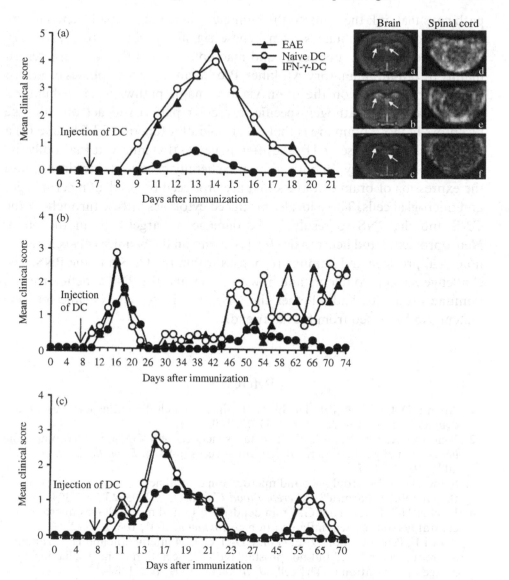

Figure 14.3. Therapeutic potential of IFN-γ DC in EAE. (a) Lewis rats were immunized with encephalitogenic peptide MBP 68–86 + complete Freund's adjevant (CFA) and were subcutaneously injected with PBS, naive DC, or IFN-γ DC; (b) SJL/J mice were immunized with the proteolipid protein PLP peptide 139–151 + CFA and were subcutaneously injected with PBS, naive DC, or IFN-γ DC; (c) B6 mice were immunized with MOG peptide 35–55 + CFA and were subcutaneously injected with PBS, naive DC, or IFN-γ DC. Insert are magnetic resonance imaging axial slices of brain (A–C) and lumbar spinal cord level (D–F) performed in Lewis rat EAE injected with PBS (A and D), naive DC (B and E), and IFN-γ DC (C and F). Note enlarged lateral ventricles and third ventricle (arrows) in (A) PBS- and (B) naive DC-injected rats, and normal size of ventricles in (C) IFN-γ DC-injected rats. Note also scattered T2 lesions in axial slices at the lumbar spinal cord level in (D) PBS- and (E) naive DC-injected rats, and normal T2 appearance in (F) IFN-γ DC-injected rats.

pathways that link the brain to the immune system are normally activated by signals from the immune system. These signals originate from accessory immune cells such as monocytes and macrophages and they are represented mainly by pro-inflammatory cytokines. Pro-inflammatory cytokines produced in the periphery act on the brain via two major pathways: (1) a humoral pathway allowing pathogen-specific molecular patterns to act on Toll-like receptors in those brain areas that are devoid of a functional BBB, and (2) a neural pathway represented by the afferent nerves that innervate the bodily site of infection and injury. In both cases, peripherally produced cytokines induce the expression of brain cytokines that are produced by resident macrophages and microglial cells. These locally produced cytokines diffuse throughout the CNS and the PNS to result in the damage of target cells in the brain. Neuroprotective and neurotoxic effects depend on the balance between immunological privilege and immune responses within the CNS and the PNS. The challenge remains to understand how the CNS and the PNS benefits from its immune properties and whether the CNS, the PNS and systemic immune system can be turned from foes to friends.

References

1. Allen DD, Lockman PR. The blood–brain barrier choline transporter as a brain drug delivery vector. *Life Sci.* 2003, **73**: 1609–1615.
2. Xiao BG, Xu LY, Yang JS. TGF-beta 1 synergizes with GM-CSF to promote the generation of glial cell-derived dendriform cells in vitro. *Brain Behav. Immun.* 2002, **16**: 685–697.
3. Schwartz M. Macrophages and microglia in central nervous system injury: are they helpful or harmful? *J. Cereb. Blood Flow Metab.* 2003, **23**: 385–394.
4. Fischer HG, Reichmann G. Brain dendritic cells and macrophages/microglia in central nervous system inflammation. *J. Immunol.* 2001, **166**: 2717–2726.
5. Aloisi F, Penna G, Polazzi E, *et al.* CD40–CD154 interaction and IFN-gamma are required for IL-12 but not prostaglandin E2 secretion by microglia during antigen presentation to Th1 cells. *J. Immunol.* 1999, **162**: 1384–1391.
6. Dong Y, Benveniste EN. Immune function of astrocytes. *Glia* 2001, **36**: 180–190.
7. Dietrich PY, Walker PR, Saas P. Death receptors on reactive astrocytes: a key role in the fine tuning of brain inflammation? *Neurology* 2003, **60**: 548–554.
8. Neumann H. Control of glial immune function by neurons. *Glia* 2001, **36**: 191–199.
9. Flugel A, Schwaiger FW, Neumann H, *et al.* Neuronal FasL induces cell death of encephalitogenic T lymphocytes. *Brain Pathol.* 2000, **10**: 353–364.
10. Buntinx M, Stinissen P, Steels P, *et al.* Immune-mediated oligodendrocyte injury in multiple sclerosis: molecular mechanisms and therapeutic interventions. *Crit. Rev. Immunol.* 2002, **22**: 391–424.
11. Bechmann I, Steiner B, Gimsa U, *et al.* Astrocyte-induced T cell elimination is CD95 ligand dependent. *J. Neuroimmunol.* 2002, **132**: 60–65.

12. Noseworthy JH, Lucchinetti C, Rodrigez M, *et al.* Multiple sclerosis. *New Engl. J. Med.* 2000, **343**: 938–952.

13. Haas J, Storch-Hagenlocher B, Biessmann A, *et al.* Inducible nitric oxide synthase and argininosuccinate synthetase: co-induction in brain tissue of patients with Alzheimer's dementia and following stimulation with beta-amyloid 1–42 in vitro. *Neurosci. Lett.* 2002, **322**: 121–125.

14. Suter T, Biollaz G, Gatto D, *et al.* The brain as an immune privileged site: dendritic cells of the central nervous system inhibit T cell activation. *Eur. J. Immunol.* 2003, **33**: 2998–3006.

15. Weiner HL, Selkoe DJ. Inflammation and therapeutic vaccination in CNS diseases. *Nature* 2002, **420**: 879–884.

16. Reina MA, Lopez A, Villanueva MC, *et al.* [The blood–nerve barrier in peripheral nerves.] *Rev. Esp. Anestesiol. Reanim.* 2003, **50**: 80–86. (In Spanish)

17. Tabuchi T, Nakao Y, Sakihama N, *et al.* Vascular permeability to fluorescent substance in human cranial nerves. *Ann. Otol. Rhinol. Laryngol.* 2002, **111**: 736–737.

18. Hirakawa H, Okajima S, Nagaoka S, *et al.* Loss and recovery of the blood–nerve barrier in the rat sciatic nerve after crush injury are associated with expression of intercellular junctional proteins. *Exp. Cell Res.* 2003, **284**: 196–210.

19. Lilje O. The processing and presentation of endogenous and exogenous antigen by Schwann cells in vitro. *Cell Mol. Life Sci.* 2002, **59**: 2191–2198.

20. Hadden RD, Gregson NA, Gold R, *et al.* Accumulation of immunoglobulin across the 'blood–nerve barrier' in spinal roots in adoptive transfer experimental autoimmune neuritis. *Neuropathol. Appl. Neurobiol.* 2002, **28**: 489–497.

21. Keswani SC, Polley M, Pardo CA, *et al.* Schwann cell chemokine receptors mediate HIV-1 gp120 toxicity to sensory neurons. *Ann. Neurol.* 2003, **54**: 287–296.

22. Molina-Holagado E, Arevalo-Martin A, Vela JM, *et al.* [Theiler's virus encephalomyelitis infection as a model for multiple sclerosis: cytokines and pathogenic mechanisms.] *Rev. Neurol.* 2002, **35**: 973–978. (In Spanish)

23. Xiao BG, Diab A, Zhu J, *et al.* Astrocytes induce hyporesponses of myelin basic protein-reactive T and B cell function. *J. Neuroimmunol.* 1998, **89**: 113–121.

24. Xu LY, Yang JS, Xiao BG. TGF-beta1-conditioned glial cell-derived dendritic cells inhibit expansion of MBP-reactive T cells in vitro. *NeuroReport* 2002, **13**: 35–39.

25. Litzenburger T, Fassler R, Bauer J, *et al.* B lymphocytes producing demyelinating autoantibodies: development and function in gene-targeted transgenic mice. *J. Exp. Med.* 1998, **188**: 169–180.

26. Mead RJ, Singhrao SK, Neal JW, *et al.* The membrane attack complex of complement causes severe demyelination associated with acute axonal injury. *J. Immunol.* 2002, **168**: 458–465.

27. Calida DM, Constantinescu C, Purev E, *et al.* Cutting edge: C3, a key component of complement activation, is not required for the development of myelin oligodendrocyte glycoprotein peptide-induced experimental autoimmune encephalomyelitis in mice. *J. Immunol.* 2001, **166**: 723–726.

28. Weerth SH, Rus H, Shin ML, *et al.* Complement C5 in experimental autoimmune encephalomyelitis (EAE) facilitates remyelination and prevents gliosis. *Am. J. Pathol.* 2003, **163**: 1069–1080.

29. Zhang GX, Ma CG, Xiao BG, *et al.* Depletion of CD8$^+$ T cells suppresses the development of experimental autoimmune myasthenia gravis in Lewis rats. *Eur. J. Immunol.* 1995, **25**: 1191–1198.

30. Zhang GX, Xiao BG, Bakhiet M, *et al.* Both CD4$^+$ and CD8$^+$ T cells are essential to induce experimental autoimmune myasthenia gravis. *J. Exp. Med.* 1996, **184**: 349–356.

31. Zhang GX, Xiao BG, Yu LY, *et al.* Interleukin 10 aggravates experimental autoimmune myasthenia gravis through inducing Th2 and B cell responses to AChR. *J. Neuroimmunol.* 2001, **113**: 10–18.

32. Saoudi A, Bernard I, Hoedemackers A, *et al.* Experimental autoimmune myasthenia gravis may occur in the context of a polarized Th1- or Th2-type immune response in rats. *J. Immunol.* 1999, **162**: 7189–7197.

33. Mackay F, Mackay CR. The role of BAFF in B-cell maturation, T-cell activation and autoimmunity. *Trends Immunol.* 2002, **23**: 113–115.

34. Mariette X, Roux S, Zhang J, *et al.* The level of BLyS (BAFF) correlates with the titre of autoantibodies in human Sjogren's syndrome. *Ann. Rheum. Dis.* 2003, **62**: 168–171.

35. Xiao BG, Duan RS, Link H, *et al.* Induction of peripheral tolerance to experimental autoimmune myasthenia gravis by acetylcholine receptor-pulsed dendritic cells. *Cell Immunol.* 2003, **223**: 63–69.

36. Lin F, Kaminski HJ, Conti-Fine BM, *et al.* Markedly enhanced susceptibility to experimental autoimmune myasthenia gravis in the absence of decay-accelerating factor protection. *J. Clin. Invest.* 2002, **110**: 1269–1274.

37. Clayton A, Harris CL, Court J, *et al.* Antigen-presenting cell exosomes are protected from complement-mediated lysis by expression of CD55 and CD59. *Eur. J. Immunol.* 2003, **33**: 522–531.

38. Evoli A, Tonali PA, Padua L, *et al.* Clinical correlates with anti-MuSK antibodies in generalized seronegative myasthenia gravis. *Brain* 2003, **126**: 2304–2311.

39. Vincent A, McConville J, Farrugia ME, *et al.* Antibodies in myasthenia gravis and related disorders. *Ann. NY Acad. Sci.* 2003, **998**: 324–335.

40. Racke MK, Ratts RB, Arredondo L, *et al.* The role of co-stimulation in autoimmune demyelination. *J. Neuroimmunol.* 2000, **107**: 205–215.

41. Cannella B, Gaupp S, Tilton RG, *et al.* Differential efficacy of a synthetic antagonist of VLA-4 during the course of chronic relapsing experimental autoimmune encephalomyelitis. *J. Neurosci. Res.* 2003, **71**: 407–416.

42. Yarilin D, Duan R, Huang YM, *et al.* Dendritic cells exposed in vitro to TGF-beta1 ameliorate experimental autoimmune myasthenia gravis. *Clin. Exp. Immunol.* 2002, **127**: 214–219.

43. Xiao BG, Wu XC, Yang JS, *et al.* Therapeutic potential of IFN-gamma-modified dendritic cells in acute and chronic experimental allergic encephalomyelitis. *Int. Immunol.* 2004, **16**: 13–22.

15

Animal models of sex differences in non-reproductive brain functions

GEORGE T. TAYLOR, JUERGEN WEISS, AND FRANK ZIMMERMANN

15.1 Overview

A neuroscientist embarking on a study of reproduction is eminently aware that an animal model chosen must consider gender differences and the endocrine factors determining them. Neuroscientists embarking on a study of function unrelated to reproduction may require the same consideration. It is now clear that gonadal hormones are important contributors to sex differences in a wide array of non-reproductive brain activities.[1,2]

This conclusion has emerged from studies with animal models, sometimes unexpectedly when the experimental paradigm has included both males and females as subjects. Other findings of sex differences were observed first in human populations that suggested further study with animal models.

This review is a sampling of the remarkable variety of sex differences uncovered in adult brain function of which a neuroscientist may be unaware. A recent personal experience serves as an example. A respected colleague mentioned a new project to be conducted in her laboratory using an animal model of neuropathic pain. The interest was on a hypothesized acute attenuation of pain from treatments with a glutamate antagonist. Because the animal colony had an abundance of female rats, the subjects were to be groups of females. The assumption was that the topic had little relevance to reproduction and reproductive hormones, and any findings could be generalized equally to both sexes. Yet, there are reasons to question both assumptions. Both pain and glutamatergic pathways are influenced by sex hormones, and males and females may respond quite differently. After further discussion, our colleague still chose to use the abundance of females. But, she will surely temper conclusions on a drug therapy for pain. If this chapter has a similar result with other neuroscientists, we will consider writing it worthwhile.

Handbook of Experimental Neurology, ed. Turgut Tatlisumak and Marc Fisher. Published by Cambridge University Press. © Cambridge University Press 2006.

We will begin with an overview of current thinking about sex differences. It will lay the groundwork for sections reviewing sexually dimorphic brain functions. Concluding each will be "Take-home points" that are just that, pointers to take away from the reading.

15.2 Background information

The typical subject in a neuroscience experiment is a normal adult laboratory animal. That is to say, the animal has undergone normal development without surgical or pharmaceutical intervention prior to implementation of the experimental protocol. Nonetheless, it is safe to state that sex hormones have already exerted a profound influence on the animal.

15.2.1 The concept

It is understandable that early biologists were tempted, upon finding a gender difference in function in normally reared adults, to assume the underlying mechanism was the type and titers of sex hormones.[3] Male-typical traits would seem to be from the androgens, mostly testosterone, and female-typical traits from estrogens and progesterone. Yet, studies now decades old revealed that administering testosterone to females or estrogen to males seldom reversed function to the other gender. Even more startling were findings that estrogen could be *more* effective than testosterone in restoring function to castrated male rodents. Finally, sensitive radioimmunoassays revealed that all adults have measurable quantities of androgens, estrogens, and progesterone in circulation, calling into question the labeling of sex steroids as "male" or "female" hormones.

With development of the organizational–activational model came the recognition that it is quite correct to identify the sex steroids as the source of most sex differences. However, sex differentiation began during prenatal development, most important being the presence or absence of testosterone that programmed brain circuitry as masculine or feminine. Sex steroidal influences lie dormant until puberty when the same sex hormones, now joined by gonadotropins and neuropeptides, activate the circuits organized during fetal development.

15.2.2 Refinement of the concept

One significant refinement to the organizational–activational model has followed observations of changes in neuronal structure in cycling female rats.

Rather than being invariant and permanent, neural morphology was shown to change with fluctuations of endogenous sex hormones in adult female rats.[4] These data highlight both the plasticity of the adult brain and the importance of hormone fluctuations on the brain during the activational phase. It is probably accurate to suggest that even neuroendocrinologists have not fully appreciated the dramatic differences between a fluctuating hormonal stimulus and a more or less constant one.

The metabolic cascade of steroidal hormones is remarkably complex and details remain unclear. However, one feature of note is that estradiol (E2), the most bioactive estrogen, is a metabolite of testosterone. Thus, testosterone can directly bind an androgen receptor or, upon conversion by aromatase to E2, bind an estrogen receptor. In adults of many non-primate species the androgenic effects are, in fact, from E2 binding estrogen receptors in the male brain.

Take-home points

- Gonadal steroidal influences on the adult brains of common laboratory animals can be from either fetal organizational effects, post-pubertal activational effects, or, most often, both effects.
- A notable neuroendocrine feature of the adult female animal is fluctuating hormone levels during the estrous cycle that can activate or reorganize a brain structure.
- An equally notable neuroendocrine feature of adult males is that testosterone can undergo conversion to estradiol and bind the estrogen receptor.

15.3 Sex differences in brain anatomy

The brains of adult males and females, nonetheless, are built differently, although the functional significance may not yet be established. The best established are regional size differences in structures involved in reproduction. Dimorphism also has been reported for non-reproductive brain structures. Most often, the difference favors the male.[5] Examples from rats include volume (amygdala, neocortex, and bed nucleus stria terminalis), cell numbers (visual cortex), and synapses (suprachiasmatic nucleus of the hypothalamus). However, there are exceptions as some female rat brain regions are larger (locus coeruleus) or have more neurons (striatum). Sex steroids are related in some way to the establishment of these structural features and others that are more difficult to identify, for example, configuration of connections between brain nuclei.

There are several excellent reviews of morphological sex differences and the organizational–activational model.[1,2,6] Here, we will only summarize data from animal models on the hippocampus and the steroid receptors.

15.3.1 Sexually dimorphic hippocampus

A great deal of attention has been directed at sex differences in the hippocampus. In many species the male hippocampus is larger than that of the female. Compared with females, male rats and mice also have more granulose cells in the dentate gyrus, the width of the granule cell layer is thicker, and there are more mossy fiber synapses in the hilus.[7]

Most likely these differences are an organizational effect. Indeed, during the period of development when testosterone is elevated in the male fetus, aromatase and estrogen receptors are transiently expressed in the hippocampus.

Still, adult levels of the steroids can induce structural changes in the hippocampus. The now classic findings are of the density of hippocampal dendritic spines changing over the few days of the estrous cycle of the female rat.[8] The result is that synapses are formed with the surge of estrogen at proestrus and then disappear with the subsequent rise of progesterone. These and other data suggest that the structural integrity of the adult hippocampus remains sensitive to environmental manipulation and hormonal modification throughout adulthood.

It is also of interest that the hippocampus may show dimorphism in hemispheric asymmetry.[6] Male brains have more lateralized functions than female brains, and some of the underlying structures have been identified. For example, width of the dentate gyrus granule cell layer is larger in the right than left hemisphere of male rats, yet females show no similar laterality. These differences provide support to an often cited, albeit controversial, hypothesis that fetal testosterone is responsible for widespread peripheral and central asymmetry.[9]

15.3.2 Steroid receptors

Sex hormones acting on steroid receptors in the brain during fetal life and after puberty are responsible for most of the observed differences between males and females. Estrogen receptors (ER) and androgen receptors (AR) are ubiquitous in the periphery and brains of common laboratory animals. Both ERs and ARs are present in presynaptic and postsynaptic neurons, in both genders, and in brain structures unrelated to reproduction.[10]

There is a single androgen receptor but two estrogen receptors. ARs are found in a fairly limited range of brain regions in males and females. Different concentrations between the sexes are detected mostly in hypothalamic nuclei and other structures related to reproduction.[11]

The two subtypes of estrogen receptor, designated as ER-alpha and ER-beta, are distributed differently in male and female brains. Their locations suggest ER-alpha is the pre-eminent subtype for co-ordinating reproductive functions, and ER-beta is the subtype involved in most non-reproductive brain functions. An example is that only ER-beta was detected in the hippocampus of male and female rats, with higher concentrations found in females.[12]

In many non-reproductive structures, however, there are surprisingly few or no sex differences in distribution and concentrations of ERs and ARs.[13] This would seem to pose interpretation problems for relating dimorphic functions to the steroid receptor. High concentrations of ERs in males can be explained, however, by the metabolism of testosterone into E2 in brain tissues to interact with ERs. Notably, amounts of aromatase are higher in many brain regions of males than of females.[11] The presence of high concentrations of ARs in the brains of females is more puzzling.

Take-home points

- The sexually dimorphic hippocampus has provided a model system for linking morphological and functional sex differences.
- The surprisingly few sex differences in locations of androgen and estrogen receptors in many brain regions has directed the explanatory focus to sex differences in steroid metabolism.

15.4 Sex hormone–neurotransmitter interactions

Perhaps the single most important influence of sex hormones on the adult brain is via neurotransmitter (NT) systems. Distribution of steroid receptors on presynaptic and postsynaptic neurons in the brainstem, midbrain, and subcortical areas provide the sex hormones ample opportunity to modulate NT activities. Despite the presence of few steroid receptors in the prefrontal cortex, the hormones also can have a profound influence on prefrontal function through NT projections from the subcortex.

A typical experiment on sex hormone–NT interactions is to administer an animal a drug that targets a particular transmitter and measure the level of the NT and metabolites in a discrete brain region. Results from non-reproductive regions have pointed to estrogen and the estrogen receptor as the key players. Alterations of acetylcholine, monoamine, and amino acid NTs through estrogen-mediated mechanisms have been reported consistently.[4]

15.4.1 Dopamine and serotonin

Because of their involvement in psychiatric disorders, considerable research effort with animal models has focused on dopamine (DA) and serotonin (5-HT). There is evidence of sex differences in both.

Basis for differences in DA pathways is likely the estrogen receptor. There are high concentrations of estrogen receptors in DA-rich areas of the brain. Changes in circulating estrogen have a dramatic effect on dopaminergic activity. Biosynthesis, concentration, degradation, uptake, and receptor density in nigrostriatal and mesocorticolimbic DA pathways fluctuate with the estrous cycle.[14] For example, drug-induced release of DA is greater during estrus than during diestrus. Exogenous estrogen also can impact DA pathways by increasing the density and sensitivity of DA receptors.[15]

Sex differences in the serotonergic system also revolve around the fluctuations in circulating estrogen. There are changes in 5-HT synthesis, release, reuptake, and metabolism during the estrous cycles of intact animals.[16] Turnover and other measures of 5-HT activity are higher in female than in male rats,[14,16] with differences most noticeable at proestrus. Ovariectomy decreases 5-HT receptor numbers in various brain regions, and estrogen replacement restores receptor concentrations to those of intact females. Estrogen treatments and, perhaps, progesterone increase 5-HT concentrations in females while testosterone decreases 5-HT activity in both males and females.[17] Nonetheless, estrogen is believed to have the greatest influence on 5-HT systems.

15.4.2 Other neurotransmitters

McEwen and colleagues have researched estrogen–acetylcholine (ACh) interactions extensively and reported that female rats typically have higher ACh activity than males, due mainly to ovarian hormones.[4] For example, changes in estrogen and progesterone with the estrous cycle influence basal forebrain cholinergic function. The mechanism appears to be the influence of estrogen on synthesis of cholinergic metabolic enzymes.

Gamma-aminobutyric acid (GABA) is a ubiquitous inhibitory neurotransmitter, and GABA activity is sexually dimorphic.[18] Depending on the brain region, there are differences of GABA turnover between male and female rats. In the hippocampus many of the GABA neurons contain receptors for estrogen where the ERs modulate enzymatic activity and synthesis of GABA. Progesterone plays a particularly important role in GABA functions. There is a well-established relation between the GABAergic neurons and neurosteroids. One of the more important neurosteroids is allopregnanolone, a progesterone metabolite.

Glutamate and the glutamate receptors amino-3-hydroxy-5-methyl-4-isoxazol proprionic acid (AMPA) and *N*-methyl-D-aspartate (NMDA) have major excitatory functions. Studies with rats suggest estrogenic activation of

AMPA and, mainly, NMDA in certain brain regions of females. Progesterone has either no influence on NMDA activity or opposes the effects of estrogen.[19]

Take-home points

- Neurotransmitter activities differ between male and female laboratory animals, with the clearest being the modulation of neurotransmission by the estrogen receptor.
- Measures of release, reuptake, metabolism, and receptor numbers of neurotransmitters are likely to depend partly on the stage of the estrous cycle at which the female is tested.

15.5 Sex differences in drug responses

Pharmacological agents are common tools in a neuroscientist's research arsenal. It is of value to point out the different responses of males and females administered the same amount of drug adjusted for body weight.

Interest has centered on sex differences in response to psychoactive drugs, especially the drugs of high abuse potential. Physiological measures in this literature have included body weights and metabolic changes, withdrawal symptoms, numbers of necrotic neurons, systemically administered drug subsequently appearing in brain tissues, neurotransmitter changes, or mortality.[20,21] Behavioral measures have included drug self-administration, cognitive behaviors, and especially motor activity.[22,23]

15.5.1 Female sensitivity

With such a wide array of outcome measures from different nuclei and different drugs, the results are not in complete agreement. However, more often than not it is the female who shows greater sensitivity.[22,24]

Female sensitivity to drugs can be observed in gross behavioral measures. Female rats exhibit more rotational behaviors, a marker of DA activation, in response to amphetamine. Female rats from Lewis, Fischer 344, spontaneously hypertensive, and Wistar Kyoto strains all experienced longer sleep times to a hypnotic dose of pentobarbital than the males.[25] Withdrawal symptoms, in the form of jerks and seizures, after flumazenil were greater in diazepam-treated female mice.[21]

Circulating testosterone appears to be important in the lesser drug response of males. Castrations left males with a female-like benzodiazepine withdrawal response.[21] Circulating ovarian steroids, on the other hand, increase the drug response. Rotational responses were increased markedly in estrogen-restored ovariectomized female rats administered cocaine. Comparisons of control males and females gonadectomized without hormone restoration in the same experiment indicated the females remained more sensitive than males,[26] suggesting an organizational influence. Still, circulating hormones in the adult are critical. In intact females, the drug response often is reported to change over the estrous cycle, with greater sensitivity during high levels of ovarian hormones. Interestingly, pregnant rats experienced high mortality to cocaine at a time in the pregnancy of unusually high levels of estrogen and progesterone.[20]

15.5.2 Sources of female sensitivity

Mechanisms for sex differences in drug sensitivity are likely to be found in the liver and in the brain. Liver metabolic capacity of cytochrome P450 isozymes is highly sensitive to the sex steroids. Androgens can increase the synthesis of hepatic enzymes with the result that more drug is metabolized in the liver before reaching the brain of a male.[27] This may explain the finding that male rats have lower blood alcohol concentrations than females after acute ethanol administration, the higher amounts of systemic amphetamine found in whole brain and striatum samples of females, and the reduced effectiveness of a serotonin-specific reuptake inhibitor that suppressed circulating steroid levels in female rats.[28,29]

A feminized brain also processes drugs differently from a masculinized brain. As a result, estrogen increases sensitivity of the same monoamine NT pathways that are the targets of many of the drugs of abuse.[14] Progesterone and allopregnanolone provide the female brain with the opportunity to modify the GABA receptor complex from benzodiazepines, barbiturates, and ethanol.

A final word is about the costs and benefits of differences in drug sensitivity. It is often pointed out, quite accurately, that elevated sensitivity places the female in greater toxicological dangers. However, that same sensitivity may underlie the enhanced effectiveness of psychotherapeutic drugs in patients and animal models.

Take-home points

- In a variety of functional measures, female animal models display greater sensitivity to the same amount of drug relative to body weight administered to a male.
- A peripheral mechanism underlying lesser male sensitivity is that circulating androgens modify hepatic enzymes so that more drug is metabolized before reaching the male brain.

- A central mechanism underlying greater female sensitivity is suggested by the capacity of progesterone and, especially, estrogen to modulate neurotransmitter systems targeted by psychoactive drugs.
- Pharmacological studies using only male animal models may underestimate the responses of physiological systems impacted by drugs.

15.6 Sex differences in basic functions

Many experiments in neuroscience either directly or indirectly employ measures that are involved with maintenance functions. It would seem useful to address the potential for gender differences and sex steroidal influences on these basic functions.

15.6.1 Ingestive behaviors

In most common animal models the male weighs more than the female. Circulating levels of gonadal steroids in the adult are intimately involved in regulating food intake and body weight.[30] Beginning at puberty, males eat more and drink more than females. Castrated adult male rats gain weight more slowly than gonadally intact male rats whereas ovariectomized females show the opposite pattern, gaining more body weight than intact females. The hormones also influence body composition. Estrogen and progesterone, for instance, act synergistically to increase fat reserves.

Other practical considerations include the potential of drugs, stimulants for example, to suppress metabolic activities differently in males and females. Also, manipulating ingestive behaviors may reveal a dimorphic influence on brain activities. An example is that a strict food deprivation regimen decreased serotonin concentrations in discrete brain nuclei of male rats but not of females.[31]

15.6.2 Locomotor activity

Female rats and mice often are observed to be more active than males in a running wheel or other apparatus allowing free movement. Female locomotor activity changes over the estrous cycle. Females become more active with the estrogenic surge that precedes ovulation or with exogenous estrogen.[32]

It is interesting that intact adult males also appear sensitive to elevated estrogen titers. Males increase their activity when administered E2 or an exogenous androgen that is converted to E2 in the brain. On the other hand, high endogenous testosterone in a fear-inducing situation may increase anxiety and suppress activity in males.[33]

15.6.3 *Circadian rhythms*

Not only are females more active, their daily patterns of activity differ from those of males.[34] The onset of activity in female rats and, especially, hamsters occurs earlier in days when endogenous estrogen titers are high. Ovariectomies have the predictable effect of delaying onset of daily activity, but castration of male hamsters has no similar effect. The suggestion is of female circadian activity patterns being more sensitive than males to circulating hormones. Interestingly, the same may apply to the rhythmic release of neurotransmitters.[35]

The circadian rhythm of steroids released into circulation of both males and females also deserves mention. Endocrine glands release pulses of hormone in a seemingly random pattern during the day. Testosterone, for instance, is released in pulses so that male laboratory animals have a notable range of testosterone levels in circulation over a 24-hr period. The patterns are notorious for their unpredictability both between and within animals.[36]

15.6.4 *Pain sensitivity*

Animal models of acute and chronic pain have provided a means to examine the endocrine basis of the reported greater response to pain by women. Reports with animals, overall, have pointed to a lower threshold for pain in female rats with sensitivity at its highest at proestrus.

More research has centered on sex differences in an analgesic response to pain-relieving drugs. Male rodents show greater analgesia than the females. Sex steroid involvement is suggested by gonadectomies leaving the animal with the analgesic response of the opposite sex.[37] Nonetheless, findings with animal models indicate the response to pain is complex, with different results depending on a number of factors unrelated to sex hormones.[38]

15.6.5 *Dimorphic immune system*

The higher incidence of autoimmune diseases in women has fueled research with animal models on sex differences in the immune system. The results have mostly confirmed the greater immune system sensitivity in females.[39] The more difficult problem has been to pinpoint the role that sex hormones play in different immune responses. Distinct immune environments in males and females underlie many of the sex differences in autoimmunity. Sex steroids can influence an array of immune system features, including T cell receptor signaling, T lymphocytes, molecular changes in cytokine genes, or lymphocyte homing. The details, however, remain murky.

A noteworthy controversy has been the effect of testosterone on the immune system. Findings that feral males with high endogenous testosterone titers also carried a high parasite load suggested the hypothesis that aggressive males were at greater health risks than other males and females. We have postulated, however, that rather than being immunosuppressive testosterone redirects an immune response toward specific regions of the body to deal with any injuries sustained.[40]

Take-home points

- Sex steroids contribute to the findings on maintenance functions so that females are generally more active and more sensitive to pain, whereas males eat more and have a better analgesic response.
- Less is known about sex hormonal influences on circadian rhythms and immune responses except that sex differences exist for both.

15.7 Sex differences in higher brain functions

So-called higher brain functions are revealed primarily in complex behaviors. These include normal cognitive behaviors and the disturbed thought processes of psychiatric disorders. It has proven far easier to model normal cognitive function than to model the dysfunction of schizophrenia or Alzheimer's disease. Nonetheless, there is evidence from animal models of sex differences in many higher brain functions and malfunctions.

15.7.1 Cognition

A consistent finding in the neuropsychological literature is of males making fewer errors than females in hippocampal-dependent spatial learning tasks. The data suggest that, largely from fetal testosterone, males use different and more effective strategies to navigate their environments.[41]

The influence of postpubertal hormones on spatial learning is more complex. Elevated titers of testosterone in adult males do not typically improve spatial performance and may impair it.[42] High estrogen titers may improve or impair spatial performance depending upon several factors, some known and some not known. Most reliable is that an intact female's performance on a spatial task is worst at mid-cycle when estrogen levels are highest.[43]

Results from experiments on sex differences in non-spatial cognitive abilities in adult animals also have been mixed. Nonetheless, a case can be made that testosterone levels in adult males have a small positive effect and progesterone in the absence of estrogen in female animals worsening non-spatial cognitive performance. Estrogen, on the other hand, has proven to be of considerable cognitive benefit to females. That aged animal models enjoy the same benefits on cognition and neurophysiological integrity has recommended estrogen as a neuroprotective agent.[44]

Finally, male rats show greater tenacity, or response "perseverance."[45] Compared to females, male rats continued to respond longer when the experimental rules to obtain reward had changed. Circulating testosterone is the suggested mechanism because castrated males showed female-like flexibility, which was reversed by testosterone restoration.

One interpretation is that perseverance is a sexually selected trait that improves the reproductive success of males. From a different perspective, flexibility could represent a fundamental cognitive feature of females being more attuned to the contingencies associated with responding. Regardless, tenacity by males in the face of non-reward has intriguing implications for more than a few experimental paradigms.

15.7.2 *Alzheimer's disease*

Healthy old animals are a common model for research on age-related dementia, including Alzheimer's disease. Declining cognitive function with "normal aging," however, is an imperfect animal model for pathological aging of the brain.

Still, there are demonstrable relations between sex hormones and aging. Aging decreases the sex differences in neurophysiology and cognitive behaviors observed in young adults.[46] Of particular note is that many of the brain regions impacted by gonadal hormones during young adulthood are the same regions affected by pathological aging.

Research with animal models of dementia has focused on estrogenic neuroprotection and neurogenesis.[47] Age-related declines in cognition and neural integrity correspond to the declines in ovarian hormones in aging female rats and monkeys. Exogenous estrogen with or without progesterone can improve cognition and reverse the neural declines in old animals, but those successes have not been duplicated in Alzheimer's patients.[48]

New paradigms based on better understanding of molecular mechanisms underlying dementia offer new hope for the development of more valid animal models. Excitotoxicity from changes in glutamate pathways is one example. Recently, we found that chronic, but not acute, E2 treatments to female rats significantly reduced excitotoxic damage to cerebrocortical neurons.[49]

15.7.3 Schizophrenia

One of the more reliable relationships in psychiatry is existence of sex differences in the incidence of major depression and in the onset and outcome of schizophrenia. Moreover, the symptoms of both diseases are worse during the menstrual cycle when ovarian hormones are at their lowest levels.[50] Nonetheless, there are surprisingly few relevant studies with animals addressing these differences.

One reason is the scarcity of valid animal models, that is, models in which the data yield a similar outcome to the gender findings in the psychiatric literature.[51] A possible exception is an animal model of hemineglect, the symptom of some schizophrenic patients to ignore a part of their attentional field.[52] Rats that consistently showed a preference for removing a nuisance stimulus – strips of surgical tape applied loosely to the forelimbs – from one paw and "neglecting" the other paw were administered anti-psychotic drugs. Neglect was more easily eliminated by drugs in females than in male rats, and females became our subjects for subsequent experiments.

These data are consistent with the literature indicating greater sensitivity to anti-psychotic drugs by female schizophrenics. However, other studies have a conceptual problem by attempting to demonstrate estrogen is neuroprotective at DA sites.[53] Excess DA activation is a key feature of schizophrenia and, as we saw earlier,[15] the animal data indicate estrogen enhances DA activity. Advancement in this area awaits new animal models and new ways of thinking of the brain pathology underlying schizophrenia.

15.7.4 Depression

The forced swimming test is a common animal model of depression. Also known as the Porsolt test, a rat or mouse is dropped into an inescapable pool of water and measured for latency and duration of immobility as a behavioral model of "despair." Both testosterone and estrogen administered to gonadectomized animals reduced immobility,[54] suggesting binding the estrogen receptor plays a key role in depression.

As with animal models of schizophrenia, validity of the Porsolt test for studies of sex differences has been questioned.[51] For example, male rodents may exhibit *longer* durations of immobility than females rather than vice versa. Also, immobility in females appears not to change with the estrous cycle.

More attention has been placed on modeling the hypothalamic–pituitary–adrenal (HPA) axis dysregulation observed in human depression, and with greater success. A sex difference exists in the response of the HPA axis in animals to stress, with females reacting more robustly than males. Testosterone can inhibit HPA function, whereas estrogen enhances HPA responses to environmental stressors.[55] More important is that HPA disruption is related to the estrous cycle.[56] A suggested mechanism is that the changing levels of ovarian hormones block estrogen from neutralizing the glucocorticoids released during stress.

15.7.5 Outcome from traumatic brain injury

A fascinating literature is the different outcomes in recovery from traumatic brain injury (TBI) in males and females. Unlike the situation with psychiatric disorders, there are well-established animal models of TBI that allow comparisons of males and females, and of the hormonal mechanisms involved. The resulting evidence points to: (1) females experiencing less damage than male animals, (2) the ovarian hormones circulating at the time of the injury as the source of neuroprotection for females, and (3) estrogen similarly protecting the males.

A common animal model of stroke is temporal middle artery occlusion with infarct lesion volume as the dependent measure. In both normatotensive and stroke-prone rodent strains gonadally intact females fared better than intact males.[57] Ovariectomies increase TBI damage and administering estrogen or progesterone restores the benefits to the females. Males may also enjoy the benefits from acute exposure to exogenous estrogen.[58] Finally, estrogen appears to continue promoting recovery long after the traumatic event.

Circulating testosterone may do the opposite. In a rodent stroke model of ischemia reperfusion injury,[59] males were castrated and restored with a testosterone pellet. Males from whom the pellet was removed 1–6 hr prior to TBI had lesions approximately half those of males still sporting the testosterone pellets. Unfortunately, few studies have also included a behavioral measure to demonstrate the ultimate measure of TBI success, improved behavioral recovery.

Take-home points

- Males learn hippocampal-dependent spatial learning tasks better than females, likely from having a masculine organized brain.
- Circulating estrogen is the best candidate for enhancing non-spatial cognitive performance in adult animals, although estrogen–cognition relations are surprisingly complex.
- Weaknesses of the available animal models limit progress in the study of sex differences in schizophrenia and depression, but the capacity of estrogen to modulate neurotransmitter activities has pointed the way to develop new animal models.

- TBI presents perhaps the most valid animal models and perhaps the best evidence for current titers of estrogen in adults serving both neuroprotective and neuronal growth-promoting roles.

15.8 Choosing an animal model for neuroscience research

One goal of this chapter has been to bring sex differences to the attention of neuroscientists working on a topic unrelated to reproduction. A second goal is to assist the neuroscientists in choosing a male or female animal model.

Obviously, the gender chosen will depend upon the interest of the researcher. It is equally obvious that with their more stable hormonal status males often are the pragmatic choice.

It is claimed that the historical preference of males as subjects in biomedical research reflected a raging sexism and concern only for the health of men. We suspect that was seldom the basis for choosing males for studies of reproductive function. Male animals avoided the potential "problems" introduced by the fluctuating hormones of females. The wisdom of that choice has been confirmed by the expansion of the influence of fluctuating hormones to an array of non-reproductive measures of brain function.

Would a neuroscientist ever want to choose a female animal model? Naturally, females are the choice when the researcher has a specific interest in sex differences or a specific interest in female brain function. Also given the large literature of sex differences, the suggestion is clear that both males and females should be included to generalize the results widely.

We also have seen examples to suggest a less obvious reason to choose females over males. Females may be more sensitive to an experimental manipulation, and a measure may reveal treatment effects more easily. Drug exposure is an excellent example. It may be easier to demonstrate a drug relation with females than with males, and the researcher can leave the clarification of male–female differences to another day, or another researcher.

References

1. Breedlove SM, Hampson E. Sexual differentiation of the brain and behavior. In Becker JB, Breedlove SM, Crews D, McCarthy MM (eds.) *Behavioral Endocrinology*, 2nd edn. Cambridge, MA: MIT Press, 2002, pp. 75–116.
2. Payne AP. Gonadal hormones and the sexual differentiation of the nervous system: mechanisms and interactions. In Stone TW (ed.) *Neurotransmitters and Neuromodulators: Neuroactive Steroids*. Boca Raton, FL: CRC Press, 1996, pp. 153–175.

3. Balthazart J, Tlemcani O, Ball GF. Do sex differences in the brain explain sex differences in the hormonal induction of reproductive behavior? What 25 years of research on the Japanese quail tells us. *Hormones Behav.* 1996, **30**: 627–661.

4. McEwen BS, Alves SE. Estrogen actions in the central nervous system. *Endocrine Rev.* 1999, **20**: 279–307.

5. Darlington C. *The Female Brain*. New York: Taylor & Francis, 2002.

6. Cooke B, Hegstrom CD, Villeneuve LS, Breedlove SM. Sexual differentiation of the vertebrate brain: principles and mechanisms. *Frontiers Neuroendocrinol.* 1999, **20**: 323–362.

7. Tabibnia G, Cooke BM, Breedlove SM. Sex difference and laterality in the volume of mouse dentate gyrus granule cell layer. *Brain Res.* 1999, **827**: 41–45.

8. Woolley CS, McEwen BS, Beatty WW. Roles of estradiol and progesterone in regulation of hippocampal dendritic spine density during the estrous cycle in the rat. *J. Comp. Neurol.* 1993, **336**: 293–306.

9. Geschwind N, Galaburda A. Cerebral lateralization: biological mechanisms, associations and pathology. *Arch. Neurol.* 1985, **42**: 428–459.

10. Don Carlos LL, Garcia-Ovejero D, Sarkey S, Garcia-Segura LM, Azcoitia I. Androgen receptor immunoreactivity in forebrain axons and dendrites in the rat. *Endocrinology* 2003, **144**: 3632–3638.

11. Lu SF, McKenna SE, Cologer-Clifford A, Nau EA, Simon NG. Androgen receptor in mouse brain: sex differences and similarities in autoregulation. *Endocrinology* 1998, **139**: 1594–1601.

12. Zhang JQ, Cai WQ, Zhou de S, Su BY. Distribution and differences of estrogen receptor beta immunoreactivity in the brain of adult male and female rats. *Brain Res.* 2002, **935**: 73–80.

13. Michael RP, Clancy AN, Zumpe D. Distribution of androgen receptor-like immunoreactivity in the brains of cynomolgus monkeys. *J. Neuroendocrinol.* 1995, **7**: 713–719.

14. Majewska MD. Sex differences in brain morphology and pharmacodynamics. In Jensvold MF, Halbreich U, Hamilton J (eds.) *Psychopharmacology and Women*. Washington, DC: American Psychiatric Press, 1996, pp. 73–83.

15. Di Paolo T. Modulation of brain dopamine transmission by sex steroids. *Revi. Neurosci.* 1994, **5**: 27–41.

16. Maswood S, Truitt W, Hotema M, Caldarola-Pastuszka M, Uphouse L. Estrous cycle modulation of extracellular serotonin in mediobasal hypothalamus: role of the serotonin transporter and terminal autoreceptors. *Brain Res.* 1999, **831**: 146–154.

17. Sundblad C, Eriksson E. Reduced extracellular levels of serotonin in the amygdala of androgenized female rats. *Eur. Neuropsychopharmacol.* 1997, **7**: 253–259.

18. Purdy RH, Paul SM. Potentiation of GABAergic neurotransmission by steroids. In Baulieu EE, Robel P, Schumacher M (eds.) *Neurosteroids: A New Regulatory Function in the Nervous System*. Totowa, NJ: Humana Press, 1999, pp. 143–153.

19. Cyr M, Calon F, Morissette M, Di Paolo T. Estrogenic modulation of brain activity: implications for schizophrenia and Parkinson's disease. *J. Psychiat. Neurosci.* 2002, **27**: 12–27.

20. Church M, Subramanian M. Cocaine's lethality increases during late gestation in the rat: a study of "critical periods" of exposure. *Am. J. Obstet. Gynecol.* 1997, **176**: 901–906.

21. Pesce ME, Acevedo X, Pinardi G, Miranda HF. Gender differences in diazepam withdrawal syndrome in mice. *Pharmacol. Toxicol.* 1994, **75**: 353–355.

22. Becker JB. Hormonal influences on sensorimotor function. In Becker JB, Breedlove SM, Crews D, McCarthy M (eds.) *Behavioral Endocrinology*, 2nd edn. Cambridge, MA: MIT Press, 2002, pp. 497–526.

23. Yilmaz O, Kanit L, Okur BE, Pogun S. Effects of nicotine on active avoidance learning in rats: sex differences. *Behav. Pharmacol.* 1997, **8**: 253–260.

24. Perrotti LI, Beck KD, Luine VN, Quinones V. Progesterone and cocaine administration affect serotonin in the medial prefrontal cortex of ovariectomized rats. *Neurosci. Lett.* 2000, **291**: 155–158.

25. Suzuki T, Koike Y, Yanaura S, George FR, Meisch RA. Sex differences in physical dependence on pentobarbital in four inbred strains of rats. *Gen. Pharmacol.* 1992, **23**: 487–492.

26. Hu M, Becker JB. Effects of sex and estrogen on behavioral sensitization to cocaine in rats. *J. Neurosci.* 2003, **23**: 693–699.

27. Nabeshima T, Yamaguchi K, Furukawa H, Kameyama T. Role of sex hormones in sex-dependent differences in phencyclidine induced stereotyped behaviors in rats. *Eur. J. Pharmacol.* 1984, **105**: 197–206.

28. Taylor GT, Farr S, Klinga K, Weiss J. Chronic fluoxetine suppresses circulating estrogen and the enhanced spatial learning of estrogen-restored ovariectomized female rats. *Psychoneuroendocrinology* 2004, **100**: 1–10.

29. Webb B, Burnett PW, Walker DW. Sex differences in ethanol-induced hypnosis and hypothermia in young Long-Evans rats. *Alcoholism: Clin. Exp. Res.* 2002, **26**: 695–704.

30. Albert D, Jonik R, Gorzalka B, *et al.* Serum estradiol concentration required to maintain body weight, attractivity, proceptivity, and receptivity in the ovariectomized female rat. *Physiol. Behav.* 1991, **49**: 225–231.

31. Haider S, Haleem DJ. Decreases of brain serotonin following a food restriction schedule of 4 weeks in male and female rats. *Med. Sci. Monit.* 2000, **6**: 1061–1067.

32. Leshner AI. *An Introduction to Behavioral Endocrinology*. New York: Oxford University Press, 1978.

33. Perrot-Sinal T, Ossenkopp KP, Kavaliers M. Influence of a natural stressor (predator odor) on locomotor activity in the meadow vole (*Microtus pennsylvanicus*): modulation by sex, reproductive condition and gonadal hormones. *Psychoneuroendocrinology* 2000, **25**: 259–276.

34. Gorman MR, Lee TM. Hormones and biological rhythms. In Becker JB, Breedlove SM, Crews D, McCarthy MM (eds.) *Behavioral Endocrinology*, 2nd edn. Cambridge, MA: MIT Press, 2002, pp. 451–494.

35. Mitsushima D, Win-Shwe TT, Kimura F. Sexual dimorphism in the GABAergic control of gonadotropin release in intact rats. *Neurosci. Res.* 2003, **46**: 399–405.

36. Robaire B, Bayly S. Testicular signaling: incoming and outgoing messages. *Ann. NY Acad. Sci.* 1988, **56**: 251–260.

37. Barrett AC, Smith ES, Picker MJ. Capsaicin-induced hyperalgesia and mu-opioid-induced antihyperalgesia in male and female Fischer 344 rats. *J. Pharmacol. Exp. Therap.* 2003, **307**: 237–245.

38. Mogil JS, Chesler EJ, Wilson SG, Juraska JM, Sternberg WF. Sex differences in thermal nociception and morphine antinociception in rodents depend on genotype. *Neurosci. Biobehav. Rev.* 2000, **24**: 375–389.

39. Whitacre CC, Reingold SC, O'Looney PA. A gender gap in autoimmunity. *Science* 1999, **283**: 1277–1278.

40. Braude S, Lacey E, Tang-Martinez Z, Taylor GT. Stress, testosterone, and the immunoredistribution hypothesis. *Behav. Ecol.* 1999, **100**: 201–210.

41. Williams CL. Hormones and cognition in nonhuman animals. In Becker JB, Breedlove SM, Crews D, McCarthy MM (eds.) *Behavioral Endocrinology*, 2nd edn. Cambridge, MA: MIT Press, 2002, pp. 527–578.
42. Galea LA, Kavalis M, Ossenkopp K, Hampson D. Gonadal hormone levels and spatial learning performance in the Morris water maze in male and female meadow voles: *Microtus pennsylvanicus. Hormones Behav.* 1995, **29**: 106–125.
43. Warren SG, Juraska JM. Spatial and nonspatial learning across the rat estrous cycle. *Behav. Neurosci.* 1997, **111**: 259–266.
44. Behl C. Oestrogen as a neuroprotective hormone. *Nature Rev. Neurosci.* 2002, **3**: 433–442.
45. van Hest A, van Haaren F, van de Poll N. Perseverative responding in male and female Wistar rat: effects of gonadal hormones. *Hormones Behav.* 1989, **23**: 57–67.
46. Lacreuse A, Herndon JG, Killiany RJ, Rosene DL, Moss MB. Spatial cognition in rhesus monkeys: male superiority declines with age. *Hormones Behav.* 1999, **36**: 70–76.
47. Brinton RD. Cellular and molecular mechanisms of estrogen regulation of memory function and neuroprotection against Alzheimer's disease: recent insights and remaining challenges. *Learning Memory* 2001, **8**: 121–133.
48. Webber KM, Bowen R, Casadesus G, *et al.* Gonadotropins and Alzheimer's disease: the link between estrogen replacement therapy and neuroprotection. *Acta Neurobiol. Exp.* 2004, **64**: 113–118.
49. Dribben WH, Nemmers BM, Nardi AR, *et al.* Chronic but not acute estradiol treatment protects against the neurodegenerative effects of NMDA receptor antagonists. *Endocrine* 2003, **21**: 53–58.
50. Stevens JR. Schizophrenia: reproductive hormones and the brain. *Am. J. Psychiat.* 2002, **159**: 713–719.
51. Weiss JM, Kilts CD. Animal models of depression and schizophrenia. In Schatzberg A, Nemeroff C (eds.) *Textbook of Psychopharmacology*, 2nd edn. Washington, DC: American Psychiatric Press, 1998, pp. 89–131.
52. Taylor GT, Bardgett M, Csernansky J, *et al.* Neuroleptic influences on a lateralized behavioral bias in unoperated rats. *Psychopharmacology* 1999, **144**: 30–37.
53. Hafner H, Behrens S, De Vry J, Gattaz W. An animal model for the effects of estradiol on dopamine-mediated behavior: implications for sex differences in schizophrenia. *Psychiat. Res.* 1991, **38**: 125–134.
54. Estrada-Camarena E, Fernandez-Guasti A, Lopez-Rubalcava C. Antidepressant-like effect of different estrogenic compounds in the forced swimming test. *Neuropsychopharmacology* 2003, **28**: 830–838.
55. Handa RJ, Burgess LH, Kerr JE, O'Keefe J. Gonadal steroid hormone receptors and sex differences in the hypothalamo-pituitary-adrenal axis. *Hormones Behav.* 1994, **28**: 464–476.
56. Karandrea D, Kittas CK. Contribution of sex and cellular context in the regulation of brain corticosteroid receptors following restraint stress. *Neuroendocrinology* 2000, **71**: 343–353.
57. Alkayed NJ, Harukuni I, Kimes AS, *et al.* Gender-linked brain injury in experimental stroke. *Stroke* 1998, **29**: 159–165.
58. Rusa R, Alkayed NJ, Crain BJ, *et al.* 17beta-estradiol reduces stroke injury in estrogen-deficient female animals. *Stroke* 1999, **30**: 1665–1670.
59. Yang SH, Perez E, Cutright J, *et al.* Testosterone increases neurotoxicity of glutamate in vitro and ischemia-reperfusion injury in an animal model. *J. Appl. Physiol.* 2002, **92**: 195–201.

16

The ependymal route for central nervous system gene therapy

ERICA BUTTI, GIANVITO MARTINO, AND ROBERTO FURLAN

16.1 Introduction

Therapies targeting the central nervous system (CNS) are a crucial challenge for future medicine. In fact, degenerative and immune-mediated disorders of the CNS are a major threat to quality of life in the elderly, but diseases affecting the brain are also not infrequent in infancy and adult life. Transfer of recent progresses in the knowledge of molecular mechanisms involved in the pathogenesis of neurological disorders into novel therapies is difficult, because penetration of molecules into the brain is extremely limited by the presence of the blood–brain barrier (BBB). The BBB is characterized by tight junctions between endothelial cells which are impermeable to macromolecules and even ions, and by reduced endothelial endocytic activity that considerably decreases the number of molecules that can cross the BBB in a non-specific fashion.[1] Most of conventional therapeutic agents effective in the CNS are supposed to cross the BBB because of their small size. However, more than 98% of small molecules cannot cross the BBB either,[1] and only the presence of specific transport mechanisms assures that molecules essential for the brain metabolism (e.g., amino acids and glucose) reach the brain parenchyma. Thus, by employing conventional administration routes (i.e., oral, intravenous, intramuscular), which share the bloodstream as the final driving force to the brain, both rate and selectivity of the drug delivery are severely hampered, resulting in limited efficacy and potential side effects. Strategies to selectively target small molecules to the brain include modification of physical or chemical properties through the addition of moieties to increase passive diffusion, modification of molecules or production of chimeric molecules to exploit BBB-specific transport mechanisms, and, finally, partial disruption of the BBB by coinjection of hyperosmolar solutions.[2] In this perspective, the delivery of therapeutic molecules through gene therapy becomes a reasonable

Handbook of Experimental Neurology, ed. Turgut Tatlisumak and Marc Fisher. Published by Cambridge University Press. © Cambridge University Press 2006.

alternative approach. Gene therapy has been initially considered as a way to replace defective genes in inherited disorders, including in the CNS, but studies on its potential as drug delivery system have followed soon after. Three crucial issues in any gene therapy approach are: (1) what is the therapeutic gene to be delivered, (2) what are the target cells of the gene transfer, and (3) what is the tool needed to achieve a successful gene transfer. The two initial questions are strictly dependent on the disease considered: for example, if you are investigating Parkinson's disease you may want to transfer the gene coding for tyrosine hydroxylase, or other enzymes in the metabolic pathway of dopamine, or even neuroprotective growth factors, and you would like to target cells in the substantia nigra. The tool used for gene transfer is a consequence of the first two points: it has to be able to accommodate the wanted gene and the corresponding regulatory sequences, to target the appropriate cell, and to express the transgene for the desired time-frame. Several types of non-biological vectors for gene transfer, i.e., liposomes, are available but due to their poor transfer efficiency and the very transient expression of delivered genes, they will not be discussed here. Biological, i.e., viral, vectors are the most successful tools used for CNS gene transfer. Viral vectors are derived from the parent virus by deleting viral genes essential for replication or pathogenicity and replacing them with the desired expression cassette(s). The engineered viral vector maintains the ability to infect the same cells as the parent virus, although it is possible to modify membrane glycoproteins to broaden the host range (pseudotyped vectors). Once inside the infected cells, viral vectors transfer their genome into the nucleus where, depending on the virus type, it may persist in episomal form or integrate into the host genome. In the latter case, the transgene is obviously transmitted to daughter cells during replication. Efficient transcription of the transgene is usually obtained using strong constitutive promoters such as viral promoters. Regulation of transcription is a critical issue, however current technology is still unsatisfactory, since the use of physiological promoters usually yields insufficient levels of expression and regulatable promoters are extremely difficult to use in vivo. Specificities of CNS gene therapy are that most of target cells replicate poorly or do not replicate at all, and that the target tissue is behind anatomical and physiological barriers. In experimental animal models of neurological diseases, viral vectors or virally modified cells have been delivered locally or systemically. Genetically modified encephalitogenic T cells have been injected systemically as therapeutic agents in experimental autoimmune encephalomyelitis (EAE),[3] the animal model for human multiple sclerosis, while genetically modified hematopoietic stem cells have been injected in metachromatic leukodystrophy and lysosomal storage diseases.[4,5,6] The advantages of this procedure are the control of in vitro gene transfer and the easy administration route, the disadvantage the limited efficiency of CNS-specific grafting of systemically injected cells leading to a relatively low amount of therapeutic molecule released into the brain. Genetically modified cells have been also directly transplanted into selected brain areas in experimental models of, for example, lysosomal storage diseases and Parkinson's disease.[7] Capsules made of biocompatible polymers and containing genetically modified cells releasing therapeutic molecules have been transplanted also in humans, for example for amyotrophic lateral sclerosis.[8] Survival of transplanted cells, and thus production of the transgene, are the major limitation of these approaches. Genetic modification of CNS resident cells by direct injection of viral vectors has also been a widely used approach. Experimental protocols include the vascular route, i.e., intracarotideal injection, which has been employed for brain tumors and ischemic brain injury,[2] and the local injection of the viral vectors into specific brain areas which has been used in a variety of experimental neurological animal models such as Parkinson's disease, ischemia, amyotrophic lateral sclerosis, metachromatic leukodystrophy, EAE, and several others.[9] A human trial employing this approach has been also approved.[10]

16.2 The ependymal route

We have developed an alternative approach to CNS gene therapy by using the ependymal route.[11] Injection into the cerebrospinal fluid (CSF) allows viral vectors to infect only cells lining liquoral spaces, like ependymal and leptomeningeal cells (Fig. 16.1). The large number of viral particles that can be delivered in this relatively small compartment ensures high infection efficiency. If the delivered gene codes for a soluble, secreted molecule, this will be released into the CSF and be able to travel through the ventricular system to reach all brain areas, remaining confined to the brain and unable to induce unwanted side effects in the periphery. This approach has been used in EAE in mice and non-human primates,[3] and in ischemic stroke,[12] but holds promise for all multifocal brain diseases.

Since ependymal and leptomeningeal cells are slow-dividing cells that are poorly renewed, their infection allows long-term (up to 6 months) expression of the delivered transgene. To summarize, the advantages of the ependymal route for CNS gene therapy are:

- the high concentration of soluble therapeutic proteins that can be achieved in the CSF;
- the possibility of reaching multiple brain areas and thus potential usefulness in multifocal CNS disorders;

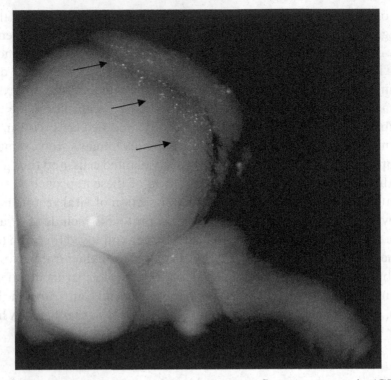

Figure 16.1. Meningeal cells infected by a green fluorescent protein (GFP)-expressing adenovirus through an intracisternal injection. A C57BL/6 mouse was intracisternally injected with 10^8 particles of a helper-dependent adenoviral vector (HD-Ad) expressing GFP. After 1 month the mouse was sacrificed, and the brain was removed and analyzed under a fluorescent stereo microscope (Leica MZ 16 FA). Fluorescent HD-Ad infected meningeal cells can be clearly seen on the external cerebellar surface (arrows).

- the ability of vectors injected in the CSF to express the transgene in the long term, which is potentially useful for chronic diseases;
- the absence of unwanted peripheral toxicity and side effects;
- the absence of an intrathecal immune response towards the viral vector which should allow repetitive injections without loss of therapeutic efficacy.

Some of these features rely on the nature of the protein encoded by the transferred gene. The therapeutic molecule has to be soluble and secreted, and its ability to travel across the brain–CSF barrier, and "soak" the brain parenchyma, depends on its physical and chemical properties and has to be assessed for each molecule. Using a herpes simplex virus type 1 (HSV-1)-derived vector expressing the cytokine interferon gamma (IFN-γ) in mice, we have been able to show that the biological effect (i.e., induction of major histocompatibility complex (MHC) class I and class II expression) of the molecule transferred by gene therapy could be detected in the brain parenchyma at least at 1 mm distance from liquoral spaces.[13] With the same type of vector, but delivering the cytokine interleukin-4 (IL-4), however, we were able to interfere with an inflammatory disease ongoing in the brain of larger mammals such as rhesus monkeys,[14] indicating that data obtained in mice were, most likely, underestimated.

16.3 Viral vectors suitable for the ependymal route

Requirements of the viral vector to be employed in the ependymal administration route are: (1) the ability to infect non-dividing cells since ependymal and leptomeningeal cells cycle at a very slow rate; (2) the possibility of obtaining very high titer viral stocks since only very small volumes can be injected; (3) low or no immunogenicity, to avoid unwanted inflammatory reactions in the brain; and (4) long-term expression of the transgene since repeated intrathecal injection of the vectors is not a feasible approach in a routine clinical setting. A brief outline of the more common viral vectors suitable for CNS gene therapy through the ependymal route follows.

16.3.1 Herpes simplex type 1-derived vectors

Herpesviruses have promise as vehicles for transfer of genes to cells in vivo based on their ability to persist after primary infection in humans in a state of latency where disease is absent in human hosts with normal immune status. HSV-1 is currently the most engineered herpesvirus for purposes of gene transfer. The HSV-1 genome comprises 152 kb of linear double-stranded DNA containing at least 84 entirely contiguous genes, approximately half of which are non-essential for virus replication in cell culture. Replication attenuated vectors, replication-incompetent vectors, or helper-dependent vectors (amplicons) derived from HSV-1 have been employed in experimental gene therapy protocols.[15] Using replication defective herpetic vectors engineered to express IL-4, IFN-γ, and fibroblast growth factor II (FGF-II), we have obtained encouraging results in both mice and non-human primates affected by EAE.[11,13,14,16,17,18,19] Advantages of herpetic vectors are the large size, the ability to infect postmitotic cells, and the ability to reach neurons by retrograde axonal transport; disadvantages are the short-term expression of the transgene, and the high immunogenicity.

16.3.2 Adenoviral vectors

Adenovirus (Ad) is a non-enveloped, icosahedral virus of 60–90 nm in diameter with a linear, double-stranded DNA genome of 30–40 kb. Two generations of vectors have been obtained deleting essential genes provided in *trans* by complementing cell lines. A "second generation" of Ad vector, called high-capacity (HC) or "gutless," was produced devoid of all coding viral genes, but contains only the inverted terminal repeats and the packaging signal (ψ) as viral elements. They can accommodate up to 36 kb of non-viral DNA so that large complementary DNA, longer tissue-specific or regulatable promoters, several expression cassettes, or even small genomic loci can be transferred. The lack of viral gene expression from these vectors has been shown to considerably reduce their toxicity and immunogenicity in vivo,[20] and long-term transgene expression in liver cells for more than 1 year has been observed in mice.[21] For the production of HC-Ad vectors, all viral gene functions except E1 are provided in *trans* by a helper virus.[22] Advantages of HC-Ad vectors are the ability to infect postmitotic cells, the ability to carry transgenes of more than 30 kb, reduced toxicity and immunogenicity, and long-term expression of the transgene (up to 6 months); disadvantages are the difficulties of obtaining high titers and of manipulating its genome.

16.3.3 Lentiviral vectors

These viruses are lipid-enveloped particles comprising a homodimer of linear, positive-sense, single-stranded RNA genomes of 7–11 kb. Following entry into target cells, the RNA genome is retro-transcribed into linear double-stranded DNA and integrated into the cell chromatin. Replication-defective vectors were originally derived from human immunodeficiency virus 1 (HIV-1) to transduce lymphocytes, but it was a vesicular stomatitis virus (VSV-G) pseudotyped lentiviral vector with expanded tropism that spurred applications for gene therapy.[23,24] Advantages of lentiviral vectors are the ability to infect non-dividing cells, as the nervous system cells, the ability to integrate into the genome of host cells, and the easy manipulation of its genome; disadvantages are the limited size of the expression cassette that can be inserted and the low, but significant risk, of activating a proto-oncogene or inactivating a crucial gene due to insertion into the host genome.

16.3.4 Adeno-associated virus vectors

Adeno-associated viruses (AAV) are human parvoviruses that normally require a helper virus, such an adenovirus, to mediate a productive infection.[25]

The viral genome is 4.68 kb in length and AAV vectors are obtained by packaging the recombinant genome into AAV particles by cotransfection of a helper plasmid providing missing genes in *trans*. AAV vectors have been shown to transduce cells both through episiomal transgene expression and by random chromosomal integration.[26,27] Advantages of AAV vectors are the lack of association with toxicity or inflammatory response, the ability to transduce postmitotic cells, the possibility of obtaining very high titers, and long-term gene expression; a disadvantage is the limited transgene capacity, about 4–5 kb.

16.4 Injection protocols for the ependymal route

The ependymal route to CNS gene therapy can be achieved in small rodents by intracerebroventricular (ICV) or intracisternal (IC) injection of the vectors. The advantages of IC over ICV injections are: (1) IC injections take 3–5 min per mouse as compared to the 15–20 min necessary to perform an ICV injection by stereotaxis, allowing to manipulate larger groups of mice; (2) in ICV injections the needle goes across the corpus callosum, and vector going back through the needle track can infect these structures; and (3) for IC injections there is no need for a costly stereotactic apparatus. On the other hand, IC injections are not more difficult than intravenous injections in the lateral tail vein, but ICV injections rely even less on the ability of the operator and may be thus more reproducible. A detailed description of IC injection procedure follows.

16.4.1 Intracisternal injection procedure

Preparation of the injecting device

The first step is to prepare the injection device necessary for IC injections as previously described.[28,29] Take flat forceps and, using a ruler and a marker, make a line at exactly 3.5 mm from the tip of the forceps (Fig. 16.2A). Use these forceps to bend a dental 27-gauge needle (21 mm in length) (Fig. 16.2A and B). Keeping the cutting edge towards the inside of the loop (Fig. 16.2B), the needle should end up J-shaped with an angle of approximately 40°. Before re-capping, the needle should be briefly flamed on a Bunsen burner. Again using the forceps, connect a 1-cm long polyethylene tubing (internal diameter 0.38 mm, external diameter 1.09 mm) (Becton Dickinson no. 427406) to the short needle that you can find at the opposite end of the dental needle. Several needles can be prepared and kept for further use. The last step for preparing the injecting device is to further connect the dental

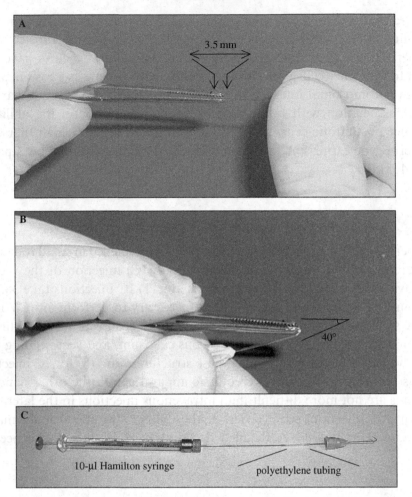

Figure 16.2. Preparation of the injection device. (A) The dental needle is held by the forceps with the tip aligned to the mark at 3.5 mm, and the cutting edge facing down. (B) The needle is bent around the forceps to obtain a J-shape and an angle of approximately 40°. (C) The bent needle is then connected to a 10-μl Hamilton syringe through a polyethylene tubing.

needle, through the polyethylene tubing, to the needle of a 10-μl Hamilton GC syringe (Fig. 16.2C).

Preparation of the working area

To be safe from the effects of the diethyl ether that is used to anesthetize mice, and to keep the area as clean as possible, it is recommended to work under a chemical or laminar flow hood. Tools that should be prepared in this area are the injecting device, a 1–20-μl pipette, a pipette tip box, a multi-channel pipette reservoir, and the vector to be injected. Most viral vectors rapidly lose their infectivity when kept at room temperature; thus we usually prepare small frozen aliquots of the viral vectors that can be thawed when needed. The viral suspension is then transferred, as a drop, to a multi-channel pipette reservoir where it is possible to put the tip of the dental needle into the drop to aspirate the solution and fill the injecting device.

Injection procedure

A good injection requires two operators, one keeping the needle in the right position, the second pushing the piston of the syringe.

Anesthetize the mouse with ether so that it will stay unconscious for approximately 1–2 min. Take the mouse and lean it on the pipette tip box, keeping forelimbs backward and the head bent slightly forward (Fig. 16.3). Run the needle along the external surface of the occiput and insert it into the cleft between the occiput and the atlas vertebra through the intact skin, muscles and ligaments in the midline at the back of the neck. Insertion of the needle tip into the cleft occurs with the needle tip in nearly vertical position. The needle is then rotated forwards so that the bent part is kept in close contact with the internal surface of the occiput for the entire length. The operator should learn to recognize the feeling of the needle being "hooked" to the mouse skull and, to practice, it is possible to inject a vital dye (e.g., trypan blue) to differentiate a successful from a failed injection. Injection of the vector should be done in approximately 10 s and the needle should be kept in place a few more seconds before extracting it. The highest volume that can be injected is 10 μl. Injection of more fluid will result in reflux along the needle track and excessive pressure will cause hydrocephalus. The same needle can be used to inject several mice. The entire injection procedure takes less than 1 min. A correct injection procedure distributes the vector throughout the ventricular and CSF space. In fact, although liquoral circulation goes from choroid plexi, where it is produced, to the cauda, the intracisternal injection will transiently revert the flux direction allowing viral vector particles to reach the whole ventricular system. If a reporter gene-containing vector (e.g., green fluorescent protein) is employed, infected cells can be easily traced in leptomeninges and in the ependymal cell layer and, in the case of fluorescent tracers, will appear as the whole mount in Fig. 16.1.

Follow-up

Mice usually recover rapidly from the injection procedure and show no evident adverse effects. A possible side effect of this procedure is ataxia due to a cerebellar lesion. The length of 3.5 mm indicated for the bent part of the needle

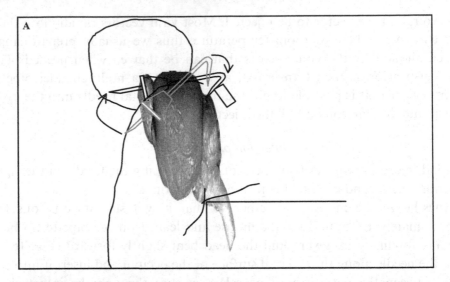

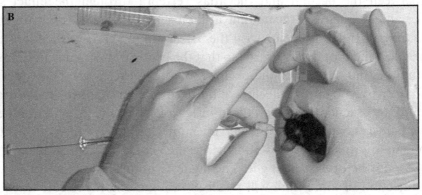

Figure 16.3. The intracisternal injection. (A) The needle of the assembled injection device is inserted in the cisterna magna through a rotating movement. The 3.5 mm long tip of the bent needle starts from a nearly vertical position, and after slipping into the cleft between occiput and atlas, is rotated to keep the needle hooked to the mouse skull. (B) Once inserted, one operator keeps the needle in place while a second operator injects in around 10 s.

should ensure that the cerebellum remains untouched in most mice strains and at different ages. In case application of this technique to small or very young mice is planned, shortening the needle length has to be considered. Mice will lose weight in the 2 days following an intracisternal injection, because of reduced food intake. After intracisternal injection, a transient local inflammatory reaction occurs, with an increase of the BBB permeability, lasting less then a week. Neuropathological signs of inflammation are, however, absent. Intracisternal injections can be repeated but at least 5 days apart.

References

1. Pardridge WM. Targeting neurotherapeutic agents through the blood–brain barrier. *Arch Neurol.* 2002, **59**: 35.
2. Pardridge WM. Drug and gene delivery to the brain: the vascular route. *Neuron* 2002, **36**: 555–558.
3. Furlan R, Pluchino S, Martino G. The therapeutic use of gene therapy in inflammatory demyelinating diseases of the central nervous system. *Curr. Opin. Neurol.* 2003, **16**: 385–392.
4. Miranda SR, Erlich S, Friedrich Jr VL, Gatt S, Schuchman EH. Hematopoietic stem cell gene therapy leads to marked visceral organ improvements and a delayed onset of neurological abnormalities in the acid sphingomyelinase deficient mouse model of Niemann–Pick disease. *Gene Ther.* 2000, **7**: 1768–1776.
5. Leimig T, Mann L, Martin M, del P, *et al.* Functional amelioration of murine galactosialidosis by genetically modified bone marrow hematopoietic progenitor cells. *Blood.* 2002, **99**: 3169–3178.
6. Matzner U, Hartmann D, Lullmann-Rauch R, *et al.* Bone marrow stem cell-based gene transfer in a mouse model for metachromatic leukodystrophy: effects on visceral and nervous system disease manifestations. *Gene Ther.* 2002, **9**: 53–63.
7. Burton EA, Fink DJ, Glorioso JC. Gene delivery using herpes simplex virus vectors. *DNA Cell Biol.* 2002, **21**: 915–936.
8. Zurn AD, Henry H, Schluep M, *et al.* Evaluation of an intrathecal immune response in amyotrophic lateral sclerosis patients implanted with encapsulated genetically engineered xenogeneic cells. *Cell Transplant.* 2000, **9**: 471–484.
9. Davidson BL, Breakefield XO. Viral vectors for gene delivery to the nervous system. *Nature Rev. Neurosci.* 2003, **4**: 353–364.
10. Janson C, McPhee S, Bilaniuk L, *et al.* Clinical protocol. Gene therapy of Canavan disease: AAV–2 vector for neurosurgical delivery of aspartoacylase gene (ASPA) to the human brain. *Hum. Gene Ther.* 2002, **13**: 1391–1412.
11. Martino G, Furlan R, Comi G, Adorini L. The ependymal route to access the central nervous system: an emerging immuno-gene therapy approach to multiple sclerosis. *Trends Immunol.* 2001, **22**: 483–490.
12. Shimamura M, Sato N, Oshima K, *et al.* Therapeutic strategy to treat brain ischemia: overexpression of hepatocyte growth factor gene reduced ischemic injury without cerebral edema in rat model. *Circulation* 2004, **109**: 424–431.
13. Furlan R, Brambilla E, Ruffini F, *et al.* Intrathecal delivery of IFNγ protects C57BL/6 mice from chronic-progressive experimental autoimmune encephalomyelitis by increasing apoptosis of CNS-infiltrating lymphocytes. *J. Immunol.* 2001, **167**: 1821–1829.
14. Poliani PL, Brok H, Furlan R, *et al.* Delivery of a non-replicative herpes simplex type-1 vector engineered with the IL-4 gene to the central nervous system protects rhesus monkeys from hyperacute autoimmune encephalomyelitis. *Hum. Gene Ther.* 2001, **12**: 905–920.
15. Burton EA, Glorioso JC, Fink DJ. Therapy progress and prospects: Parkinson's disease. *Gene Ther.* 2003, **10**: 1721–1727.
16. Martino G, Furlan R, Galbiati F, *et al.* A gene therapy approach to treat demyelinating diseases using non-replicative herpetic vectors engineered to produce cytokines. *Mult. Scler.* 1998, **4**: 222–227.

17. Furlan R, Poliani PL, Galbiati F, *et al.* Central nervous system delivery of Interleukin-4 by a non replicative Herpes Simplex Type I viral vector ameliorates autoimmune demyelination. *Hum. Gene Ther.* 1998, **9**: 2605–2617.
18. Ruffini F, Furlan R, Poliani PL, *et al.* Fibroblast growth factor-II gene therapy reverts the clinical course and the pathological signs of chronic experimental autoimmune encephalomyelitis in C57BL/6 mice. *Gen Ther.* 2001, **8**: 1207–1213.
19. Furlan R, Poliani PL, Marconi PC, *et al.* Interleukin-4 gene delivery in the central nervous system at the time of disease onset inhibits progression of autoimmune demyelination. *Gen. Ther.* 2001, **8**: 13–19.
20. Thomas CE, Schiedner G, Kochanek S, Castro MG, Lowenstein PR. Peripheral infection with adenovirus causes unexpected long-term brain inflammation in animals injected intracranially with first generation, but not with high-capacity, adenovirus vectors: towards realistic long-term neurological gene therapy for chronic diseases. *Proc. Natl Acad. Sci. USA* 2000, **97**: 7482–7487.
21. Schiedner G, Morral N, Parks RJ, *et al.* Genomic DNA transfer with a high-capacity adenovirus vector results in improved in vivo gene expression and decreased toxicity. *Nature Genet.* 1998, **18**: 180–183.
22. Parks RJ, Chen L, Anton M, *et al.* A helper-dependent adenovirus vector system: removal of helper virus by Cre mediated excision of the viral packaging signal. *Proc. Natl Acad. Sci. USA* 1996, **93**: 13565–13570.
23. Bukovsky AA, Song JP, Naldini L. Interaction of human immunodeficiency virus-derived vectors with wild-type virus in transduced cells. *J. Virol.* 1999, **73**: 7087–7092.
24. High KA. Gene transfer as an approach to treating hemophilia. *Circ. Res.* 2001, **88**: 137–144.
25. Muzyczka N. Use of adeno-associated virus as a general transduction vector for mammalian cells. *Curr. Top. Microbiol. Immunol.* 1992, **158**: 97–129.
26. Duan D, Li Q, Kao AW, *et al.* Circular intermediates of recombinant adeno-associated virus have defined structural characteristic responsible for long-term episomial persistence in muscle tissue. *J. Virol.* 1999, **73**: 8568–8577.
27. Nakai H, Iwaki Y, Kay MA, Couto LB. Isolation of recombinant adeno-associated virus vector-cellular DNA junction from mouse liver. *J. Virol.* 1999, **73**: 5438–5447.
28. Ueda H, Amano H, Shiomi H, Takagi H. Comparison of the analgesic effects of various opioid peptides by a newly devised intracisternal injection technique in conscious mice. *Eur. J. Pharmacol.* 1979, **56**: 265–268.
29. Furlan R, Pluchino S, Marconi PC, Martino G. Cytokine gene delivery into the central nervous system using intrathecally injected nonreplicative viral vectors. *Methods Mol. Biol.* 2003, **215**: 279–289.

17

Neural transplantation

STEPHEN B. DUNNETT, EDUARDO M. TORRES, MONTE A. GATES,
AND ROSEMARY A. FRICKER-GATES

17.1 Introduction

In spite of early attempts at neural transplantation as long ago as the late
nineteenth century, throughout most of the twentieth century it was widely
believed that the mammalian brain was relatively fixed and immutable in
adulthood, incompatible with receiving and supporting viable transplants.[1]
However, at the end of the 1960s, two discoveries challenged this received
view: the demonstration that sprouting and reorganization of axons can
indeed take place after damage in adult central nervous system (CNS) pathways;[2] and new experimental methods for transplanting nerve cells that were
remarkably successful in yielding surviving grafts.[3,4]

In the first decade after these pioneering studies, attention focused on
understanding the basic cellular and developmental biology of neural transplantation in a variety of model systems. Cells were transplanted into the CNS
of adult rats using a wide variety of experimental model systems – anterior
eye chamber, spinal cord, cerebellum, and diverse forebrain sites including
cortex, hypothalamus, striatum, and hippocampus. In the first wave of studies
(as illustrated in Fig. 17.1), pieces of neural tissue were implanted into natural
cavities such as the anterior chamber of the eye,[5] the brain ventricles[6,7] or
choroidal fissure.[8,9] In the search for a greater flexibility of graft placement,
other studies introduced inoculation of tissue fragments directly into brain
parenchyma,[10,11] although such grafts did not survive well, or the creation of
artificial cavities with a rich vascular lining that would nourish newly grafted
tissues.[12,13] However, the development of the dissociated cell suspension
method in the early 1980s[14,15] has – by virtue of its simplicity and reliability –
presaged a more widespread adoption of neural transplantation as a powerful
experimental tool in restorative neurology and neuroscience.

The cell suspension method has a number of distinct advantages over
previous methods: it is simple and reliable, and so found to yield good graft

Handbook of Experimental Neurology, ed. Turgut Tatlisumak and Marc Fisher. Published by Cambridge
University Press. © Cambridge University Press 2006.

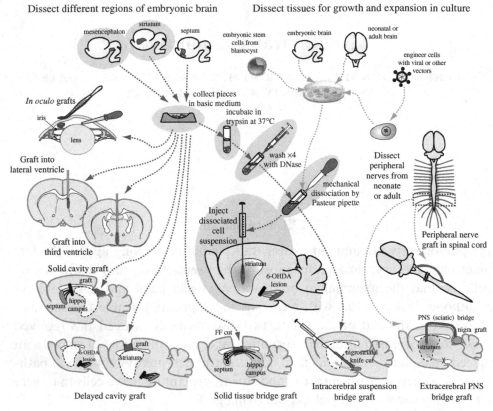

Figure 17.1. Schematic illustration of the variety of techniques used for neural transplantation in the rat nervous system. The methods described in detail in the present chapter are highlighted by back-shading. The sources of other methods are referenced in the text. PNS, peripheral nervous system.

survival in many laboratories; it is flexible, allowing multiple sources of cells and virtually any CNS target; the grafts can be placed at multiple sites, and in multiple deposits comprising one, mixed, or different cells in each; graft placements are made with stereotaxic accuracy; and the implantation method is relatively atraumatic, not requiring separate cavities or large implantation implements. For these reasons, the present protocols will focus on the preparation and implantation of dissociated cell suspension transplants in adult rat CNS. Of course, there remain experimental purposes for which solid tissue transplants are favored. Thus for example it may be necessary to locate the graft tissue in vivo for implanting an electrode or injecting an anatomical tracer. Alternatively, the transplant may be made with the purpose of providing space-occupying or bridging tissue, such as in the repair of spinal cord damage. Thirdly, some experiments require the maintenance of internal organization within the grafted tissues, as in lamination of cortical or retinal tissues, whereas in other studies it is important to determine if that level of organization can develop within dissociated cells. These specific purposes are however beyond the general scope of the present account, and we will focus on the more widely applicable methods that have application for diverse experimental purposes in different systems of the CNS.

17.2 Factors in successful neural transplantation

From early studies, several key principles have emerged that must be considered in determining the selection of an appropriate transplantation method for the particular experimental system under investigation.

17.2.1 Source, dissection, and age of donor tissue

The single most important factor in successful neural transplantation is the age of the donor tissue. In general, CNS neurons only survive transplantation if derived from early embryos or neonatal donors. Although this principle was first determined empirically, it turns out that optimal graft survival is achieved when the donors are selected at an age close to the period of peak neurogenesis for the neuronal population under investigation. Thus, a single donor age is not optimal for all tissues, but will depend on the birth dates of the proposed populations of neuron to be transplanted. In essence, with a 22–23 day gestation, early developing populations such as the diffusely projecting brainstem regulatory systems (dopamine, norepinephrine, serotonin) develop early and give best survival when taken from younger embryos (e.g., E12–E14 days of embryonic age*), other forebrain nuclei are better harvested a day or two later (e.g., striatum, septum: E14–E16), and some late developing nuclei (e.g., hippocampus, neocortex) survive well when taken from late embryonic development or even from a neonatal donor. Whereas there is a restricted time window in early development for harvesting CNS neurons from donor embryos, corresponding to the period of peak neurogenesis, other neural tissues are not so restricted. Peripheral neurons (e.g., dorsal root or sympathetic cervical ganglia), neuroendocrine cells (e.g., the chromaffin cells of the adrenal medulla), and central and peripheral glia (e.g., astrocytes, oligodendrocytes, or Schwann cells) all undergo division throughout life,

---

* According to current interpretation of UK legislation, in the UK embryos >E11 days of age must be killed according to a "Schedule 1" method. This is achieved by taking embryos from a dam which had been terminally anesthetized with barbiturate overdose, followed by a single direct incision through the brainstem.

and can similarly survive transplantation when harvested from more mature donors.

How should one determine, then, the age of the donor for the particular transplant tissues of experimental interest? There are essentially three sources of information. Firstly, the developmental literature can usually provide information on the timing of final mitosis, based on thymidine or bromodeoxyuridine (BrDU) labeling methods. Systematic accounts of birth dates of different populations in the rodent fore- and midbrain are provided by Altman, Bayer, and colleagues.[16–19] Secondly, there is now a large empirical neural transplantation literature, in which the viability of many, if not most, sources of primary cells have been documented at different developmental ages. Tables of optimal ages for different neuronal populations from rat embryonic donors have been published in several places,[20–22] one of which is reproduced in Table 17.1. Thirdly, the optimal ages suitable for growth in tissue culture[23] typically translate directly to similar ages being suitable for cell transplantation. Finally, any new experimental programs should include pilot studies to determine whether the selected parameters are appropriate, and in the case of neural transplantation such pilots may need to include a determination of optimal donor age as a key parameter.

17.2.2 Status of the host target

Several factors need to be considered relating to the status of the target sites in the host brain. Early studies of neural transplantation based on placement of solid pieces of tissue into the host brain found that grafts did not survive well unless positioned in a richly vascularized location in the host brain.[12] The grafts become incorporated into the host circulation within a few days of implantation[24,25] and their survival is presumably dependent upon their rapid establishment of this critical source of nutrition. A limited number of highly vascularized surfaces are available naturally in the adult brain, such as the endothelial lining of the ventricles, the pial surface of the brain, and the anterior chamber of the eye, whereas a freshly aspirated cavity is not suitable without further artificial preparation such as provision of co-grafts[12] or delayed transplantation.[13] However, a further advantage of dissociated cell suspension grafts over earlier methods is that they survive well when injected directly into the host neuropil, which may perhaps be due to the better apposition between, and closer integration of, the graft and host tissues.

In contrast to the age of the donor, the age of the host is less critical. Neuronal grafts can survive transplantation throughout host life, whether

Table 17.1. *Optimal ages and stages for transplanting embryonic rat tissues*

Region	Gestation day[a]	Crown–rump length (mm)[a]	Carnegie stage[b]	Expected growth (%)[a]
Parietal cortex	17–19	18–24	F	200–500
Entorhinal cortex	15–19	14–25	21–23	200–400
Hippocampus	19–21	26–34	F	200–600
Dentate gyrus	20–22	30–36	F/N	300–600
Cerebellum	14–15	11–13	19–21	400–800
Olfactory bulb	17–19	19–25	F	0–100
Spinal cord	15–17	14–20	21–23	100–400
Caudate nucleus[c]	15–16	12–16	20–22	200–300
Septum[c]	15–16	12–16	20–22	0–100
Substantia nigra[c]	14–15	10–14	18–21	100–200
Locus coeruleus[c]	14–15	10–14	18–21	50–200
Dorsal raphé[c]	14–15	10–14	18–21	100–200

Notes:

[a] Based on Table II in Olson *et al.*,[20] including all data on expected percentage growth following transplantation in oculo. The day following mating is defined as day E0.

[b] Carnegie stages based on Butler and Juurlink;[54] F, fetal; N, 1–2 days postnatal.

[c] Our present experience of monoamine-rich intracerebral grafts indicates that the optimal age for these tissues is somewhat younger than suggested in the original account of Olson *et al.*,[20] and the day, crown–rump length, and stage data are corrected accordingly. The comparative data on growth remains based on their in oculo experiments.

Source: Reproduced from Dunnett and Björklund,[22] with permission.

implanted in utero, into the neonate, in adulthood, or into the aged brain. Nevertheless, grafts typically survive better and show better differentiation and integration when implanted in younger than in aged hosts.[26–28] Differences can be even more marked when implants are made in immature hosts, and in the embryonic brain the grafted cells can be seen to differentiate and migrate much further than ever seen in adulthood, providing far greater dispersal and integration into the host neural circuitry.[29]

Should the host brain be previously lesioned? Clearly, when the purpose of an experiment is to investigate processes of repair and functional recovery then a preceding lesion associated with the relevant dimension of brain damage or disease is required.[30] However, in other studies on the basic neurobiology of cell transplantation, for example where the study involves factors promoting graft survival,[31,32] it may be argued that lesions are not required; indeed they may simply add variability. However, caution is required, since a preceding lesion can markedly promote graft survival, integration, and function. Thus for example, striatal grafts grow to only about one-third of the size when implanted into the intact striatum than when implanted into the site of a preceding striatal lesion.[33] This is likely to be attributable to positive survival signals induced by the lesion rather than simply the increased space available for growth since even a small lesion provides as great a stimulation of graft growth as a large lesion.[33] In a different model system, although similar numbers of dopamine neurons are seen to survive in nigral grafts whether or not the animals had previously received dopamine-denervating 6-hydroxydopamine (6-OHDA) lesions, fiber outgrowth into the denervated striatum was approximately double that seen into the intact brain.[34] Again, survival and fiber outgrowth need not be dependent upon synaptic space associated with lesion of the homotypic system in the host brain, since quite different lesions can activate survival- and growth-promoting factors that act upon diverse populations of grafted neurons.[35,36]

17.2.3 Hypothesized mechanism of graft function

When replacement of a specific cell type can yield functional recovery in animals with a lesion in the same system – e.g., recovery of rotation after transplantation of embryonic nigral neurons into animals in which the intrinsic nigrostriatal dopamine system has been lesioned with the dopamine-specific toxin 6-OHDA[6,37] – it is natural to assume that specific cell replacement provides the basis for the observed recovery. However it has become apparent that this need not be the case; a variety of other less-specific mechanisms may also promote recovery without repair.[38,39] Some of these alternative routes to recovery are illustrated in Table 17.2.

Thus over and above the questions of selecting an appropriate donor tissue and host lesion model, the hypothesized mechanism of action of a graft needs to be considered when designing an appropriate transplantation strategy. For some cell types it may be sufficient to implant a secretory cell close to its target receptors. Such has been the logic of neuroendocrine grafts in the hypothalamus,[7,40] and may apply also to dopaminergic grafts in the striatum,[6,37] although in both cases there is evidence that the process may be more specific.[37,41] However in other circumstances, the reformation of connected circuits in the host brain may be critical to functional activity, which is most obvious in situations where the lesions disconnect functional neural circuits, such as are involved in corticostriatal[42] or spinal cord[43] systems.

Table 17.2. *Mechanisms of graft function*

Mechanism	Description	Example
Non-specific	Non-specific effects of surgery	Placebo effects and psychosurgical lesions
Physical	Space-occupying tissue prevents progress of degeneration	Spinal cord tissues inhibit syrinx formation
Trophic		
Protective	Diffuse release of molecules that protect against degenerative disease processes	Cells that secrete trophic factors, antiapoptotic or antioxidant molecules
Support	Provide target support for host axons	Cortical cells support host thalamocortical axons from retrograde degeneration
Plasticity	Diffuse release of trophic agents that promote active reorganization and plasticity in the damaged CNS	Cells that secrete trophic factors, substrates for axonal growth, chemoattractant molecules, etc.
Pharmacological	Diffuse release of deficient neurochemicals ("biological minipumps")	Hypothalamic grafts secreting neurohormones or engineered secretory grafts
Reinnervation	Graft cells innervate host brain providing tonic control, but probably not regulated control	Nigral grafts restore synaptic dopaminergic activation of their striatal targets
Circuit reconstruction	Graft receives host input, transduces the signal, and connects back to host circuits	Striatal grafts establish functional graft–host–graft circuits in the nigro- and cortico-striato-pallidal system
Full repair		Not achieved

Source: Reproduced from Dunnett[118] with permission.

17.2.4 Immunological compatibility of donor and host

In contrast to what we might expect from the history of organ transplantation, immunological rejection is not a major issue for neural transplants, at least when considering allografts (i.e., grafts between genetically different members of the same species). Several factors contribute to the brain being one of the few "immunologically privileged sites" of the body; there is a low expression of histocompatibility antigens by neurons, immune cells and molecules are excluded by the blood–brain barrier, and the brain has sparse lymphatic drainage. As a consequence, standard allografts typically do survive well within the brains of outbred rat or monkey strains. Nevertheless, the privilege is only partial: T cells and immunoglobulins can enter when the blood–brain barrier is breached, as happens not only with lesions but at the time of transplantation; astrocytes do express larger complements of histocompatibility antigens, especially when activated by injury; and activated macrophages and other immune cells can penetrate the blood–brain barrier.[44] Consequently, if an immune response is specifically triggered (e.g., by a peripheral skin graft), or if the donor and host differ widely in major and minor histocompatibility antigens (e.g., in a xenograft, i.e., between a donor and host of different species), then a full immune rejection is typically seen, with both T-cell mediated and antibody-mediated attack. Even so, the very rapid hyperacute rejection response, triggered when circulating antibodies recognize the foreign blood vessel walls in organ xenografts, does not arise in neural suspension grafts in the brain, presumably because the blood vessels in suspension grafts are reconstituted primarily from host-derived rather than donor-derived endothelial cells,[25] promoting the prospect that the brain may provide a suitable target for xenotransplantation if combined with effective immunosuppression.[45]

If the graft is likely to reject, standard organ immunosuppression strategies work equally well for protection of neural grafts. The most widely used strategy for rats involves giving the drug cyclosporin A (Sandimmune).[46,47] It has unfortunately not proved possible to devise acceptable protocols for oral self-administration via the food or water, which the animals reject because of the bitter taste, so the drug must be injected daily 10 mg/kg intraperitoneally (i.p.). Such treatment typically yields 70–90% survival of mouse-, human-, or pig-to-rat xenografts; not as good as allografts, but significantly better than the close to 100% rejection without treatment.[48] More complex triple treatments of cyclosporin, prednisolone, and azathioprine, as derived from human organ transplantation, yield only limited further improvement.[49] Conversely, there is currently widespread interest in novel immunosuppression strategies that might render the host specifically tolerant to the grafts.[50] These include monoclonal antibodies directed against specific components of the rejection response, such as CD3, CD4, or interleukin-2 (IL-2) receptor,[51,52] and would in principle require only single treatment for long-term protection. However, none of these strategies has yet been proved to the point of widespread acceptance as a more efficient alternative to long-term administration of daily cyclosporin.

17.3 A standard dissociated cell suspension protocol

These factors together will determine, for any particular experiment, the specific selection of donor tissue, method of tissue preparation, and the method and target site for transplantation. For the purposes of elaborating general methods of cell transplantation, we shall outline in detail the protocol used in our laboratory for the preparation of a standard dissociated cell suspension of embryonic nigra. This protocol is applicable for the stereotaxic transplantation of a wide variety of CNS tissues from embryonic donors into the adult host brain. First the standard method for transplanting dopamine-rich embryonic nigra tissue into the adult rat brain is summarized right through, from beginning to end. This is then followed by further consideration of particular components, alternative tissues, other hosts, and specific additional protocols.

17.3.1 Preparation

Facilities and equipment

Three separate laboratory areas are required, approved as required by local and national health, safety, and animal welfare regulations:

- *Procedure room*: an appropriate procedure room in the animal house or laboratory, for killing the pregnant donor and harvesting the embryos. The procedure room needs to be equipped with general anesthesia, a guillotine, and appropriate facilities for carcass disposal.
- *Cell preparation laboratory*: a clean laboratory for dissecting the embryonic tissues and preparing the dissociated cell suspensions. Although we have in the past undertaken these procedures on an open laboratory bench, the chance of contamination or infection of the tissue is markedly reduced if the work can be undertaken with a laminar flow hood. The laboratory needs to be provided with the following equipment:

  Autoclave for advance sterilization of instruments and glassware
  Category 1 hood (e.g., Astec Microflow horizontal laminar flow workstation)
  Binocular stereo dissecting microscope, ideally with zoom and transmitted light base (e.g., Leica MZ6 or MZ7.5)
  Fiberoptic incident light source for dissection microscope stage (e.g., Schott KL1500)
  Hot bead sterilizer or alcohol and spirit burner for resterilizing instruments in use
  Heating block or water bath, suitable to incubate 1.5 ml Eppendorf tubes at $37 \pm 1\,°C$
  20, 200, and 1000 μl Gilson pipettes
  Bench-top centrifuge (e.g., Beckman Microfuge)

Hemocytometer and simple bright field laboratory microscope with ×10 objective for cell counting and viability estimates (e.g., Leica Laborlux).

- *Surgery*: a surgical area or room for transplantation into the host animals. This room should be fully equipped for stereotaxic surgery under general anesthesia:

  Stereotaxic frame (e.g., Kopf Model 900 for rats or mice) with syringe holder

  Syringes for transplantation. A 10 µl glass microsyringe, preferably with guided plunger and removable needle (e.g., SGE Model 10-RN-GP or Hamilton 801-RN). The syringe should best be fitted with wide-bore needle (outer diameter 0.5 mm, inner diameter 0.25 mm), cut down to approx 2 cm length to reduce vibration, and the tip cut square and domed to increase accuracy of the depth of injection

  General anesthesia: we prefer the greater safety and control of gaseous anesthesia, which requires cylinders of O_2 and NO, flow regulators, an isofluorane atomizer, induction chamber, stereotaxic delivery mask, a scavenging system, and appropriate tubing and connectors (e.g., International Market Supplies); appropriate injectable anesthetics can also be suitable, subject to local veterinary advice and guidelines

  Surgical microscope (e.g., Zeiss OPMI mounted on bench or floor stand)

  Fiberoptic or other surgical light source (e.g., Schott KL1500)

  Animal shavers, dental drill, heated recovery blankets

  Refrigerator for storing the cell suspension during surgery (a simple domestic model is suitable); alternatively, if space or costs are an issue, the tissue may be held for the duration of the surgical session in a polystyrene bucket containing crushed ice.

Media

Four solutions are required. Each should be prepared sterile and filtered.

- *Base solution*: sterile DMEM/F12 (Gibco 21331–046). Store at 4 °C. Aliquot into 50 ml centrifuge tubes for use.
- *Dissection solution*: DMEM/F12 base solution (Gibco 21331–046) containing 0.6% glucose (Sigma G7021), 0.125% $NaHCO_3$ (Gibco 11810–025) and 0.005M HEPES (Gibco 15630–056). The dissection solution is prepared as stock and may be stored for up to a month at 4 °C. Aliquot into 50 ml centrifuge tubes for use.
- *Trypsin solution*: low Ca and Mg $HBSS^{--}$ (Gibco 14170–138) containing 0.1% bovine trypsin (Worthington 3703) and 0.05% DNase (Sigma DN-25). Prepare in batches and store as 1 ml aliquots in 1.5 ml Eppendorf tubes at −20 °C.
- *DNase solution*: 0.05% DNase in dissection solution. Prepare in batches and store in 1 ml aliquots in 1.5 ml Eppendorf tubes at −20 °C.

Instruments, disposables, and glassware

Separate sets of instruments are required for each stage of the preparation. They are kept in separate kits and sterilized on each occasion before use.

- *Procedure room*: the kit for the procedure room contains large and medium scissors, and large toothed and medium serrated forceps. Also available are: Euthetal, 1 ml and 2 ml syringes and needles for euthanasia; sterile cotton surgical swabs, Betadine, and 70% alcohol for sterilizing the abdomen of the pregnant rat(s); 50 ml centrifuge tube(s) containing base medium, for collecting the embryos from each mother. Sterile disposable gloves
- *Cell preparation laboratory*: the dissection kit contains small pointed scissors, small forceps, small scalpel handle, 3 × Dumont No. 5 forceps, Dumont No. 7 forceps, ultrafine Vannas spring iridectomy scissors, 3 × single cavity glass microscope slides. Also in the laminar flow hood are the dissection microscope and hot bead sterilizer, sterile 100 mm diameter Petri dishes, the three Gilson pipettes and sterile pipette tips, sterile fine pointed scalpel blades (Beaver No. 65 blades are preferred, but standard No. 11 blades will suffice), and sterile dissection, trypsin and DNase solutions (a thawed 1.5 ml Eppendorf of each for each brain region to be dissected). Also available in the cell preparation laboratory are sterile disposable gloves, 70% alcohol and swabs, filtered 1M HCl solution in a glass-stoppered bottle, the hemocytometer, a 0.4% trypan blue solution (Sigma), an ice bucket containing crushed ice
- *Surgery*: each person will have their own preferred selection of instruments for inclusion in the surgery kit. Ours contain large round-tipped scissors, small pointed scissors, large and medium forceps, 1 × No. 5 Dumont forceps, 1 × No. 7 Dumont forceps, 2 × hemostats, large and medium scalpel handle. Also available are sterile disposable gloves, sterile distilled water, 70% alcohol and swabs, 1 ml syringes and syringe needles, Sizes ½ and 3 dental drill bits, sterile cotton buds.

Preparation

On the day before surgery, time-mated rats are checked for pregnancy and the stage of pregnancy estimated (see below). If the pregnancy is at a stage suitable for transplantation, prepare for surgery on the following day; otherwise tissue collection and surgery may be put back one or two days as required:

(1) Confirm the availability of all solutions, instruments, and equipment.
(2) Sterilize the three instrument kits and other glassware, either using an autoclave or by heating in an oven at 160 °C for 1 hr.
(3) Delicate instruments such as the transplantation microlitre syringes and the Vannas scissors should not be autoclaved – sterilize by immersion in 70% alcohol overnight.
(4) Clean and lay out the procedure room, cell preparation laboratory, and surgery facilities.

17.3.2 Staging pregnant rats

As indicated above, harvesting donor tissues at the optimal stage of fetal development is critical for graft viability. Accurate staging of the pregnancy is therefore an important adjunctive procedure. Ideally, this is achieved by accurate and reliable mating being provided by the animal supplier or your own animal house. However, even if this source is reliable, two additional cautions are required. Firstly, different laboratories and authors variously describe the day following overnight pairing of the receptive female with a stud male and confirmation of a vaginal plug in the morning as either embryonic day E0, day E0.5, or day E1, with up to 1 day difference in all subsequent statements on embryonic age. Secondly, depending on strain and litter size, the embryonic development and physical growth of embryos can progress at slightly different rates. Therefore rather than embryonic age per se, what is required is an accurate estimate of the size and stage of embryonic development. This has been studied in great morphological detail in particular for human embryos[53] but also for a wide variety of other laboratory species.[54] This information allows graded stages of fetal development to be determined, not only with reference to embryonic age but also in terms of the size of the embryo and the appearance of critical morphological features.[54] Consequently, the stage of donor development should always be determined and reported not only in terms of 'E*n*' days of embryonic age but also with reference to the size, determined from the crown–rump length (CRL) (Fig. 17.2A).

Although accurate estimation of CRL requires killing of the dam and removal of the embryos for direct measurement, fetal size can be estimated

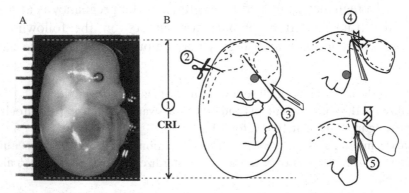

Figure 17.2. Measurement and dissection of embryos. (A) Photograph of E15 embryo illustrating the dimension for measurement of crown–rump length (CRL). (B) Steps in removing the brain from the cranium (see text for details).

Table 17.3. *Estimation of length of pregnancy in rats by palpation under ether anesthesia*

Age (days)	Crown–rump length (CRL) (mm)[a]	Carnegie stage[b]	Signs at palpation[a]
4–7		3–5	Uterine horns are difficult to find and have variable thickness
8–9		6–9	Uterine horns have small, closely spaced, distinct swellings
10		10–11	
11		12–13	
12	8	14–15	
13	9	16–17	Small, distinct, firm spheres with an increasing diameter which approximates the corresponding CRL stage
14	10–11	18–19	
15	12–14	20–21	
16	15–16	22–23	
17	17–19	Fetal	Elastic, somewhat ovoid enlargements; width less than CRL
18	21–23	Fetal	Fetal structures begin to become palpable; head becomes identifiable; small distinct borders between adjacent fetuses; softer than at day 17
19	24–25	Fetal	Fetal indurations appear
20		Fetal	Uterine horns are thick, soft continuous tubes if litter is large
22	45	Neonatal	Day of birth

Notes:
[a] The CRL and palpation signs are based on Table I from Olson *et al.*[20] for live embryos in vivo, with the morning following overnight mating defined as E0.
[b] The Carnegie stages at each age are based on Butler and Juurlink.[54] Note that they define the morning of vaginal plug as E1, which has been modified to E0 in the table above. Also, the CRL measurements given here do not correspond accurately with their report since the latter were based on fixed tissues.

Source: Reproduced from Dunnett and Björklund[22] with permission.

in vivo by palpation of the pregnant rat under light gaseous anesthesia.[20,22] This is especially important if there is any doubt about the reliability of the mating, pregnancy, or estimate of embryonic age. The anesthetised dam is laid out belly down and with head away from you; then place either hand around the body, thumbs along the flank, and palpate the abdomen with the fingers. The uterine horns can be clearly felt, the individual embryos identified, and their size and firmness estimated (Table 17.3). With practice and experience an accuracy of 1–2 mm in the estimate of CRL can readily be achieved, sufficient in each case to determine/confirm the optimum day for transplantation.

17.3.3 Harvesting embryos

On the day of surgery:

(1) Overdose the pregnant rat with barbiturate anesthesia (0.5–1 ml Euthetal® i.p.), and then cervically dislocate or decapitate to kill.
(2) Lay the corpse on its back on paper towels, and swab the abdomen with Betadine followed by 70% alcohol.
(3) Open the peritoneum with a midline incision using the large blunt scissors and large toothed forceps. First cut the skin away from the site, then make a midline incision in the fascia of the abdomen (approx 3 cm).
(4) Using clean forceps and scissors, expose and lift out the uterine horns in turn, ensuring they do not touch the outside skin and hair, trimming away tissues attaching to the abdomen, and remove intact. Transfer the uterine horns (still containing the embryos) to the 50 ml centrifuge tube containing the base medium for transfer to the cell preparation laboratory.
(5) Dispose of the corpse and clean the preparation room.

17.3.4 Removing the embryo brains

All tissue handling is undertaken in the laminar flow hood. Sterilize all instruments in the bead sterilizer for 10–15 s, immediately prior to use.

(1) Transfer each uterine horn, typically containing 5–8 embryos, with the medium forceps to a clean Petri dish containing several milliliters of dissection medium.
(2) Using the pointed scissors and forceps, open the uterus with a longitudinal incision to expose the individual embryos. Separate each embryo from its amniotic sac and placenta and transfer using the No. 7 Dumont forceps into a second Petri dish containing 2–4 ml dissection medium. All embryos from the two horns of one dam can be collected into the second Petri dish before commencing the brain removal and tissue dissection.
(3) Inspect the embryos and discard any obvious runts. Measure the CRL of two or three of the embryos by placing a graduated rule beneath the Petri dish (Fig. 17.2B(1)).
(4) Remove the embryonic brain from each embryo. There are different approaches to removing the embryonic brain but a simple and reliable lateral approach for younger embryos (E17 or less) is illustrated in Fig. 17.2B. Using the pointed scalpel blade make a single incision into the mesencephalic flexure just above the eye and below the base of the skull (Fig. 17.2B(3)). Overlying skin and

cartilage may then be peeled away using Dumont No. 5 forceps (Fig. 17.2B(4)), and the brain is removed from any further attachments at the neck (Fig. 17.2B(5)). More detailed descriptions of this dissection are provided elsewhere.[21]

Visualization of the dissection is easiest using a transmitted light base for the microscope, alongside incident illumination, since brain structures can be visualized through the semitranslucent superficial tissues. If this is not available, position the fiberoptic light source to provide oblique illumination with as good contrast as possible.

For older embryos or neonates, after decapitation, the skull may be removed by a midline cut from the spine to the snout, along the dorsal surface over the brain using small scissors. The tissue can then be peeled back each side to remove the brain, akin to the procedure for brain removal from adult rats.

17.3.5 Dissecting embryonic tissues

Many alternative dissections are possible depending on purpose. We here describe preparation of a standard nigral dissection (Fig. 17.3). Several other dissections used in the laboratory are summarized in Section 17.5.1.

(1) Place ~0.5 ml dissection solution into a clean single cavity glass microscope slide, and transfer two or three embryonic brains at a time for dissection.
(2) Lay the brain on its side and, using Dumont No. 5 forceps and the iridectomy scissors, make two cuts (1 and 2) perpendicular to the ventral surface of the brain at the anterior and posterior ends of the mesencephalic flexure (Fig. 17.3A and B).

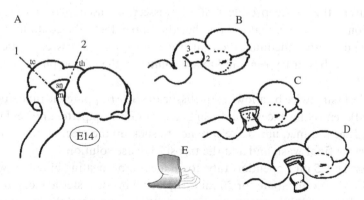

Figure 17.3. Nigral grafts. Schematic illustration of the steps (A–E) in dissecting the ventral mesencephalon from an E14 brain (see text for details). m, mesencephalic flexure; sn, substantia nigra; tc, tectum; th, thalamus.

(3) Slide the point of the iridectomy scissors into the mesencephalic tube and make a longitudinal cut (3) between cuts 1 and 2, about one-third of the distance between the ventral and dorsal surfaces (Fig. 17.3B and C).

(4) Fold open the exposed ventral mesencephalon and separate from the rest of the brain with a further longitudinal cut (4) on the ventral surface of the mesencephalic tube (Fig. 17.3C and D).

(5) Tease away the meninges from the external surface of the dissected piece (Fig. 17.3E).

(6) Collect dissected pieces from all embryos into a 1.5 ml Eppendorf tube containing ~1 ml sterile dissection medium.

When dissecting embryonic tissues, the essential principle is to minimize trauma to the target tissue itself. Therefore it is important to avoid touching the target tissue with the scalpel blade, forceps, or scissors, at all times gripping and stabilizing the dissection by contact with other parts of the embryo, and always cutting or prising away from the target itself. The removal of meninges from the surface of the tissue can be tricky, but is important, since its inclusion in the suspension can give rise to non-neural tissues developing within the grafts. This is best achieved by grasping the relatively resilient meninges with one pair of Dumont No. 5 forceps, and drawing it through the almost closed jaws of the second pair to leave the neural tissue behind. Again, do not pinch the dissected piece directly but transfer it to the collection Eppendorf tube either by scooping it from below with the curved tips of the Dumont No. 7 forceps or by bracketing the piece between the partly closed tips of the No. 5 forceps and lifting it by surface tension in the meniscus of trapped medium.

17.3.6 *Preparing dissociated cell suspensions*

(1) Clear away the waste products of the dissection, used plastic ware, and the dissection microscope. Gather together the Eppendorf tube containing dissected pieces in dissection medium, the centrifuge tube of extra dissection medium, the Eppendorf tubes of trypsin and DNase solutions, the Gilson pipettes, and sterile pipette tips.

(2) Wash the tissue twice by allowing the tissue to settle (tapping the tube side gently if required), removing excess fluid using a 1 ml Gilson pipette, and replacing with sterile dissection medium. Take care not to suck up the pieces into the pipette.

(3) Remove the final wash and add the trypsin/DNase solution.

(4) Transfer the 1.5 ml Eppendorf tube to an incubator, heating block, or water bath set at 37 °C, and incubate for 20 min. If placing inside a sterile incubator, loosen the cap slightly. Halfway through the incubation, resuspend the pieces once: close the cap firmly, make a single rapid inversion of the tube; loosen the cap again once upright, and return to the incubator.

(5) While the pieces are incubating, adjust the pH of the DNase solution using 1M HCl to approximately pH 7.4. The pH in a small-volume Eppendorf tube may most conveniently be tested by using a needle tip to transfer small amounts of the solution and spotting onto pH paper.

(6) Remove the trypsin solution and wash twice with 200 µl DNase solution using a Gilson pipette. Replace the final wash with 200 µl of DNase solution.

(7) Mechanically triturate the tissue into single cells using Gilson pipettes. First take a 1 ml pipette set to 180 µl and gently break up the tissue with 10 strokes. Then repeat the trituration using a 200 µl Gilson pipette set to 180 µl, using a maximum of 15 strokes. If the cells do not form a single cell suspension (which is a common problem with ventral mesencephalic tissue) allow any lumps to settle out then remove the supernatant to a fresh Eppendorf tube. Replace 200 µl DNase solution on top of the remaining pieces and triturate with a 200 µl Gilson pipette a further 15 strokes. Repeat this step as necessary until all cells are in suspension. Mix all aliquots together into a single Eppendorf tube.

(8) Remove an aliquot of suspension for cell counting (see Section 17.3.7 below) then place the Eppendorf tube in the centrifuge and spin at 600 *g* for 3 min.

(9) Remove the supernatant and replace with DNase solution to a final volume calculated from the cell counting procedure (usually a known volume of solution per piece of tissue, e.g., 1 ventral mesencephalon piece per 5 µl). Make the volume up to the maximum required using a second Eppendorf tube containing the known volume as a blank against which to measure. Resuspend the cells and store on crushed ice or transfer directly to the surgery refrigerator until ready for surgery.

17.3.7 Counting cell viability

The viability and final density of the suspension is determined using a vital dye stain in a hemocytometer counting chamber. A combination of acridine orange and ethidium bromide can provide independent counts of live and dead cells,[55] but this method does require an appropriately equipped fluorescence microscope to be available in, or close to, the cell preparation laboratory. A simpler strategy is to use the trypan blue exclusion principle – whereby dead cells accumulate but live cells exclude the dye – and counting stained and unstained cells in the counting chamber in a simple bright-field laboratory microscope.

(1) To set up the hemocytometer, breathe on the cover-slip to attach it to the base and check for "Newton's rings."

(2) Resuspend the cell suspension in its 1.5 ml Eppendorf tube using a sterile yellow tip in a 200 µl Gilson pipette set at 160 µl.

(3) For a 1 : 10 dilution, use Gilson pipettes to transfer 5 µl cell suspension to 45 µl trypan blue solution in a small glass well or small centrifuge tube, and mix by further resuspension.

(4) Transfer 10 µl to the hemocytometer's engraved counting platform under the attached cover-slip, ensuring that the platform is entirely covered.

(5) Count live and dead cells under the microscope. The grid has 5×5 square sectors, with each sector subdivided into 4×4 smaller squares. It is necessary to count 100–200 cells in total to get an accurate estimation. With a 10-fold dilution, this typically requires sampling the whole grid, counting the number of cells in each of the 16 small squares in each of the 25 sectors. (If the density is very much greater, count only every nth cell in each sector of the grid ($n = 2, 4, 8, 16$) to bring the total count into the required range). When counting the number of cells in each square, apply an inclusion/exclusion rule whereby all cells touching the upper or right hand edges of the square are counted, whereas any cells touching the left or lower edge are excluded from the count. Accumulate separate counts of white (live) cells and blue (dead) cells over all 25 sampled squares, TL and TD, respectively.

(6) Calculate cell viability (V) as a percentage according to the formula:

$$V = 100 \times \frac{TL}{(TL + TD)}\%$$

(7) Calculate the density (D) of live cells according to the formula:

$$D = 10 \times TL \times 10 \, \text{cells}/\mu l$$

based on counting every square in the grid with a 10-fold dilution of the suspension, the dimensions of a standard hemocytometer comprising a 1 mm square grid, the depth of the space between the cover-slip and counting frame is 1/10 mm, and $1 \, \mu l = 1 \, \text{mm}^3$.

If only every nth cell is counted, add an additional component into the formula:

$$D = 10 \times TL \times 10 \, n \, \text{cells}/\mu l$$

(8) A typical experiment will seek to control the amount of grafted tissue according to one of two principles:

> a standard number and density of cells (e.g., inject 3 µl of a 200 000 cells/µl suspension)
>
> a standard amount of donor tissue (e.g., inject 1 donor ventral mesencephalon per host in a final volume of 5 µl).

(9) Based on the number of tissue pieces, the estimated live cell density, and volume of cells and media within the sampled Eppendorf tube, adjust the volume of DNase medium added to the spun cell suspension to give the final working density (step 9 in the preceding protocol of Section 7.3.6).

Cell viability may be expected to decline across a surgical session lasting several hours.[55] We routinely set a pragmatic limit of 3 hr from the completion of cell preparation to the last transplant injection for nigral tissues, although longer periods up to 6 hr are feasible for more robust cells such as striatal cell suspensions, or by dividing the cells into aliquots for surgery (see Section 17.4 below). A cell viability measurement should be taken both prior to and after the transplantation surgery session to allow an estimate of decline during the session, since this may affect subsequent graft survival. When there is more than one transplant group in an experiment, it is important to counterbalance the order of operations on the animals from each group to ensure that additional treatment effects are not confounded with the order of surgery during the surgical session.

17.3.8 Transplantation surgery

The prepared cells are transplanted into the rodent brain using standard stereotaxic surgical technique, as described in many places. As such, it should not be necessary to provide a full step-by-step protocol, and details of the anesthetic regimes, stereotaxic equipment, and procedures will be well worked out already for each laboratory. However, there are specific components of the surgical procedures – related to the selection, handling, and stereotaxic positioning of the injection syringe, injection parameters, and postoperative care – that may need to be adapted for cell transplantation.

Surgical sterility

In contrast to most other mammalian species, rats and mice are robust to surgical infection and full sterile technique may not be required. However, cell suspensions can be an effective route for surgical infection, compromising graft survival, and good sterile technique during surgery is advised.

The suspension microsyringe

We have routinely found a 10 µl glass microsyringe suitable. We favor syringes with removable needles and guided plungers. The removable needle allows a wide-bore needle to be selected, the syringe needle to be shortened to allow less movement during implantation, and the bevel of the needle tip reduced, cut square, or domed in order to improve accuracy of the depth measurement and symmetry of the injection. Standard needles can be difficult to load without clogging which is aided by the wide bore. The ease of cleaning will also decline with repeated cellular loading and sterilization, and although reused they can be readily discarded and replaced if removable. The glass syringe is mounted on the vertical electrode carrier of the stereotaxic gantry; this is best achieved using a universal holder (Kopf Model 1772) and a section of polyethylene tubing spliced around the glass syringe barrel to protect it from direct pressure from the metal clamp. A guided plunger design of the syringe is favored, both for its robustness and for ease of mounting vertically without the plunger falling under its own weight. Both Hamilton and SGE make suitable syringes, as detailed in Section 17.3.1.

Note that although we use fine glass and stainless steel cannulae attached via polyethylene tubing to a syringe in a microdrive pump for smooth delivery of toxin solutions when making lesions, this approach is not suitable for transplants; both the reduced dead space and the pulsatile delivery achieved with direct syringe injection together serve to reduce the incidence of clogs in the injection cannulae, which is a much greater problem when injecting dense cell suspensions than when injecting solutions.

Loading the syringe

It is preferable to load the syringe separately for each injection, to avoid cells settling out between injections. Once the host animal is anesthetized and mounted in the frame, the stereotaxic co-ordinates are determined from the mounted syringe tip positioned against an external landmark, such as bregma, and the skull burr holes drilled and prepared for penetration. Then:

  raise the syringe in the gantry;
  take the vial of cell suspension from the refrigerator or ice bucket, and briefly resuspend using a 200 µl Gilson with sterile yellow tip;
  if the syringe has not already been cleaned, flush the syringe and use cotton buds to wipe the external tip of the needle first with 70% alcohol followed by sterile distilled water;
  draw the cell suspension up into the syringe by raising the plunger;
  check that there are no air bubbles in the syringe (back illumination with the fiberoptic light source helps visualization).

The suspension injection

The stereotaxic injection itself should proceed as follows:

  Positioning. Lower the syringe needle to the surface of the dura. Nick the dura with a disposable needle tip, and further lower the syringe needle slowly to the stereotaxic target.
  Injection. The suspension should be injected gradually over several minutes to allow the suspension to diffuse slowly into the host neuropil. The injection should proceed in a pulsatile manner, slowly extending or twisting the plunger by, e.g., 0.25 µl every 15 s, to inject 3 µl over 3 min.

Withdrawal. A further 2–5 min should be allowed for the suspension to settle before withdrawing the needle, which should also be done slowly over 10 s or longer. If the diffusion time is too short or the needle is withdrawn too rapidly, suspension is sucked back up the needle track, losing tissue from the target site, yielding instead vertically elongated grafts and leakage back out over the cortical surface. The rat brain can readily accommodate injections of 2–3 µl but larger volumes give additional problems of graft vascularization and survival alongside the problem of back extrusion of tissue. It is preferable to flush and clean the needle at the end of each injection rather than prior to the following injection, as this reduces the likelihood of remaining cells congealing to block the needle between animals.

Perioperative care

Grafted animals are provided with the same postoperative care as applied for all neurosurgery, being given fluid and glucose replacement, analgesics, and antibiotics as advised by local regulations and veterinary advice. Neural transplantation is typically an innocuous procedure; we see a response in host animals similar to that seen after sham lesions involving injections of saline, and considerably fewer adverse symptoms than many experimental lesion procedures such as aspiration or excitotoxic injections.

The long-term prospects of the grafts are also typically innocuous from a welfare perspective; indeed the purpose of many transplantation procedures is to alleviate symptoms associated with previous lesion treatments. Nevertheless, the animals should be closely monitored for adverse consequences, some of which may take months or even years to develop, as illustrated by the dyskinesias that have developed in some Parkinson's disease patients receiving nigral transplants.[56] Attention should be paid to the possibility of the animals developing tumors, in particular when using a novel tissue source or when the experimenter is not yet well experienced with embryonic tissue dissection.

17.4 Refinements in the cell suspension protocols

Preparation of the cell suspension and its storage prior to implantation are important parameters for obtaining healthy grafts, and considerable attention was paid in the early development of the method to issues of enzyme digestion, tissue dissociation, media used, etc.[57–59] The protocol provided above incorporates the basic technical refinements without detailed discussion.

One important parameter is the delay between preparation and implantation. Brundin and colleagues showed that the viability of cell suspensions

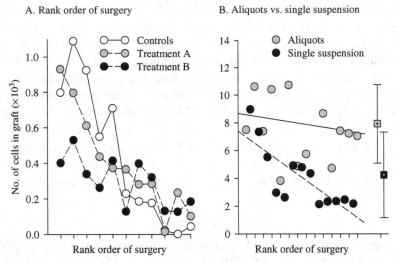

Figure 17.4. Effect of time since preparation on survival of tyrosine hydroxylase (TH) cells in nigral grafts. All rats received identical unilateral nigrostriatal lesions and identically prepared nigral grafts. (A) Notwithstanding three different drug treatments that had no effect on graft survival, the number of surviving cells in animals of each group declines similarly the longer the interval between cell preparation and implantation (33 rats implanted over a 5-hr surgery session). (B) The single cell suspension was on preparation divided in half, one half kept as a single suspension, which was repeatedly resuspended each time a subsequent sample was taken for implantation, the other half divided into six small aliquots, each used for only two consecutive hosts (25 rats received grafts alternatively between the two conditions over a 4-hr surgery session). Note that the standard deviation of the cell numbers in the aliquots group is slightly less than that in the single suspension group, even though the mean survival is approximately double. Note also that up to 14 000 TH-positive cells have survived in some of the grafts (implanted at the density of one donor ventral mesencephalon (VM) to one host) using present preparation methods, compared with approximately 40 000–48 000 in total in the adult VM.

prepared from E14 donor embryos, determined using vital dyes, remained at greater than 90% for up to 3 hr after trypsinization; thereafter viability dropped to 80% at the 5-hr time point and just 50% at 9 hr.[55] The deterioration of graft suspension can similarly be seen in vivo when a single nigral cell suspension has been used to implant a large group of animals. Using tyrosine hydroxylase (TH) immunohistochemistry to label surviving dopamine cells, the number of TH-positive cells seen in the host declines with time, such that rats which received implanted tissue from the fresh nigral cell suspension contain more TH-positive cells than those which received implants at a later time in the surgical session (Fig. 17.4A). It is important therefore that, once prepared, the suspension is implanted rapidly into the host brain, preferably within 3 hr of dissociation. With large groups of animals this may necessitate two operators to carry out the implantation procedure.

Of course, it may be that it is not the passage of time per se that leads to declining viability, but that cells are subjected to cumulative stress pending surgery. Over the course of a surgery session, the graft suspension is conventionally kept in a single Eppendorf tube, stored in a container of crushed ice. Cells in the suspension have a tendency to settle and aggregate at the bottom of the tube. Thus, each time the grafting syringe is reloaded cells need to be dissociated and resuspended. It is therefore likely that repeated trituration of a cell suspension exposes the cells to a cumulative detrimental degree of trauma, hastening the decline in cell viability. We have tested this by dividing the cells into multiple small aliquots immediately following preparation of the final cell suspension so that each aliquot need only be resuspended once or twice prior to implantation. When 25 animals are implanted over a 5-hr session alternating between a single large suspension and multiple smaller aliquots, we see a progressive decline in the numbers of TH-positive cells surviving in the former case but stable cell survival in the latter (Fig. 17.4B). As well as improving viability, using multiple smaller aliquots also allows the cell suspension to be divided more accurately between animals and may decrease the variability of graft size between animals in the same experimental group. Thus, the standard deviation is smaller as a proportion of the mean in the multiple aliquots group than in the single suspension group (Fig. 17.4B).

Nevertheless, one never sees 100% cell survival, and many studies find that only 1–10% of nigral dopamine cells survive in nigral grafts,[60] which has turned out to be a major issue in clinical trials of neuronal transplants in Parkinson's disease.[61] A variety of factors contribute to the cell death, including physical trauma during preparation and implantation, lack of positive trophic support for the embryonic cells in the adult brain, and oxidative stress and other toxic assaults on the newly grafted cells in the host brain. Systematic review of the variety of factors compromising viability has led to the search for additional neuroprotective and trophic agents to add to the grafts,[32] including antioxidants such as lazaroids,[62] calcium channel antagonists such as nimodipine,[63] antiapoptotic agents such as caspases,[31] broad-acting and specific trophic factor supplements such as fibroblast growth factor (FGF) and glial-derived neurotrophic factor (GDNF), respectively,[64–66] and variations in preparation and implantation protocols.[58,67] Each of these factors has been seen to have significant – but typically small – effects. The mechanisms are relatively specific since other neuroprotective agents have not proved effective, including treatment with the free-radical scavenger alpha-phenyl-*N*-tert-butyl nitrone,[68] with the glutamate receptor antagonist MK-801[69] or with other neurotrophins.[70] Nevertheless, in our experience, the greatest single factor in promoting good survival is the application of care in tissue handling, dissociation and implantation. Thus, in our latest experiments, we are achieving a mean of ~20% survival of TH neurones in the grafts, and >30% in some animals, in the absence of additional supplements (EM. Torres, unpublished data; see Fig. 17.4B).

17.5 Specific variations

The preceding discussion has described standard protocols for injecting dissociated cell suspensions of nigral tissues. Other sources of embryonic and adult central and peripheral tissues are available; some further considerations apply when seeking to inject a cell suspension into neonatal or embryonic hosts; and other methods apply when transplanting tissue as solid pieces. These variations are here considered, briefly, in turn.

17.5.1 *Alternative fetal tissue dissections*

Whatever the brain tissue to be dissected, the same procedures will apply to mating, staging the pregnancy, harvesting the embryos, and removing the brains (Sections 17.3.1–4).

The precise dissection of individual brain regions for any particular experiment will be determined from several sources. The logical sequence progresses from anatomical studies of the distribution of the specific cells and systems of experimental interest in the adult brain; developmental studies of early markers for these cells, their site and sequence of development in the embryonic brain; developing an embryonic dissection protocol for embryos of a particular age validated, first anatomically, then by the survival, differentiation, and growth of the cells in vitro; and finally by transplantation into a relevant animal model. These stages of development are already well established for many different cell types, so that when developing a new application the starting point will be to review both the developmental literature, and specific in vitro and transplantation studies, to guide the general dissection. The value of those previous studies will be determined not only by whether a particular dissection protocol is effective in yielding surviving cells; more important is information from systematic empirical variation of the age of the donor (Section 17.2.1), the borders of the tissue dissection, and cell handling protocols. Fortunately, detailed validated descriptions for the most widely used embryo dissection protocols are now published in a number of neuronal culture[23] and neural transplantation handbooks.[21,22,71]

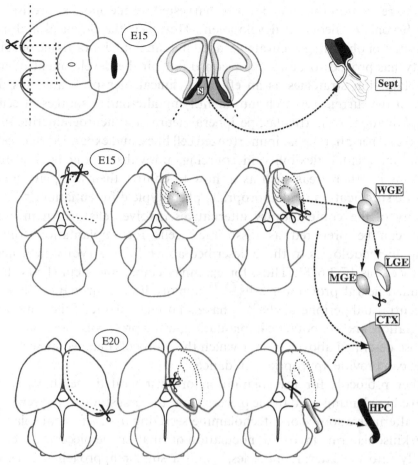

Figure 17.5. Schematic illustration of alternative tissue dissections for septum (Sept), cortex (CTX), hippocampus (HPC), and the whole, medial, and lateral ganglionic eminence (WGE, MGE, LGE). The ringed numbers indicate embryonic age for the different dissections.

The dissections used in our laboratory for nigral dopamine neurons are described above in Section 17.3.5, and illustrated in Fig. 17.3. Other widely used brain tissue dissections include brainstem locus coeruleus and raphé nuclei, cerebellum, septal cholinergic neurons, striatal ganglionic eminence, cortex, and hippocampus. Several of these, as used in our laboratory, are illustrated in Fig. 17.5, and described in detail elsewhere.[21,22]

17.5.2 Peripheral, adult, and non-neuronal sources

As described above, the major donor source for neuronal repair in the adult mammalian brain has been grafts of appropriately specified CNS neurons, with the restriction that they must be harvested from donors at precise stages of embryonic or neonatal development. However, the practical and ethical difficulties of obtaining accurately staged human fetal donor tissue of suitable quality has proved to be a major constraint on the development of neural transplantation strategies as an effective clinical therapy,[61] and this drives much of the current research into identifying alternative sources of cells for transplantation. In particular, peripheral neural and neuroendocrine tissues, central and peripheral glia, immortalized cell lines, and expanded stem cells all exhibit far greater flexibility in sourcing, notwithstanding having greater problems in other areas such as in how to control their adequate survival, accurate specification, and appropriate phenotypic differentiation.[72]

Many of the contemporary alternatives involve cells grown in culture. These can be prepared as dissociated cells for implantation following similar methodologies to those described above for embryonic neuronal tissues (Sections 17.3.6–8). Thus, for example, embryonic stem (ES) cells,[73,74] expanded neural progenitor cells,[75–77] immortalized neuronal cell lines,[78–80] and central and peripheral glia[81–83] have all been implanted following culture, dissociation, and stereotactic implantation, using protocols essentially similar to those described above, and for which the protocols detailed in Section 17.3 above can provide appropriate guidance.

Other protocols for transplantation of peripheral tissues have typically involved implanting solid tissue pieces. Thus, the first studies of adrenal grafts as an alternative source of catecholamine-secreting tissues for transplantation in Parkinsonian rats involved inoculation of small tissue pieces via a cannula directly into the lateral ventricles,[84] and a similar approach was used for inoculating hypothalamic tissues into the third ventricle of the Brattleboro rat and hypogonadal mice with their different neuroendocrine deficiencies.[7,40] Nevertheless, most other tissues can equally be dissociated. Adrenal grafts appear to survive just as well after stereotaxic injection as dissociated cell suspensions into the striatum,[25,85,86] brainstem and spinal cord,[87] or periphery,[88] although some studies still favor the solid approach for hypothalamic tissues.[89]

Other protocols clearly require solid tissues, in particular where the goal is to reconstruct overt areas of tissue cavitation. Even in such cases cell suspension may still prove preferable, in particular where diffusion is constrained such as in a site of focal ischemia or syrinx formation in the spinal cord.[90] However, for bridging spinal or peripheral nerve injuries, solid grafts are typically still required; although such grafts may readily survive with appropriate technique, quite complex protocols can be required to maintain tissues integrity and ensure adequate connectivity.[91]

17.5.3 Labeling cells for transplantation

A common issue is how can one best track cells after transplantation and identify the grafts in the post mortem brain. There are a very wide variety of methods that have been used to label and identify grafted cells, and several good reviews comparing the alternative methods are available.[92–94] The field is complex, and none of the available methods is ideal for all circumstances, but the main approaches are summarized in Table 17.4.

The simplest circumstance is where there are features of the grafted cells or tissues that are distinct and not expressed by the host brain. Thus for example if an animal has a lesion that eliminates all cells of a specific phenotype that are replaced in the transplant, then a histological stain that allows visualization of that phenotype can provide a simple way of visualizing the grafted cells. Examples are provided by the visualization of dopamine cells by catecholamine fluorescence[14,37] or immunohistochemistry[95,96] after transplantation of embryonic nigra into the dopamine-depleted brain – the main method detailed

Table 17.4. *Labels for transplanted cells*

Method	Strategy	Examples[a]
Intrinsic markers of cell phenotype	Catecholamine fluorescence	Locus coeruleus or nigral grafts
	Immunohistochemistry	TH, ChAT or AChE
	Cellular morphology	Schwann cells or oligodendrocytes
Cytoplasmic markers	Enzyme labels	Horseradish peroxidase
	Fluorescent dyes	DiI or bisbenzamide
	Metallic particles or colloids	Gold particles
	Fluorescent microbeads	Propidium iodide beads
	Retrograde neuronal labeling	DiI or granular blue
Dividing cells	[^{3}H] Thymidine	
	BrDU	
Genetic markers	Species-specific antibodies	Mouse or human grafts in rats
	Other strain-specific markers	Allelic forms of Thy-1
	Sex-specific markers	Y-chromosome probes
	Genetic labels	*LacZ* or *GFP*
Imaging labels	Positron emission tomography	F-DOPA or raclopride
	Magnetic resonance imaging	Ferrite particles, gadolinium labeling or magnetodendromers

Note:
[a] See references 93, 94.

in this chapter – or visualization of myelin basic protein expressing cells after transplantation of oligodendrocytes into the myelin-deficient mutant.[97,98] The problems of this approach are that only the specific cells are identified, and it is more difficult to identify all cells from the graft, especially when they may have migrated into the brain; there are many situations where a lesion is not required and we need to distinguish graft- and host-derived cells of similar phenotype; and it can be easy to confuse the grafted cells with induction of expression of the lost marker or the sprouting of axons by the host neurons.[99] Consequently there has been a search to find ways to select, mark, or label cells with distinctive features that will be retained.

The most obvious strategy is to seek to label the cell with a marker or dye. A wide variety of compounds have been tried, some of which are identified in Table 17.4. However, a number of common difficulties remain. Can we establish that the label is retained and expressed permanently in the cell? If it leaches out, can the label be taken up by – and hence falsely label – host cells? Does the presence of the label compromise the survival of grafted cells, and if grafted cells die can the label be incorporated into host macrophages removing the debris?

These are recurrent problems, which have led on to alternative methods of seeking to label cells genetically. This includes taking cells from a different sex, strain or species such that the use of sex-specific (e.g., Y chromosome), strain-specific (e.g., the surface antigen Thy-1), or species-specific (e.g., rodent-, rabbit-, or human-specific neurofilaments) labels can be identified as cellular markers of cells of graft origin in the host brain. This might appear a more straightforward approach in identifying stable cellular markers that are unlikely to be expressed by host cells if the grafted cells die, but other concerns remain: does a cell from a genetically different animal integrate normally into the host brain – perhaps the grafted cells do not recognize all host signals for differentiation and growth; genetic differences between donor and host increase the problems of immunological rejection; and many of the available antibodies for species-specific antigens are not very sensitive and can be quite unreliable.

Some of the best methods combine these approaches by incorporating a genetic label, by introducing a marker transgene (e.g., *lacZ* or the green fluorescent protein, *GFP*) into a strain of mice that can be used as donors[100] into wild-type hosts – or vice versa[101] – or by using a viral vector to transfect the gene into the donor cells.[102–104] Retroviruses are the most common vector in such studies, provided the grafts are taken from early donors and rich in dividing cells, but adenovirus, herpesvirus, and lentivirus can be used to label neurons that have already differentiated at the time of transplantation. At the same time there are concerns that with some vectors the rates of infection of the cells for grafting can be quite low, that the viruses can become toxic when used at higher concentration, and that virus components can be effective antigens for raising an immune response in the host if expressed or if the grafted cell dies.

Finally, there is a rapidly growing interest in the search for methods that will allow the fate of the implanted cells to be tracked in vivo by direct imaging. By and large, unless the grafted tissues aggregate as a large and distinct mass, conventional X-ray-based images give rather little information other than the site of placement from disruption caused by the implantation track. Positron emission tomography (PET) has been used for more than a decade for tracking grafts in Parkinson's patients where fluorodopa uptake into dopamine cells and their terminals appears to yield a clear and distinct signal associated with the specific survival of dopamine cells – the essential functional component – in the grafts,[105,106] and fluorodeoxyglucose (FDG) imaging of metabolic activity is beginning to provide important information on graft function.[107] Nevertheless, the spatial and temporal resolution is limited even at the scale of the human brain and provides extremely low resolution in the rodent.[108] Consequently, there are now considerable efforts being directed at the development of new contrast agents that allow grafted cells to be identified in magnetic resonance imaging (MRI) with the potential for much higher spatial and temporal resolution,[109–111] and that may eventually allow visualization of single labeled cells in the living brain.

From this very brief summary it can be seen that a variety of approaches are available for labeling cells prior to transplantation or identifying them following transplantation; each can work quite well in some circumstances, but raise significant concerns of toxicity, stability, or specificity in others. The most appropriate method will need to be selected – with help of the available reviews[92–94] for each particular circumstance.

17.5.4 Neonatal transplantation

Both we and others have developed the basic transplantation procedure to include implantation of cell suspensions to the developing rodent brain in the early neonatal period between postnatal day 0 (P0) and postnatal day 4 (P4).[112–114] Neonatal surgery requires three modifications of the basic transplantation technique: adaptation of the stereotaxic restraint, alternative anesthesia protocols, and modification of the delivery device for the cells.

Stereotaxic neonatal surgery requires a specialized Teflon-coated neonatal adaptor (Stoelting) which attaches directly to the stereotaxic frame.[115] In this device the neonates are restrained using a nose cone and rubber-tipped ear bars that allow the head to be positioned correctly and held gently in place. Using a flat head position between bregma and lambda, co-ordinates for specific regions can be obtained using reference to the developing rat brain atlas.[116]

Anesthesia can be induced by chilling on ice, with low body temperature maintained during the surgery by cooling the Teflon-coated platform using a mixture of dry ice and 70% ethanol placed in the freezing chamber at the front.* Pups are then warmed to normal body temperature on a heated pad, and on full recovery are returned to the dam. Alternatively, gaseous anesthesia using a mixture of 2–4% isofluorane, in a mixture of $2:1$ $O_2:NO$ may be utilized.[117] Early neonates are fairly resistant to anesthetic gases and require both a high concentration of anesthetic and an extended period of induction to ensure full anesthesia. However, recovery from gaseous anesthesia is rapid, and therefore minimizes time away from the dam, limiting the possibility for rejection of the pup.

To minimize trauma to the neonate brain, cells are delivered via a fine-bore glass capillary, with an outer diameter of 70 μm or less, similar to that adopted for adult rats by Nikkhah and colleagues.[58] This can be attached directly to a transplantation syringe (described above) using polyethylene tubing or silicone, ensuring that the connection is airtight. Alternatively, a nano/micro-injector may be used (e.g., Nanoject II, Drummond Scientific). Both devices can be attached to the stereotaxic frame. To penetrate the skull, a fine hole may be drilled, taking care not to penetrate the soft tissues below.

A number of other issues should be taken into account when handling neonates. Rejection of the pup by the dam can be a problem, but is prevented by wearing protective gloves at all times when handling pups, minimizing time away from the dam, and minimizing stress to the dam, e.g., by removing only half a litter at a time. Pups should be kept on a heated pad to maintain body heat during time away from the litter. Over-cleaning of the head wound, particularly by mouse dams, may lead to reopening of the incision and then to cannibalism. This can be prevented by suturing with extremely fine thread, using tight but very small knots, or using a veterinary adhesive to reseal the incision. Finally, conventional ear or tail marking systems may not be sufficient for individual recognition. Alternative permanent labeling of the toes can be carried out using the Aramis microtattoo system (Lillico, Betchworth, UK).

---

* In the UK, recent rulings of the Home Office Inspectorate no longer allow cooling as an approved mode of anesthesia in neonatal rodents, requiring that the gaseous anesthetic method be used.

17.5.5 *In utero transplantation*

Cell transplants can be placed into the ventricles or parenchyma of rats between E13-E19 days of gestation (day of plugging here is designated as embryonic day – E0) without the aid of an ultrasound devise. Before this developmental stage, an ultrasound device is essential for such surgeries as the embryonic sac is not yet translucent enough to visualize the embryo with white light alone.

Surgery

Time-mated rats are anesthetized in an induction chamber using isofluorane gas (or equivalent). After a dam is suitably anesthetized, the animal is placed (belly up) on a pre-warmed heating pad, and the nose/mouth slid into a nose cone attached to an anesthetic gas flow unit. A 3–4 cm wide vertical strip of the abdominal midline is shaved free of fur from a point just above the vaginal crease to about 1 cm below the sternum. After the skin surface is cleaned with sterilizing surgical scrub (e.g., Betadine), a rounded scalpel blade (e.g., no. 23) is used to make a 3–4 cm vertical incision in the dermis along the abdominal midline. This incision is centred so that it extends from about 1 cm above the vaginal crease to about 2 cm below the xiphoid process of the sternum. Next, the abdominal muscle is lifted slightly from the abdominal cavity and a similar incision made (either with a scalpel blade or very sharp fine scissors) vertically along the linea alba. The embryos can subsequently be exposed by massaging the dorsal–lateral portion of the dam's abdomen until they emerge through this abdominal opening.

Upon exposure, manipulate the pups into a correct orientation with sterilized gloved hands only (do not use instruments). For visualization, place a fiberoptic light behind the uterine sac and transilluminate the embryos through the uterine lining. The transilluminated embryo has obvious features for orientation, and the forebrain ventricles show as rounded grey regions deep within each cerebral hemisphere. For injections, a fine glass capillary (outside diameter approximately $100\,\mu m$) is attached to a nanolitre injection pump (with a foot-pedal delivery switch) mounted onto the stereotaxic frame (e.g., Nanoject II, Drummond Scientific). The needle is lowered to within $0.5\,cm$ of the embryo, and injections made by raising the embryo into the needle and pulse injecting the cell suspension. When the procedure is complete on each embryo from one side of the abdomen, tuck the uterine horn back into the cavity and repeat the procedure for the uterine horn on the other side. It is important not to expose too many embryos at once. The uterine horn must be keep moist by application of sterile saline throughout surgery, since the uterine muscle can contract slightly if it begins to dry, making visualization of the pups and the ability to expose the uterine horn much more difficult.

Upon completing the injections of the embryos on both sides, replace all into the abdominal cavity and administer 5 ml of a prewarmed sterile (5%) sucrose/ saline solution (Aquapharm) with a 5 ml syringe without an attached needle. Suture the muscle and skin layers separately with a "box" stitch using 2–0 mersilk suture. Subsequently, the dam is dried and lain, belly down, in a tissue-lined cage set upon a prewarmed heating pad.

17.6 Conclusions

Neural transplantation is a powerful tool in experimental neuroscience. This applies not just to the obvious clinical development of novel therapeutics for "brain repair," but also as a means to manipulate cells, pathways, and neural networks for the experimental analysis of neuronal development, regeneration, and function. The purpose of this chapter is to describe the core techniques for experimental neural transplantation. We have provided a detailed description for the basic methods in the most commonly used paradigm as applied to one of the commonest model systems, stereotaxic implantation of dissociated embryonic nigral cell suspensions in the rat. This method of cell preparation and implantation is widely applicable by direct translation to other sources of cells, to other model systems of the brain, to other mammalian species, and to neonatal and embryonic as well as adult hosts. Many of these variations have equally been described in some detail. However, there are other applications that will require specialist adaptation on a case-by-case basis, such as delivery in other systems outside the brain (e.g., spinal cord, the retina, the anterior eye chamber, or repair of peripheral nerves), and these fall outside the scope of the present review.

Acknowledgments

The Medical Research Council, the Wellcome Trust, and the Parkinson's Disease Society of Great Britain has funded our own studies, on which this review is based.

References

1. Björklund A, Stenevi U. Intracerebral neural grafting: a historical perspective. In Björklund A, Stenevi U (eds.) *Neural Grafting in the Mammalian CNS.* Amsterdam: Elsevier, 1985, pp. 3–14.

2. Raisman G. Neuronal plasticity in the septal nuclei of the adult brain. *Brain Res.* 1969, **14**: 25–48.
3. Olson L, Malmfors T. Growth characteristics of adrenergic nerves in the adult rat: fluorescence histochemical and 3H-noradrenaline uptake studies using tissue transplantation to the anterior chamber of the eye. *Acta Physiol. Scand. (Suppl.)* 1970, **348**: 1–112.
4. Das GD, Altman J. Transplanted precursors of nerve cells: their fate in the cerebellums of young rats. *Science* 1971, **173**: 637–638.
5. Olson L, Björklund H, Hoffer BJ. Camera bulbi anterior: new vistas on a classical locus for neural tissue transplantation. In Sladek JR, Gash DM (eds.) *Neural Transplants: Development and Function*. New York: Plenum Press, 1984, pp. 125–165.
6. Perlow MJ, Freed WJ, Hoffer BJ, *et al.* Brain grafts reduce motor abnormalities produced by destruction of nigrostriatal dopamine system. *Science* 1979, **204**: 643–647.
7. Gash DM, Sladek JR, Sladek CD. Functional development of grafted vasopressin neurons. *Science* 1980, **210**: 1367–1369.
8. Björklund A, Stenevi U, Svendgaard N-A. Growth of transplanted monoaminergic neurones into the adult hippocampus along the perforant path. *Nature* 1976, **262**: 787–790.
9. Lund RD, Hauschka SD. Transplanted neural tissue develops connections with host rat brain. *Science* 1976, **193**: 582–585.
10. Das GD, Hallas BH, Das KG. Transplantation of neural tissues into the brains of laboratory mammals: technical details and comments. *Experientia* 1979, **35**: 143–153.
11. Smith LM, Ebner FF. The differentiation of non-neuronal elements in neocortical transplants. In Das GD, Wallace RB (eds.) *Neural Transplantation and Regeneration*. New York: Springer-Verlag, 1986, pp. 81–101.
12. Stenevi U, Björklund A, Svendgaard N-A. Transplantation of central and peripheral monoamine neurons to the adult rat brain: techniques and conditions for survival. *Brain Res.* 1976, **114**: 1–20.
13. Stenevi U, Kromer LF, Gage FH, *et al.* Solid neural grafts in intracerebral transplantation cavities. In Björklund A, Stenevi U (eds.) *Neural Grafting in the Mammalian CNS*. Amsterdam: Elsevier, 1985, pp. 41–49.
14. Björklund A, Schmidt RH, Stenevi U. Functional reinnervation of the neostriatum in the adult rat by use of intraparenchymal grafting of dissociated cell suspensions from the substantia nigra. *Cell Tiss. Res.* 1980, **212**: 39–45.
15. Schmidt RH, Björklund A, Stenevi U. Intracerebral grafting of dissociated CNS tissue suspensions: a new approach for neuronal transplantation to deep brain sites. *Brain Res.* 1981, **218**: 347–356.
16. Altman J, Bayer SA. Development of the brain stem in the rat. V. Thymidine-radiographic study of the time of origin of neurons in the midbrain tegmentum. *J. Comp. Neurol.* 1981, **198**: 677–716.
17. Das GD, Altman J. Postnatal neurogenesis in the caudate nucleus and nucleus accumbens septi in the rat. *Brain Res.* 1970, **21**: 122–127.
18. Altman J, Bayer SA. *Atlas of Prenatal Rat Brain Development*. Boca Raton, FL: CRC Press, 1995.
19. Bayer SA, Wills KV, Triarhou LC, *et al.* Time of neuron origin and gradients of neurogenesis in midbrain dopaminergic neurons in the mouse. *Exp. Brain Res.* 1995, **105**: 191–199.

20. Olson L, Seiger Å, Strömberg I. Intraocular transplantation in rodents: a detailed account of the procedure and examples of its use in neurobiology with special reference to brain tissue grafting. *Adv. Cell Neurobiol.* 1983, **4**: 407–442.

21. Dunnett SB, Björklund A. Dissecting embryonic neural tissues for transplantation. In Dunnett SB, Boulton AA, Baker GB (eds.) *Neural Transplantation Methods.* Totowa, NJ: Humana Press, 2000, pp. 3–25.

22. Dunnett SB, Björklund A. Staging and dissection of rat embryos. In Dunnett SB, Björklund A (eds.) *Neural Transplantation: A Practical Approach.* Oxford: IRL Press, 1992, pp. 1–19.

23. Shahar A, De Vellis J, Vernadakis A, *et al. A Dissection and Tissue Culture Manual of the Central Nervous System.* New York: A. R. Liss, 1989.

24. Lawrence JM, Huang SK, Raisman G. Vascular and astrocytic reactions during establishment of hippocampal transplants in adult host brain. *Neuroscience* 1984, **12**: 745–760.

25. Broadwell RD, Charlton HM, Ebert P, *et al.* Angiogenesis and the blood–brain barrier in solid and dissociated cell grafts within the CNS. *Prog. Brain Res.* 1990, **82**: 95–101.

26. Collier TJ, Sortwell CE, Daley BF. Diminished viability, growth, and behavioral efficacy of fetal dopamine neuron grafts in aging rats with long-term dopamine depletion: an argument for neurotrophic supplementation. *J. Neurosci.* 1999, **19**: 5563–5573.

27. Gage FH, Björklund A, Stenevi U, *et al.* Intracerebral grafting of neuronal cell suspensions. VIII. Survival and growth of implants of nigral and septal cell suspensions in intact brains of aged rats. *Acta Physiol. Scand. (Suppl.)* 1983, **522**: 67–75.

28. Eriksdotter-Nilsson M, Gerhardt GA, Seiger Å, *et al.* Age-related alterations in noradrenergic input to the hippocampal formation: structural and functional studies in intraocular transplants. *Brain Res.* 1989, **478**: 269–280.

29. Brüstle O, Choudhary K, Karram K, *et al.* Chimeric brains generated by intraventricular transplantation of fetal human brain cells into embryonic rats. *Nature Biotechnol.* 1998, **16**: 1040–1044.

30. Dunnett SB, Björklund A. *Functional Neural Transplantation*, vol. 2, *Novel Cell Therapies for CNS Disorders.* Amsterdam: Elsevier Science, 2000.

31. Schierle GS, Hansson O, Leist M, *et al.* Caspase inhibition reduces apoptosis and increases survival of nigral transplants. *Nature Med.* 1999, **5**: 97–100.

32. Brundin P, Karlsson J, Emgård M, *et al.* Improving the survival of grafted dopaminergic neurons: a review over current approaches. *Cell Transplant.* 2000, **9**: 179–195.

33. Watts C, Dunnett SB. Effects of severity of host striatal damage on the morphological development of intrastriatal transplants in a rodent model of Huntington's disease: implications for timing of surgical development. *J. Neurosurg.* 1998, **89**: 367–374.

34. Doucet G, Brundin P, Descarries L, *et al.* Effect of prior dopamine denervation on survival and fiber outgrowth from intrastriatal fetal mesencephalic grafts. *Eur. J. Neurosci.* 1990, **2**: 279–290.

35. Gage FH, Björklund A, Stenevi U. Denervation releases a neuronal survival factor in adult rat hippocampus. *Nature* 1984, **308**: 637–639.

36. Gage FH, Björklund A. Denervation-induced enhancement of graft survival and growth: a trophic hypothesis. *Ann. NY Acad. Sci.* 1987, **495**: 378–395.

37. Björklund A, Dunnett SB, Stenevi U, *et al*. Reinnervation of the denervated striatum by substantia nigra transplants: functional consequences as revealed by pharmacological and sensorimotor testing. *Brain Res.* 1980, **199**: 307–333.
38. Björklund A, Lindvall O, Isacson O, *et al*. Mechanisms of action of intracerebral neural implants: studies on nigral and striatal grafts to the lesioned striatum. *Trends Neurosci.* 1987, **10**: 509–516.
39. Dunnett SB, Björklund A. Mechanisms of function of neural grafts in the adult mammalian brain. *J. Exp. Biol.* 1987, **132**: 265–289.
40. Krieger DT, Perlow MJ, Gibson MJ, *et al*. Brain grafts reverse hypogonadism of gonadotropin releasing hormone deficiency. *Nature* 1982, **298**: 468–471.
41. Charlton HM. Neural grafts and the restoration of pituitary and gonadal function in hypogonadal (HPG) mice. *Ann. Endocrinol.* 1987, **48**: 378–384.
42. Dunnett SB. Functional repair of striatal systems by neural transplants: evidence for circuit reconstruction. *Behav. Brain Res.* 1995, **66**: 133–142.
43. Bregman BS. Recovery of function after spinal cord injury: transplantation strategies. In Dunnett SB, Björklund A (eds). *Functional Neural Transplantation*. New York: Raven Press, 1994, pp. 489–529.
44. Ohmoto Y, Wood K. Immunology: mechanisms of rejection. In Dunnett SB, Boulton AA, Baker GB (eds.) *Neural Transplantation Methods*. Totowa, NJ: Humana Press, 2000, pp. 461–475.
45. Brevig T, Holgersson J, Widner H. Xenotransplantation for CNS repair: immunological barriers and strategies to overcome them. *Trends Neurosci.* 2000, **23**: 337–344.
46. Strömberg I, Bygdeman M, Goldstein M, *et al*. Human fetal substantia nigra grafted to the dopamine-denervated striatum of immunosuppressed rats: evidence for functional reinnervation. *Neurosci. Lett.* 1986, **71**: 271–276.
47. Brundin P, Strecker RE, Widner H, *et al*. Human fetal dopamine neurons grafted in a rat model of Parkinson's disease: immunological aspects, spontaneous and drug-induced behavior, and dopamine release. *Exp. Brain Res.* 1988, **70**: 192–208.
48. Björklund A, Stenevi U, Dunnett SB, *et al*. Cross-species neural grafting in a rat model of Parkinson's disease. *Nature* 1982, **298**: 652–654.
49. Pedersen EB, Zimmer J, Finsen B. Triple immunosuppression protects murine intracerebral, hippocampal xenografts in adult rat hosts: effects on cellular infiltration, major histocompatibility complex antigen induction and blood–brain barrier leakage. *Neuroscience* 1997, **78**: 685–701.
50. Watts C, Dunnett SB. Immunoprotection of cell and tissue implants in the central nervous system. In Dunnett SB, Boulton AA, Baker GB (eds.) *Neural Transplantation Methods*. Totowa, NJ: Humana Press, 2000, pp. 477–501.
51. Honey CR, Clarke DJ, Dallman MJ, *et al*. Human neural graft function in rats treated with anti-interleukin II receptor antibody. *NeuroReport* 1990, **1**: 247–249.
52. Honey CR, Charlton HM, Wood KJ. Rat brain xenografts reverse hypogonadism in mice immunosuppressed with anti-CD4 monoclonal antibody. *Exp. Brain Res.* 1991, **85**: 149–152.
53. O'Rahilly R, Müller F. *Developmental Stages in Human Embryos*. Washington, DC: Carnegie Institute, 1987.
54. Butler H, Juurlink BHJ. *An Atlas for Staging Mammalian and Chick Embryos*. Boca Raton, FL: CRC Press, 1987.

55. Brundin P, Isacson O, Björklund A. Monitoring of cell viability in suspensions of embryonic CNS tissue and its use as a criterion for intracerebral graft survival. *Brain Res.* 1985, **331**: 251–259.
56. Freed CR, Greene PE, Breeze RE, *et al.* Transplantation of embryonic dopamine neurons for severe Parkinson's disease. *New Engl. J. Med.* 2001, **344**: 710–719.
57. Brundin P. Dissection, preparation, and implantation of human embryonic brain tissue. In Dunnett SB, Björklund A (eds.) *Neural Transplantation: A Practical Approach.* Oxford: IRL Press, 1992, pp. 139–160.
58. Nikkhah G, Olsson M, Eberhard J, *et al.* A microtransplantation approach for cell suspension grafting in the rat Parkinson model: a detailed account of the methodology. *Neuroscience* 1994, **63**: 57–72.
59. Barker RA, Fricker RA, Abrous DN, *et al.* A comparative study of the preparation techniques for improving the viability of nigral grafts using vital stain, in vitro cultures and in vivo grafts. *Cell Transplant.* 1995, **4**: 173–200.
60. Castilho RF, Hansson O, Brundin P. Improving the survival of grafted embryonic dopamine neurons in rodent models of Parkinson's disease. *Prog. Brain Res.* 2000, **127**: 203–231.
61. Björklund A. Better cells for brain repair. *Nature* 1993, **362**: 414–415.
62. Nakao N, Frodl EM, Duan W-M, *et al.* Lazaroids improve the survival of grafted rat embryonic dopamine neurons. *Proc. Natl. Acad. Sci. USA* 1994, **91**: 12408–12412.
63. Finger S, Dunnett SB. Nimodipine enhances growth and vascularization of neural grafts. *Exp. Neurol.* 1989, **104**: 1–9.
64. Mayer E, Fawcett JW, Dunnett SB. Basic fibroblast growth factor promotes the survival of embryonic ventral mesencephalic dopaminergic neurons. II. Effects on neural transplants in vivo. *Neuroscience* 1993, **56**: 389–398.
65. Rosenblad C, Martinez-Serrano A, Björklund A. Glial cell line-derived neurotrophic factor increases survival, growth and function of intrastriatal fetal nigral dopaminergic grafts. *Neuroscience* 1996, **75**: 979–985.
66. Sinclair SR, Svendsen CN, Torres EM, *et al.* GDNF enhances dopaminergic cell survival and fibre outgrowth in embryonic nigral grafts. *NeuroReport* 1996, **7**: 2547–2552.
67. Sinclair SR, Zietlow R, Fawcett JW, *et al.* Delayed implantation of nigral grafts improves survival of dopamine neurones and rate of functional recovery. *NeuroReport* 1999, **10**: 1263–1267.
68. Karlsson J, Emgård M, Rosenblad C, *et al.* Treatment with the spin trap agent α-phenyl-*N*-tert-butyl nitrone does not enhance the survival of embryonic or adult dopamine neurons. *Brain Res.* 1998, **805**: 155–168.
69. Schierle GS, Karlsson J, Brundin P. MK-801 does not enhance dopaminergic cell survival in embryonic nigral grafts. *NeuroReport* 1998, **9**: 1313–1316.
70. Haque NSK, Hlavin M-L, Fawcett JW, *et al.* The neurotrophin NT-4/5, but not NT-3, enhances the efficacy of nigral grafts in a rat model of Parkinson's disease. *Brain Res.* 1996, **712**: 45–52.
71. Brundin P, Strecker RE. Preparation and intracerebral grafting of dissociated fetal brain tissue in rats. In Conn PM (ed.) *Lesions and Transplantation.* New York: Academic Press, 1991, pp. 305–326.
72. Fawcett JW, Rosser AE, Dunnett SB. *Brain Damage, Brain Repair.* New York: Oxford University Press, 2001.
73. Björklund L, Sanchez-Pernaute R, Chung S, *et al.* Embryonic stem cells develop into functional dopaminergic neurons after transplantation in a Parkinson rat model. *Proc. Natl. Acad. Sci. USA* 2002, **99**: 2344–2349.

74. Kim JH, Auerbach JM, Rodriguez-Gomez JA, *et al.* Dopamine neurons derived from embryonic stem cells function in an animal model of Parkinson's disease. *Nature* 2002, **418**: 50–56.
75. Gage FH, Coates PW, Palmer TD, *et al.* Survival and differentiation of adult neuronal progenitor cells transplanted to the adult brain. *Proc. Natl. Acad. Sci. USA* 1995, **92**: 11879–11883.
76. Winkler C, Fricker RA, Gates MA, *et al.* Incorporation and glial differentiation of mouse EGF-responsive neural progenitor cells after transplantation into the embryonic rat brain. *Mol. Cell Neurosci.* 1998, **11**: 99–116.
77. Svendsen CN, Clarke DJ, Rosser AE, *et al.* Survival and differentiation of rat and human EGF responsive precursor cells following grafting into the lesioned adult CNS. *Exp. Neurol.* 1996, **137**: 376–388.
78. Sinden JD, Rashid-Doubell F, Kershaw TR, *et al.* Recovery of spatial learning by grafts of a conditionally immortalized hippocampal neuroepithelial cell line into the ischaemia-lesioned hippocampus. *Neuroscience* 1997, **81**: 599–608.
79. Shihabuddin LS, Hertz JA, Holets VR, *et al.* The adult CNS retains the potential to direct region-specific differentiation of a transplanted neuronal precursor cell line. *J. Neurosci.* 1995, **15**: 6666–6678.
80. Broadwell RD, Charlton HM, Ebert PS, *et al.* Allografts of CNS tissue possess a blood–brain barrier. II. Angiogenesis in solid tissue and cell suspension grafts. *Exp. Neurol.* 1991, **112**: 1–28.
81. Groves AK, Barnett SC, Franklin RJM, *et al.* Repair of demyelinated lesions by transplantation of purified O-2A progenitor cells. *Nature* 1993, **362**: 453–455.
82. Duncan ID, Aguayo AJ, Bunge RP, *et al.* Transplantation of rat Schwann cells grown in tissue culture into the mouse spinal cord. *J. Neurol. Sci.* 1981, **49**: 241–252.
83. Brook GA, Lawrence JM, Raisman G. Morphology and migration of cultured Schwann cells transplanted into the fimbria and hippocampus in adult rats. *Glia* 1993, **9**: 292–304.
84. Freed WJ, Morihisa JM, Spoor E, *et al.* Transplanted adrenal chromaffin cells in rat brain reduce lesion-induced rotational behavior. *Nature* 1981, **292**: 351–352.
85. Patel-Vaidya U, Wells MR, Freed WJ. Survival of dissociated adrenal chromaffin cells of rat and monkey transplanted into rat brain. *Cell Tiss. Res.* 1985, **240**: 281–285.
86. Brown VJ, Dunnett SB. Comparison of adrenal and fetal nigral grafts on drug-induced rotation in rats with 6-OHDA lesions. *Exp. Brain Res.* 1989, **78**: 214–218.
87. Pappas GD, Sagen J. Fine structural correlates of vascular permeability of chromaffin cell transplants in CNS pain modulatory regions. *Exp. Neurol.* 1988, **102**: 280–289.
88. Scheumann GF, Hiller WF, Schroder S, *et al.* Adrenal cortex transplantation after bilateral total adrenalectomy in the rat. *Henry Ford Hosp. Med. J.* 1989, **37**: 154–156.
89. Boer GJ, Griffioen HA, Saeed P. Grafted fetal suprachiasmatic nucleus cells survive much better in tissue pieces than in suspension. *Rest. Neurol. Neurosci.* 1992, **4**: 261–269.
90. Falci S, Holtz A, Åkesson E, *et al.* Obliteration of a posttraumatic spinal cord cyst with solid human embryonic spinal cord grafts: first clinical attempt. *J. Neurotrauma* 1997, **14**: 875–884.

91. Cheng H, Cao YH, Olson L. Spinal cord repair in adult paraplegic rats: partial restoration of hind-limb function. *Science* 1996, **273**: 510–513.
92. Cadusseau J, Peschanski M. Identifying grafted cells. In Dunnett SB, Björklund A (eds.) *Neural Transplantation: A Practical Approach*. Oxford: IRL Press, 1992, pp. 177–201.
93. Whittemore SR, Holets VR. Labeling and identification of cells for CNS transplantation. In Ricordi C (ed.) *Methods in Cell Transplantation*. Austin, TX: R. G. Landes, 1995, pp. 333–344.
94. Harvey AR. Labeling and identifying grafted cells. In Dunnett SB, Boulton AA, Baker GB (eds.) *Neural Transplantation Methods*. Totowa, NJ: Humana Press, 2000, pp. 319–361.
95. Jaeger CB. Cytoarchitectonics of substantia nigra grafts: a light and electron microscopic study of immunocytochemically identified dopaminergic neurons and fibrous astrocytes. *J. Comp. Neurol.* 1985, **231**: 121–135.
96. Freund TF, Bolam JP, Björklund A, *et al.* Efferent synaptic connections of grafted dopaminergic-neurons reinnervating the host neostriatum: a tyrosine hydroxylase immunocytochemical study. *J. Neurosci.* 1985, **5**: 603–616.
97. Gumpel M, Baumann N, Raoul M, *et al.* Survival and differentiation of oligodendrocytes from neural tissue transplanted into newborn mouse brain. *Neurosci Lett.* 1983, **37**: 307–311.
98. Baulac M, Lachapelle F, Gout O, *et al.* Transplantation of oligodendrocytes in the newborn mouse brain: extension of myelination by transplanted cells – anatomical study. *Brain Res.* 1987, **420**: 39–47.
99. Bohn MC, Cupit L, Marciano F, *et al.* Adrenal grafts enhance recovery of striatal dopaminergic fibers. *Science* 1987, **237**: 913–916.
100. Bahn S, Wisden W, Dunnett SB, *et al.* The intrinsic specification of γ-amino-butyric acid type A receptor α6 subunit gene expression in cerebellar granule cells. *Eur. J. Neurosci.* 1999, **11**: 2194–2198.
101. Gates MA, Laywell ED, Fillmore H, *et al.* Astrocytes and extracellular matrix following intracerebral transplantation of embryonic ventral mesencephalon or lateral ganglionic eminence. *Neuroscience* 1996, **74**: 579–597.
102. Shimohama S, Rosenberg MB, Fagan AM, *et al.* Grafting genetically modified cells into the rat brain: characteristics of *Escherichia coli* β-galactosidase as a reporter gene. *Mol. Brain Res.* 1989, **5**: 271–278.
103. Quintana JG, Lopez-Colberg I, Cunningham LA. Use of GFAP-*lacZ* transgenic mice to determine astrocyte fate in grafts of embryonic ventral midbrain. *Devel. Brain Res.* 1998, **105**: 147–151.
104. Aboody-Guterman KS, Pechan PA, Rainov NG, *et al.* Green fluorescent protein as a reporter for retrovirus and helper virus-free HSV-1 amplicon vector-mediated gene transfer into neural cells in culture and in vivo. *NeuroReport* 1997, **8**: 3801–3808.
105. Lindvall O, Brundin P, Widner H, *et al.* Grafts of fetal dopamine neurons survive and improve motor function in Parkinson's disease. *Science* 1990, **247**: 574–577.
106. Sawle GV. [^{18}F]-6-L-fluorodopa PET studies of graft and host dopaminergic function following fetal mesencephalic transplantation. *Adv. Neurol.* 1993, **60**: 715–720.
107. Piccini P, Lindvall O, Björklund A, *et al.* Delayed recovery of movement-related cortical function in Parkinson's disease after striatal dopaminergic grafts. *Ann. Neurol.* 2000, **48**: 689–695.

108. Torres EM, Fricker RA, Hume S, *et al.* Assessment of striatal graft viability in the rat in vivo using a small diameter PET scanner. *NeuroReport* 1995, **6**: 2017–2021.

109. Bulte JWM, Zhang SC, Van Gelderen P, *et al.* Neurotransplantation of magnetically labeled oligodendrocyte progenitors: magnetic resonance tracking of cell migration and myelination. *Proc. Natl. Acad. Sci. USA* 1999, **96**: 15256–15261.

110. Bulte JWM, Douglas T, Witwer B, *et al.* Magnetodendrimers allow endosomal magnetic labeling and in vivo tracking of stem cells. *Nature Biotechnol.* 2001, **19**: 1141–1147.

111. Bulte JWM, Duncan ID, Frank JA. In vivo magnetic resonance tracking of magnetically labeled cells after transplantation. *J. Cereb. Blood Flow Metab.* 2002, **22**: 899–907.

112. Gates MA, Olsson M, Bjerregaard K, *et al.* Region-specific migration of embryonic glia grafted to the neonatal brain. *Neuroscience* 1998, **84**: 1013–1023.

113. Englund U, Fricker-Gates RA, Lundberg C, *et al.* Transplantation of human neural progenitor cells into the neonatal rat brain: extensive migration and differentiation with long-distance axonal projections. *Exp. Neurol.* 2002, **173**: 1–21.

114. Lund RD, Yee KT. Intracerebral transplantation to immature hosts. In Dunnett SB, Björklund A (eds.) *Neural Transplantation: A Practical Approach.* Oxford: IRL Press, 1992, pp. 79–91.

115. Cunningham MG, McKay RDG. A hypothermic miniaturized stereotaxic instrument for surgery in newborn rats. *J. Neurosci. Methods* 1993, **47**: 105–114.

116. Paxinos G, Ashwell KWS, Törk I. *Atlas of the Developing Rat Nervous System,* 2nd edn. San Diego, CA: Academic Press, 1994.

117. Danneman PJ, Mandrell TD. Evaluation of five agents/methods for anesthesia of neonatal rats. *Lab. Anim. Sci.* 2003, **47**: 386–395.

118. Dunnett SB. Brain grafts. In Adelman G (ed.) *Encyclopaedia of Neuroscience.* New York: Elsevier Science, 2004, pp. 1–9.

Part II

Experimental models of major
neurological diseases

18

Focal brain ischemia models in rodents

FUHAI LI AND TURGUT TATLISUMAK

18.1 Introduction

Stroke is the second leading cause of mortality worldwide[1] and the third leading cause of death in the United States.[2] Approximately 80% of strokes are ischemic in origin. Stroke ranked as the sixth leading cause of disability-adjusted life years in 1990 and is estimated to rank fourth by the year 2020.[3] Of the stroke survivors about one-half are left with a permanent handicap.[4] It is estimated that 731 000 new strokes per year, 4 000 000 stroke survivors, and 160 000 stroke deaths cost approximately $50 billion (direct and indirect costs) in the USA alone.[5] Given this epidemiological evidence and the magnitude of the problem, it is clear that stroke is a major public health issue and requires urgent effort for developing novel remedies. Experimental focal brain ischemia models serve this purpose.

Experimental focal cerebral ischemia models have been developed with significant effort to mimic closely the changes that occur during and after human stroke. Models help us learn about the pathogenesis of stroke and to define the biochemical changes in tissue during ischemia, thereby discovering mechanisms involved in the evolution of ischemic injury and infarction. This can lead to the development of novel molecules that may reduce the consequences of ischemia and these same animal models can be utilized to test whether these novel molecules have beneficial anti-ischemic effects in vivo. Since human ischemic stroke is often caused by occlusion of the middle cerebral artery (MCA) or one of its branches,[6] most focal cerebral ischemia models were developed to induce ischemia within the MCA territory. Ideally, an ischemic stroke animal model should satisfy the following criteria:[7] (1) the ischemic processes and pathophysiological changes should be relevant to human ischemic stroke, (2) the ischemic lesion should be reproducible, (3) the technique used to induce ischemia should be relatively easy to perform and minimally invasive, (4) physiologic variables should be monitored and maintained within normal ranges, (5) brain samples should be readily available for outcome measurements such as histopathological, biochemical, and molecular biological evaluation, and (6) the cost and effort should be reasonable.

Handbook of Experimental Neurology, ed. Turgut Tatlisumak and Marc Fisher. Published by Cambridge University Press. © Cambridge University Press 2006.

18.2 Selection of animal

Although higher species animals such as cats, rabbits, dogs, pigs, and non-human primates can be used in focal ischemia models, small animals such as rats, mice, and gerbils are more commonly used. Rats are the most commonly used animals in stroke studies because of: (1) their resemblance to humans in cerebrovascular anatomy and physiology, (2) their moderate size which allows researchers to easily monitor the physiologic parameters and collect the brain specimens, (3) the low cost of animals, regarding transportation, storage, and feeding, (4) the relative homogeneity within strains owing to inbreeding, (5) their small brain size that is well suited to fixation procedures, microscopic, and macroscopic examination, (6) the ease of conducting reproducible studies, (7) the greater acceptability (compared to non-human primates and pet animals) from ecological and ethical perspectives.[8-10] Mice have been of increasing interest because of the availability of transgenic technology, which offers new insights into the molecular mechanisms involved in ischemic stroke. The gerbil may not be a good candidate for testing potential neuroprotective agents, since many neuroprotective agents effective in the gerbil failed to protect against ischemic damage in other species.[11] Because of the relatively higher cost and difficulty in experimental procedures, the higher species of animals are used in a more limited manner. However, it may be reasonable and necessary to consider testing neuroprotective agents in larger animal stroke models to determine if the compound is broadly effective before clinical trials begin.[11]

18.3 Approaches inducing focal cerebral ischemia

Focal cerebral ischemia can be induced by many approaches, including intra-luminal suture insertion, thromboembolus injection, direct surgical occlusion of the MCA, embolization of microspheres, photochemical thrombosis, and endothelin-1 infusion. Here we are focused on the intraluminal suture MCA occlusion model, thromboembolic models, and direct surgical MCA occlusion models because of their increasing popularity in developing neuroprotective, thrombolytic, and restorative drugs.

18.3.1 Intraluminal suture (monofilament) MCA occlusion model

This model is the most commonly used one in focal brain ischemia studies, likely because of its relatively easy performance and less invasiveness compared to other models. In this model, the MCA is occluded by inserting a monofilament suture into the internal carotid artery to block blood flow to the

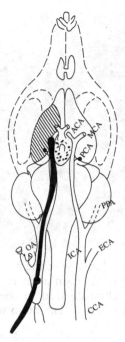

Figure 18.1. Monofilament suture occlusion of the middle cerebral artery. The shaded area in the brain hemisphere represents the typical infarct induced by the occlusion. CCA, common carotid artery; ICA, internal carotid artery; ECA, external carotid artery; OA, occipital artery; PPA, pterygopalatinal artery; PCA, posterior cerebral artery; MCA, middle cerebral artery; ACA, anterior cerebral artery.

MCA (Fig. 18.1). Either permanent or transient MCA occlusion can be simply achieved by maintaining or withdrawing the monofilament suture.

This suture MCA occlusion model was originally described in rats by Koizumi and his colleagues[12] in 1986 and then modified by others. Usually, a 3–0 or 4–0 monofilament suture is used as the occluder. The monofilament can be coated with silicone[12,13] or poly-L-lysine,[14] or can be used without coating.[15,16] The suture occluder can be inserted through the common carotid artery, the external carotid artery, or the internal carotid artery. The length of suture inserted from the bifurcation of the common carotid artery is approximately 17–22 mm depending on body weight, size of the suture tip, rat strain, and location of the bifurcation.[17–19]

The typical infarct areas induced by this model include both the lateral caudoputamen and frontoparietal cortex (Fig. 18.2). It is established that there exists a substantial ischemic penumbra in this model early after ischemia[20] and the infarct size induced by prolonged ischemia (>90 min) is relatively reproducible, making this suture model appropriate for testing

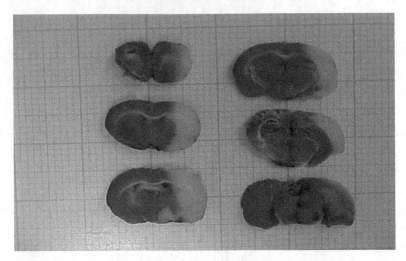

Figure 18.2. Typical infarct induced with the monofilament suture occlusion model in the rat brain. The dark brain areas represent intact tissue stained with triphenyl tetrazolium chloride (red in the original image) and pale (white) regions represent the infarct. The brain was cut into six 2-mm-thick slices.

neuroprotective agents. However, it must be remembered that many factors may affect infarct size. Firstly, one study showed that slight differences of the monofilament (i.e., diameter, tensile strength, and extensibility) may cause a significant difference in infarct volume.[21] Secondly, the ischemia induced by a silicone-coated suture is likely more substantial and less variable,[14,15] consequently the infarct volume is more reproducible and larger than that induced by an uncoated suture.[15,16] Thirdly, a longer insertion distance of the monofilament suture may give rise to larger infarction because the deeper insertion of the suture can also obstruct blood flow in some branches of the anterior cerebral artery.[18] Lastly, inadvertent premature reperfusion is another factor that may cause variability of infarct volume.[22] It is therefore important that consistent and standardized surgical procedures and techniques be used in order to generate a reproducible lesion.

This suture MCA occlusion method was also successfully applied to mice because transgenic or knockout mice provide a unique way for basic research into the molecular mechanisms contributing to ischemic cell damage and development of novel therapeutic interventions.[23–25] Usually, a 5–0 monofilament nylon suture or 8–0 suture coated with silicone is used to occlude blood flow to the MCA territory. The insertion depth from the bifurcation of common carotid artery is approximately 9–11 mm.[24,25] The lesion is reproducible and its distribution is similar to that in the rat (Fig. 18.3).

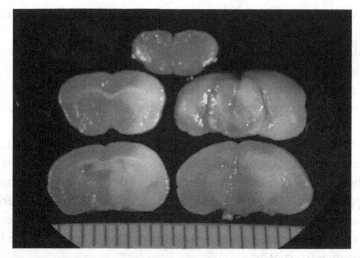

Figure 18.3. Mouse brain with infarction in the monofilament suture occlusion model; white area represents the infarct. (Courtesy of Dr. Jun Li, Trinity College, Dublin, Ireland.)

Another important role of this suture MCA occlusion method is that it can also be modified to induce ischemia in a magnetic resonance imaging (MRI) unit by remotely advancing the suture occluder (so-called in-bore suture MCA occlusion model).[19,26–28] Combined with new MRI techniques, this in-bore occlusion method enables researchers to monitor in vivo ischemic changes at a very early time point after the onset of ischemia and to acquire both pre- and post-ischemic data for later pixel-by-pixel comparison. This in-bore MCA occlusion method has been improved recently and achieved a high success rate.[19]

There are some disadvantages and complications with the intraluminal suture MCA occlusion model. Firstly, subarachnoid hemorrhage may occur because of inadvertent arterial rupture caused by the suture. This complication is likely to have a higher incidence with uncoated sutures than with silicone-coated sutures.[14,22] Secondly, spontaneous hyperthermia occurs when the ischemic duration lasts more than 2 hr.[29,30] This is most likely due to ischemic damage of the hypothalamus which is caused by blockage of small branches to the hypothalamus by suture insertion.[30] Finally, the inner surface of vessels may be mechanically injured by the suture, which may complicate reperfusion.

18.3.2 Thromboembolic model

Focal ischemia induced by thromboemboli is of great interest because of its resemblance to human ischemic stroke approximately 80% of which are

caused by thromboembolism[31] and its role in seeking and evaluating thrombolytic therapy. Thrombolytic therapy with recombinant tissue plasminogen activator (rt-PA) administered intravenously within 3 hr after onset of
ischemic stroke in human improves neurological outcome[32] and has already
become a standard therapy in carefully selected patients. Thromboembolic
animal models are therefore playing an increasingly important role in these
aspects.

Thromboembolic ischemia can be produced by a photochemical approach
or by injection of autologous or heterologous thrombi. The photochemical
method gives rise to an arterial lesion in the common carotid artery which
results in platelet-rich thrombus formation. This thrombus can then dislodge
and thus embolize to distal vessels.[33,34] The photochemically induced thromboemboli are platelet-rich and they therefore may not be amenable to thrombolytic therapy with rt-PA.

The most commonly used thromboembolic model is blood clot injection
(Fig. 18.4). This model was first described in the dog by Hill and colleagues[35]
and then was applied to the rat.[36,37] In the early versions of this model, a
suspension of microembolic clot was injected, causing diffuse and inhomogeneous infarction in the MCA territory because of peripheral branch micro-
embolization. Scattered, multifocal lesions were also observed in the territories
of the anterior cerebral artery and posterior cerebral artery and even in the
contralateral hemisphere.[36,37] In addition, early spontaneous recanalization
frequently occurred, which made evaluation of thrombolytic therapy difficult.
The early autolysis of blood clots may be due to a more fragile red thrombus
formed in vitro by whole blood. In order to overcome these problems, a more
resistant white thrombus was produced by using a moving high-pressure
closed compartment system (PE-10 polyethylene tube with 0.28 mm in inner
diameter).[38] Using white thrombi, Overgaard demonstrated a substantial
reduction of cerebral blood flow (CBF) in the affected region and no spontaneous recanalization at 2 hr after embolization, a condition necessary for
studying thrombolytic treatment.[38]. However, infarct size was variable and
ischemia caused by multiple small clots does not mimic typical clinical
ischemic stroke. An ideal thromboembolic model should entail a blood clot
that appropriately lodges in the proximal segment of the MCA, but the distal
branches remain open. Smaller clots embolize into the end-arterial trees, while
larger clots may lodge in vessel too proximal from the origin of MCA to
occlude MCA. Therefore, size (length and diameter) as well as the characteristics of blood clots (i.e., more rigid fibrin-rich clot) is crucial in this model.
Recently, Busch and colleagues developed a rat clot model in which 12
medium-sized (1.5 × 0.35 mm), fibrin-rich autologous clots formed in a

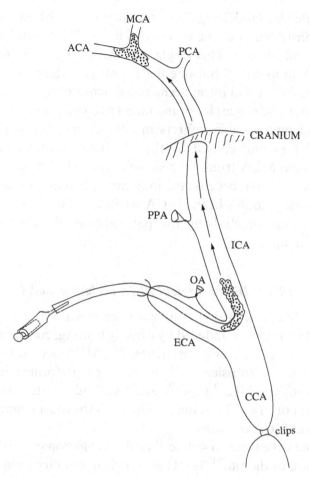

Figure 18.4. Thromboembolic occlusion of the middle cerebral artery in the rat. CCA, common carotid artery; ECA, external carotid artery; OA, occipital artery; ICA, internal carotid artery; PPA, pterygopalatinal artery; PCA, posterior cerebral artery; MCA, middle cerebral artery; ACA, anterior cerebral artery.

PE-50 polyethylene catheter (0.58 mm in inner diameter) were injected to produce reliable occlusion of the proximal MCA.[39] A consistent reduction of CBF and histological damage in the MCA territory were observed. Visual inspection demonstrated no early spontaneous clot lysis in the ipsilateral vessels at 3 hr after injection and no clots in the contralateral vessels. Thrombolytic therapy with rt-PA[39] or prourokinase[40] can recanalize the occluded MCA. By using a modified tube that was inserted into internal carotid artery 2–3 mm proximal to the MCA origin, a single fibrin-rich clot (25 × 0.1 mm) can also be selectively introduced into the proximal part of the MCA[41] or a thrombosis can be induced at the origin of the MCA,[42] thus causing typical MCA occlusion.

Using this single clot model, significant reduction of CBF in the MCA territory was demonstrated, and the blood clot in the MCA trunk was found at 24 hr after embolization.[42] This single clot was also applied to occlude the proximal MCA in mouse,[43] but one disadvantage is the relatively high incidence of subarachnoid and intraparenchymal hemorrhage.

In conclusion, these single clot or medium-sized multiple clot models induce predictable and reproducible infarcts in both extent and size in the MCA territory, similar to that caused by the intraluminal suture model. Embolizing the proximal MCA trunk by a single fibrin-rich clot bears similarity to human embolic ischemia, because the majority of human ischemic strokes are caused by a single embolus in the MCA territory.[6] Therefore, the single clot model is promising for studying the pathogenesis of ischemic stroke and thrombolytic therapy.

18.3.3 Direct surgical MCA occlusion model

Direct surgical MCA occlusion is invasive, as it requires a craniectomy. In this model, ischemia can be induced by directly ligating, coagulating, clipping, or snaring the MCA trunk or its branches. The MCA occlusion in this model can be permanent or transient.[44–46] It has been performed in non-human primates,[47] dogs,[48] rabbits,[49] cats,[50] rats,[51] and mice.[52] It can also be done under anesthesia or in awake animals. The rat is the most common species to undergo surgical MCA occlusion.

Robinson and colleagues first described direct ligation of the distal MCA at the rhinal fissure in the rat.[51] The typical ischemic injury induced by such a method is in the frontoparietal cortex, but the extent of lesion is quite variable. Through a subtemporal craniectomy, Albanese[53] and Tamura[54] performed surgical occlusions more proximally in the MCA trunk. Occluding the main trunk of the MCA proximal to the lenticulostriatel branches that supply the lateral caudoputamen results in an infarction involving both the cortex and caudoputamen. The infarction areas induced by a proximal MCA occlusion appear to be larger and less variable, compared with those induced by distal MCA occlusion. This model is appropriate for investigating cerebrovascular function after focal ischemia.[55] Since focal occlusion of the MCA may not always produce infarction even when the occlusion was performed at the proximal MCA trunk, Bederson further refined this model and demonstrated that both the site and extent of MCA occlusion affect the neuropathological outcome and are critical factors to produce reproducible infarction.[56] Occlusion of a very short segment (1–2 mm) of the MCA results in greater variability of infarction and the rate of infarction is low when focal MCA occlusion was performed at the origin of MCA. This may relate to the persistence of abundant collateral circulation. Furthermore, since MCA branching is variable,[57] such a focal occlusion at one point may not really involve both the lenticulostriatel and cortical branches. Interestingly, in the young (36 days) rat, MCA occlusion beyond the point of origin of the lenticulostriate branches does not cause neuronal injury, probably because of better collateral supply in the young rat.[9]

Extensive (3 or 6 mm) MCA occlusion, however, induces uniform infarction in both extent and location. This extensive occlusion involves the lenticulostriate and small cortical branches, and therefore produces reproducible infarction. Direct MCA occlusion can be combined with unilateral (two-vessel method) or bilateral CCA occlusion (three-vessel method). Studies have demonstrated that these combined two-vessel or three-vessel occlusions give rise to larger and more reproducible infarcts.[58] The ischemic penumbra in this model may be small[59] and it may be less amenable to testing neuroprotective compounds. Because of higher long-term survival of rats due to the relatively small lesion, this model is a good option for screening stroke restorative drugs.[11]

There are some disadvantages with direct surgical MCA occlusion models. Firstly, performing this model is more difficult and requires more experience and technical skill due to varying MCA anatomical patterns.[54] Secondly, direct exposure of brain to air after craniectomy may change intracranial pressure and blood–brain barrier permeability.[9] Thirdly, a small amount of subarachnoid hemorrhage around the MCA trunk may occur.[54] Although these models were extensively used, they have been largely replaced by the intraluminal suture MCA occlusion model.

18.3.4 Embolus model

Many materials such as carbon, plastic microspheres, silicone cylinders, and air can be injected to induce ischemic injury as emboli via the common carotid artery or the internal carotid artery.[60–62] The magnitude and severity of ischemic damage induced by these embolic models depends on the number and size of the embolic particles injected.[63] Previously, diffuse distribution and inhomogeneous infarction were the neuropathological hallmarks of these models, making histological evaluation difficult. However, these models have recently been refined and injection of six ceramic spheres of 0.3–0.4 mm in diameter into the common carotid artery via the external carotid artery led to reproducible infarcts.[64] The advantage of this model is the lack of potential hyperthermia, but the disadvantage is that it does not allow reperfusion.

18.3.5 Photochemically induced thrombosis model

In this model, the ischemic injury is induced by vascular injection of a photo-active dye, such as rose Bengal[65] or photofrin,[66] in combination with irradiation with a light beam at a specific wavelength. It has been shown that a reaction between the circulating dye and the light engenders free radicals, leading to platelet aggregation and thrombosis.[65] The location and extent of photochemically induced lesions can be well controlled by selectively illuminating the brain tissue and by using different intensities of light and different doses of dye. A typical lesion in this model is a sharply circumscribed infarct that involves only the cortex. It is likely that there is only a small penumbra. In addition, breakdown of the blood–brain barrier and vasogenic edema occur very early in this model.[67,68] It is debatable whether the lesion induced by this model is secondary to an ischemic event. Although this model was used to test neuroprotective agents,[69] its usefulness is limited, because it is believed that the pathophysiological processes induced in this model are less likely relevant to those in human ischemic stroke.

18.3.6 Endothelin-induced MCA occlusion model

Endothelin-1 is a 21-amino acid peptide that has a potent vasoconstrictor effect.[70] Application of endothelin-1 to the exposed MCA induces a significant decrease in CBF. Furthermore, microinjection of endothelin-1 into areas near the MCA through a cannula also decreases CBF in the MCA territory. The distribution of ischemic infarct induced by this method is similar to that following permanent surgical ligation of the MCA.[71] Interestingly, CBF around the ischemic core significantly increases in this model. The advantage of this model is that ischemia can be induced in conscious rats, which excludes the confounding situation that anesthesia may cause. However, the ischemic damage is variable due to different responses of vessels to endothelin-1,[70] and the duration of ischemia is not controllable since endothelin-1-mediated vaso-constriction may gradually disappear.[72] These limitations inhibit its use in drug development although this model was used to test drug efficacy.[71]

18.4 Why do drugs work in animals but not in humans?

Although animal modeling has provided invaluable information about ischemic mechanisms and potential treatment of ischemic stroke, the relevance of animal stroke models to human stroke has been increasingly questioned, because many compounds showing neuroprotective effects in animal models have failed to show efficacy in stroke patients. There are several concerns or problems that need attention.

18.4.1 Age

Most animal stroke models are performed in young adult animals, although some studies used aged rats.[73,74] In aged animals, the immune system, neurochemistry, and vascular structure and morphology may differ from those in young rats, and the neurochemical, morphological, and behavioral changes to ischemia may also be different.[75] Recent evidence demonstrated that the infarct size is larger in older rats and that the lesion distribution is different between young and old rats,[76] although one study did not demonstrate bigger infarct size with aging.[77] It may be important to determine whether a compound is still effective in the aged animals in addition to younger animals. However, it is not known what age in animals is comparable to the typical human stroke population.

18.4.2 Health status

Animals used in most experimental stroke models are young and healthy, which is in contrast to most human stroke patients who may also have diabetes mellitus, chronic arterial hypertension, and hyperlipidemia.[78] These complicating factors may preclude response to therapy in humans. Therefore, experimental data from healthy animals may not be extrapolatable to sick and fragile patients. Some attempts have been made to model "unhealthy status" such as by using animals with atherosclerosis, hypertension, or diabetes mellitus.

18.4.3 Gender

One study demonstrated that infarct volume in stroke models is sex-related, and that female rats typically have smaller infarct size than male rats.[79] Because of difference in physiological status, it is possible that response to treatment is different between the two genders. In preclinical assessments, male rats are predominantly used and only a few studies have used female rats. It is important to know if the neuroprotective effect of compounds exists in both male and female animals.

18.4.4 Mortality

Most experimental studies do not report mortality rates. Mortality may be due to a number of reasons such as adverse effects of a drug (hypotension, toxicity) or due to bleeding (such as with thrombolytic agents), but also may occur for reasons not related to drug effects (surgical complications, bleeding during surgery, or extensive infarction and severe brain edema). Mortality should not be overlooked in experimental studies.

18.4.5 Outcome measures and time points

In experimental studies, the most precise outcome measure used is the infarct volume. Most experimental studies ended within 24 hr. In contrast, outcome is measured in terms of neurological scores and at much later time points (typically at 3 months) in clinical trials. More sophisticated behavioral tests should be incorporated into experimental studies and both behavioral outcome and infarct volumes should be determined at later time points. There is a chance that some neuroprotective agents might delay infarct evolution at early stage, but infarct volumes enlarge later. Late evaluation rules out this possibility. On the other hand, measurement of infarct volumes (by means of diffusion-weighted MRI at early stages and T2-weighted MRI at later time points) should be incorporated into clinical trials, enforcing the results and diminishing the number of patients required. Such trials have already been undertaken.[80,81]

18.4.6 Dosing, dose-finding studies, and adverse effects

Experimental studies use higher doses than clinical trials. For instance, thrombolytic agents such as tissue plasminogen activator (t-PA) and pro-urokinase were used at 10-fold doses in experimental studies compared with clinical trials.[32,39,40,82] Most adverse effects, especially behavioral ones, remain unnoticed in experimental studies. MK801 caused severe psychomimetic adverse effects in clinical trials and could never have been given at doses similar to those found to be effective in experimental studies. Therefore, a wide range of doses should be tried in experimental studies to accurately find the range of effective doses with the least adverse effects.

18.4.7 Treatment initiation time point and time window studies

In most experimental studies, treatment is started before induction of ischemia or only shortly after that. In contrast, early clinical trials used a time window of up to 24 hr. Recent clinical trials prefer a time window of 3–6 hr. While every effort should be made to shorten the time window in clinical trials, time window studies should be performed in animals to find out the latest time point when the drug is still beneficial.

18.4.8 Publication bias

Experimental studies with negative results are usually not published, so that what appears in the literature often can be mistakenly interpreted as over-whelmingly positive results. On the other hand, negative clinical trials are often published or as most of them are large multi-center trials, their results become widely known.

18.4.9 Model-related neuroprotection

It is possible that neuroprotection may be model-related, because ischemic characteristics in different models may be different and some models may not produce ischemic regions amenable to therapeutic regimens. This is confirmed by one recent study in which neuroprotection was positive in one but negative in the other animal model.[83] Therefore, choosing the most appropriate model or several animal models including permanent and transient ischemia models is important for developing novel drugs.

18.4.10 Strain- or species-related neuroprotection

One reason for failure of data transition from the laboratory to bedside may be that neuroprotective effects may be strain- or species-related. At least one study demonstrated that reduction in infarct size with calcium or *N*-methyl-D-aspartate (NMDA) antagonists depends on the rat strains used.[84] Although the reasons and mechanisms are not clear, it is essential that testing drug efficacy be performed in animal models with different strains and species. If efficacy can be demonstrated in lower species, similar experiments should be performed in one or more higher species.

18.4.11 Lack of sufficient data

Moreover, it is likely that for many drugs which were tested in experimental studies, the data were not sufficiently robust to warrant the expectations placed on them.[85] All experimental evidence should be gathered and criti-cally reviewed by experimental and clinical scientists before proceeding to clinical trials.

All in all, focal ischemia models and experimental stroke drug development work have had a huge impact on our understanding of stroke and on devel-opment of novel therapies during the last two decades, but results from experimental work must be interpreted with caution. Experimental and clinical studies have developed interactively regarding the various demands, design, time window, and attempts have been made to establish outcome measures and uniform standards.[11,86,87] A recent major impact of the experimental models on clinical stroke care and research has been the development of diffusion and perfusion MRI in experimental models, and the recent progression of this superb technology to clinical trials and routine use.

Acknowledgments

We thank Dr. Daniel Strbian (Helsinki, Finland) for his technical help with the figures and Dr. Jun Li (Dublin, Ireland) for providing Figure 18.3.

References

1. Bonita R. Stroke prevention: global perspective. In Norris JW, Hachinski V (eds.) *Stroke Prevention*. New York: Oxford University Press, 2001, pp. 259–274.
2. Saxena R, Lewis S, Berge E, Sandercock PA, Koudstaal PJ. Risk of early death and recurrent stroke and effect of heparin in 3169 patients with acute ischemic stroke and atrial fibrillation in the International Stroke Trial. *Stroke* 2001, **32**: 2333–2337.
3. Sacco RL, Wolf PA, Gorelick PB. Risk factors and their management for stroke prevention: outlook for 1999 and beyond. *Neurology* 1999, **53**: S15–S24.
4. Kaste M, Fogelholm R, Rissanen A. Economic burden of stroke and the evaluation of new therapies. *Public Health* 1998, **112**: 103–112.
5. Sacco RL, Boden-Albala B. Stroke risk factors: identification and modification. In Fisher M (ed.) *Stroke Therapy*, 2nd edn. Woburn, MA: Butterworth-Heinemann, 2001, pp. 1–24.
6. del Zoppo GJ, Poeck K, Pessin MS, *et al.* Recombinant tissue plasminogen activator in acute thrombotic and embolic stroke. *Ann. Neurol.* 1992, **32**: 78–86.
7. Hsu CY. Criteria for valid preclinical trials using animal stroke models. *Stroke* 1993, **24**: 633–636.
8. Yamori Y, Horie R, Handa H, Sato M, Fukase M. Pathogenetic similarity of strokes in stroke-prone spontaneously hypertensive rats and humans. *Stroke* 1976, **7**: 46–53.
9. Coyle P. Middle cerebral artery occlusion in the young rat. *Stroke* 1982, **13**: 855–859.
10. Ginsberg MD, Busto R. Rodent models of cerebral ischemia. *Stroke* 1989, **20**: 1627–1642.
11. STAIR (Stroke Therapy Academic Industry Roundtable) Recommendations for standards regarding preclinical neuroprotective and restorative drug development. *Stroke* 1999, **30**: 2752–2758.
12. Koizumi J, Yoshida Y, Nakazawa T, Ooneda G. Experimental studies of ischemic brain edema. I. A new experimental model of cerebral embolism in which recirculation can be introduced in the ischemic area. *Jap. J. Stroke* 1986, **8**: 1–8.
13. Takano K, Tatlisumak T, Bergmann AG, Gibson DGI, Fisher M. Reproducibility and reliability of middle cerebral artery occlusion using a silicon-coated suture (Koizumi) in rats. *J. Neurol. Sci.* 1997, **153**: 8–11.

14. Bclayev L, Alonso OF, Busto R, Zhao W, Ginsberg MD. Middle cerebral artery occlusion in the rat by intraluminal suture: neurological and pathological evaluation of an improved model. *Stroke* 1996, **27**: 1616–1623.

15. Longa EZ, Weinstein PR, Carlson S, Cummins R. Reversible middle cerebral artery occlusion without craniectomy in rats. *Stroke* 1989, **20**: 84–91.

16. Laing RJ, Jakubowski J, Laing RW. Middle cerebral artery occlusion without craniectomy in rats: which method works best? *Stroke* 1993, **24**: 294–298.

17. Nagasawa H, Kogure K. Correlation between cerebral blood flow and histological changes in a new rat model of middle cerebral artery occlusion. *Stroke* 1989, **20**: 1037–1043.

18. Zarow GJ, Karibe H, States BA, Graham SH, Weinstein PR. Endovascular suture occlusion of the middle cerebral artery in rats: effect of suture insertion distance on cerebral blood flow, infarct distribution and infarct volume. *Neurol. Res.* 1997, **19**: 409–416.

19. Li F, Han S, Tatlisumak T, *et al.* A new method to improve in-bore middle cerebral artery occlusion in rats: demonstration with diffusion- and perfusion-weighted imaging. *Stroke* 1998, **29**: 1715–1720.

20. Meng X, Fisher M, Shen Q, Sotak CH, Duong TQ. Characterizing the diffusion/perfusion mismatch in experimental focal cerebral ischemia. *Ann. Neurol.* 2004, **55**: 207–212.

21. Kuge Y, Minematsu K, Yamaguchi T, Miyake Y. Nylon monofilament for intraluminal middle cerebral artery occlusion in rats. *Stroke* 1995, **26**: 1655–1658.

22. Schmid-Elsaesser R, Zausinger S, Hungerhuber E, Baethmann A, Reulen H-J. A critical reevaluation of the intraluminal thread model of focal cerebral ischemia: evidence of inadvertent premature reperfusion and subarachnoid hemorrhage in rats by laser-Doppler flowmetry. *Stroke* 1998, **29**: 2162–2170.

23. Kinouchi H, Epstein CJ, Mizui T, *et al.* Attenuation of focal cerebral ischemic injury in transgenic mice overexpressing CuZn superoxide dismutase. *Proc. Natl Acad. Sci. USA* 1991, **88**: 11158–11162.

24. Yang G, Chan PH, Chen J, *et al.* Human copper-zinc superoxide dismutase transgenic mice are highly resistant to reperfusion injury after focal cerebral ischemia. *Stroke* 1994, **25**: 165–170.

25. Hata R, Mies G, Wiessner C, *et al.* A reproducible model of middle cerebral artery occlusion in mice: hemodynamic, biochemical, and magnetic resonance imaging. *J. Cereb. Blood Flow Metab.* 1998, **18**: 367–375.

26. Roussel SA, van Bruggen N, King MD, *et al.* Monitoring the initial expansion of focal ischemic changes by diffusion-weighted MRI using a remote controlled method of occlusion. *Nucl. Magn. Res. Biomed.* 1994, **7**: 21–8.

27. Kohno K, Back T, Hoehn-Berlage M, Hossmann K-A. A modified rat model of middle cerebral artery thread occlusion under electrophysiological control for magnetic resonance investigations. *Magn. Reson. Imaging* 1995, **13**: 65–71.

28. Röther J, de Crespigny AJ, D'Arceuil H, Moseley ME. MRI detection of cortical spreading depression immediately after focal ischemia in the rat. *J. Cereb. Blood Flow Metab.* 1996, **16**: 214–220.

29. Zhao Q, Memezawa H, Smith ML, Siesjö BK. Hyperthermia complicates middle cerebral artery occlusion induced by an intraluminal filament. *Brain Res.* 1994, **649**: 253–259.

30. Li F, Omae T, Fisher M. Spontaneous hyperthermia and its mechanism in the intraluminal suture middle cerebral artery occlusion model of rats. *Stroke* 1999, **30**: 2464–2471.

31. Albers GW. Antithrombotic agents in cerebral ischemia. *Am. J. Cardiol.* 1995, **75**: 348–388.
32. National Institute of Neurological Disorders and Stroke rt-PA Stroke Study Group T. Tissue plasminogen activator for acute ischemic stroke. *New Engl. J. Med.* 1995, **333**: 1581–1587.
33. Futrell N, Watson BD, Dietrich WD, *et al.* A new model of embolic stroke produced by photochemical injury to the carotid artery in the rat. *Ann. Neurol.* 1988, **23**: 251–257.
34. Futrell N. An improved photochemical model of embolic cerebral infarction in rats. *Stroke* 1991, **22**: 225–232.
35. Hill NC, Millikan CH, Wakim KG, Sayre GP. Studies in cerebrovascular disease. VII. Experimental production of cerebral infarction by intracarotid injection of homologous blood clot: preliminary report. *Mayo Clin. Proc.* 1955, **30**: 625–633.
36. Kudo M, Aoyama A, Ichimori S, Fukunaga N. An animal model of cerebral infarction: homologous blood clot emboli in rats. *Stroke* 1982, **13**: 505–508.
37. Kaneko D, Nakamura N, Ogawa T. Cerebral infarction in rats using homologous blood emboli: development of a new experimental model. *Stroke* 1985, **16**: 76–84.
38. Overgaard K, Sereghy T, Boysen G, *et al.* A rat model of reproducible cerebral infarction using thrombotic blood clot emboli. *J. Cereb. Blood Flow Metab.* 1992, **12**: 484–490.
39. Busch E, Kruger K, Hossmann K-A. Improved model of thromboembolic stroke and rt-PA induced reperfusion in the rat. *Brain Res.* 1997, **778**: 16–24.
40. Takano K, Carano RAD, Tatlisumak T, *et al.* Efficacy of intra-arterial and intravenous prourokinase in an embolic stroke model evaluated by diffusion-perfusion magnetic resonance imaging. *Neurology* 1998, **50**: 870–875.
41. Zhang RL, Chopp M, Zhang ZG, Jiang Q, Ewing JR. A rat model of focal embolic cerebral ischemia. *Brain Res.* 1997, **766**: 83–92.
42. Zhang Z, Zhang R, Jiang Q, *et al.* A new rat model of thrombotic focal cerebral ischemia. *J. Cereb. Blood Flow Metab.* 1997, **17**: 123–135.
43. Zhang ZG, Chopp M, Zhang RL, Goussev A. A mouse model of embolic focal cerebral ischemia. *J. Cereb. Blood Flow Metab.* 1997, **17**: 1081–1088.
44. Shigeno T, Teasdale GM, McCulloch J, Graham DI. Recirculation model following MCA occlusion in rats: cerebral blood flow, cerebrovascular permeability, and brain edema. *J. Neurosurg.* 1985, **63**: 272–277.
45. Shigeno T, McCulloch J, Graham DI, Mendelow AD, Teasdale GM. Pure cortical ischemia versus striatal ischemia. *Surg. Neurol.* 1985, **24**: 47–51.
46. Takizawa S, Hakim AM. Animal models of cerebral ischemia. II. Rat models. *Cerebrovasc. Dis.* 1990, **1**(Suppl. 1): 16–21.
47. Hudgins WR, Garcia JH. Transorbital approach to the middle cerebral artery of the squirrel monkey: a technique for experimental cerebral infarction applicable to ultrastructural studies. *Stroke* 1970, **1**: 107–111.
48. Suzuki J, Yoshimoto T, Tanaka S, Sakamoto T. Production of various models of cerebral infarction in the dog by means of occlusion of intracranial trunk arteries. *Stroke* 1980, **11**: 337–341.
49. Slivka A, Pulsinelli W. Hemorrhagic complications of thrombolytic therapy in experimental stroke. *Stroke* 1987, **18**: 1148–1156.
50. Hayakawa T, Waltz AG. Immediate effects of cerebral ischemia: evolution and resolution of neurological deficits after experimental occlusion of one middle cerebral artery in conscious cats. *Stroke* 1975, **6**: 321–327.

51. Robinson RG, Shoemaker WJ, Schlumpf M, Valk T, Bloom FE. Effect of experimental infarction in rat brain on catecholamines and behaviour. *Nature* 1975, **255**: 332–334.
52. Backhauss C, Karkoutly C, Welsch M, Krieglstein J. A mouse model for focal cerebral ischemia for screening neuroprotective drug effects. *J. Pharmacol. Toxicol. Methods* 1992, **27**: 27–32.
53. Albanese V, Tommasino C, Sparado A, Tomasello F. A transbasisphenoidal approach for selective occlusion of the middle cerebral artery in rats. *Experientia* 1980, **36**: 1302–1304.
54. Tamura A, Graham DI, McCulloch J, Teasdale GM. Focal cerebral ischemia in the rat. I. Description of technique and early neuropathological consequences following middle cerebral artery occlusion. *J. Cereb. Blood Flow Metab.* 1981, **1**: 53–60.
55. Tamura A, Graham DI, McCulloch J, Teasdale M. Focal cerebral ischaemia in the rat. II. Regional cerebral blood flow determined by [^{14}C] iodoantypyrine autoradiography following middle cerebral artery occlusion. *J. Cereb. Blood Flow Metab.* 1981, **1**: 61–69.
56. Bederson JB, Pitts LH, Tsuji M, *et al*. Rat middle cerebral artery occlusion: evaluation of the model and development of a neurologic examination. *Stroke* 1986, **17**: 472–476.
57. Fox G, Gallacher D, Shevde S, Loftus J, Swayne G. Anatomic variation of the middle cerebral artery in the Sprague-Dawley rat. *Stroke* 1993, **24**: 2087–2093.
58. Chen ST, Hsu CY, Hogan EL, Maricq H, Balentine JD. A model of focal ischemic stroke in the rat: reproducible extensive cortical infarction. *Stroke* 1986, **17**: 738–743.
59. Tyson GW, Teasdale GM, Graham DI, McCulloch J. Focal cerebral ischemia in the rat: topography of hemodynamic and histopathological changes. *Ann. Neurol.* 1984, **15**: 559–567.
60. Siegel BA, Meidinger R, Elliott AJ, *et al*. Experimental cerebral microembolism: Multiple tracer assessment of brain edema. *Arch. Neurol.* 1972, **26**: 73–77.
61. Garcia JH. Experimental ischemic stroke: a review. *Stroke* 1984, **15**: 5–14.
62. Takeda T, Shima T, Okada Y, Yamane K, Uozumi T. Pathophysiological studies of cerebral ischemia produced by silicone cylinder embolization in rats. *J. Cereb. Blood Flow Metab.* 1987, **7**(Suppl.): S66.
63. Fukuchi K, Kusuoka H, Watanabe Y, Nishimura T. Correlation of sequential MR images of microsphere-induced cerebral ischemia with histologic changes in rats. *Invest. Radiol.* 1999, **34**: 698–703.
64. Gerriets T, Li F, Silva MD, *et al*. The macrosphere model: evaluation of a new stroke model for permanent middle cerebral artery occlusion in rats. *J. Neurosci. Methods* 2003, **122**: 201–211.
65. Watson BD, Dietrich WD, Busto R, Wachtel MS, Ginsberg MD. Induction of reproducible brain infarction by photochemically initiated thrombosis. *Ann. Neurol.* 1985, **17**: 497–504.
66. Yoshida Y, Dereski MO, Garcia JH, Hetzel FW, Chopp M. Neuronal injury after photoactivation of photofrin II. *Am. J. Pathol.* 1992, **141**: 989–997.
67. Dietrich WD, Watson BD, Busto R, Ginsberg MD, Bethea JR. Photochemically induced cerebral infarction. I. Early microvascular alterations. *Acta Neuropathol. (Berlin)* 1987, **72**: 315–325.
68. Dietrich W, Watson B, Busto R, *et al*. Photochemically induced cerebral infarction. II. Edema and blood–brain barrier disruption. *Acta Neuropathol. (Berlin)* 1987, **72**: 326–334.

69. de Ryck M. Animal models of cerebral stroke: pharmacological protection of function. *Eur. J. Neurol.* 1990, **3**(Suppl.): 21–27.

70. Robinson MJ, Macrae IM, Todd M, Read JL, McCulloch J. Reduction of local cerebral blood flow to pathological levels by endothelin-1 applied to the middle cerebral artery in the rat. *Neurosci. Lett.* 1990, **118**: 269–272.

71. Sharkey J, Ritchie IM, Kelly PAT. Perivascular microapplication of endothelin-1: a new model of focal cerebral ischaemia in the rat. *J. Cereb. Blood Flow Metab.* 1993, **13**: 865–871.

72. Sharkey J, Butcher SP, Kelly JS. Endothelin-1 induced middle cerebral artery occlusion: pathological consequences and neuroprotective effects of MK801. *J. Autonom. Nerv. Syst.* 1994, **49**: S177–S185.

73. Wang LC, Futrell N, Wang DZ, *et al.* A reproducible model of middle cerebral infarcts, compatible with long-term survival, in aged rats. *Stroke* 1995, **26**: 2087–2090.

74. Sutherland GR, Dix GA, Auer RN. Effect of age in rodent models of focal and forebrain ischemia. *Stroke* 1996, **27**: 1663–1668.

75. Millikan CH. Animal stroke models. *Stroke* 1992, **23**: 795–797.

76. Davis M, Mendelow AD, Perry RH, Chambers IR, James OFW. Experimental stroke and neuroprotection in the aging rat brain. *Stroke* 1995, **26**: 1072–1078.

77. Duverger D, MacKenzie ET. The quantification of cerebral infarction following focal ischemia in the rat: influence of strain, arterial pressure, blood glucose concentration, and age. *J. Cereb. Blood Flow Metab.* 1988, **8**: 449–461.

78. Wiebers DO, Adams HPJ, Whisnant JP. Animal models of stroke: are they relevant to human disease? *Stroke* 1990, **21**: 1–3.

79. Alkayed NJ, Harukuni I, Kimes AS, *et al.* Gender-linked brain injury in experimental stroke. *Stroke* 1998, **29**: 159–165.

80. Warach S, Kaste M, Fisher M. The effect of GV150526 on ischemic lesion volume: the GAIN Americas and GAIN International MRI Substudy. *Neurology* 2000, **54**(Suppl. 3): A87.

81. Warach S, Pettigrew LC, Dashe JF, *et al.* Effect of citicoline on ischemic lesions as measured by diffusion-weighted magnetic resonance imaging. *Ann. Neurol.* 2000, **48**: 713–722.

82. Furlan A, Higashida R, Wechsler L, *et al.* Intra-arterial prourokinase for acute ischemic stroke: the PROACT (Prolyse in Acute Cerebral Thromboembolism) II study – a randomized controlled trial. *J. Am. Med. Ass.* 1999, **282**: 2003–2011.

83. Takamatsu H, Kondo K, Ikeda Y, Umemura K. Neuroprotective effects depend on the model of focal ischemia following middle cerebral artery occlusion. *Eur. J. Pharmacol.* 1998, **362**: 137–142.

84. Sauter A, Rudin M. Strain-dependent drug effects in rat middle cerebral artery occlusion model of stroke. *J. Pharmacol. Exp. Ther.* 1995, **274**: 1008–1013.

85. Jonas S, Ayigari V, Viera D, Waterman P. Neuroprotection against cerebral ischemia: A review of animal studies and correlation with human trial results. *Ann. NY Acad. Sci.* 1999, **890**: 2–3.

86. STAIR (Stroke Therapy Academic Industry Roundtable) II Recommendations for clinical trial evaluation of acute stroke therapies. *Stroke* 2001, **32**: 1598–1606.

87. Fisher M (for Stroke Therapy Academic Industry Roundtable) Recommendations for advancing development of acute stroke therapies. *Stroke* 2003, **34**: 1539–1546.

19

Rodent models of global cerebral ischemia

JULIA KOFLER AND RICHARD J. TRAYSTMAN

19.1 Introduction

Each year, about 500 000 people in the USA suffer a cardiac arrest, an event that is associated with high mortality and poor neurological outcome[1,2] Survival rates range from 1% to 33%,[3] and up to 60% of survivors have moderate to severe cognitive deficits 3 months after resuscitation.[1] Frequent neuropsychological sequelae include anterograde memory deficits, learning difficulties, changes in emotional and social behavior, and depression.[4,5] Despite improvements in resuscitation techniques, survival rates have not changed for decades.[6,7] One reason for this disappointing development is the lack of effective treatment options to ameliorate reperfusion injury in the post resuscitation period despite promising results of a variety of agents in animal studies.[1,8] However, recent clinical trials showed that induction of mild hypothermia in unresponsive cardiac arrest survivors can improve neurological outcome and 6-month survival.[9] This was the first demonstration in humans that the development of brain injury after cardiac arrest can be positively influenced by a post-ischemic intervention, even with delayed onset of treatment.

This exciting evidence that ischemic human brain tissue is potentially salvageable has renewed interest in global cerebral ischemia research. In the following review we will describe the most commonly used rodent models of transient global or forebrain ischemia and summarize their advantages and disadvantages. The use of small animals for research studies presents some clear advantages over large animals. Rodents are much less costly to obtain and maintain for longer periods of time. They are genetically homogenous, and genetic modifications can be made relatively easily to reproduce many different transgenic and knockout strains, particularly in mice. In addition, there are fewer animal welfare concerns over the use of rats and mice than of dogs, cats, or monkeys. These smaller animals, however, have lissencephalic brains and thus may be quite different in anatomy and functional aspects from

Handbook of Experimental Neurology, ed. Turgut Tatlisumak and Marc Fisher. Published by Cambridge University Press. © Cambridge University Press 2006.

human brain, a clear disadvantage. Physiological monitoring is also considerably more challenging in small animals, and concurrent measurements over time are limited or may not be possible.

Rodent global cerebral ischemia models can be divided into two major groups. In the first type of injury model, isolated brain or forebrain ischemia is produced via occlusion of major cerebral vessels, whereas in the second, in cardiac arrest models, cessation of brain circulation is produced via induction of cardiac standstill and cerebral ischemia is accompanied by whole-body ischemia. We will focus on these two major groups of injury models, but will also mention alternate techniques.

19.2 Vessel occlusion models

19.2.1 Gerbils

Gerbils have been widely used in global ischemia studies because of their convenient cerebral vasculature. The unique anatomical feature of gerbils is an incomplete circle of Willis lacking a posterior communicating artery which connects the carotid and vertebrobasilar arterial systems. Thus, forebrain ischemia in gerbils can be induced by bilateral common carotid artery occlusion (BCCAO) or two-vessel occlusion (2-VO). Occlusion for 5 min results in delayed, near complete cell loss in the CA1 subfield of the hippocampus.[10,11] However, no or only minimal neuronal damage is usually seen in other forebrain regions,[12] although some groups also report severe damage outside the hippocampus.[13] A variety of interventions has been shown to prevent ischemia-induced neuronal degeneration in the gerbil hippocampus.[12,14–16] The advantages of the gerbil model are the relative simplicity of the surgical procedure, permitting many animals to be studied, and the availability of several behavioral tests as outcome measures which have been extensively studied and shown to correlate with severity of ischemic cell loss.[13,17] Some of the disadvantages are the susceptibility of the gerbil to seizures, which offers a confounding variable into the assessment of ischemic outcome, and the limited physiological monitoring because of the animal's small size.

19.2.2 Rat

In contrast to the gerbil, rats and mice have uni- or bilateral posterior communicating arteries and thus collateral blood flow at the circle of Willis. Therefore, bilateral occlusion of the common carotid arteries is not sufficient to reduce cerebral blood flow to forebrain below a critical threshold to produce ischemic cell death. In 1979, a four-vessel occlusion (4-VO) model was developed to provide a method of reversible forebrain ischemia in rats.[18] This often-used model can be produced in awake, freely moving rats, but it involves a two-stage procedure. On the first day, atraumatic clasps are placed loosely around each common carotid artery. The vertebral arteries are then electro-cauterized via the alar foramina of the first cervical vertebra. Unfortunately, it is impossible to visualize these vessels directly, but this occlusion of vertebral vessels is critical to the success of the model (for a detailed description of this procedure see reference[19]). A modification of this surgical step involves occlusion of vertebral arteries at the level of the second cervical vertebra[20] or in the soft tissue between the first and second vertebrae but this is associated with a higher incidence of hemorrhage.[19] Another variation of the original model involves electrocauterization of the basilar artery via a transcervical–transcli-val approach (three–vessel occlusion) instead of occlusion of the vertebral arteries, but this procedure itself causes neurological deficits in about 20–30% of rats.[21] On the second day, the common carotid arteries are occluded while the animal is awake, and ischemia is produced. This procedure must result in a complete loss of the righting reflex for the animal to be included in the study that usually occurs within 15–30 s after occlusion and can be achieved in approximately 75% of rats.[18] Dilatation of the pupils with occlusion of the carotid arteries or the rapid appearance of an isoelectric electroencephalogram (EEG) are alternative criteria that can be employed to assure successful occlusion.[22]

Four-vessel occlusion markedly decreases perfusion of cerebral hemispheres but does not produce complete ischemia.[18,23] Perfusion of brainstem and cerebellum is usually preserved probably due to collateral filling via the anterior spinal artery. Still, some animals die during the occlusion period from respiratory failure due to brainstem ischemia.[18,24] On the other hand, about 15% of rats fail to become unresponsive following occlusion of carotid and vertebral arteries. The source of continued cerebral blood flow in these rats is collateral arteries in cervical and paravertebral muscles. Variable collateral blood flow is also held accountable for the differences seen in response to 4-VO between rats of different strains or even different shipments of rats from the same supplier.[19,25] A modification of the original 4-VO model was described to increase the percentage of rats that meet the criteria of successful occlusion. A suture is placed in the cervical region anterior to cervical and paravertebral muscles and tightened after occlusion of the carotid arteries to occlude collateral blood vessels in the neck muscles.[19,26] However, overtightening of this suture may lead to death from respiratory arrest and brainstem ischemia. The issue of collateral cerebral blood flow (CBF) was also addressed in another modification of the model, which includes temporary or permanent occlusion of both external carotid arteries, both pterygopalatine branches of the internal carotid artery, and electrocauterization of the basilar artery followed by reversible occlusion of the common carotid arteries (seven-vessel occlusion model).[27]

The grade of damage after 4-VO in rats varies among regions and is proportional to the duration of ischemia. The most vulnerable structures are the CA1 sector of hippocampus, thalamus, cortical layers 3, 5, and 6, and small to medium-sized neurons in striatum.[19] With 10 and 20 min of ischemia, vulnerable zones of the hippocampus show ischemic cell change in approximately 40% and 85%, respectively, after 3 days of survival. Consistent neuronal injury to the striatum requires at least 20–30 min of ischemia, and these changes are maximally expressed by 24 hr.[25,28]

One major advantage of the 4-VO model is that occlusion can be produced in awake animals, thus avoiding use of anesthetics during the ischemic phase which may depress cerebral energy metabolism and modify brain damage.[18] It also allows observation of the behavioral response of the animal subjected to ischemia. The major disadvantages of the 4-VO model are that it requires a preparatory operative procedure that may increase the risk of extraneous factors confounding the response to the ischemic insult itself, and that the procedure is only partly reversible with the vertebral arteries remaining permanently occluded.[29] The lack of anesthesia can also be considered disadvantageous since it does not allow physiological monitoring during ischemia. Therefore other groups have modified the original model by performing both steps of the procedure under anesthesia.[24,30,31]

The 2-VO model overcomes some of the disadvantages of the 4-VO model since it is a fully reversible procedure with bilateral occlusion of the common carotid arteries without the need for the technically challenging procedure of vertebral artery occlusion. However, it requires a simultaneous intervention to reduce systemic blood pressure in order to induce a sufficient reduction in cerebral blood flow.[32] Hypotension can be achieved by controlled exsanguination and subsequent reinfusion of blood upon reperfusion,[33,34] by administration of vasodilators (trimetaphan, phentolamine)[32], a combination of both,[35,36] by increasing the level of a vasoactive anesthetic (halothane),[37] or by inducing negative lower body pressure (hypobaric hypotension) using a suction device.[38,39] In general, injury after 2-VO is similar in size and location[34] to the damage observed after 4-VO with the exception of slightly higher injury scores in the cerebellum after 4-VO[29] suggesting that in the 2-VO model impairment of blood flow to hindbrain structures is less severe than in 4-VO with permanent occlusion of the vertebral arteries. Preservation of blood flow to respiratory centers in the brainstem is also the most likely explanation why animals recovering from 2-VO have reportedly fewer respiratory problems.[29] However, to allow for better control of ventilatory parameters and avoid respiratory insufficiency, anesthetized animals are usually intubated or tracheotomized and mechanically ventilated during occlusion and reperfusion.[32,36] Advantages of the 2-VO model are the one-stage surgical preparation, the rapid induction of ischemia and reperfusion, and the suitability for chronic survival studies. On the other hand, the need for anesthetics and drugs to induce hypotension may complicate the interpretation of outcome. The model cannot be used in awake animals, so behavioral alterations immediately after occlusion cannot be assessed.[25]

19.2.3 Mouse

While earlier global cerebral ischemia experiments were predominantly performed in gerbils and rats, the availability of increasing numbers of transgenic and knockout mouse strains have made the development of appropiate mouse models necessary. Since attempts of 3-VO and 4-VO were associated with technical difficulty and high mortality,[40–43] most groups focused on the 2-VO model without blood pressure manipulations.[43–46] However, some groups adapted the rat 2-VO + hypotension model for the mouse and lowered blood pressure with pharmacologic agents (trimetaphane) and controlled exsanguination,[42,47] or blood pressure lowering doses of anesthetic agents (chloral hydrate) combined with controlled ventilation to avoid hypercapnia.[40] In general, 2-VO in the mouse can be performed with or without intubation and mechanical ventilation, but ventilation allows for better control of respiratory parameters and prevents respiratory problems during ischemia. In an attempt to compare models, it was found that 2-VO + hypotension produced a more uniform and reliable insult and more consistent reduction in CBF than 2-VO alone, but also requires more complex surgical preparations including vascular cannulation for blood pressure monitoring and blood withdrawal.[47]

Similar to rats, mice usually have communicating arteries at the circle of Willis with a high degree of variability between mouse strains. Based on their different degree of patency of these vessels, mouse strains show high variability in neuronal damage after similar ischemic periods.[40,43,48] Some strain differences seen after 2-VO were not reproduced when the basilar artery was also occluded[41] or even reversed after cardiac arrest.[49] However, there also appears to be other factors than vascular anatomy to attribute to strain-related differences in neuronal vulnerability.[47–49] Since genetically engineered mice are often bred on a mixed background, it is important to compare vascular anatomy between experimental groups before making a statement about differences in ischemic susceptibility. Side differences in vascular anatomy are also held responsible for the often observed variability of injury between hemispheres.[43] Lack of collateral blood flow in some mice explains the high mortality associated with 4-VO since occlusion of the vertebral arteries causes severe hindbrain ischemia and respiratory arrest in these mice.[43] To avoid the confounding problem of collateral blood flow, many groups perform experiments with unilateral or even bilateral laser Doppler flow (LDF) monitoring to assure adequate reduction in CBF.[50–52] Animals without a drop of LDF below a certain threshold are excluded from the experiment.

Another modification of the 2-VO model allows vessel occlusion in conscious mice by using a two-step procedure. On day 1, a loose thread is placed around both common carotid arteries and exteriorized at the back of the neck which is then tightened some days later to induce ischemia.[53] A similar modification has also been described for gerbils.[54]

The disadvantages of the mouse model are the vascular variability and the small size of the animal which makes physiologic monitoring challenging and excludes repeated measurements of blood gases or metabolic parameters. On the other hand, the small size of the mouse can reduce the costs of an experiment since smaller amounts of drugs or radioactive tracers for autoradiographic CBF studies are needed. Housing costs for mice are also less than for larger animals. Another advantage of mice is the low susceptibility to post-ischemic seizures.[42]

Interestingly, while in gerbils and rats, the region most vulnerable to ischemia seems to be the hippocampus,[28,33,35,55] many groups reported injury to be more variable in the mouse hippocampus while the caudoputamen appears to be the area most consistently injured in mice.[43–44,46,51–52,56] This variability in hippocampal injury in the murine models must be taken into consideration when designing experiments involving electrophysiological or behavioral measurements. While some groups report neuropathological damage after short periods of ischemia, most studies in rats and mice use ischemia periods of 10–20 min with a wide range from 3 to 75 min. Some of the variability is probably due to different experimental protocols, different strains of animals, and variable accuracy in controlling physiological parameters such as body and head temperatures.

19.3 Cardiac arrest models

While all vessel occlusion and cardiac arrest models produce global or forebrain ischemia and similar neuronal injury in selectively vulnerable brain regions, there are several important differences that should be addressed.

Firstly, vessel occlusion does not cause complete ischemia since residual CBF occurs via communicating arteries as outlined above. Considerable blood flow to hindbrain structures is usually maintained, and therefore respiration and state of consciousness might be altered differently than after a true cardiac arrest. Secondly, chest compressions during CPR and impaired post-ischemic cardiac function cause a low-flow period that can further increase neuronal damage by aggravating the no-reflow phenomenon.[57] Thirdly, vessel occlusion produces isolated brain ischemia, whereas in cardiac arrest the whole organism is affected. Metabolic acidosis, systemic inflammation, and impaired function of coagulation and extracerebral organs (post resuscitation syndrome) can impair post-ischemic reperfusion and affect cerebral functions causing secondary brain damage in cardiac arrest survivors.[58-60] Fourthly, resuscitation of cardiac arrest patients usually requires administration of supplemental oxygen and a vasopressor such as epinephrine, both of which have been shown to adversely affect neurological outcome.[61,62]

Since all these factors can confound experimental results and complicate data analysis, many investigators use vessel occlusion models for elucidating injury pathways and potential therapeutic targets. However, in transitional research, it is important to mimic the clinical situation as closely as possible, and therefore many groups attempted to incorporate these confounding intra- and post-ischemic factors into their experimental setup and developed rodent cardiac arrest models.

19.3.1 Rats

A variety of cardiac arrest protocols have been developed in rats. All models usually require controlled mechanical ventilation after endotracheal intubation or tracheostomy, electrocardiogram (EKG) monitoring, venous cannulation for drug administration, and arterial cannulation for blood pressure and blood gas monitoring. The models differ from each other by the way cessation of circulation is induced. CPR generally includes chest compressions, ventilation with 100% oxygen, administration of epinephrine, and sometimes bicarbonate with some variations and specifics depending on experimental protocol.

The most common cause of cardiac arrest in human adults is ventricular fibrillation (VF). VF can be induced in rats by electrical stimulation of the heart via an esophageal electrode and reversed by external defibrillation as part of the CPR procedures.[57,63,64] Some groups observed that VF tends to reverse spontaneously in rats,[65] while others did not encounter this problem.[57]

Asphyxia from upper airway obstruction or apnea is another frequent cause of cardiac arrest in adults and even more so in children. Asphyxia in experimental animals is induced by administration of a muscle relaxant followed by disconnecting the ventilator and clamping the endotracheal tube at end exhalation. Transient hypertension is observed followed by progressive bradycardia, hypotension, and pulselessness starting at about 3–4 min of apnea.[65,66] By using an 8-min asphyxiation period, animals are therefore only about 5 min in true cardiac arrest which is considerably shorter than in most vessel occlusion studies but long enough to produce widespread injury. The disadvantage of this model is that timing of cardiac arrest is not precisely uniform which can potentially influence the consistency of outcome values. An important feature of asphyxial cardiac arrest is the progression from incomplete ischemia to complete ischemia before cardiovascular collapse.[66] The result is a different and more severe pattern of central nervous system injury when compared with sudden complete ischemia as occurs with ventricular fibrillation.[67] Interestingly, there seem to be significant differences between rat strains not only with respect to neuronal injury, but also in their cardiovascular system as seen in different "time to cardiac arrest" and CPR periods.[68] Mortality rates using this model vary, but some laboratories are able to achieve a high percentage of animals surviving for several days while still producing significant histopathological injury.[65]

An interesting modification of the asphyxial cardiac arrest model was developed by one group to allow magnetic resonance imaging during CPR without interference from the resuscitation efforts. This so-called remote resuscitation is performed without chest compressions and includes intra-aortic infusion of oxygenated blood and a resuscitation cocktail containing heparin, sodium bicarbonate, and epinephrine achieving resuscitation success rates of 95%.[69]

Another frequently used method to induce cardiac standstill involves administration of (cold) potassium chloride via central venous or percutaneous intracardiac injection which leads to immediate arrest.[70–74] Although hyperkalemia can lead to cardiac arrest in humans, it is not one of the major causes. However, this model has the advantages of an immediate, precisely timed onset of ischemia similar to the VF model, and it requires less surgery than most other models. A possible concern with this model is the potential impact of hyperkalemia on cerebral electrophysiology. Due to the immediate cardiac standstill after injection, it is likely that most of the potassium stays within the heart during ischemia, but with restoration of spontaneous circulation (ROSC) some of it will reach the brain. In a similar mouse model, systemic potassium levels were still elevated 5 min after CPR, but returned to normal within 15 min.[49]

Cardiac arrest can also be simulated non-invasively by hydraulic compression of the chest. This maneuver restricts excursions of the chest and blocks ventricular filling leading to electromechanical dissociation and cessation of arterial flow,[75–77] but variations up to 1 min until flattening of the EEG occurs are reported. This model can be performed without vascular cannulation thus minimizing surgical preparations.

Compression of major cardiac vessels is the underlying principle of a more invasive model which includes the insertion of a hook-shaped device into the mediastinum. By lifting the device and simultaneously applying pressure from the outside, the bundle of major cardiac vessels is occluded thus interrupting circulation.[78–80]

All cardiac arrest models have in common that there is usually some variability in ischemia length due to different CPR periods necessary to achieve ROSC. Therefore animals that exceed a certain pre-set time limit without ROSC are usually excluded from further analysis. Another feature that is unique to the cardiac arrest models, is the observation of spastic hind-leg paralysis in many resuscitated rats which is often only temporary and possibly due to spinal cord ischemia.[63,65,71,77] This finding has to be taken into consideration when analyzing and comparing behavioral and neurological deficit scores since it may not be related to brain injury.

19.3.2 Mouse

In recent years, several groups have tried with varying success to adopt different rat cardiac arrest models for mice. One group evaluated 5 min of VF-induced cardiac arrest and was able to achieve high ROSC and survival rates, but found only minimal histopathological evidence of hippocampal injury. Despite the lack of widespread cell death, they described a marked upregulation of various immediate early genes in hippocampal neurons.[81]

Other groups transferred the hook model from rats to mice which uses compression of the cardiac vessel bundle to induce cessation of circulation. While in one study, most animals were successfully resuscitated, only about 50% survived for 7 days and only one showed histological injury in the hippocampus.[82] In contrast, another group found many degenerating neurons in CA1 using the same experimental paradigm with 5 min ischemia.[83] However, different strains were used in these studies and no information was provided about duration of resuscitation procedures and thus total length of ischemia.

Our group succeeded in developing a KCl-induced cardiac arrest model in mice. Since we did not see any significant histopathological injury with short ischemia periods, we modified the original model in several ways to ensure consistent behavioral and histopathological damage in several brain regions including caudoputamen and, to a lesser degree, hippocampus.[49,84] To reduce mortality and the chance of spinal cord ischemia, we lower body temperature during cardiac arrest to 27–28 °C while simultaneously raising head temperature to 39–40° to produce brain damage. This model has a high success rate in achieving ROSC of almost 100% and is associated with a 3-day survival period of about 70% after 10 min of cardiac arrest. A major advantage of this model is that it requires only minimal surgery and can be performed without arterial cannulation. In this case, successful induction of cardiac arrest and ROSC is ensured by EKG monitoring and observation of the chest for visible cardiac contractions to ascertain that electrical activity of the heart is accompanied by appropiate mechanical activity. One disadvantage of this model is the necessity for very tight control of temperatures to reduce variability in insult severity. Also, we cannot exclude the possibility that different or additional injury pathways are activated in hyperthermia-aggravated ischemia compared to a pure ischemia paradigm.

19.4 Other global cerebral ischemia models

One of the easiest methods to produce global ischemia without recirculation is decapitation. This technique was used many years ago in small animals to study biochemical mechanisms and pathways in global ischemia[85,86] but it does not allow any modulations, and the effect of severing nervous connections between excised tissue and the rest of the nervous system is not known.

The use of a neck tourniquet to produce global ischemia in rats has also been used for many years,[87–89] but with this technique there are complicating factors such as venous congestion and vagal nerve compression, which can lead to variable ischemic outcome.

Global brain ischemia can also be induced by infusing artificial cerebrospinal fluid (CSF) into the cisterna magna to elevate CSF pressure above arterial blood pressure by 20–70 mm Hg. Reflex hypertension can be prevented by administration of the ganglionic blocker trimetaphan. This model has been used to study various metabolic pathways and tissue acidosis.[90,91] However, analysis of the results obtained by this technique is complicated by the effects of increased intracranial pressure on brain tissue. Elevation of CSF pressure to different levels was also used in combination with 2-VO and induced hypotension to compare the sequelae of complete and incomplete ischemia.[25,92]

19.5 Concluding remarks

This article provides a review of the most frequently used rodent models of global cerebral ischemia. All of these models offer an opportunity to investigate mechanisms, prevention, and treatment options of ischemic brain injury. Whatever model one uses for investigation, however, requires care in measuring and controlling important physiological conditions such as blood pressure, brain temperature, blood gases, and cerebral blood flow so that tissue injury is reproducible and consistent.

We have learned much from these ischemic models concerning our understanding of complex cellular cascades underlying the development of ischemic injury. However, it may be that none of the animal models discussed in this review actually closely reflects human global cerebral ischemia.[93] In addition, the animals used in models are usually young and healthy, whereas patients are usually of advanced age and may have other existing pathologies, such as diabetes, hypertension, and coronary vascular disease. These underlying diseases may alter the way global ischemia presents in humans and change the response to therapeutic interventions. Despite these reservations, the described rodent models are the best in vivo experimental preparations we have at the moment to screen for potential therapeutic targets, and to learn more about the underlying mechanisms of global cerebral ischemia and neuroprotection.

Acknowledgments

This work was supported by US Public Health Service Grants NS20020 and NS46072.

References

1. Roine RO, Kajaste S, Kaste M. Neuropsychological sequelae of cardiac arrest. *J. Am. Med. Ass.* 1993, **269**: 237–242.
2. Eisenberg MS, Mengert T. Primary care: cardiac resuscitation. *New Engl. J. Med.* 2001, **344**: 1304–1313.
3. Becker LB, Ostrander MP, Barrett J, Kondos GT. Outcome of CPR in a large metropolitan area: where are the survivors? *Ann. Emerg. Med.* 1991, **20**: 355–361.
4. Reich P, Regestein QR, Murawski BJ, DeSilva RA, Lown B. Unrecognized organic mental disorders in survivors of cardiac arrest. *Am. J. Psychiat.* 1983, **140**: 1194–1197.
5. Nunes B, Pais J, Garcia R, *et al.* Cardiac arrest: long-term cognitive and imaging analysis. *Resuscitation* 2003, **57**: 287–297.

6. Rea TD, Eisenberg MS, Becker LJ, Murray JA, Hearne T. Temporal trends in sudden cardiac arrest: a 25-year emergency medical services perspective. *Circulation* 2003, **107**: 2780–2785.
7. Herlitz J, Rundqvist S, Bång A, *et al*. Is there a difference between women and men in characteristics and outcome after in hospital cardiac arrest? *Resuscitation* 2001, **49**: 15–23.
8. Jastremski M, Sutton-Tyrrell K, Vaagenes P, *et al*. Glucocorticoid treatment does not improve neurological recovery following cardiac arrest (Brain Resuscitation Clinical Trial I Study Group). *J. Am. Med. Ass.* 1989, **262**: 3427–3430.
9. Hypothermia after Cardiac Arrest Study Group. Mild therapeutic hypothermia to improve the neurologic outcome after cardiac arrest. *New Engl. J. Med.* 2002, **346**: 549–556.
10. Kirino T. Delayed neuronal death in the gerbil hippocampus following ischemia. *Brain Res.* 1982, **239**: 57–69.
11. Welsh FA, Harris VA. Postischemic hypothermia fails to reduce ischemic injury in gerbil hippocampus. *J. Cereb. Blood Flow Metab.* 1991, **11**: 617–620.
12. Gill R, Foster AC, Woodruff GN. Systemic administration of MK-801 protects against ischemia-induced hippocampal neurodegeneration in the gerbil. *J. Neurosci.* 1987, **7**: 3343–3349.
13. Mileson BE, Schwartz RD. The use of locomotor activity as a behavioral screen for neuronal damage following transient forebrain ischemia in gerbils. *Neurosci. Lett.* 1991, **128**: 71–76.
14. Colbourne F, Auer RN, Sutherland GR. Characterization of postischemic behavioral deficits in gerbils with and without hypothermic neuroprotection. *Brain Res.* 1998, **803**: 69–78.
15. Jover T, Tanaka H, Calderone A, *et al*. Estrogen protects against global ischemia-induced neuronal death and prevents activation of apoptotic signaling cascades in the hippocampal CA1. *J. Neurosci.* 2002, **22**: 2115–2124.
16. Uyama O, Matsuyama T, Michishita H, Nakamura H, Sugita M. Protective effects of human recombinant superoxide dismutase on transient ischemic injury of CA1 neurons in gerbils. *Stroke* 1992, **23**: 75–81.
17. Corbett D, Nurse S. The problem of assessing effective neuroprotection in experimental cerebral ischemia. *Prog. Neurobiol.* 1998, **54**: 531–548.
18. Pulsinelli WA, Brierley JB. A new model of bilateral hemispheric ischemia in the unanesthetized rat. *Stroke* 1979, **10**: 267–272.
19. Pulsinelli WA, Buchan AM. The four-vessel occlusion rat model: method for complete occlusion of vertebral arteries and control of collateral circulation. *Stroke* 1988, **19**: 913–914.
20. Sugio K, Horigome N, Sakaguchi T, Goto M. A model of bilateral hemispheric ischemia: modified four-vessel occlusion in rats. *Stroke* 1988, **19**: 922.
21. Kameyama M, Suzuki J, Shirane R, Ogawa A. A new model of bilateral hemispheric ischemia in the rat: three-vessel occlusion model. *Stroke* 1985, **16**: 489–493.
22. Pulsinelli WA, Levy DE, Duffy TE. Cerebral blood flow in the four-vessel occlusion model. *Stroke* 1983, **14**: 832–833.
23. Pulsinelli WA, Levy DE, Duffy TE. Regional cerebral blood flow and glucose metabolism following transient forebrain ischemia. *Ann. Neurol.* 1982, **11**: 499–509.
24. Schmidt-Kastner R, Paschen W, Ophoff BG, Hossmann KA. A modified four-vessel occlusion model for inducing incomplete forebrain ischemia in rats. *Stroke* 1989, **20**: 938–946.

25. Ginsberg MD, Busto R. Rodent models of cerebral ischemia. *Stroke* 1989, **20**: 1627–1642.
26. Pulsinelli WA, Duffy TE. Regional energy balance in rat brain after transient forebrain ischemia. *J. Neurochem.* 1983, **40**: 1500–1503.
27. Shirane R, Shimizu H, Kameyama M, Weinstein PR. A new method for producing temporary complete cerebral ischemia in rats. *J. Cereb. Blood. Flow Metab.* 1991, **11**: 949–956.
28. Pulsinelli WA, Brierley JB, Plum F. Temporal profile of neuronal damage in a model of transient forebrain ischemia. *Ann. Neurol.* 1982, **11**: 491–498.
29. McBean DE, Kelly PAT. Rodent models of global cerebral ischemia: a comparison of two-vessel occlusion and four-vessel occlusion. *Gen. Pharmacol.* 1998, **30**: 431–434.
30. Alps BJ, Hass WK. The potential beneficial effect of nicardipine in a rat model of transient forebrain ischemia. *Neurology* 1987, **37**: 809–814.
31. Zoli M, Grimaldi R, Ferrari R, Zini I, Agnati LF. Short- and long-term changes in striatal neurons and astroglia after transient forebrain ischemia in rats. *Stroke* 1997, **28**: 1049–1059.
32. Eklöf B, Siesjö BK. The effect of bilateral carotid artery ligation upon the blood flow and the energy state of the rat brain. *Acta Physiol. Scand.* 1972, **86**: 155–165.
33. Chan PH, Kawase M, Murakami K, *et al.* Overexpression of SOD1 in transgenic rats protects vulnerable neurons against ischemic damage after global cerebral ischemia and reperfusion. *J. Neurosci.* 1998, **18**: 8292–8299.
34. Larsson E, Lindvall O, Kokaia Z. Stereological assessment of vulnerability of immunocytochemically identified striatal and hippocampal neurons after global cerebral ischemia in rats. *Brain Res.* 2001, **913**: 117–132.
35. Smith ML, Auer RN, Siesjö BK. The density and distribution of ischemic brain injury in the rat following 2–10 min of forebrain ischemia. *Acta Neuropathol.* 1984, **64**: 319–332.
36. Smith ML, Bendek G, Dahlgren N, *et al.* Models for studying long-term recovery following forebrain ischemia in the rat. 2. A 2-vessel occlusion model. *Acta Neurol. Scand.* 1984, **69**: 385–401.
37. McBean DE, Winters V, Wilson AD, *et al.* Neuroprotective efficacy of lifarizine (RS-87476) in a simplified rat survival model of two-vessel occlusion. *Br. J. Pharmacol.* 1995, **116**: 3093–3098.
38. Dirnagl U, Thorén P, Villringer A, *et al.* Global forebrain ischemia in the rat: controlled reduction of cerebral blood flow by hypobaric hypotension and two-vessel occlusion. *Neurol. Res.* 1993, **15**: 128–130.
39. Noppens R, Christ M, Körner IP, Brambrink AM, Kempski O. Hypertonic/hyperoncotic solution improves long-term functional and histopathological outcome after global cerebral ischemia in rats. *J. Cereb. Blood Flow Metab.* 2003, **23**: 56.
40. Murakami K, Kondo T, Kawase M, Chan PH. The development of a new mouse model of global ischemia: focus on the relationships between ischemia duration, anesthesia, cerebral vasculature, and neuronal injury following global ischemia in mice. *Brain Res.* 1998, **780**: 304–310.
41. Panahian N, Yoshida T, Huang PL, *et al.* Attenuated hippocampal damage after global cerebral ischemia in mice mutant in neuronal nitric oxide synthase. *Neuroscience* 1996, **72**: 343–354.
42. Sheng H, Laskowitz DT, Pearlstein RD, Warner DS. Characterization of a recovery global cerebral ischemia model in the mouse. *J. Neurosci. Methods* 1999, **88**: 103–109.

43. Yang G, Kitagawa K, Matsushita K, *et al.* C57Bl/6 strain is most susceptible to cerebral ischemia following bilateral common carotid artery occlusion among seven mouse strains: selective neuronal death in the murine transient forebrain ischemia. *Brain Res.* 1997, **752**: 209–218.

44. Horsburgh K, Macrae IM, Carswell H. Estrogen is neuroprotective via an apolipoprotein E-dependent mechanism in a mouse model of global ischemia. *J. Cereb. Blood Flow Metab.* 2002, **22**: 1189–1195.

45. Kawase M, Murakami M, Fujimura M, *et al.* Exacerbation of delayed cell injury after transient global ischemia in mutant mice with CuZn superoxide dismutase deficiency. *Stroke* 1999, **30**: 1962–1968.

46. Wu C, Zhan RZ, Qi S, *et al.* A forebrain ischemic preconditioning model established in C57Bl/Crj6 mice. *J. Neurosci. Methods* 2001, **107**: 101–106.

47. Wellons III JC, Sheng H, Laskowitz DT, *et al.* A comparison of strain-related susceptibility in two murine recovery models of global cerebral ischemia. *Brain Res.* 2000, **868**: 14–21.

48. Fujii M, Hara H, Meng W, *et al.* Strain-related differences in susceptibility to transient forebrain ischemia in SV-129 and C57Bl/6 mice. *Stroke* 1997, **28**: 1805–1811.

49. Kofler J, Hattori K, Sawada M, *et al.* Histopathological and behavioral characterization of a novel model of cardiac arrest and cardiopulmonary resuscitation in mice. *J. Neurosci. Methods* 2004, **136**: 33–44.

50. Brambrink AM, Hey B, Körner IP, Noppens R, Kempski O. Validation of global cerebral ischemia using a noninvasive method to continuously monitor cerebral blood flow is an important tool to reduce variability in the 2-vessel occlusion model in mice. *J. Cereb. Blood Flow Metab.* 2003, **23**(Suppl. I): 50.

51. Olsson T, Wieloch T, Smith ML. Brain damage in a mouse model of global cerebral ischemia: effect of NMDA receptor blockade. *Brain Res.* 2003, **982**: 260–269.

52. Yang G, Kitagawa K, Ohtsuki T, *et al.* Regional differences of neuronal vulnerability in the murine hippocampus after transient forebrain ischemia. *Brain Res.* 2000, **870**: 195–198.

53. Himori N, Watanabe H, Akaike N, *et al.* Cerebral ischemia model with conscious mice. *J. Pharmacol. Methods* 1990, **23**: 311–327.

54. Chandler MJ, DeLeo J, Carney JM. An unanesthetized-gerbil model of cerebral ischemia-induced behavioral changes. *J. Pharmacol. Methods* 1985, **14**: 137–146.

55. Gionet TX, Thomas JD, Warner DS, *et al.* Forebrain ischemia induces selective behavioral impairments associated with hippocampal injury in rats. *Stroke* 1991, **22**: 1040–1047.

56. Terashima T, Shobu N, Hoshimaru M, *et al.* Consistent injury in the striatum of C57Bl/6 mice after transient bilateral common carotid artery occlusion. *Neurosurgem* 1998, **43**: 900–908.

57. Böttiger BW, Krumnikl JJ, Gass P, *et al.* The cerebral "no-reflow" phenomenon after cardiac arrest in rats: influence of low-flow perfusion. *Resuscitation* 1997, **34**: 79–87.

58. Burne-Taney MJ, Kofler J, Yokota N, *et al.* Acute renal failure after whole body ischemia is characterized by inflammation and T cell-mediated injury. *Am. J. Physiol. Renal Physiol.* 2003, **285**: F87–F94.

59. ECC Guidelines. Part 6: Advanced cardiovascular life support. *Circulation* 2000, **102**(Suppl. I): I86–I171.

60. Papadopoulos MC, Davies DC, Moss RF, Tighe D, Bennett ED. Pathophysiology of septic encephalopathy: a review. *Crit. Care Med.* 2000, **28**: 3019–3024.

61. Behringer W, Kittler H, Sterz F, *et al.* Cumulative epinephrine dose during cardiopulmonary resuscitation and neurologic outcome. *Ann. Intern. Med.* 1998, **129**: 450–456.
62. Zwemer CF, Whitesall SE, D'Alecy LG. Cardiopulmonary–cerebral resuscitation with 100% oxygen exacerbates neurological dysfunction following nine minutes of normothermic cardiac arrest in dogs. *Resuscitation* 1994, **27**: 159–170.
63. Krep H, Brinker G, Schwindt W, Hossmann KA. Endothelin type A-antagonist improves long-term recovery after cardiac arrest in rats. *Crit. Care Med.* 2000, **28**: 2873–2880.
64. Vogel P, van den Putten H, Popp E, *et al.* Improved resuscitation after cardiac arrest in rats expressing the baculovirus caspase inhibitor protein p35 in central neurons. *Anesthesiology* 2003, **99**: 112–121.
65. Katz L, Ebmayer U, Safar P, Radovsky A, Neumar R. Outcome model of asphyxial cardiac arrest in rats. *J. Cereb. Blood Flow Metab.* 1995, **15**: 1032–1039.
66. Hickey RW, Ferimer H, Alexander HL, *et al.* Delayed, spontaneous hypothermia reduces neuronal damage after asphyxial cardiac arrest in rats. *Crit. Care Med.* 2000, **28**: 3511–3516.
67. Vaagenes P, Safar P, Moossy J, *et al.* Asphyxiation versus ventricular fibrillation cardiac arrest in dogs. Differences in cerebral resuscitation effects: a preliminary study. *Resuscitation* 1997, **35**: 41–52.
68. Ebmayer U, Keilhoff G, Wolf G, Röse W. Strain-specific differences in a cardiopulmonary resuscitation rat model. *Resuscitation* 2002, **53**: 189–200.
69. Liachenko S, Tang P, Hamilton RL, Xu Y. A reproducible model of circulatory arrest and remote resuscitation in rats for NMR investigation. *Stroke* 1998, **29**: 1229–1239.
70. Badylak SF, Babbs CF, Kougias C, Blaho K. Effect of allopurinol and dimethylsulfoxide on long-term survival in rats after cardiorespiratory arrest and resuscitation. *Am. J. Emerg. Med.* 1988, **4**: 313–318.
71. Blomqvist P, Wieloch T. Ischemic brain damage in rats following cardiac arrest using a long-term recovery model. *J. Cereb. Blood Flow Metab.* 1985, **5**: 420–431.
72. Crumrine RC, LaManna JC. Regional cerebral metabolites, blood flow, plasma volume, and mean transit time in total cerebral ischemia in the rat. *J. Cereb. Blood Flow Metab.* 1991, **11**: 272–282.
73. Garrison HG, Hansen AR, Palladino GW, Fillipo DC, Proctor HJ. Effect of nifedipine on cerebral high-energy phosphates after cardiac arrest and resuscitation in the rat. *Ann. Emerg. Med.* 1986, **15**: 685–691.
74. Jaw SP, Su DD, Truong DD. Astrocyte-derived growth factor (S100β) and motor function in rats following cardiac arrest. *Pharmacol. Biochem. Behav.* 1994, **52**: 667–670.
75. Dhooper A, Young C, Reid KH. Ischemia-induced anxiety following cardiac arrest in the rat. *Behav. Brain Res.* 1997, **84**: 57–62.
76. Li MM, Payne RS, Reid KH, *et al.* Correlates of delayed neuronal damage and neuroprotection in a rat model of cardiac-arrest-induced cerebral ischemia. *Brain Res.* 1999, **826**: 44–52.
77. Wauquier A, Melis W, Jansen PAJ. Long-term neurological assessment of the post-resuscitative effects of flunarizine, verapamil and nimodipine in a new model of global complete ischemia. *Neuropharmacology* 1989, **28**: 837–846.
78. Kawai K, Nitecka L, Ruetzler CA, *et al.* Global cerebral ischemia associated with cardiac arrest in the rat. I. Dynamics of early neuronal changes. *J. Cereb. Blood Flow Metabol.* 1992, **12**: 238–249.

79. Pluta R, Lossinsky AS, Mossakowski MJ, Faso L, Wiśniewski HM. Reassessment of a new model of complete cerebral ischemia in rats: method of induction of clinical death, pathophysiology and cerebrovascular pathology. *Acta Neuropathol.* 1991, **83**: 1–11.

80. Ross DT, Brasko J, Patrikios P. The AMPA anatagonist NBQX protects thalamic reticular neurons from degeneration following cardiac arrest in rats. *Brain Res.* 1995, **683**: 117–128.

81. Böttiger BW, Teschendorf P, Krumnikl JJ, *et al.* Global cerebral ischemia due to cardiocirculatory arrest in mice causes neuronal degeneration and early induction of transcription factor genes in the hippocampus. *Mol. Brain Res.* 1999, **65**: 135–142.

82. Kawahara N, Kawai K, Toyoda T, *et al.* Cardiac arrest cerebral ischemia model in mice failed to cause delayed neuronal death in the hippocampus. *Neurosci. Lett.* 2002, **322**: 91–94.

83. Mizushima H, Zhou CJ, Dohi K, *et al.* Reduced postischemic apoptosis in the hippocampus of mice deficient in interleukin-1. *J. Comp. Neurol.* 2002, **448**: 203–216.

84. Neigh GN, Kofler J, Meyers JL, *et al.* Cardiac arrest/cardiopulmonary resuscitation increases anxiety-like behavior and decreases social interaction. *J. Cereb. Blood Flow Metab.* 2004, **24**: 372–382.

85. Lowry OH, Passoneau JV, Hasselberger FX, Schulz DW. Effect of ischemia on known substrates and cofactors of the glycolytic pathway in the brain. *J. Biol. Chem.* 1964, **249**: 18–30.

86. Abe K, Yoshida S, Watson BD, *et al.* Alpha-tocopherol and ubiquinones in rat brain subjected to decapitation ischemia. *Brain Res.* 1983, **273**: 166–169.

87. Siemkowicz E, Hansen AJ. Clinical restitution following cerebral ischemia in hypo-, normo-, and hyperglycemic rats. *Acta Physiol. Scand.* 1978, **58**: 1–8

88. Siemkowicz E, Gjedde A. Post-ischemic coma in rat: effect of different pre-ischemic blood glucose levels on cerebral metabolic recovery after ischemia. *Acta Physiol. Scand.* 1980, **110**: 225–232.

89. Singh NC, Kochanek PM, Schiding JK, Melick JA, Nemoto EM. Uncoupled cerebral blood flow and metabolism after severe global ischemia in rats. *J. Cereb. Blood Flow Metab.* 1992, **12**: 802–808.

90. Kagstrom E, Smith ML, Siesjo BK. Recirculation in the rat brain following incomplete ischemia. *J. Cereb. Blood Flow Metab.* 1983, **3**: 183–192.

91. Ljunggren B, Schutz H, Siesjö BK. Changes in energy state amd acid-base parameters of the rat brain during complete compression ischemia. *Brain Res.* 1974, **73**: 277–289.

92. Yoshida S, Busto R, Watson BD, Santiso M, Ginsberg MD. Postischemic cerebral lipid peroxidation in vitro: modification by dietary vitamin E. *J. Neurochem.* 1985, **44**: 1593–1601.

93. Traystman RJ. Animal models of focal and global cerebral ischemia. *Inst. Anim. Lab. Res. J.* 2003, **44**: 85–95.

20

Rodent models of hemorrhagic stroke

FATIMA A. SEHBA AND JOSHUA B. BEDERSON

20.1 Introduction

Under normal physiological conditions, neurons do not come in direct contact with blood. The blood–brain barrier, consisting of astrocyte end feet, extracellular matrix, and endothelial cells, forms an elaborate meshwork that surrounds blood vessels and regulates the selective passage of blood elements and nutrients to the neurons. When an artery in the brain ruptures, blood envelopes cells in the surrounding tissue, upsets the blood supply provided by the injured vessel and disturbs the delicate chemical equilibrium essential for neurons to function. This is called hemorrhagic stroke and accounts for approximately 20% of all strokes.

Hemorrhagic stroke has been less investigated than ischemic stroke although it represents a significant clinical problem. Direct tissue destruction, tissue compression around the hematoma, and an inflammatory response lead to neuronal injury and neurological deficits after hemorrhagic strokes. The size of the hematoma has a direct relationship with the clinical outcome. The hematoma causes mass effect and compresses the surrounding tissue, contributing to the neuronal death at the margin of the hematoma and in the penumbral region around the hematoma. Decreasing the space-occupying effect by aspiration of the hematoma[1] and decreasing inflammation[2,3] ameliorate the neurological deficits after hemorrhagic stroke.

A number of experimental cerebral hemorrhagic models have been developed to study the mechanisms underlying cerebral bleeding and resulting pathophysiology. The knowledge gained has helped in identifying many factors that contribute to rupture of an artery or an aneurysm. This research has also helped in defining various novel pharmacological therapies that would protect against cerebral injury and improve quality of life when used within the window of therapeutic activity. In this review we will discuss some of the commonly used animal models developed to study hemorrhagic strokes.

Handbook of Experimental Neurology, ed. Turgut Tatlisumak and Marc Fisher. Published by Cambridge University Press. © Cambridge University Press 2006.

20.2 General properties of a good experimental cerebral hemorrhagic model

An ideal experimental cerebral hemorrhagic model would have the following characteristics: (1) blood deposition in a distribution consistent with the type of hemorrhage desired, (2) uniform degree of hemorrhage, (3) a mechanism of hemorrhage which closely simulates the human condition, (4) easily performed, and (5) reasonable cost.

Although a variety of species have been used to develop cerebral hemorrhagic models (see below), rats have been preferred by a majority of investigators[4–11] because they are relatively inexpensive, easy to manipulate in a laboratory setting, and have been extensively studied. Recently developed transgenic technologies in the mouse have created the need to develop mouse models of existing diseases as well.

In this chapter we will discuss the rodent models of hemorrhagic stroke. We defined the term stroke in its broad meaning so that subdural bleeding that is conventionally not considered a hemorrhagic stroke could be included in this review. The following types of hemorrhagic stroke are discussed:

(1) intracerebral hemorrhage (ICH)
(2) intraventricular hemorrhage (IVH)
(3) subarachnoid hemorrhage (SAH)
(4) subdural hemorrhage (SDH).

20.2.1 Intracerebral hemorrhage

Intracerebral hemorrhage (ICH) accounts for approximately 10% of all strokes in Western populations and a considerably higher proportion in Asian populations. Mortality rate after ICH is 32% to 55% during the first month, and recovery after ICH is poor, with most survivors experiencing some kind of neurological deficits. Approximately half of the clinical cases of ICH are associated with hypertension. The most common sites of human ICH are caudate putamen, thalamus, cerebellum, and pons. Acute neurological deficits are due to direct tissue destruction, space-occupying effect of the hematoma with potential ischemic damage to adjacent tissue, and cerebral edema. Few pharmaceutical therapies have been evaluated for treating clinical ICH; neither glycerol nor dexamethasone for edema management was found to be of any benefit.

Several animal models of ICH have been developed to identify the mechanisms underlying neuronal injury after ICH (for review see reference 12).

A number of species have been used for establishing these models including mouse,[13] rat,[4-6] cat,[14] dog,[15] rabbit,[16] baboon,[17] pig,[18] and primates.[19] Two widely used methods of producing ICH are the injection model and collagenase model. Since their introduction these models have been modified and refined over the time. Each has advantages and disadvantages that are discussed below:

(1) blood injection model
(2) bacterial collagenase injection model
(3) balloon inflation model.

Blood injection model

This model uses infusion of autologous blood into the brain parenchyma. The model is designed to mimic the natural events that occur with spontaneous ICH. Some of the important considerations for this model are site of blood injection, volume of injection, reproducibility of the hematoma size and end points.

Site of injection Although basal ganglia is the most common site of blood injection other brain regions such as left frontal lobe,[20] paramedian white matter,[21] and foreleg area of the motor cortex[22] have occasionally also been used. However, based on the most common human ICH blood distribution basal ganglia is still considered the favorite site of blood injection.[4,23]

Volume of blood The volume of blood injected varies from 10 to 100 μl.[4,24] Most investigators agree that 50 μl is best suited for injection in the rat since it provides a suitable size hematoma without risk of leakage of blood into the subdural, subarachnoid or intraventricular space.[23-25] Others have used as much as 100 μl of blood without apparent leakage; however, it has also been argued that a blood volume of 100 μl in rats causes increased intracranial pressure and complicates ICH pathophysiology due to systemic effects.[25]

Reproducibility of hematomas One of the major problems in the rat model of ICH is that size and extension of hematomas are not reproducible.[20,24] A number of reasons for irreproducibility of hematoma size in ICH model exist: (1) ventricular rupture, (2) backflow of infused blood along the needle track and (3) excess of blood volume injected. Deinsberger *et al.* introduced in 1996 a variant double-injection protocol in which desired volume of blood is injected at slow rate over a time period separated by a 7-min break.[23] A smaller volume of blood is injected first and is followed by injection of the rest of the blood after 7 min. The break allows blood to clot along the needle track so that when the rest of the blood is infused it creates a reproducible hematoma without leakage into subarachnoid space. This model has been used in rat[26] and has been adapted in other species with good results.[27,28]

Pathophysiology Like any other experiment a well-defined end point is important for an experimental model to provide useful information. Some of the end points studied using ICH injection model include cerebral hypoperfusion, edema formation, infarction volume, neuronal injury, neurodegeneration, neurological deficits and hemorrhagic transformation.[12] Intracranial pressure rises at ICH and can be related to the volume of hemorrhage.[24] Cerebral blood flow (CBF) falls markedly on the side of blood injection at ICH and may or may not return to basal levels 24 hr later.[29] The volume of tissue perfused at ischemic CBF threshold corresponds closely to the volume of hemorrhage.[24] Brain edema reaches a maximum 24 hr after ICH, remains elevated for several days,[30] and contributes to neurological deficits.[31] Thrombin and erythrocytes are the major components of hematoma responsible for edema formation after ICH.[31] Pharmacological inhibition of thrombin is associated with decreased edema formation in rats.[32] Microglia are activated within 24 hr[33] and inflammation and cell death reach a maximum 42–72 hr after ICH.[34] Apoptotic neuronal death is seen as early as at 6 hr, peaks at 3 days, and continues for at least 2 weeks after ICH.[35]

Bacterial collagenase injection model

In this model ICH is induced by injection of bacterial collagenase in striatum, which degrades collagen IV of microvascular basal lamina. Since collagen IV is the major protein of the basal lamina and is important for its integrity, its loss opens the blood–brain barrier and leads to intraparenchymal bleeding which mimics human spontaneous ICH. This model was introduced by Rosenberg and colleagues in rat in 1990[5] but has since been adapted to other species.[13,18] The simplicity of the procedure and induction of hemorrhage without significant blood leakage along the needle track makes this model very attractive. However, a major disadvantage of this model is that collagenase injection induces an inflammatory reaction that is more intense than using the autologous blood injection model or in human ICH. As a result the hematoma is degraded much earlier, possibly by inflammatory cells that migrate from the periphery.[2]

Site of injection In rat striatum remains the primary site of collagenase injection for inducing ICH. The only other site used was in the swine model in which ICH was induced by injecting collagenase in primary somatosensory cortex.[18]

Amount of bacterial collagenase used Originally Rosenberg *et al.* used 0.1–1 units of bacterial collageanse in 2 μl of saline for ICH induction and reported that 0.5 units gave expected results and 1 unit limited 24-hr survival.[5] Del Bigio modified the amount of collagenase injected to 0.14 unit in 0.7 μl saline and added 1.4 unit of heparin to this combination as a carrier and reported that this combination gave rise to a rapidly forming hematoma of uniform shape and reproducible size, minimizing the possible confounding effects due to tissue compression and "infusion edema" after solution injection.[2] Another consideration to injection/infusion technique was added by Mun-Bryce *et al.*, who placed 5 μl of saline in the tip of the injection pipette used for injecting the collagenase to ensure that base-line data were not influenced by collagenase leaking into the brain tissue environment.[18]

Reproducibility of hematomas Most investigators report that this model develops reproducible hemorrhage with volumes that correlate with the amount of collagenase injected.[5,36]

Pathophysiology Intrastriatal bleeding is seen 10 min after collagenase infusion and increases with time and develops into full hematoma 4–24 hr later.[5] Cerebral edema develops within 4 hr and is resolved 48 hr later.[5] Behavioral deficits are observed 4 hr after collagenase injection and begin to improve 48 hr later.[5] A pronounced inflammatory response, with neutrophil infiltration around the hematoma, is observed within 12 hr of onset of ICH and is followed by macrophage infiltration 1–2 days later.[2] Fucoidan, which inhibits neutrophil extravasation, reduces inflammation after ICH.[3] Development of brain injury after ICH in part involves a role of free radicals and their inhibition can improve the outcome of ICH.[37] Neuronal death through apoptosis that can be inhibited by caspase-3 inhibition is seen within 24 hr after ICH.[38]

Balloon inflation model

Introduced in 1987 by Sinar *et al.*, this is a pure mechanical model of ICH[6] which mimics the space-occupying effect of a hematoma and its removal and studies the pathophysiology of these events. A microballoon mounted on a 25-gauge blunted needle is inserted into caudate to a depth of 5.5 mm and inflated to a 50 μl volume over a period of 20 s with a radiopaque contrast medium. Inflation is confirmed by X-ray fluoroscopy and the balloon is deflated 10 min later.[6] Since its introduction the balloon model has been modified for the volume and duration of inflation.[4,39] Although rat remains the primary species for this model, cats have also been used.[40]

Reproducibility Since inflation of balloon is performed mechanically the lesion produced is reproducible. Moreover, reproducibility of results and the extent of CBF fall and ischemia in this model can be controlled by the volume and the duration of balloon inflation.

Pathophysiology At balloon inflation, CBF falls, and it continues to fall for the next 4 hr regardless of the time of balloon deflation. Ischemia develops 4 hr after balloon inflation. Mendelow and Valdes *et al.*, in two separate studies, have used this model to show that early deflation of the balloon (or removal of a mass lesion) limits the intensity of ischemic brain injury.[4,39] Cell death is found in the mass lesion 6–24 hr after deflation and involves apoptosis.[41] Basic fibroblast growth factor injected locally into the cavity left by balloon deflation protects against neuronal injury.[42]

20.2.2 Intraventricular hemorrhage

Intraventricular hemorrhage (IVH) is a major complication of preterm birth and spontaneous ICH that independently contributes to poor outcome and disability. Extensive research in understanding IVH during the last 20 years has decreased the number of infants who would develop IVH from 35–50% to around 15%.[10,43] However, this number will rise with the increase in survival of premature infants in developed countries. In adults the most common causes of IVH include hypertensive hemorrhage, trauma, and ruptured aneurysm.

IVH accounts for 3–10% of total hemorrhagic strokes and can be divided into primary and secondary subtypes.[44] Primary IVH (30% of total) is confined to the ventricles. Secondary IVH (70% of total) represents extension of intracerebral or subarachnoid hemorrhages.

The major factor contributing to IVH in preterm infants is developmental anatomy at the end of the second trimester and the pathophysiology associated with preterm birth.[43] Other causes of IVH include hypoxia, hypercarbia, alkali therapy, arterial hypotension and hypertension, loss of autoregulation, alveolar rupture, volume expansion, and dehydration of the brain. Factors leading to poor clinical outcome after IVH include obstruction of flow of cerebrospinal fluid due to intraventricular blood clots, ventricular dilation, increased intra-cranial pressure, and hydrocephalous. A number of treatment regimens have been tested both antenatally and postnatally to prevent IVH. There is some indication that corticosteroid given before preterm delivery reduces IVH and may decrease disability.[45] Indomethacin reduces mortality but there is little indication on its ability to decrease disability.[46] Intraventricular fibrinolysis to prevent or inhibit post-hemorrhagic ventricular dilatation is recommended for adults[47] but not for preterm infants after IVH.[48]

Two classes of animal models of IVH have been developed to study this clinical problem and are explained below:

(1) hemodynamic IVH models
(2) injection model.

Hemodynamic IVH models

Goddard and colleagues defined a number of experimental techniques to induce IVH by creating hemodynamic changes that affect CBF and predispose animals to hemorrhage.[49–51] In these models IVH is induced by making animals hypertensive by infusion of phenylephrine,[49] or hypotensive by intra-peritoneal injection of 50% glycerol,[51] by inducing respiratory stress such as hypercapnia,[50] or by inducing hypovolemic hypotension followed by volume re-expansion.[52] The most extensively used IVH model is the hemorrhagic hypotension/volume re-expansion model, introduced in 1981 and since adapted and extensively used by others.[53,54] In this model IVH is induced by rapid venous (femoral vein) withdrawal of 20–25% of the animal's estimated blood volume in a heparinized syringe until mean arterial blood pressure falls to 50% of its basal value; 5 min later the blood is reinfused along with 1 mg of protaminesulfate for each 100 units of heparin.[55]

Since a large number of IVH cases are observed in newborn or preterm infants, these hemodynamic models use newborn or preterm animals to produce IVH.[49–51,53] Rabbits and beagle puppy are considered most suitable animals to study IVH as temporal development of their brain and germinal matrix prior to birth parallels that of infants and hence, as with infants, predisposes them to developing spontaneous germinal matrix and intraventricular hemorrhage.[51,53,56]

Reproducibility Most hemodynamic models rely on spontaneous induction of IVH and suffer from a low incident of IVH.[49,50] The hemorrhagic hypotension/volume re-expansion model is the most reliable among hemodynamic models of IVH in which up to 75–100% of the animals develop IVH.[52,53]

Pathophysiology In hypotension/re-expansion model of IVH systemic blood pressure falls during hypotension and rises to a peak following volume re-expansion.[53] Cerebral blood flow is maintained or is increased during hypertension in brain and elevates significantly after volume re-expansion.[55,57] Ment and colleagues have used this model extensively to examine mechanisms underlying CBF changes and ischemia after IVH.[57,58] They found that prostaglandin E_2 levels increased significantly in response to hemorrhagic hypotensive insult[57] and that prior to of ethamsylate or indomethacin protects against decreases in CBF, and can reduce mortality.[59]

Injection model of IVH

As the name indicates this model is based on injection of autologous blood into lateral ventricles of adults rats or rat pups using stereotaxic co-ordinates.[9,10] Intraventricular injection of artificial cerebrospinal fluid or saline is used for sham controls.

Volume of blood In the adult rat model of IVH 30 µl of blood made viscous by 1–3-min incubation at 25 °C was infused at a rate of 4 µl/min.[9] In rat pups IVH models 80 µl blood was injected over 10 min.[9] Once again rat is the species commonly used for studying IVH.[9,10]

Reproducibility This can be maintained by careful selection of blood injection volume (see above). Use of large volumes of blood can cause a leak around the needle tract and subdural accumulation.[10]

Pathophysiology Cerebral blood flow decreases immediately after IVH induction and is still decreased 24 hr later.[9] Wang *et al.* have shown that tissue plasminogen activator administered after IVH can ameliorate reductions in CBF without any effect on ventricular dilation.[9] Intracranial pressure increases at injection and returns to basal levels soon after. Cherian *et al.* showed that ventricular dilation after IVH is accompanied by loss of ependyma, astrocytic gliosis, variable rarefaction of the periventricular white matter, and in some cases edema.[10]

20.2.3 Subarachnoid hemorrhage

Aneurysmal subarachnoid hemorrhage (SAH) accounts for 5–10% of yearly stroke cases[60] and kills approximately 50% of patients within 30 days, with two-thirds of the deaths occurring within 48 hr.[61] Acute brain injury after SAH is primarily ischemic in nature and is associated with major decreases in CBF. The causes of acutely decreased CBF after SAH involve not only reductions in cerebral perfusion pressure upon aneurysm rupture[62,63] but a number of additional interrelated processes including release of vasoactive substances during platelet aggregation,[64] unopposed sympathetic activity,[65] alterations in the NO/NOS pathways,[66–68] and lipid peroxidation[69] (for review see reference 70). Elucidation of these processes could lead to new treatment paradigms for acute cerebral ischemia, which is the most important determinant of outcome after SAH.

A variety of animal models of SAH have been developed to investigate the mechanisms of brain injury (see below). Several species have been employed including monkeys,[71] baboons,[72] pigs,[73] rabbits,[74] dogs,[75] cats,[76] rats,[77] and mice.[78] We have reviewed advantages and disadvantages of the major variations.[79] The most commonly used experimental models of SAH are described below:

(1) endovascular filament model of SAH
(2) blood injection model.

Endovascular filament model of SAH

This model exerts a direct puncture of the basilar artery using a tungsten wire to puncture the basilar artery via a transclival approach.[77,80] More recently, we have used an endovascular filament to perforate the intracranial internal carotid artery bifurcation,[7] and others have published a similar technical approach.[8] This non-craniotomy model, in theory, more closely resembles the mechanism of acute aneurysmal rupture. Since its development this model has extensively been used to investigate mechanisms underlying both acute and chronic pathophysiology of SAH. This technique has been adapted to mouse but as the mouse version lacks continuous physiological recording which makes this technique extremely attractive it has lesser applicability.[81,82] Nevertheless, this endovascular model has been used to determine importance of certain genes and their products using transgenic mice.[81,82]

Reproducibility A major drawback of this model is the lack of effective control over the intensity of hemorrhage. Although in clinical settings increased intracranial pressure after rupture of an aneurysm varies widely between patients,[83] in the laboratory such deviations between animals introduce statistical noise. Veelken *et al.* tried occluding the ipsilateral common carotid artery or leaving the endovascular filament in situ to control SAH intensity.[8] These maneuvers hinder normal arterial perfusion superimposing regional ischemia on the SAH model. Recently we manipulated SAH severity by varying the size of the endovascular filament used to perforate the internal carotid artery bifurcation.[79] This study demonstrated that filament size is proportionate to SAH intensity. For a review of experimental models of cerebral vasospasm see reference 84.

Pathophysiology An immediate increase in intracranial pressure and fall in CBF is observed at SAH induction.[7,85-88] Peak intracranial pressure values are related primarily to the amount of blood released into the subarachnoid space and by the rate of hemorrhage.[7,65,79,85] In our studies using the rat, intracranial pressure peaks approximately 60 s after SAH onset and returns to values near or above base-line.[7] Cerebral blood flow decreases immediately at the onset of SAH while intracranial pressure is rising, and continues to drop as it returns towards base-line, with CBF reaching a nadir approximately 3 min after SAH onset. After reaching its nadir, CBF returns towards base-line and 60 min later settles at a value that can predict the outcome of SAH 24 hr later.[85] We noted that reductions of CBF to < 40% of base-line 60 min after SAH predict a 100% mortality rate at 24 hr while 81% of animals survive when CBF was >40% 60 min after SAH.[85] We have previously used the rat endovasuclar model to document acute changes in the NO pathway after SAH.[66-68] Others have used it for investigating mechanisms contributing to cerebral injury after SAH as well as to test the effectiveness of various therapies against these mechanisms.[89-91,92]

Blood injection model

In this model blood is introduced into the subarachnoid space to simulate human SAH. In addition to fresh blood, blood products and blood clots have also been used for injection.[93,94] Since its introduction, this model has been adapted and modified in a number of ways to give better control over the intensity and reproducibility of SAH. These variations include double injection, in which the same volume of blood is injected twice through the same injection site 24 or 48 hr apart,[95,96] pressure infusion, in which a preselected volume of blood is infused at a preselected pressure, and more commonly used volume infusion, in which preselected blood is injected at an arbitrary pressure.[78,97] Because of its simplicity, this technique which was originally developed in rats has been adapted into the mouse to take advantage of transgenic technology.[98,99]

The advantages that the blood injection model offers over the endovascular model are investigator control of hemorrhage intensity and the use of saline or artificial cerebrospinal fluid injection as a positive control. A disadvantage of the injection technique is that blood is dispersed primarily dorsally in the intracranial space and into the spinal canal, which is less representative of aneurysmal rupture.

Site of injection The most common site of blood injection is cisterna magna, which is approached either through the atlanto-occipital membrane[100] or transoccipitally.[101] Other sites used include the prechiasmatic cistern[97] or next to an intracranial[102] or extracranial artery.[103,104]

Volume of blood A number of different volumes of autologous blood have been tested for injection into mouse or rat cisterna magna for producing consistent SAH. A volume of 50–60 µl is found to be most appropriate in the mouse[78] and 200–300 µl autologous blood in the rat[97,105] without a risk of leakage from the injection site.

Reproducibility In this model reproducibility can be ensured in two ways: (1) controlling for the volume of the blood injection (see above) and (2) immediate placement of animals in a head-down (75° vertical) position for 10 min after blood injection to facilitate the diffusion of injected blood in the basal cisterns and discourage its leakage.

Pathophysiology Similar hemodynamic changes (increased intracranial pressure and fall in CBF) occur upon injection of blood in the cisterna magna are the same as in the endovascular model of SAH. The hemorrhages produced using blood injection models are however of lesser intensity as compared to those of the endovascular model.[96,105] Nevertheless, the ability to have a proper sham-operated control and investigator control on hemorrhage intensity has made this model quite popular and extensively used. It has been used to examine upregulation of molecular markers for neuronal stress response in reaction to SAH[78] and to establish apoptotic neuronal death within 24 hr after experimental SAH.[98] A number of knockout mice have also been used to study importance of genes and their products in pathophysiology of SAH.[98,99]

20.2.4 Subdural hemorrhage

Subdural hemorrhages (SDH) accounts for a majority of deaths in head injury patients. Both acute SDH (ASDH) and chronic SDH (CSDH) occur. ASDH occurs in young and old alike and can result from direct laceration of cortical arteries and veins with penetrating injuries lacerating the brain, or large contusions upon closed head injury causing subdural bleeding or most commonly occurring tearing of veins that bridge the subdural space.[106] The occurrence of ASDH does not necessarily require a direct head injury as strain-rate acceleration due to brisk head movements, or more commonly violent shaking of infants, can lead to it.[106] CSDH is a common disease of the elderly with high incidence in persons older than 65 years of age. The risk factors of CSDH include alcoholism, concomitant diseases such as kidney or liver dysfunction, hemodialysis, diabetes, dementia, coagulopathy, or use of anti-coagulants or platelet aggregation inhibitors.

A number of animal models for studying ASDH and CSDH have been established and are described below. Recently more attention has been given to studying acute SDH as opposed to chronic SDH.

ASDH models include the following:

(1) Blood injection model
(2) Non-missile head injury model.

Blood injection model

In this model blood is placed over the cerebral convexity. The two main variations of this model are the open cranium and the closed cranium models.[107] As the name indicates open cranium is a craniotomy model in which the dura is opened and fresh autologous blood is placed on the cortical surface.[107–110] In parietal craniotomy closed cranium model blood is placed on the cortex through a cranial window that is made leaving the dura intact.[107] Originally established in the rat, the craniotomy model is widely used and has been adapted to a number of other species including mice,[109] beagle dogs,[110] and pigs.[111] An advantage of this model is that it allows the use of sham-operated, saline, or artificial cerebrospinal fluid injected animals as true controls.

Site of blood injection A number of stereotaxic co-ordinates have been used in rats to create ASDH. The most common of these remain the ones originally used by Miller *et al.*: 2 mm left of the sagittal suture and 1 mm posterior to the coronal suture.[108] Other lesser commonly used stereotaxic coordinates for creating ASDH in rat are: 1 mm caudal and 2.8 mm lateral to bregma,[112] and 4.5 mm posterior to bregma and 3.0 mm lateral from the midline.[113] In mouse parietal region 2 mm from sagittal suture and 1 mm anterior to the lambdoid suture is used for creating ASDH.[109]

Volume of blood The most commonly used volume of non-heparanized fresh venous autologous blood for ASDH creation in rat is 400 μl injected slowly over a period of 7–8 min.[108] However, 100–300 μl volume has also been used in a rat.[112,114] In mouse 30–50 μl blood is tested and 20 μl is found to be optimum for creating an adequate size ASDH without excessive mortality.[109]

Reproducibility Besides the volume of blood injection the speed of its delivery seems to be an important factor in getting consistent ASDH. Miller *et al.* have demonstrated that a slow injection (over a period of 5–7 min) would create a consistent ASDH and that a fast injection of the same amount of blood would lead to spreading into the basal cisterns and convexities of both ipsilateral cerebral and cerebellar hemispheres.[108] In mouse injection of 20 μl blood over 1 min creates reproducible ASDH.

Pathophysiology Intracranial pressure rises at ASDH and declines to values above base-line 1 hr later.[108] Cerebral blood flow falls in the ipsilateral hemisphere but this reduction is confined to the cerebral cortex and not found in subcortical regions.[115] The greatest CBF reductions occur in the cortical regions immediately underlying the hematoma.[115] A shift of glycolysis to anaerobic and increase in glutamate occur after ASDH[116,117] and may contribute to ischemic injury. Occlusion of local microvessels occurs and presence of red blood cells and platelets in the cortical vessels beneath ASDH are noted.[115] Electron microscopy studies show swelling of astrocytes leading to massive perivascular spaces.[115] Infarction develops in the cortical area underlying the hematoma.[115] A number of agents have been tested for their neuroprotective effects against ischemic injury after ASDH.[112,118,119]

Subdural balloon model

In this lesser craniotomy model a metallic cylinder containing a rubber stopper and a collapsed rubber balloon is placed subdurally and a controlled bleeding from the aorta into the balloon is performed to simulate SDH. This model was originally developed in pigs by Zwetnow and colleagues,[111] and has been adapted to dogs.[110]

Chronic SDH

Research in CSDH at present has progressed from animals to clinics such that most if not all recent studies examining pathophysiology of CSDH are performed using human tissues rather than animal models of CSDH. Nevertheless a number of experimental models exist and were established during the 1970s and 1980s to simulate human CSDH and to study changes in composition and morphology of hematoma as a function of time.[120–122] The majority of these models used dogs, cats, or primates and created CSDH by blood inoculation into the subdural or subcutaneous space. The main difference between the blood-injected models of ASDH and CSDH is the frequent use of clotted rather than fresh blood for the creation of CSDH and its examination at times later than those used for ASDH.

An exception to the blood/clot injection model of CSDH is the more recently developed model of spontaneous CSDH.[11] This model uses intraperitoneal injection of 6-aminonicotinamide (6AN), a niacin antagonist to create CSDH over the next 20 days in 5-day-old mice by inhibiting activities of nicotinamide adenine dinucleotide phosphate (NADP)-dependent enzymes.[11,123] Aikawa *et al.* have used this model to study the true location and microscopic and ultrastructural composition of subdural hematoma.[11,123]

20.3 Summary

Most hemorrhagic stroke models were developed during the span of 20–25 years, starting in the 1970s. A number of species were used to study hemorrhagic stroke; however, rodents, especially the rat, remained the species of choice due to the ease of handling and availability. Research using the rat models of hemorrhagic strokes has been productive in elucidating the mechanisms and pathways underlying the pathophysiology of ischemic cerebral injury. However, the recent advances in transgenic technology that allow us to investigate the role of specific genes and their products in a disease state in the mouse makes urgent the task of adapting existing experimental techniques to the mouse. This need has already been recognized in other disease state models including cerebral ischemia models, and a number of transgenic mice that overexpress or lack genes whose products are considered important in cerebral ischemic injury have been studied. Moreover, the list of transgenic mice is growing daily. Adapting rat-based hemorrhagic stroke techniques to the mouse will allow us to take advantage of advances and may prove to be an important step towards the development of therapeutic interventions against cerebral injury following these catastrophes.

References

1. Altumbabic M, Peeling J, Del Bigio MR. Intracerebral hemorrhage in the rat: effects of hematoma aspiration. *Stroke* 1998, **29**: 1917–1922; discussion 1922–1923.
2. Del Bigio MR, Yan HJ, Buist R, Peeling J. Experimental intracerebral hemorrhage in rats: magnetic resonance imaging and histopathological correlates. *Stroke* 1996, **27**: 2312–2319; discussion 2319–2320.
3. Del Bigio MR, Yan HJ, Campbell TM, Peeling J. Effect of fucoidan treatment on collagenase-induced intracerebral hemorrhage in rats. *Neurol Res.* 1999, **21**: 415–419.

4. Mendelow AD. Mechanisms of ischemic brain damage with intracerebral hemorrhage. *Stroke* 1993, **24**: 1115–1117; discussion 1118–1119.
5. Rosenberg GA, Mun-Bryce S, Wesley M, Kornfeld M. Collagenase-induced intracerebral hemorrhage in rats. *Stroke* 1990, **21**: 801–807.
6. Sinar EJ, Mendelow AD, Graham DI, Teasdale GM. Experimental intracerebral hemorrhage: effects of a temporary mass lesion. *J. Neurosurg.* 1987, **66**: 568–576.
7. Bederson JB, Germano IM, Guarino L. Cortical blood flow and cerebral perfusion pressure in a new noncraniotomy model of subarachnoid hemorrhage in the rat. *Stroke* 1995, **26**: 1086–1091.
8. Veelken JA, Laing RJ, Jakubowski J. The Sheffield model of subarachnoid hemorrhage in rats. *Stroke* 1995, **26**: 1279–1283; discussion 1284.
9. Wang YC, Lin CW, Shen CC, Lai SC, Kuo JS. Tissue plasminogen activator for the treatment of intraventricular hematoma: the dose–effect relationship. *J. Neurol. Sci.* 2002, **202**: 35–41.
10. Cherian SS, Love S, Silver IA, *et al.* Posthemorrhagic ventricular dilation in the neonate: development and characterization of a rat model. *J. Neuropathol. Exp. Neurol.* 2003, **62**: 292–303.
11. Aikawa H, Suzuki K. Experimental chronic subdural hematoma in mice: gross morphology and light microscopic observations. *J. Neurosurg.* 1987, **67**: 710–716.
12. Andaluz N, Zuccarello M, Wagner KR. Experimental animal models of intracerebral hemorrhage. *Neurosurg. Clin. N. Am.* 2002, **13**: 385–393.
13. Clark W, Gunion-Rinker L, Lessov N, Hazel K. Citicoline treatment for experimental intracerebral hemorrhage in mice. *Stroke* 1998, **29**: 2136–2140.
14. Kobari M, Gotoh F, Tomita M, *et al.* Bilateral hemispheric reduction of cerebral blood volume and blood flow immediately after experimental cerebral hemorrhage in cats. *Stroke* 1988, **19**: 991–996.
15. Coulter DM, Gooch WM. Falling intracranial pressure: an important element in the genesis of intracranial hemorrhage in the beagle puppy. *Biol. Neonate* 1993, **63**: 316–326.
16. Kaufman HH, Pruessner JL, Bernstein DP, *et al.* A rabbit model of intracerebral hematoma. *Acta Neuropathol. (Berlin)* 1985, **65**: 318–321.
17. Del Zoppo GJ, Copeland BR, Waltz TA, *et al.* The beneficial effect of intracarotid urokinase on acute stroke in a baboon model. *Stroke* 1986, **17**: 638–643.
18. Mun-Bryce S, Wilkerson AC, Papuashvili N, Okada YC. Recurring episodes of spreading depression are spontaneously elicited by an intracerebral hemorrhage in the swine. *Brain Res.* 2001, **888**: 248–255.
19. Bullock R, Brock-Utne J, van Dellen J, Blake G. Intracerebral hemorrhage in a primate model: effect on regional cerebral blood flow. *Surg. Neurol.* 1988, **29**: 101–107.
20. Masuda T, Dohrmann GJ, Kwaan HC, Erickson RK, Wollman RL. Fibrinolytic activity in experimental intracerebral hematoma. *J. Neurosurg.* 1988, **68**: 274–278.
21. Cossu M, Dorcaratto A, Pau A, *et al.* Changes in infratentorial blood flow following experimental cerebellar haemorrhage: a preliminary report. *Ital. J. Neurol. Sci.* 1991, **12**: 69–73.
22. Kleiser B, Van Reempts J, Van Deuren B, *et al.* Favourable effect of flunarizine on the recovery from hemiparesis in rats with intracerebral hematomas. *Neurosci. Lett.* 1989, **103**: 225–228.
23. Deinsberger W, Vogel J, Kuschinsky W, Auer LM, Boker DK. Experimental intracerebral hemorrhage: description of a double injection model in rats. *Neurol. Res.* 1996, **18**: 475–477.

24. Nath FP, Jenkins A, Mendelow AD, Graham DI, Teasdale GM. Early hemodynamic changes in experimental intracerebral hemorrhage. *J. Neurosurg.* 1986, **65**: 697–703.

25. Kingman TA, Mendelow AD, Graham DI, Teasdale GM. Experimental intracerebral mass: description of model, intracranial pressure changes and neuropathology. *J. Neuropathol. Exp. Neurol.* 1988, **47**: 128–137.

26. Hickenbottom SL, Grotta JC, Strong R, Denner LA, Aronowski J. Nuclear factor-kappa B and cell death after experimental intracerebral hemorrhage in rats. *Stroke* 1999, **30**: 2472–2477; discussion 2477–2478.

27. Belayev L, Saul I, Curbelo K, *et al.* Experimental intracerebral hemorrhage in the mouse: histological, behavioral, and hemodynamic characterization of a double-injection model. *Stroke* 2003, **34**: 2221–2227.

28. Thiex R, Kuker W, Muller HD, *et al.* The long-term effect of recombinant tissue-plasminogen-activator (rt-PA) on edema formation in a large-animal model of intracerebral hemorrhage. *Neurol. Res.* 2003, **25**: 254–262.

29. Ropper AH, Zervas NT. Cerebral blood flow after experimental basal ganglia hemorrhage. *Ann. Neurol.* 1982, **11**: 266–271.

30. Yang GY, Betz AL, Chenevert TL, Brunberg JA, Hoff JT. Experimental intracerebral hemorrhage: relationship between brain edema, blood flow, and blood–brain barrier permeability in rats. *J. Neurosurg.* 1994, **81**: 93–102.

31. Hua Y, Keep RF, Schallert T, Hoff JT, Xi G. A thrombin inhibitor reduces brain edema, glioma mass and neurological deficits in a rat glioma model. *Acta Neurochir. (Suppl.)* 2003, **86**: 503–506.

32. Kitaoka T, Hua Y, Xi G, *et al.* Effect of delayed argatroban treatment on intracerebral hemorrhage-induced edema in the rat. *Acta Neurochir. (Suppl.)* 2003, **86**: 457–461.

33. Gong C, Hoff JT, Keep RF. Acute inflammatory reaction following experimental intracerebral hemorrhage in rat. *Brain Res.* 2000, **871**: 57–65.

34. Xue M, Del Bigio MR. Intracerebral injection of autologous whole blood in rats: time course of inflammation and cell death. *Neurosci. Lett.* 2000, **283**: 230–232.

35. Gong C, Boulis N, Qian J, *et al.* Intracerebral hemorrhage-induced neuronal death. *Neurosurgery* 2001, **48**: 875–882; discussion 882–883.

36. Terai K, Suzuki M, Sasamata M, Miyata K. Amount of bleeding and hematoma size in the collagenase-induced intracerebral hemorrhage rat model. *Neurochem. Res.* 2003, **28**: 779–785.

37. Peeling J, Yan HJ, Chen SG, Campbell M, Del Bigio MR. Protective effects of free radical inhibitors in intracerebral hemorrhage in rat. *Brain Res.* 1998, **795**: 63–70.

38. Matsushita K, Meng W, Wang X, *et al.* Evidence for apoptosis after intercerebral hemorrhage in rat striatum. *J. Cereb. Blood Flow Metab.* 2000, **20**: 396–404.

39. Lopez Valdes E, Hernandez Lain A, Calandre L, *et al.* Time window for clinical effectiveness of mass evacuation in a rat balloon model mimicking an intraparenchymatous hematoma. *J. Neurol. Sci.* 2000, **174**: 40–46.

40. Ichimi K, Kuchiwaki H, Inao S, Shibayama M, Yoshida J. Responses of cerebral blood flow regulation to activation of the primary somatosensory cortex during electrical stimulation of the forearm. *Acta Neurochir. (Suppl.)* 1997, **70**: 291–292.

41. Nakashima K, Yamashita K, Uesugi S, Ito H. Temporal and spatial profile of apoptotic cell death in transient intracerebral mass lesion of the rat. *J. Neurotrauma* 1999, **16**: 143–151.

42. Kawakami N, Kashiwagi S, Kitahara T, Yamashita T, Ito H. Effect of local administration of basic fibroblast growth factor against neuronal damage caused by transient intracerebral mass lesion in rats. *Brain Res.* 1995, **697**: 104–111.

43. Whitelaw A. Intraventricular haemorrhage and posthaemorrhagic hydrocephalus: pathogenesis, prevention and future interventions. *Semin. Neonatol.* 2001, **6**: 135–146.

44. Engelhard HH, Andrews CO, Slavin KV, Charbel FT. Current management of intraventricular hemorrhage. *Surg. Neurol.* 2003, **60**: 15–21; discussion 21–22.

45. van der Heide-Jalving M, Kamphuis PJ, van der Laan MJ, *et al.* Short- and long-term effects of neonatal glucocorticoid therapy: is hydrocortisone an alternative to dexamethasone? *Acta Paediatr.* 2003, **92**: 827–835.

46. Pleacher MD, Vohr BR, Katz KH, Ment LR, Allan WC. An evidence-based approach to predicting low IQ in very preterm infants from the neurological examination: outcome data from the indomethacin Indomethacin Intraventricular Hemorrhage Prevention Trial. *Pediatrics* 2004, **113**: 416–419.

47. Naff NJ, Williams MA, Rigamonti D, Keyl PM, Hanley DF. Blood clot resolution in human cerebrospinal fluid: evidence of first-order kinetics. *Neurosurgery* 2001, **49**: 614–619; discussion 619–621.

48. Yapicioglu H, Narli N, Satar M, Soyupak S, Altunbasak S. Intraventricular streptokinase for the treatment of posthaemorrhagic hydrocephalus of preterm. *J. Clin. Neurosci.* 2003, **10**: 297–299.

49. Goddard J, Lewis RM, Armstrong DL, Zeller RS. Moderate, rapidly induced hypertension as a cause of intraventricular hemorrhage in the newborn beagle model. *J. Pediatr.* 1980, **96**: 1057–1060.

50. Goddard J, Lewis RM, Alcala H, Zeller RS. Intraventricular hemorrhage: an animal model. *Biol. Neonate* 1980, **37**: 39–52.

51. Conner ES, Lorenzo AV, Welch K, Dorval B. The role of intracranial hypotension in neonatal intraventricular hemorrhage. *J. Neurosurg.* 1982, **58**: 204–209.

52. Goddard J, Lewis RM, Armstrong DL, Zeller RS. Intraventricular and subependymal cell plate hemorrhages following hypovolemic hypotension and volume expansion in the newborn beagle: relationship to hemodynamic changes. *Ann Neurol. (Abstract)* 1980, **8**: 224.

53. Ment LR, Stewart WB, Duncan CC, Lambrecht R. Beagle puppy model of intraventricular hemorrhage. *J. Neurosurg.* 1982, **57**: 219–223.

54. Pasternak JF, Groothuis DR, Fischer JM, Fischer DP. Regional cerebral blood flow in the beagle puppy model of neonatal intraventricular hemorrhage: studies during systemic hypertension. *Neurology* 1983, **33**: 559–566.

55. Goddard J, Armstrong DL, Michael L. Regional cerebral blood flow in the beagle model of intraventricular hemorrhage during volume expansion following acute hemorrhagic hypotension. *Ann Neurol. (Abstract)* 1981, **10**: 305.

56. Lorenzo AV, Welch K, Conner S. Spontaneous germinal matrix and intraventricular hemorrhage in prematurely born rabbits. *J. Neurosurg.* 1982, **56**: 404–410.

57. Ment LR, Stewart WB, Duncan CC, *et al.* Beagle puppy model of perinatal cerebral infarction: acute changes in cerebral blood flow and metabolism during hemorrhagic hypotension. *J. Neurosurg.* 1985, **63**: 441–447.

58. Ment LR, Stewart WB, Duncan CC. Beagle puppy model of intraventricular hemorrhage: effect of superoxide dismutase on cerebral blood flow and prostaglandins. *J. Neurosurg.* 1985, **62**: 563–569.

59. Ment LR, Stewart WB, Duncan CC. Beagle puppy model of intraventricular hemorrhage: ethamsylate studies. *Prostaglandins* 1984, **27**: 245–256.

60. Le Roux PD, Winn HR. Management of the ruptured aneurysm. *Neurosurg. Clin. N. Am.* 1998, **9**: 525–540.

61. Broderick JP, Brott TG, Duldner JE, Tomsick T, Leach A. Initial and recurrent bleeding are the major causes of death following subarachnoid hemorrhage. *Stroke* 1994, **25**: 1342–1347.

62. Fisher CM. Clinical syndromes in cerebral thrombosis, hypertensive hemorrhage, and ruptured saccular aneurysm. *Clin. Neurosurg.* 1975, **22**: 117–147.

63. Nornes H. The role of intracranial pressure in the arrest of hemorrhage in patients with ruptured intracranial aneurysm. *J. Neurosurg.* 1973, **39**: 226–234.

64. Clower BR, Yoshioka J, Honma T, Smith R. Blood platelets and early intimal changes in cerebral arteries following experimental subarachnoid hemorrhage. In Wilkins RL (ed.) *Cerebral Vasospasm*. New York: Ravens Press, 1988, pp. 335–341.

65. Furuichi S, Endo S, Haji A, *et al.* Related changes in sympathetic activity, cerebral blood flow and intracranial pressure, and effect of an alpha-blocker in experimental subarachnoid haemorrhage. *Acta Neurochir.* 1999, **141**: 415–423.

66. Sehba FA, Ding WH, Chereshnev I, Bederson JB. Effects of *S*-nitrosoglutathione on acute vasoconstriction and glutamate release after subarachnoid hemorrhage. *Stroke* 1999, **30**: 1955–1961.

67. Sehba FA, Schwartz AY, Chereshnev I, Bederson JB. Acute decrease in cerebral nitric oxide levels after subarachnoid hemorrhage. *J Cereb. Blood Flow Metab.* 2000, **20**: 604–611.

68. Schwartz AY, Sehba FA, Bederson JB. Decreased nitric oxide availability contributes to acute cerebral ischemia after subarachnoid hemorrhage. *Neurosurgery* 2000, **47**: 208–214; discussion 214–215.

69. Hall ED, Travis MA. Effects of the nonglucocorticoid 21-aminosteroid U74006 F on acute cerebral hypoperfusion following experimental subarachnoid hemorrhage. *Exp. Neurol.* 1988, **102**: 244–248.

70. Sehba FA, Bederson JB. Mechanisms of injury after acute subarachnoid hemorrhage (SAH). *Proceedings of the 17th Spasm Symposium, Osaka* 2001, **17**: 4–23.

71. Echlin FA. Spasm of basilar and vertebral arteries caused by experimental subarachnoid hemorrhage. *J. Neurosurg.* 1965, **23**: 1–11.

72. Dorsch N, Branston NM, Symon L, Jakubowski J. Intracranial pressure changes following primate subarachnoid haemorrhage. *Neurol. Res.* 1989, **11**: 201–204.

73. Mayberg MR, Okada T, Bark DH. The significance of morphological changes in cerebral arteries after subarachnoid hemorrhage. *J. Neurosurg.* 1990, **72**: 626–633.

74. Johshita H, Kassell NF, Sasaki T. Blood–brain barrier disturbance following subarachnoid hemorrhage in rabbits. *Stroke* 1990, **21**: 1051–1058.

75. Lougheed WM, Tom M. A method of introducing blood into the subarachnoid space in the region of the circle of Willis in dogs. *J. Neurosurgery* 1961, **4**: 329–337.

76. Kapp J, Mahaley MS, Odom GL. Cerebral arterial spasm. I. Evaluation of experimental variables affecting the diameter of the exposed basilar artery. *J. Neurosurg.* 1968, **29**: 331–338.

77. Barry KJ, Gogjian MA, Stein BM. Small animal model for investigation of subarachnoid hemorrhage and cerebral vasospasm. *Stroke* 1979, **10**: 538–541.

78. Matz PG, Copin JC, Chan PH. Cell death after exposure to subarachnoid hemolysate correlates inversely with expression of CuZn-superoxide dismutase. *Stroke* 2000, **31**: 2450–2459.

79. Schwartz AY, Masago A, Sehba FA, Bederson JB. Experimental models of subarachnoid hemorrhage in the rat: a refinement of the endovascular filament model. *J. Neurosci. Methods* 2000, **96**: 161–167.

80. Kader A, Krauss WE, Onesti ST, Elliott JP, Solomon RA. Chronic cerebral blood flow changes following experimental subarachnoid hemorrhage in rats. *Stroke* 1990, **21**: 577–581.

81. Parra A, McGirt MJ, Sheng H, *et al.* Mouse model of subarachnoid hemorrhage associated cerebral vasospasm: methodological analysis. *Neurol. Res.* 2002, **24**: 510–516.

82. Kamii H, Kato I, Kinouchi H, *et al.* Amelioration of vasospasm after subarachnoid hemorrhage in transgenic mice overexpressing CuZn-superoxide dismutase. *Stroke* 1999, **30**: 867–871; discussion 872.

83. Nornes H, Magnaes B. Intracranial pressure in patients with ruptured saccular aneurysm. *J. Neurosurg.* 1972, **36**: 537–547.

84. Megyesi JF, Vollrath B, Cook DA, Findlay JM. In vivo animal models of cerebral vasospasm: a review. *Neurosurgery* 2000, **46**: 448–460; discussion 460–461.

85. Bederson JB, Levy AL, Ding WH, *et al.* Acute vasoconstriction after subarachnoid hemorrhage. *Neurosurgery* 1998, **42**: 352–360.

86. Kamiya K, Kuyama H, Symon L. An experimental study of the acute stage of subarachnoid hemorrhage. *J. Neurosurg.* 1983, **59**: 917–924.

87. Rasmussen G, Hauerberg J, Waldemar G, Gjerris F, Juhler M. Cerebral blood flow autoregulation in experimental subarachnoid haemorrhage in rat. *Acta Neurochir.* 1992, **119**: 128–133.

88. Travis MA, Hall ED. The effects of chronic two-fold dietary vitamin E supplementation on subarachnoid hemorrhage-induced brain hypoperfusion. *Brain Res.* 1987, **418**: 366–370.

89. Matz PG, Sundaresan S, Sharp FR, Weinstein PR. Induction of HSP70 in rat brain following subarachnoid hemorrhage produced by endovascular perforation. *J. Neurosurg.* 1996, **85**: 138–145.

90. Sayama T, Suzuki S, Fukui M. Role of inducible nitric oxide synthase in the cerebral vasospasm after subarachnoid hemorrhage in rats. *Neurol. Res.* 1999, **21**: 293–298.

91. Saito A, Kamii H, Kato I, *et al.* Transgenic CuZn-superoxide dismutase inhibits NO synthase induction in experimental subarachnoid hemorrhage. *Stroke* 2001, **32**: 1652–1657.

92. Marshman LA, Morice AH, Thompson JS. Increased efficacy of sodium nitroprusside in middle cerebral arteries following acute subarachnoid hemorrhage: indications for its use after rupture. *J. Neurosurg Anesthesiol.* 1998, **10**: 171–177.

93. Echlin F. Experimental vasospasm, acute and chronic, due to blood in the subarachnoid space. *J. Neurosurg.* 1971, **35**: 646–656.

94. Peterson JW, Roussos L, Kwun BD, *et al.* Evidence of the role of hemolysis in experimental cerebral vasospasm. *J. Neurosurg.* 1990, **72**: 775–781.

95. Meguro T, Clower BR, Carpenter R, Parent AD, Zhang JH. Improved rat model for cerebral vasospasm studies. *Neurol. Res.* 2001, **23**: 761–766.
96. Gules I, Satoh M, Clower BR, Nanda A, Zhang JH. Comparison of three rat models of cerebral vasospasm. *Am. J. Physiol. Heart Circ. Physiol.* 2002, **283**: H2551–H2559.
97. Hansen-Schwartz J, Hoel NL, Zhou M, *et al.* Subarachnoid hemorrhage enhances endothelin receptor expression and function in rat cerebral arteries. *Neurosurgery* 2003, **52**: 1188–1194; discussion 1194–1195.
98. Matz PG, Fujimura M, Lewen A, Morita-Fujimura Y, Chan PH. Increased cytochrome *c*-mediated DNA fragmentation and cell death in manganese-superoxide dismutase-deficient mice after exposure to subarachnoid hemolysate. *Stroke* 2001, **32**: 506–515.
99. McGirt MJ, Parra A, Sheng H, *et al.* Attenuation of cerebral vasospasm after subarachnoid hemorrhage in mice overexpressing extracellular superoxide dismutase. *Stroke* 2002, **33**: 2317–2323.
100. Ram Z, Sahar A, Hadani M. Vasospasm due to massive subarachnoid haemorrhage: a rat model. *Acta Neurochir.* 1991, **110**: 181–184.
101. Solomon RA, Antunes JL, Chen RY, Bland L, Chien S. Decrease in cerebral blood flow in rats after experimental subarachnoid hemorrhage: a new animal model. *Stroke* 1985, **16**: 58–64.
102. Tsuji T, Cook DA, Weir BK, Handa Y. Effect of clot removal on cerebrovascular contraction after subarachnoid hemorrhage in the monkey: pharmacological study. *Heart Vessels* 1996, **11**: 69–79.
103. Pickard JD, Walker V, Perry S, *et al.* Arterial eicosanoid production following chronic exposure to a periarterial haematoma. *J. Neurol. Neurosurg. Psychiatr.* 1984, **47**: 661–667.
104. Megyesi JF, Findlay JM, Vollrath B, Cook DA, Chen MH. In vivo angioplasty prevents the development of vasospasm in canine carotid arteries: pharmacological and morphological analyses. *Stroke* 1997, **28**: 1216–1224.
105. Prunell GF, Mathiesen T, Diemer NH, Svendgaard NA. Experimental subarachnoid hemorrhage: subarachnoid blood volume, mortality rate, neuronal death, cerebral blood flow, and perfusion pressure in three different rat models. *Neurosurgery* 2003, **52**: 165–175; discussion 175–176.
106. Gennarelli TA, Thibault LE. Biomechanics of acute subdural hematoma. *J. Trauma* 1982, **22**: 680–686.
107. Duhaime AC, Gennarelli LM, Yachnis A. Acute subdural hematoma: is the blood itself toxic? *J. Neurotrauma* 1994, **11**: 669–678.
108. Miller JD, Bullock R, Graham DI, Chen MH, Teasdale GM. Ischemic brain damage in a model of acute subdural hematoma. *Neurosurgery* 1990, **27**: 433–439.
109. Sasaki M, Dunn L. A model of acute subdural hematoma in the mouse. *J. Neurotrauma* 2001, **18**: 1241–1246.
110. Orlin JR, Thuomas KA, Ponten U, Bergstrom K, Zwetnow NN. MR imaging of experimental subdural bleeding: correlates of brain deformation and tissue water content, and changes in vital physiological parameters. *Acta Radiol.* 1997, **38**: 610–620.
111. Zwetnow NN, Orlin JR, Wu WH, Tajsic N. Studies on supratentorial subdural bleeding using a porcine model. *Acta Neurochir.* 1993, **121**: 58–67.

112. Mauler F, Hinz V, Augstein KH, Fassbender M, Horvath E. Neuroprotective and brain edema-reducing efficacy of the novel cannabinoid receptor agonist BAY 38–7271. *Brain Res.* 2003, **989**: 99–111.

113. Jiang ZW, Gong QZ, Di X, Zhu J, Lyeth BG. Dicyclomine, an M1 muscarinic antagonist, reduces infarct volume in a rat subdural hematoma model. *Brain Res.* 2000, **852**: 37–44.

114. Patel TR, Fujisawa M, Schielke GP, *et al.* Effect of intracerebral and subdural hematomas on energy-dependent transport across the blood–brain barrier. *J. Neurotrauma* 1999, **16**: 1049–1055.

115. Fujisawa H, Maxwell WL, Graham DI, Reasdale GM, Bullock R. Focal microvascular occlusion after acute subdural haematoma in the rat: a mechanism for ischaemic damage and brain swelling? *Acta Neurochir. (Suppl.)* 1994, **60**: 193–196.

116. Bullock R, Butcher SP, Chen MH, Kendall L, McCulloch J. Correlation of the extracellular glutamate concentration with extent of blood flow reduction after subdural hematoma in the rat. *J. Neurosurg.* 1991, **74**: 794–802.

117. Inglis FM, Bullock R, Chen MH, *et al.* Ischaemic brain damage associated with tissue hypermetabolism in acute subdural haematoma: reduction by a glutamate antagonist. *Acta Neurochir. (Suppl.)* 1990, **51**: 277–279.

118. Di X, Bullock R. Effect of the novel high-affinity glycine-site N-methyl-D-aspartate antagonist ACEA-1021 on 125I-MK-801 binding after subdural hematoma in the rat: an in vivo autoradiographic study. *J. Neurosurg.* 1996, **85**: 655–661.

119. Kuroda Y, Fujisawa H, Strebel S, Graham DI, Bullock R. Effect of neuroprotective N-methyl-D-aspartate antagonists on increased intracranial pressure: studies in the rat acute subdural hematoma model. *Neurosurgery* 1994, **35**: 106–112.

120. Glover D, Labadie EL. Physiopathogenesis of subdural hematomas. II. Inhibition of growth of experimental hematomas with dexamethasone. *J. Neurosurg.* 1976, **45**: 393–397.

121. Apfelbaum RI, Guthkelch AN, Shulman K. Experimental production of subdural hematomas. *J. Neurosurg.* 1974, **40**: 336–346.

122. Watanabe S, Shimada H, Ishii S. Production of clinical form of chronic subdural hematoma in experimental animals. *J. Neurosurg.* 1972, **37**: 552–561.

123. Aikawa H, Suzuki K. Experimental chronic subdural hematoma: ultrasound studies on the neomembrane. *Ann. Neurol.* 1988, **24**: 479–480.

21

In vivo models of traumatic brain injury

RONEN R. LEKER AND SHLOMI CONSTANTINI

21.1 Introduction

Yearly, about 2 million patients will suffer traumatic brain injury (TBI).[1,2] Much research has been conducted in the field of TBI over the past decades, yet no specific therapy is available. Different experimental models of TBI have been devised over the past years.[3] Since TBI is a heterogeneous condition no single model can depict the actual pathophysiological changes associated with its entire spectrum.[4] Therefore, each model can be seen as representing a subset of injury. Thus, some models are more akin to represent diffuse axonal injury[5] whereas others are more representative of closed head injury with contusions[6] and still others involve traumatic skull fractures with secondary brain impact.[7] Of note, although some in vitro models for TBI exist (for review see reference 8) this chapter will limit itself to discussion of in vivo models. Using each of these models the interested reader may evaluate the physiological,[6,9] neurochemical,[10–15] behavioral–cognitive,[16,17] histological,[18] and pathologi-cal[9,10,19] sequelae of TBI. Using these methods one can also assess new diagnostic tools and new therapeutic options for neurotrauma.[16,20–23] Furthermore, new diagnostic tools such as magnetic resonance imaging (MRI)[24–26] or MR spectroscopy[27,28] can be used to further outline TBI pathophysiology.

21.2 Closed head injury

TBI is induced in this model by dropping a weight on top of the exposed skull leading to closed head injury (CHI)[7,10] Adjusting the height and weight of the free-falling weight can modify the severity of the injury. This model mimics closed (non-penetrating) head injury and since the location of the injury can be altered (e.g., parietal or frontal) different brain zones can be subjected to injury and the effects of TBI on different areas of the brain can be investigated. This highly reproducible easy-to-implement model can be used in different spe-cies[10,11,29] allowing for investigations of transgenic animals,[15,29,30] and closely

Handbook of Experimental Neurology, ed. Turgut Tatlisumak and Marc Fisher. Published by Cambridge University Press. © Cambridge University Press 2006.

mimics the physiological and pathological changes observed in human trauma. Furthermore, to minimize variability in this model, animals can be tested with the neurological severity score (NSS) scale and only animals with a severity of more than a given value can be included. Ten different tasks are used to evaluate motor ability, balancing, and alertness of the tested animal. Importantly, it should be noted that skull fractures are commonly observed in severe CHI.

The pathological changes observed following CHI include hemorrhagic necrosis, edema, axonal injury, and neuronal loss with secondary gliosis.[7,10] The pathological scores correlate very well with clinical disability scores and with the degree of brain edema.[7,26] NSS at 1 hr is predictive of both mortality and morbidity and it also correlates with the extent of radiological damage seen on MRI. Moreover, in areas identified by MRI as displaying reduced apparent diffusion coefficients (ADCs), a marked reduction in the regional cerebral blood volume (r-CBV) was also observed.[25] These observations may indicate the formation of cytotoxic edema probably due to initiation of ischemic processes. Indeed, reductions in ATP and glucose levels were also noted at the same time points using bioluminescence techniques.[31]

21.3 Fluid percussion

In this model TBI is achieved by rapid injection of fluids into the cranial cavity, along the intact dura mater over the brain[6] to induce a rapid increase in intracranial pressure (ICP). The resulting neuronal damage is secondary to the rapid increase in ICP.[32,33] Different severities of TBI can be induced by controlling the amount and pressure of the injected fluids and the rate at which they are injected.[6]

The clinical correlates of this injury are transient apnea or death (depending upon the severity of TBI), suppression of postural and non-postural function and locomotor and behavioral abnormalities.[6] These changes are accompanied by hypertension, bradycardia, and hyperglycemia, simulating to an extent the changes observed in humans with TBI.[6] Post-traumatic seizures are rare with this model eliminating another possible source of pathological changes.[6]

The gross pathological correlates of this damage include hemorrhage at the site of injury (e.g., contusion), thalamus, hippocampus, and corpus callosum as well as subarachnoid hemorrhage[34] and tissue tears in the white matter.[35] The cellular correlates include neuronal and axonal loss as well as cortical cavitation with reactive gliosis.[34]

This model is well standardized and highly reproducible and can be applied to induce a wide range of severities of brain damage.[6,34] Importantly, fluid percussion may also be combined with other forms of damage such as ischemia or hypoxia allowing for better simulation of the actual conditions observed in humans with TBI. This model can be performed in mice allowing for the investigation of knockouts or overexpressers of any given gene[36] and also in other species including cats, pigs, dogs, and sheep.[33,37,38]

The disadvantages of this invasive and labor-intensive model include a high mortality rate associated with the more severe forms of TBI induced (~50%) which leads to an increase in the number of animals needed.[6] Moreover, although some of the clinical, physiological, pathological, and neurochemical changes observed with this model are similar to those observed in human severe head trauma, this model does not replicate the mechanistic features of human TBI.

21.4 Controlled cortical impact

In the controlled cortical impact (CCI) model TBI is induced by placing animals on foam bed of known spring constant when subjected to an impact delivered to the skull.[39,40] A metal helmet-like device is used to protect from fracture formation. The metal disk usually prevents skull fracturing and also allows for an even distribution of the pressure impact onto the brain below. The weight and height can be adjusted so as to cause mild, moderate, or severe injury with and without edema or contusions.[9] This is a highly reproducible model of TBI and can be used to study the effects of TBI on different brain regions as the damage can be applied to different locations. The injury results in motor and behavioral disabilities,[41] which tend to be persistent over time[42–45] and vary according to lesion site. However, CCI usually results in a severe injury with a high mortality rate. The CCI model has been applied in various species including rats and mice.[46,47] The pathological findings following CCI include intraparenchymatous and subarachnoid hemorrhages, edema, and gray and white matter damage.[46,48,49]

21.5 Rotational injury

In this model TBI is induced by exposing animals to impulsive centroidal rotation of 110° in 4–6 ms.[5] The model appears to have a high reproducibility rate and is relatively simple. It was originally developed in the mini-swine.[5,50]

The pathological correlates of this model include diffuse axonal injury in combination with gliosis that usually affects the interface between gray and white matter and the bases of gyri.[5] This model also leads to minor neuronal damage that is mostly confined to the hippocampus.[5] Notably, no bone fractures, hemorrhage, or focal contusions are noted. Since these pathological changes are similar to those observed in humans this model is used for the investigation of diffuse axonal injury (DAI).

21.6 Rigid indentation

In this group of TBI models the neural damage is induced with rigid impactor that injures the dura and the brain. Most currently used modifications of this technique use a pneumatically driven impactor. The pendulum striker model is one of the variants of this model in which a pendulum striker is used to hit the skull.[51] The model is easy to apply and can be used in many species. The severity of the resulting trauma and clinical syndrome as well as the location of the injury can be modified so as to cause mild, moderate, or severe TBI. The pathological correlates of RI include neuronal loss without contusions or skull fractures.[51]

The dynamic cortical deformation model is another variant of this model[19] in which rats are exposed to transient non-ablative vacuum pulse that lasts 25 ms.[19] This results in a rapid deformation of the cortex and the formation of a cerebral contusion. The severity of injury can be modified by using different pressure pulses.[19]

The pathological changes observed in this model are similar to those observed with human cerebral contusions and include neuronal loss at the site of injury with secondary changes in the subcortical white matter and diffuse astrogliosis of the involved hemisphere.[19] No fractures or axonal injury to the non-involved hemisphere could be discerned.[19]

21.7 Cryogenic injury

In this model TBI is induced by applying cold fluids[52,53] or metal rods[54] to the exposed brain surface. This leads to the formation of cold injury with early and delayed sequelae[52,54,55] the most important of which is brain edema. The model can be used in different species including rats,[52,54] rabbits,[55] and mice.[56,57] It has been used to evaluate neurochemical, metabolic, and blood flow changes[53,57–64] after lesioning the brain and also to evaluate therapeutic modalities targeting brain edema.[55,65,66] However, this model is not widely used since it is does not mimic human TBI.

In summary multiple in vivo models of TBI that are designed to investigate the pathophysiology of traumatic brain injury and to offer therapy to its victims exist (Table 21.1). This variety of true to form models is implied by the great variety in human TBI. Thus, different models can be used to study

Table 21.1. *Characteristics of experimental models of traumatic brain injury (TBI)*

Model	Species[a]	Technical difficulty	Reproducibility	Severity of TBI	Main pathological features[b]	Applicability to human TBI pathology[c]
Closed head injury	M/R	Low	High	Mild–severe	GM + WM	High
Rotational injury	Mini-swine	Medium	High	Mild–severe	WM	High
Controlled cortical impact	M/R	Medium	High	Severe	GM + WM	Medium
Rigid indentation	M/R	Medium	High	Severe	GM + WM	High
Cryogenic injury	M/R/Rab	Medium	High	Moderate	Edema	NA

Notes:
[a] M, mice; R, rats; Rab, rabbits.
[b] GM, gray matter; WM, white matter.
[c] NA, not applicable.

different aspects of human TBI. For example rotational injury models can be used to study DAI, and CCI or CHI models can be used to study contusion with or without skull fractures. Many of these models can be used in more than one species allowing for their use in transgenic mice. However, it should be remembered that animal models mimic only in part the clinical situations and they should be refined to better represent the human condition. Nevertheless, it is only with the use of these and other in vivo models of human disease that we can hope for the emergence of future therapies that would possibly lessen the socioeconomic burden associated with TBI.

References

1. Waxweiler RJ, Thurman D, Sniezek J, Sosin D, O'Neil J. Monitoring the impact of traumatic brain injury: a review and update. *J. Neurotrauma* 1995, **12**: 509–516.
2. Sosin DM, Sniezek JE, Waxweiler RJ. Trends in death associated with traumatic brain injury, 1979 through 1992: success and failure. *J. Am. Med. Ass.* 1995, **273**: 1778–1780.
3. Laurer HL, McIntosh TK. Experimental models of brain trauma. *Curr. Opin. Neurol.* 1999, **12**: 715–721.
4. Povlishock JT, Hayes RL, Michel ME, McIntosh TK. Workshop on animal models of traumatic brain injury. *J. Neurotrauma* 1994, **11**: 723–732.
5. Smith DH, Chen XH, Xu BN, *et al.* Characterization of diffuse axonal pathology and selective hippocampal damage following inertial brain trauma in the pig. *J. Neuropathol. Exp. Neurol.* 1997, **56**: 822–834.
6. Dixon CE, Lyeth BG, Povlishock JT, *et al.* A fluid percussion model of experimental brain injury in the rat. *J. Neurosurg.* 1987, **67**: 110–119.
7. Shapira Y, Shohami E, Sidi A, *et al.* Experimental closed head injury in rats: mechanical, pathophysiologic, and neurologic properties. *Crit. Care Med.* 1988, **16**: 258–265.
8. Morrison B 3rd, Saatman KE, Meaney DF, McIntosh TK. In vitro central nervous system models of mechanically induced trauma: a review. *J. Neurotrauma* 1998, **15**: 911–928.
9. Adelson PD, Robichaud P, Hamilton RL, Kochanek PM. A model of diffuse traumatic brain injury in the immature rat. *J. Neurosurg.* 1996, **85**: 877–884.
10. Chen Y, Constantini S, Trembovler V, Weinstock M, Shohami E. An experimental model of closed head injury in mice: pathophysiology, histopathology, and cognitive deficits. *J. Neurotrauma* 1996, **13**: 557–568.
11. Chen Y, Lomnitski L, Michaelson DM, Shohami E. Motor and cognitive deficits in apolipoprotein E-deficient mice after closed head injury. *Neuroscience* 1997, **80**: 1255–1262.
12. Genis L, Chen Y, Shohami E, Michaelson DM. Tau hyperphosphorylation in apolipoprotein E-deficient and control mice after closed head injury. *J. Neurosci. Res.* 2000, **60**: 559–564.
13. Shohami E, Shapira Y, Cotev S. Experimental closed head injury in rats: prostaglandin production in a noninjured zone. *Neurosurgery* 1988, **22**: 859–863.
14. Shohami E, Gallily R, Mechoulam R, Bass R, Ben-Hur T. Cytokine production in the brain following closed head injury: dexanabinol (HU-211) is a novel

TNF-alpha inhibitor and an effective neuroprotectant. *J. Neuroimmunol.* 1997, **72**: 169–177.

15. Shohami E, Kaufer D, Chen Y, *et al.* Antisense prevention of neuronal damages following head injury in mice. *J. Mol. Med.* 2000, **78**: 228–236.

16. Sinson G, Perri BR, Trojanowski JQ, Flamm ES, McIntosh TK. Improvement of cognitive deficits and decreased cholinergic neuronal cell loss and apoptotic cell death following neurotrophin infusion after experimental traumatic brain injury. *J. Neurosurg.* 1997, **86**: 511–518.

17. Dietrich WD, Alonso O, Busto R, Ginsberg MD. Widespread metabolic depression and reduced somatosensory circuit activation following traumatic brain injury in rats. *J. Neurotrauma* 1994, **11**: 629–640.

18. Baskaya MK, Dogan A, Temiz C, Dempsey RJ. Application of 2,3,5-triphenyltetrazolium chloride staining to evaluate injury volume after controlled cortical impact brain injury: role of brain edema in evolution of injury volume. *J. Neurotrauma* 2000, **17**: 93–99.

19. Shreiber DI, Bain AC, Ross DT, *et al.* Experimental investigation of cerebral contusion: histopathological and immunohistochemical evaluation of dynamic cortical deformation. *J. Neuropathol. Exp. Neurol.* 1999, **58**: 153–164.

20. Raghupathi R, McIntosh TK. Pharmacotherapy for traumatic brain injury: a review. *Proc. West. Pharmacol. Soc.* 1998, **41**: 241–246.

21. McIntosh TK, Saatman KE, Raghupathi R, *et al.* The Dorothy Russell Memorial Lecture. The molecular and cellular sequelae of experimental traumatic brain injury: pathogenetic mechanisms. *Neuropathol. Appl. Neurobiol.* 1998, **24**: 251–267.

22. McIntosh TK, Juhler M, Wieloch T. Novel pharmacologic strategies in the treatment of experimental traumatic brain injury: 1998. *J. Neurotrauma* 1998, **15**: 731–769.

23. Belayev L, Alonso OF, Huh PW, *et al.* Posttreatment with high-dose albumin reduces histopathological damage and improves neurological deficit following fluid percussion brain injury in rats. *J. Neurotrauma* 1999, **16**: 445–453.

24. Albensi BC, Knoblach SM, Chew BG, *et al.* Diffusion and high resolution MRI of traumatic brain injury in rats: time course and correlation with histology. *Exp. Neurol.* 2000, **162**: 61–72.

25. Assaf Y, Holokovsky A, Berman E, *et al.* Diffusion and perfusion magnetic resonance imaging following closed head injury in rats. *J. Neurotrauma* 1999, **16**: 1165–1176.

26. Beni Adani L, Gozes I, Cohen Y, *et al.* A peptide derived from activity-dependent neuroprotective protein (ADNP) ameliorates injury response in closed head injury in mice. *J. Pharmacol. Exp. Ther.* 2001, **296**: 57–63.

27. Cecil KM, Lenkinski RE, Meaney DF, McIntosh TK, Smith DH. High-field proton magnetic resonance spectroscopy of a swine model for axonal injury. *J. Neurochem.* 1998, **70**: 2038–2044.

28. Smith DH, Cecil KM, Meaney DF, *et al.* Magnetic resonance spectroscopy of diffuse brain trauma in the pig. *J. Neurotrauma* 1998, **15**: 665–674.

29. Stahel PF, Shohami E, Younis FM, *et al.* Experimental closed head injury: analysis of neurological outcome, blood–brain barrier dysfunction, intracranial neutrophil infiltration, and neuronal cell death in mice deficient in genes for pro-inflammatory cytokines. *J. Cereb. Blood Flow Metab.* 2000, **20**: 369–380.

30. Sabo T, Lomnitski L, Nyska A, *et al.* Susceptibility of transgenic mice expressing human apolipoprotein E to closed head injury: the allele E3 is neuroprotective whereas E4 increases fatalities. *Neuroscience* 2000, **101**: 879–884.

31. Mautes AE, Thome D, Steudel WI, *et al.* Changes in regional energy metabolism after closed head injury in the rat. *J. Mol. Neurosci.* 2001, **16**: 33–39.
32. Lindgren S, Rinder L. Production and distribution of intracranial and intraspinal pressure changes at sudden extradural fluid volume input in rabbits. *Acta Physiol. Scand.* 1969, **76**: 340–351.
33. Pfenninger EG, Reith A, Breitig D, Grunert A, Ahnefeld FW. Early changes of intracranial pressure, perfusion pressure, and blood flow after acute head injury. I. An experimental study of the underlying pathophysiology. *J. Neurosurg.* 1989, **70**: 774–779.
34. Dixon CE, Lighthall JW, Anderson TE. Physiologic, histopathologic, and cineradiographic characterization of a new fluid-percussion model of experimental brain injury in the rat. *J. Neurotrauma* 1988, **5**: 91–104.
35. Graham DI, Raghupathi R, Saatman KE, Meaney D, McIntosh TK. Tissue tears in the white matter after lateral fluid percussion brain injury in the rat: relevance to human brain injury. *Acta Neuropathol. (Berlin)* 2000, **99**: 117–124.
36. Carbonell WS, Maris DO, McCall T, Grady MS. Adaptation of the fluid percussion injury model to the mouse. *J. Neurotrauma* 1998, **15**: 217–229.
37. Millen JE, Glauser FL, Fairman RP. A comparison of physiological responses to percussive brain trauma in dogs and sheep. *J. Neurosurg.* 1985, **62**: 587–591.
38. Sullivan HG, Martinez J, Becker DP, *et al.* Fluid-percussion model of mechanical brain injury in the cat. *J. Neurosurg.* 1976, **45**: 521–534.
39. Marmarou A, Foda MA, van den Brink W, *et al.* A new model of diffuse brain injury in rats. I. Pathophysiology and biomechanics. *J. Neurosurg.* 1994, **80**: 291–300.
40. Lighthall JW. Controlled cortical impact: a new experimental brain injury model. *J. Neurotrauma* 1988, **5**: 1–15.
41. Adelson PD, Dixon CE, Robichaud P, Kochanek PM. Motor and cognitive functional deficits following diffuse traumatic brain injury in the immature rat. *J. Neurotrauma* 1997, **14**: 99–108.
42. Fox GB, Fan L, LeVasseur RA, Faden AI. Effect of traumatic brain injury on mouse spatial and nonspatial learning in the Barnes circular maze. *J. Neurotrauma* 1998, **15**: 1037–1046.
43. Fox GB, Fan L, LeVasseur RA, Faden AI. Sustained sensory/motor and cognitive deficits with neuronal apoptosis following controlled cortical impact brain injury in the mouse. *J. Neurotrauma* 1998, **15**: 599–614.
44. Fox GB, Faden AI. Traumatic brain injury causes delayed motor and cognitive impairment in a mutant mouse strain known to exhibit delayed Wallerian degeneration. *J. Neurosci. Res.* 1998, **53**: 718–727.
45. Dixon CE, Kochanek PM, Yan HQ, *et al.* One-year study of spatial memory performance, brain morphology, and cholinergic markers after moderate controlled cortical impact in rats. *J. Neurotrauma* 1999, **16**: 109–122.
46. Dixon CE, Clifton GL, Lighthall JW, Yaghmai AA, Hayes RL. A controlled cortical impact model of traumatic brain injury in the rat. *J. Neurosci. Methods* 1991, **39**: 253–262.
47. Smith DH, Soares HD, Pierce JS, *et al.* A model of parasagittal controlled cortical impact in the mouse: cognitive and histopathologic effects. *J. Neurotrauma* 1995, **12**: 169–178.
48. Foda MA, Marmarou A. A new model of diffuse brain injury in rats. II. Morphological characterization. *J. Neurosurg.* 1994, **80**: 301–313.

49. Kochanek PM, Marion DW, Zhang W, *et al*. Severe controlled cortical impact in rats: assessment of cerebral edema, blood flow, and contusion volume. *J. Neurotrauma* 1995, **12**: 1015–1025.
50. McGowan JC, McCormack TM, Grossman RI, *et al*. Diffuse axonal pathology detected with magnetization transfer imaging following brain injury in the pig. *Magn. Reson. Med*. 1999, **41**: 727–733.
51. Morehead M, Bartus RT, Dean RL, *et al*. Histopathologic consequences of moderate concussion in an animal model: correlations with duration of unconsciousness. *J. Neurotrauma* 1994, **11**: 657–667.
52. Husz T, Joo F, Antal A, Toldi J. Late consequences of cryogenic brain lesion in rat: an electrophysiological study. *NeuroReport* 1992, **3**: 51–54.
53. James HE, Schneider S. Cryogenic brain oedema: loss of cerebrovascular autoregulation as a cause of intracranial hypertension – implications for treatment. *Acta Neurochir. (Suppl.)* 1990, **51**: 79–81.
54. Todd MM, Weeks JB, Warner DS. A focal cryogenic brain lesion does not reduce the minimum alveolar concentration for halothane in rats. *Anesthesiology* 1993, **79**: 139–143.
55. Wilson JT, Gross CE, Bednar MM, Shackford SR. U83836E reduces secondary brain injury in a rabbit model of cryogenic trauma. *J. Trauma* 1995, **39**: 473–477.
56. Morita Fujimura Y, Fujimura M, Kawase M, Chan PH. Early decrease in apurinic/apyrimidinic endonuclease is followed by DNA fragmentation after cold injury-induced brain trauma in mice. *Neuroscience* 1999, **93**: 1465–1473.
57. Murakami K, Kondo T, Yang G, *et al*. Cold injury in mice: a model to study mechanisms of brain edema and neuronal apoptosis. *Prog. Neurobiol*. 1999, **57**: 289–299.
58. Darby JM, Nemoto EM, Yonas H, *et al*. Local cerebral blood flow measured by xenon-enhanced CT during cryogenic brain edema and intracranial hypertension in monkeys. *J. Cereb. Blood Flow Metab*. 1993, **13**: 763–772.
59. Hermann DM, Mies G, Hossmann KA. Effects of a traumatic neocortical lesion on cerebral metabolism and gene expression of rats. *NeuroReport* 1998, **9**: 1917–1921.
60. Maeda M, Akai F, Yanagihara T. Neuronal integrity and astrocytic reaction in cold injury: an immunohistochemical investigation. *Acta Neuropathol. (Berlin)* 1997, **94**: 116–123.
61. Schneider GH, Hennig S, Lanksch WR, Unterberg A. Dynamics of posttraumatic brain swelling following a cryogenic injury in rats. *Acta Neurochir. (Suppl.)* 1994, 60437–60439.
62. Siren AL, Knerlich F, Schilling L, *et al*. Differential glial and vascular expression of endothelins and their receptors in rat brain after neurotrauma. *Neurochem. Res*. 2000, **25**: 957–969.
63. Nag S. Cold-injury of the cerebral cortex: immunolocalization of cellular proteins and blood–brain barrier permeability studies. *J. Neuropathol. Exp. Neurol*. 1996, **55**: 880–888.
64. Vinas FC, Dujovny M, Hodgkinson D. Early hemodynamic changes at the microcirculatory level and effects of mannitol following focal cryogenic injury. *Neurol. Res*. 1995, **17**: 465–468.
65. Hartl R, Schurer L, Goetz C, *et al*. The effect of hypertonic fluid resuscitation on brain edema in rabbits subjected to brain injury and hemorrhagic shock. *Shock* 1995, **3**: 274–279.
66. Yamamura H, Hiraide A, Matsuoka T, *et al*. Effect of growth hormone on brain oedema caused by a cryogenic brain injury model in rats. *Brain Inj*. 2000, **14**: 669–676.

22

Experimental models for the study
of CNS tumors

TAICHANG JANG AND LAWRENCE RECHT

22.1 Introduction

Despite several decades of intensive study, the treatment of brain tumors, whether they have arisen primarily within the central nervous system (CNS) or spread there from elsewhere, represents a formidable challenge for the clinician. Several reasons underlie the difficulties in brain tumor treatment including delivering enough therapy through a blood–brain barrier (BBB), circumventing the relative immunosuppression that occurs both as a result of the brain tumor and due to its development in a relatively immunologically protected area, and the need to preserve the normal surrounding CNS. Such obstacles underscore the importance of accurate preclinical models both to understand the processes by which tumors develop and are sustained as well as to test the effectiveness of various treatments.

While in vitro systems are frequently used to assess both biology and treatment of tumors, the importance of the tumor–normal tissue relationships can only be addressed with in vivo models. Several years ago, Peterson et al. proposed criteria by which to judge the validity of such a model, including:[1] (1) the growth rate of the tumor and its malignancy characteristics should be predictable and reproducible; (2) the species used should be small and inexpensively maintained so that large numbers may be evaluated; (3) the time to tumor induction should be relatively short and the survival time after induction should be standardized; (4) the tumor should have the same characteristics as the clinical tumor in terms of intraparenchymal growth, invasiveness, angiogenesis; (5) tumors should be maintainable in culture and should be safe for laboratory personnel; and (6) therapeutic responsiveness must imitate that of the clinical tumor being tested.

Not surprisingly, despite dozens of such models that have been developed, each with its own attributes, none is perfect. Therefore, the investigator needs to carefully choose his/her model, based on the questions that they want to

Handbook of Experimental Neurology, ed. Turgut Tatlisumak and Marc Fisher. Published by Cambridge University Press. © Cambridge University Press 2006.

address. In this short review, we will approach these issues by first outlining the particular reasons for needing a brain tumor model and then assessing how some of the more common approaches meet these needs.

22.2 Rationale for using an in vivo CNS tumor model

An ideal brain tumor model should closely mimic the clinical situation, as well as be consistently reproducible from animal to animal. As a corollary, it should respond to external influences (i.e., therapies) similar to what is encountered clinically. Because we do not know exactly how brain tumors arise, an ideal model remains elusive. Therefore the investigator needs to choose a model that is optimally suited to the experimental objectives. From the aspect of choosing a model, two objectives can be envisioned:

• assessment of a particular treatment or a diagnostic test
• assessment of the development of a primary CNS tumor or a biological aspect of the relationships between tumor and normal brain (i.e., angiogenesis, invasion, immune function, etc.).

Each of these objectives requires particular properties from the model. Thus, if the objective is to assess a treatment or diagnostic test, it would be more important to have a model where tumors grow predictably in all test animals and survivals are relatively short, with little variation between experimental subjects. Less important would be the particular method (i.e., implantation of a line, induction by viruses, etc.) used to ensure these requirements.

On the other hand, the method used to induce tumors is a key aspect for studying tumor biology, especially since one is trying to assess those biological aspects that most closely resemble the clinical situation. Here, the very artificial method of implanting established tumor lines would seem to be far removed from the clinical situation. The investigator would therefore readily sacrifice such parameters as predictable growth and short survival for models that more truly reflect the clinical situation (in fact, one would want a model that is a bit stochastic so that it mimics the clinical situation better).

22.3 Models that are best utilized for assessing therapeutics and diagnostics

The usual paradigm for developing a model to assess a particular therapy involves implantation of a tumor cell line that has been established from a resected tumor (which might be a specimen removed during surgery or a tumor induced by one of the methods described below). The particular line has usually been cultivated in vitro for several passages (although models in which freshly isolated tumor specimens have been used have also been described[2]). To ensure that the model is "valid," the line utilized is generally derived from the tumor that one wants to study, although it is well known that the longer these cells are passaged in culture, the less they resemble the original tumor. Moreover, the investigator has to choose whether he/she wants to study a human cell line, which would require the utilization of an immunosuppressed animal or a tumor line isolated from another species, which could be implanted without immunosuppression but then might be too far removed from the clinical situation to be clinically useful. Finally, although the brain would seem an optimal location to assess therapies, it is less than optimal if growth measurements are needed; thus, dozens of studies assess treatments after injecting cells into other body areas. We will address each of these issues – the inoculum, the location inoculated, and the types of species utilized – below.

22.3.1 Tumor cell lines

Cell lines that are used in studies on CNS tumors can be classified into those that are syngeneic and those that are heterologous. The latter lines are generally derived from human tumors, while the former represent tumors that have arisen in various species after chemical carcinogenesis or viral infection.

Literally dozens of lines exist (the interested reader can refer to the American Tissue Culture Facility's catalog[3]). Many tumor cell lines involved in syngeneic transplantation have been derived from tumors that have been induced either by chemical carcinogenesis or after inoculation of tumorigenic viruses (see below). One of the more commonly utilized lines of this type is the C6 line because its documented astrocytic morphology, including expression of glial fibrillary acidic protein (GFAP) and S-100 protein, has made it an attractive model, not only for neurooncologists but for neurobiologists as well. Interestingly, however, although it is known that it was isolated from a tumor that developed after transplacental exposure to *N*-nitrosourea, the strain of rat utilized was never identified[4]. It is unclear whether this in some way relates to the fact that although this line grows readily in many types of rat strains, there exist reports noting that growth in Wistar rats results in a tumor more analogous to the clinical situation, i.e., with characteristic invasiveness, marked angiogenesis, etc., than in other strains such as Sprague-Dawley, where tumors tend to grow as sharply demarcated, encapsulated tumors.[5–8]

The 9L gliosarcoma cell line is also frequently used by investigators. It was also derived from a nitrosourea-exposed rat, in this case Wistar and Fisher strains. Several other clonal tumor cell lines have been developed with purported glial morphology and biological characteristics,[9,10] However, sarcomatous changes tend to occur with serial passage and its growth in vivo resembles more that of a metastatic tumor, i.e., encapsulated, poorly invasive.[11]

A number of cell lines have also been developed from human tumors and are commercially available. While their use was originally expected to provide workers with models that more closely resembled the clinical situation, it has become apparent that there are several limitations to their use.[12] For example, human brain tumors are extremely heterogeneous, and over time will show variability in mitotic rates and transformation potential. Furthermore, they frequently demonstrate sarcomatous degeneration.[13,14] Thus, variability can be observed even in the most carefully controlled transplant studies.

Besides glioma, there are also cell lines derived from clinical medullo-blastoma specimens. Such lines, such as DAOY, have been extensively studied although some workers have questioned whether they in fact retain any similarity to the tumor that is encountered in situ. Recently, a model of primary CNS lymphoma involving inoculation of cell suspensions of Epstein–Barr vious (EBV)-transformed human lymphoblastoid B cell lines into caudate nucleus of nude rats has been reported.[15]

22.3.2 Location

For intracranial modeling, tumor cells are generally injected into a defined area of the brain using a stereotactic apparatus to ensure consistent place-ment.[16] For mice, however, the investigator may want to avoid the difficulties associated with placing mice in headholders; in this instance an implantable guide screw system allows rapid and reproducible tumor engraftments.[17] Generally, the striatum is used by convention. To ensure a high percentage of tumor takes as well as reproducing what occurs clinically, care must be taken to prevent injected cells from flowing back along the shaft of the needle into the arachnoid space. Otherwise, tumor cells may be carried away into the normal brain parenchyma, the ventricles, or even the systemic circulation.

Alternatively, if one wants to observe tumor growth in situ, as is sometimes the case when analyzing angiogenesis, one can implant cells under the pial surface using direct visualization. Another possible placement location is into the leptomeninges, especially if one is interested in assessing therapeutic deliv-ery into this site.[18]

Most orthotopic animal models of human glioblastoma multiforme (GBM) are performed via use of cell suspensions, which have the advantage of limited surgical trauma.[19–27] Tumor growth occurs in approximately 70% of animals using these methods. GBMs have also been transplanted as spheroids from precultured biopsy specimens with a somewhat better engraftment.[28] A more recent report notes that GBMs could always be transplanted when the tumors were grown within the mouse abdominal walls before being heterotransplanted into the brain.[2] Interestingly, in this latter study, the abdominal tumors grew as expansive masses while the intracranial tumors were more invasive, suggesting both that the environment plays an important role in determining tumor phenotype and that different therapeutic results may be encountered depending on the site tested.

In studies where visualization of cells is required, such as in studies of tumor cell migration and invasion, a number of methods exist for tumor cell labeling. In the past, a number of methods have been used including *Phaseolus vulgaris* leukoagglutinin (PHAL), cell labeling dyes such as fast blue or DiI/DiO and transfection with the *lacZ* gene. One disadvantage of using PHAL or DiI/DiO which externally label cells, however, is that long-term studies lasting multiple cell divisions are difficult due to decrease in signal over time. Furthermore, even though transfection with the *lacZ* gene is stable, it requires post-processing using a chromogenic substrate for the β-galactosidase marker enzyme. A more optimal method that has become more widely available recently is to transfect cells with the green fluorescent protein (GFP) marker gene which enables monitoring for long periods without the need for histochemical or immunochemical treatment (Fig. 22.1).[29–31]

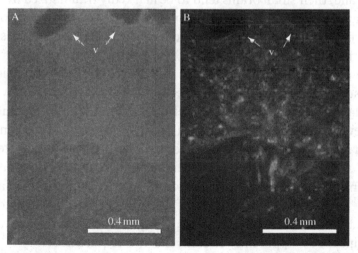

Figure 22.1. Fluorescent micrograph of C6 glioma cells labeled with green fluorescent protein (GFP) after implantation into rat striatum. Cells were labeled with a retroviral vector controlling GFP expression. (A) 4′-6-Diamidino-2-phenylindole (DAPI) stain which highlights nuclei showing increased cellularity associated with growing tumor. (B) Green fluorescence reveals invading margin of tumor cells inferiorly. V, blood vessels.

The goal of an assay system is to reproduce as closely as possible the clinical situation. Nevertheless, while intracranial implantation is a more logical site for the study of glioma, it is difficult to assess any outcome measure other than illness and death. Therefore, a rationale exists for producing tumors in areas that are easy to assess frequently so that size can be measured. Thus, although subcutaneous implantation seems much less representative of the clinical situation, it does allow for serial monitoring and measurements, thus offering the possibility of detecting more subtle changes that might be caused by a therapy. If such a route is chosen, it is important to remember that tumors grow more quickly if they are implanted nearer the abdominal wall than more distally in the lower extremity. This underlies a very important point in using any of these models for survival or growth analysis: it is very important to use identical conditions, including inoculum size, location of transplant, and even amount of media delivered, to prevent the unintentional skewing of results.

22.3.3 Species

Usually, small rodents, mostly mice and rats, are used to study in vivo brain tumor behavior since they are easier to handle and less expensive than larger animals. Mice are the least expensive and there are available numerous strains that are immunosuppressed, thus allowing engraftment of human cell lines. On the other hand, their small brains tend to be markedly traumatized by the tumor cell inoculations and the relative lack of white matter relative to that of humans render them less than ideal for assessing effects on normal CNS tissues. Rats are larger and more suited for studies on CNS. Furthermore, several of the most commonly used cell lines such as C6 and 9L are derived from rats, which creates a suitable substrate for growth of these cells. Moreover, there are now commercially available nude strains that are useful for engrafting human xenografts.

Some new treatment approaches such as convection delivery or gene therapy may require animal models of larger sizes to better indicate anticipated human responses. A few larger animal brain tumor models have been reported in the literature including allogenic rat gliomas in cats,[32] virus-induced primary canine tumors,[33,34] and monkey brain tumors.[35] They are generally difficult to generate and use and have the disadvantage of requiring immunosuppression, although a recent canine model apparently circumvents this requirement.[36]

22.4 Models that are better for assessing biological issues

The process of tumor formation results from a series of genetic and epigenetic "hits" that result in disruptions of cell cycle control, unchecked proliferation, and apoptotic resistance. Implantation of established tumor cells, such as described in the models above, is obviously not an ideal way to assess these issues. For this analysis, other strategies are necessary and essentially fall into one of three overlapping categories: chemical carcinogenesis, viral induction, and transgenic model systems.

22.4.1 Chemical carcinogenesis

Brain tumors can be reliably induced by exposing mice or rats to certain chemicals. One of the first models was developed in the 1940s using aromatic polycyclic hydrocarbons to produce experimental brain tumors in adult mice.[37,38] These tumors, which develop 125–400 days following the surgical implantation of small crystalline carcinogenic pellets, simulated various histological features seen in human brain tumors.[39–41] An inflammatory reactive gliosis, involving macrophages and virus-like particles in reactive cells, was associated with pellets that formed tumors, which occurred in approximately 50% of mice.[37,38] The requirement of an indwelling pellet, however, made an assessment of the early events underlying tumor formation impossible since it could not be distinguished whether a pathologic change represented part of the tumor process or a response to injury.

Another method for inducing brain tumors is via systemic administration of chemical carcinogens. Two general methods exist. In the first, described over three decades ago by Druckrey and colleagues,[42–45] rats are exposed during late gestation to a single dose of N-ethyl-N-nitrosourea (ENU). Although pups appear normal at birth, brain tumors of variable types including mixed oligo-astrocytomas, oligodendrogliomas, astrocytomas, and neurinomas develop in virtually all several months later (Fig. 22.2).[46] Since ENU is cleared rapidly (its half-life is only 8 min),[47,48] initiation must occur rapidly, a contention supported by the observation that brain cells isolated from recently exposed rats occasionally transform.[49,50] Despite this, pathologic changes, even subtle ones, are not seen before 30 days of age,[51] thus making this an attractive model to assess early events in the tumor process.

Although tumors are reliably formed after ENU administration, it is notable that the glioblastoma phenotype is not produced. If weaned rats are administered small doses of a similar agent (methylnitrosourea) for several weeks, GBMs develop at a very high frequency.[52]

Interestingly, there is a marked variation in the penetrance of this effect; certain rat strains, such as Sprague-Dawley and Fisher344, are very susceptible to this effect while others, such as the BD-IV strain, are much less so. Furthermore, mice do not seem readily susceptible to this effect,

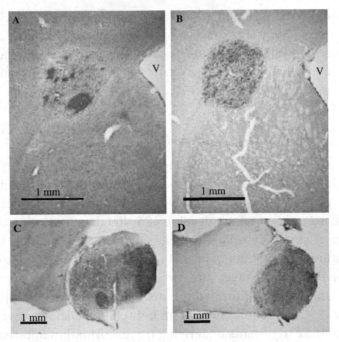

Figure 22.2. Brain sections obtained from a 150-day-old rat who was exposed to *N*-ethyl-*N*-nitrosourea (ENU) (50 mg/ml) at embryonic day 20. (A) and (B) are adjacent sections stained with hematoxylin–eosin and the neural marker nestin, respectively, of an astrocytic neoplasm located in the corpus callosum. (C) and (D) represent similarly stained sections of a trigeminal neurinoma.

although ENU can produce a high rate of tumor formation in p53 knockout mice.[53]

While the long incubation period provides a window in which to observe early events in the glioma process, there are several drawbacks to this model including the length of time it takes to form tumors, the uncertainty of the genetic injuries produced, the variable tumors that develop, and the restriction of this effect to rats (i.e., normal mice do not develop brain tumors).

22.4.2 Virus-induced tumors

Both RNA and DNA viruses can be used to create CNS tumors. Retroviruses are most commonly used, particularly the avian sarcoma viruses.[54] The type of tumor depends on the site of inoculation and the age of the animal, neonatal animals being much more susceptible.[55] A superficial cerebral or vermian location of inoculation favors sarcomas, whereas inoculation in the subependymal region results in glial type tumors.[56] A well-characterized model of this type was used to produce gliomas in newborn beagles; as little as 0.01 ml of a concentrated suspension of the Schmidt–Ruppin strain of the Rous sarcoma virus consistently resulted in the production of gliomas.[34]

DNA viruses have also been utilized. Human adenovirus 12 induces neuroblastoma and retinoblastoma after inoculation in mice, rats, and hamsters and permanent cell lines have been established using this model.[57] Papovavirus, the causative agent of progressive multifocal leukoencephalopathy (PML) produces a variety of tumors types including medulloblastoma, glioma, and ependymomas after inoculation into newborn hamsters.[58,59] In addition, the similan vacuolating virus SV40, although not oncogenic in its permissive host, the monkey, can produce dose-dependent tumorigenesis of choroid plexus papillomas and ependymomas after intracranial inoculation into newborn Syrian hamsters.[60,61]

Virus-induced tumors can be predictably produced with minimal damage to brain tissue, develop in situ with a natural blood supply, and can be cultured in vitro. Nevertheless, the viruses are difficult to maintain in the laboratory and produce tumors of a wide variety, making them difficult to use for therapeutic studies. In addition, they usually require increased safety precautions for laboratory personnel. Their study has nevertheless provided not only insights into neurooncogenesis, but also the foundation for many of the more "cutting edge" tools used by transgenic mouse modelers.

22.4.3 Murine transgenic models

It may be argued that the only way to distinguish between those genetic aberrations that are crucial to brain tumor development as opposed to merely being a bystander is by recreation of these mutations in animal models. One can do this by generating mice with either gains or losses of function (or both). The first models using transgenic strategies expressed SV40 early region genes, including large T- and small t-antigens regulated by its own promoter, in all cells. In this model, choroid plexus tumors reproducibly developed.[62–64] Varying the promoter expressing T-antigen resulted in other neural tumors. Fusion of large T to the β-subunit of luteinizing hormone generated pituitary adenomas. In addition, one founder mouse developed retinoblastomas and midline primitive neuroectodermal tumors.[65,66] When fused to the promoter sequence for the human cystic fibrosis transmembrane conductance regulator, intraventricular ependymomas were noted.[67]

Producing a mouse with a germline mutation is not optimal for investigating the development of brain tumors, however, since every cell expresses the mutation, making the exclusive development of a specific intracranial tumor unlikely. Furthermore, many mutations produce lethal phenotypes if expressed in all cells. Conditional gene aberrations in which genes are either deleted or amplified in only selected neural cells are a more optimal method for the study of brain tumor development. One of the first successful applications of this strategy was the linkage of the SV40 large T-antigen to the GFAP promoter with the resultant production of malignant gliomas.[68]

Over the last decade, several additional strategies have been used to gain insight into the process of glioma formation. Most of these aimed to address either the cell of origin of brain tumor or pathways involved in this process (Table 22.1). Genes have been activated or inactivated using either transgenic strategies where the gene is knocked in or out in an embryonic stem cell to make a founder line or by delivering genes using viral vectors. Concerning the latter, genes may be delivered non-specifically using a replication-competent Moloney murine leukemia virus (MMLV) to induce gene transfer into pro-liferating cells[69] or by a more selective delivery system using an avian leukosis virus-based (ALV) replication competent system. In this latter system, genes are delivered by injecting virus into the brain of transgenic mice expressing the RCAS receptor, tv-a, on target cells.[70,71] In this way, only cells that express the receptor (i.e., behind a cell-specific promoter) will be infected, allowing assess-ment of specific cell type involvement in tumor formation. Using this strategy, Holland and colleagues have demonstrated that tumors develop more readily from progenitor-like cells (i.e., those expressing nestin) than from astrocytic ones (expressing GFAP).[70,71]

Using these various methodologies, investigators have been able to model astrocytomas,[71–77] oligodendrogliomas,[69,78–80] and medulloblastomas.[81–85]

In most of these studies, pathologic and molecular correlations were noted between model and clinical situation. For example, in a study in which low-grade oligodendrogliomas were induced, murine tumors contained chromosomal dele-tions orthologous to human 1p.[78] Nevertheless, in other cases the parallels were less clear such as in the case of medulloblastomas, where p53 and Rb abnorm-alities play important roles in the murine models[84] but are not frequently activated in the clinical situation.[86] Presumably this results from some as yet unknown critical function for these pathways in the mouse that is due to an as yet unknown equivalent in the human. It also suggests that despite its power, the use of murine models to infer what is happening clinically must be done carefully.

The results from the above studies provide many useful insights into the development and biology of brain tumors and it is notable that the patterns of tumor occurrence in these models mimic more closely the infiltrative nature and other pathological properties of the corresponding human tumors. However, compared with some of the other models, especially tumors that

Table 22.1. *A representative survey of recent studies using transgenic murine strategies to produce brain tumors*

Reference	Strategy	Tumors produced	Comments
Danks et al.[68]	Murine glial fibrillary acidic protein (GFAP) promoter-SV40 T antigen	Astrocytomas	
Weissenberger et al.[76]	Murine GFAP promoter-*v-src* kinase	Astrocytomas	At later stages, tumors highly malignant suggesting progression over time
Holland et al.[70]	RCAS vectors expressing mutant epidermal growth factor receptor (EGFr) to nestin- and GFAP-*tv-a* expressing mice crossed with INK4a/ARF nulls	Gliomas	
Uhrbom et al.[69]	Platelet-derived growth factor (PDGF) B-chain/*c-sis* MoMuLV	Glioblastoma multiforme (GBM), peripheral neuroectodermal tumor	Tumors coexpressed PDGF B-chain and α-receptor
Reilly et al.[77]	*Nf1*/*Trp53* mutations on same chromosome (NP-*cis* mice)	Astrocytomas, including GBM	Strain-specific effect
Holland et al.[74]	RCAS vectors expressing *ras* and *akt* genes to nestin- and GFAP-*tv-a* expressing mice	GBM	Tumors formed only in nestin mice; neither Ras or Akt sufficient alone
Ding et al.[72]	GFAP promoter-V12Ha-*ras* oncogene	Low- and high-grade astrocytomas	Grade *ras* dose-dependent
Dai et al.[80]	RCAS vectors overexpressing PDGF-B to nestin- and GFAP-*tv-a* expressing mice	Oligodendrogliomas and oligoastrocytomas	Expression on *INK4a*/*ARF*[−/−] background promoted tumor progression
Xiao et al.[90]	Conditional expression of GFAP promoter-T$_{121}$ (pRb, p107, and p130 inactivator) using *Cre/Lox*	High-grade astrocytoma	Tumor regions expressed activated Akt; accelerated development on *PTEN*[+/−] background

Table 22.1. (cont.)

Reference	Strategy	Tumors produced	Comments
Ding et al.[79]	GFAP promoter-V12Ha-ras × GFAP promoter-EGFrvIII	Oligodendrogliomas and oligoastrocytomas	GFAP promoter-EGFRvIII by itself did not produce tumor
Jensen et al.[75]	GFAP promoter-c-Myc	Malignant astrocytomas	EGFr upregulation in tumors; no cooperating transgenes
Weiss et al.[78]	S100β promoter-verbB; S100β promoter-verbB × p53[+/−] or INK4a/ARF[−/−]	Oligodendroglioma; high-grade oligodendroglioma	Comparative genomic hybridization (CGH) revealed loss of region orthologous to human chromosome 1p
Bajenaru et al.[73]	GFAPCre; NF1[flox/mut]	Optic nerve gliomas	Mice in which NF1 knocked out in astrocytes only did not develop tumor suggesting role for NF[+/−] background
Goodrich et al.[85]	PTC[+/−] transgenics	Medulloblastomas	Homozygotes embryonic lethal
Marino et al.[84]	GFAP-Cre; Rb[LoxP/LoxP]; p53[−/−] or [LoxP/LoxP]	Medulloblastomas	No astrocytic tumors; GFAP-Cre expression must occur in external granular layer cells at some time
Weiner et al.[81]	Shh-expressing retrovirus into murine embryos	Medulloblastomas	Tumors also formed in Gli1 null mice
Lee & McKinnon[83]	Lig4[−/−] × p53[−/−] mice	Medulloblastomas	Lig4[−/−] embryonic lethal
Tong et al.[82]	Poly(ADP-ribose) polymerase (PARP)[−/−] × p53[−/−]	Medulloblastoma	PARP-1 senses and repairs DNA double-stranded breaks

develop after orthotopic transplantation, these tumors arise largely in unpredictable locations of the CNS and at unpredictable times. Furthermore, they are costly, both in terms of model construction and maintaining the breeding colonies, thus making their use for therapeutic studies still a bit impractical. In terms of their unpredictable development, however, recent technological advances in imaging may make this problem more manageable. Thus, several reports have appeared recently that demonstrate the power of magnetic imaging technology in facilitating assessment, and recent technical reports have demonstrated methods to correlate images with stereotaxic co-ordinates that can be used for obtaining biopsies[87] as well as increasing throughput so as to be feasible for use in therapeutic studies.[88]

22.5 Summary

Since no ideal model exists, the investigator must choose one that best fits his/her needs. From the standpoint of assessing a therapy, one would prefer a model whose sensitivities to the particular agent closely mimics the clinical situation. Some would argue, therefore, that only human lines should be utilized. This is countered, however, by the fact that tumors formed after inoculation with human glioma lines do not resemble the histologic characteristics seen in the clinical situation. Furthermore, the tendency for all established lines to increasingly deviate from the original phenotype and genotype as they are passaged in culture makes comparing studies from different laboratories even using identical lines difficult. For therapeutic studies, therefore, it is probably reasonable to recommend that the investigator make one model the laboratory's standard and focus efforts both on optimizing the delivery of tumor cells (nearly 100% takes should occur) and ensuring a small standard deviation in terms of outcomes. Care should also be taken to ensure that the model is an appropriate one for examining the particular therapy. For example, in retrospect, a widely cited study demonstrating the promise of gene therapy for brain tumors[89] was probably flawed because the line chosen (9L) is immunogenic in itself and produces a non-invasive phenotype.

The promise of transgenic strategies is the opportunity to assess the effects of therapy on specific signaling pathways as well as the hope of eventually developing a model that is closer to the ideal. Currently, their expense makes them a bit impractical for large-scale therapeutic studies; however, with the parallel development of imaging technologies and other ways to monitor tumor growth, it might be anticipated that these obstacles will be overcome in the near future and that this strategy may eventually yield the elusive gold standard model.

References

1. Peterson DL, Sheridan PJ, Brown WE. Animal models for brain tumors: historical perspectives and future directions. *J. Neurosurg.* 1994, **80**: 865–876.
2. Antunes L, Angioi-Duprez KS, Bracard SR, *et al.* Analysis of tissue chimerism in nude mouse brain and abdominal xenograft models of human glioblastoma multiforme: what does it tell us about the models and about glioblastoma biology and therapy? *J. Histochem. Cytochem.* 2000, **48**: 847–858.
3. American Tissue Culture Facility. *Catalog* 2005, available online at http://www.atcc.org
4. Benda P, Lightbody J, Sato G, *et al.* Differentiated rat glial strain in tissue culture. *Science* 1968, **161**: 370–371.
5. Cohen JD, Robins HI, Javid MJ, *et al.* Intracranial C6 glioma model in adult Wistar-Furth rats. *J. Neuro-oncol.* 1990, **8**: 95–96.
6. Farrell CL, Stewart PA, Del Maestro RF. A new glioma model in the rat: The C6 spheroid implantation technique permeability and vascular characterization. *J. Neuro-oncol.* 1987, **4**: 403–415.
7. San-Galli F, Vrignaud P, Robert J. Assessment of the experimental model of transplanted C6 glioblastoma in Wistar rats. *J. Neuro-oncol.* 1989, **7**: 299–304.
8. Nagano N, Sasaki H, Asyagi M, Hirakama K. Invasion of experimental rat brain tumor: early morphological changes following microinjection of C6 glioma cells. *Acta Neuropathol.* 1993, **86**: 117–125.
9. Schubert D, Heinemann S, Carlisle W, *et al.* Clonal cell lines from the rat central nervous system. *Nature* 1974, **249**: 224–227.
10. Benda P, Someda K, Messer J, *et al.* Morphological and immunochemical studies of rat glial tumors and clonal strains propagated in culture. *J. Neurosurg.* 1971, **34**: 310–323.
11. Pilkington GJ, Bjerkvig R, De Ridder C, Kaaijk P. In vitro and in vivo models for the study of brain tumor invasion. *Anticancer Res.* 1997, **17**: 4107–4110.
12. Rama B, Spoerri O, Holzgraefe M, *et al.* Current brain tumor models with particular consideration of the transplantation techniques: outline of literature and personal primary results. *Acta Neurochir.* 1986, **79**: 35–41.
13. Paulus W, Huettner C, Tonn JC. Collagens, integrins and the mesenchymal drift in glioblastomas: a comparison of biopsy specimens, spheroid and early monolayer cultures. *Int. J. Cancer* 1994, **58**: 841–846.
14. McKeever PE, Chronwall BM. Early switch in glial protein and fibronectin markers on cells during the culture of human gliomas. *Ann NY Acad. Sci.* 1985, **435**: 457–459.
15. Roychowdhury S, Peng R, Baiocchi RA, *et al.* Experimental treatment of Epstein–Barr virus-associated primary central nervous system lymphoma. *Cancer Res.* 2003, **63**: 965–971.
16. Kobayashi N, Allen N, Clendenon N, *et al.* An improved rat brain-tumor model. *J. Neurosurgery.* 1980; **53**: 808–815.
17. Lal S, Lacroix M, Tofilon P, *et al.* An implantable guide-screw system for brain tumor studies in small animals. *J. Neurosurg.* 2000, **92**: 326–333.
18. Rewers AB, Redgate ES, Deutsch M, *et al.* A new rat brain tumor model: glioma disseminated via the cerebral spinal fluid pathways. *J. Neuro-oncol.* 1990, **8**: 213–219.
19. Basler GA, Shapiro WR. Brain tumor research with nude mice. In Fogh J, Giovanella BC (eds.) *The Nude Mouse in Experimental and Clinical Research.* New York: Academic Press, 1982, pp. 475–490.

20. Bradley NJ, Bloom JG, Dawies AJS, Swift SM. Growth of human gliomas in immune-deficient mice: a possible model for preclinical therapy studies. *Br. J. Cancer* 1978, **38**: 263–272.

21. Bullard DE, Schold SC, Bigner S, Bigner DD. Growth and chemotherapeutic response in athymic mice of tumors arising from human glioma-derived cell lines. *J. Neuropathol. Exp. Neurol.* 1981, **40**: 410–427.

22. De Armond SJ, Stowring L, Amar A, *et al*. Development of a non-selecting, non-perturbing method to study human brain tumor cell invasion in murine brain. *J. Neuro-oncol.* 1994, **20**: 27–34.

23. Horten BC, Basler GA, Shapiro WR. Xenograft of human malignant glial tumors into brains of nude mice. *J. Neuropathol. Exp. Neurol.* 1981, **40**: 493–511.

24. Jones TR, Bigner S, Schold SC, Eng LF, Bigner DD. Anaplastic human gliomas grown in athymic mice: morphology and glial fibrillary acidic protein expression. *Am. J. Pathol.* 1981, **105**: 3274–3280.

25. Marno K, Neyama Y, Kuwahara Y, *et al*. Human tumour xenografts in athymic rats and their age dependence. *Br. J. Cancer* 1982, **45**: 786–789.

26. Rana MW, Pinkerton H, Thornton H, Nagy D. Heterotransplantation of human glioblastoma multiforme and meningioma to nude mice. *Proc. Soc. Exp. Biol. Med.* 1977, **155**: 85–88.

27. Shapiro WR, Basler GA, Chernik NA, Posner JB. Human brain tumor transplantation into nude mice. *J. Natl Cancer Inst.* 1979, **62**: 447–453.

28. Engebraaten O, Hjortland GO, Hirschbert H, Fodstad O. Growth of precultured glioma specimens in nude rat brain. *J. Neurosurg.* 1999, **90**: 125–132.

29. Chishima T, Miyagi Y, Wang X, *et al*. Cancer invasion and micrometastasis visualized in live tissue by green fluorescent protein expression. *Cancer Res.* 1997, **5**: 2042–2047.

30. Gubin AN, Reddy B, Njoroge JM, Miller JL. Long-term stable expression of green fluorescent protein in mammalian cells. *Biochem. Biophys. Res. Comm.* 1997, **262**: 347–350.

31. Fillmore HL, Shurm J, Fuqueron P, *et al*. An in vivo rat model for visualizing glioma tumor cell invasion using stable persistent expression of the green fluorescent protein. *Cancer Lett.* 1999, **141**: 9–19.

32. Ernestus RI, Wilmess LJ, Hoehn-Berlage M. Identification of intracranial liquor metastasis of experimental stereotactically implanted brain tumors by the tumor-selective MRI contrast agent MNTPPS. *Clin. Exp. Metas.* 1992, **10**: 345–350.

33. Haguenau F, Rabotti GF, Lyon G, Moraillon A. Gliomas induced by Rous sarcoma virus in the dog: an ultrastructural study. *J. Natl Cancer Inst.* 1971, **46**: 539–559.

34. Bigner DD, Odom GL, Mahaley MS, *et al*. Brain tumors induced in dogs by the Schmidt–Ruppin strain of Rous sarcoma virus: neuropathological and immunological observations. *J. Neuropathol. Exp. Neurol.* 1969, **28**: 648–680.

35. Tabuchi K, Nushimoto A, Matsumoto K, *et al*. Establishment of a brain tumor model in adult monkeys. *J. Neurosurg.* 1985, **63**: 912–916.

36. Rainov NG, Koch S, Sena-Esteves S, Berens ME. Characterization of a canine glioma cell line as related to established experimental brain tumor models. *J. Neuropathol. Exp. Neurol.* 2000, **59**: 607–613.

37. Zimmerman HM, Arnold H. Experimental brain tumors. I. Tumors produced with methylcholanthrene. *Cancer Res.* 1941, **1**: 919–938.

38. Arnold H, Zimmerman HM. Experimental brain tumors. III. Tumors produced with dibenzanthracene. *Cancer Res.* 1943, **10**: 682–685.

39. Crafts D, Wilson CB. Animal models of brain tumors. *Natl Cancer Inst. Monogr.* 1977, **46**: 11–17.
40. Rubinstein LJ. Correlation of animal brain tumor models with human neuro-oncology. *Natl Cancer Inst. Monogr.* 1977, **46**: 43–49.
41. Zimmerman HM. Brain tumors: their incidence and classification in man and their experimental production. *Ann NY Acad. Sci.* 1969, **159**: 337–359.
42. Druckrey H, Landschütz C, Ivankovic S. Transplacental induction of malignant tumors of the nervous system. II. Ethylnitrosourea in 10 genetically defined strains of rats. *Z. Krebsforsch.* 1970, **73**: 371–386.
43. Druckrey H, Ivankovic S, Preussmann R. Teratogenic and carcinogenic effects in the offspring after a single injection of ethylnitrosourea to pregnant rats. *Nature* 1966, **210**: 1378–1379.
44. Druckrey H. Genotypes and phenotypes of ten inbred strains of BD-rats. *Arzneim-Forsch.* 1971, **21**: 1274–1278.
45. Ivankovic S, Druckrey H. Transplazentare erzeugung maligner Tumoren des Nervensystems. I. Äthyl-nitroso-harnstoff (änh) in BD-ix Ratten. *Z. Krebsforsch.* 1968, **71**: 320–360.
46. Zook BC, Simmens SJ, Jones RV. Evaluation of ENU-induced gliomas in rats: nomenclature, immunohistochemistry, and malignancy. *Toxicol. Pathol.* 2000, **28**: 193–201.
47. Swann PF, Magee PN. Nitrosamine-induced carcinogenesis: the alkylation of N-7 of guanine of nucleic acids of the rat by diethylnitrosamine, N-ethyl-N-nitrosourea and ethyl methanesulphonate. *Biochem J.* 1971, **125**: 841–847.
48. Müller R, Rajewsky MF. Elimination of O-6-ethylguanine from the DNA of brain, liver and other rat tissues exposed to ethylnitrosourea at different stages of prenatal development. *Cancer Res.* 1983, **43**: 2897–2904.
49. Laerum OD, Rajewsky MF. Neoplastic transformation of fetal rat brain cells in culture after exposure to ethylnitrosourea in vivo. *J. Natl Cancer Inst.* 1975, **55**: 1177–1187.
50. Roscoe JP, Claisse PJ. Analysis of N-ethyl-N-nitrosourea-induced brain carcinogenesis by sequential culturing during the latent period. I. Morphology and tumorigenicity of the cultured cells and their growth in agar. *J. Natl Cancer Inst.* 1978, **61**: 381–390.
51. Jang T, Litofsky NS, Smith TS, Ross A, Recht L. Aberrant nestin expression during ethylnitrosourea-(ENU)-induced neurocarcinogenesis. *Neurobiol. Disease* 2004, **15**: 544–552.
52. Rushing EJ, Watson ML, Schold C, Land KJ, Kokkinakis DM. Glial tumors in the MNU rat model: induction of pure and mixed gliomas do not require typical missense mutations of p53. *J. Neuropathol. Exp. Neurol.* 1998, **57**: 1053–1060.
53. Oda H, Zhang Z, Tsurutani N, *et al.* Loss of p53 is an early event in induction of brain tumors in mice by transplacental carcinogen exposure. *Cancer Res.* 1997, **57**: 646–650.
54. Bullard DE, Bigner DD. Animal models and virus induction of tumors. In Thomas DGT, Graham DI (eds.) *Brain Tumors: Scientific Basis, Clinical Investigation, and Current Therapy*. Boston, MA: Butterworths, 1980: pp. 51–84.
55. Copeland DD, Bigner DD. Influence of age at inoculation on avian oncornavirus-induced tumor incidence, tumor morphology, and postinoculation survival in F344 rats. *Cancer Res.* 1977, **37**: 1657–1661.

56. Copeland DD, Bigner DD. The role of the subependymal plate in avian sarcoma virus brain tumor induction: comparison of incipient tumors in neonatal and adult rats. *Acta Neuropathol.* 1977, **38**: 1–6.

57. Mukai N, Kobayashi S. Primary brain and spinal cord tumors induced by human adenovirus type 12 in hamsters. *J. Neuropathol. Exp. Neurol.* 1973, **32**: 523–541.

58. Padgett BL, Walker DL, ZuRhein GM. Jc papovavirus in progressive multifocal leukoencephalopathy. *J. Infect. Dis.* 1976, **133**: 686–690.

59. Padgett BL, Walker DL, ZuRhein GM. Differential neurooncogenicity of strains of JC virus, a human polyoma virus, in newborn Syrian hamsters. *Cancer Res.* 1977, **37**: 718–720.

60. Eddy BE. Simian virus 40 (SV-40): an oncogenic virus. *Prog. Exp. Tumor Res.* 1964, **4**: 1–26.

61. Duffell D, Hinz R, Nelson E. Neoplasms in hamsters induced by simian virus 40: light and electron microscopic observations. *Am. J. Pathol.* 1964, **44**: 59–73.

62. Palmiter RD, Chen HY, Messing A, *et al.* SV40 enhancer and large-T antigen are instrumental in development of choroid plexus tumours in transgenic mice. *Nature* 1985, **316**: 457–460.

63. Marks JR, Lin J, Hinds P, *et al.* Cellular gene expression in papillomas of the choroid plexus from transgenic mice that express the simian virus 40 large T antigen. *J. Virol.* 1989, **63**: 790–797.

64. Brinster RL, Chen HY, Messing A, *et al.* Transgenic mice harboring SV40 t-antigen genes develop characteristic brain tumors. *Cell* 1984, **37**: 367–379.

65. O'Brien JM, Marcus DM, Bernands R, *et al.* Trilateral retinoblastoma in transgenic mice. *Trans. Am. Ophthalmol. Soc.* 1989, **87**: 301–326.

66. Marcus DM, Carpenter JL, O'Brien JM, *et al.* Primitive neuroectodermal tumor of the midbrain in a murine model of retinoblastoma. *Invest. Ophthalmol. Vis. Sci.* 1991, **32**: 293–301.

67. Perraud F, Yoshimura K, Louis B, *et al.* The promoter of the human cystic fibrosis transmembrane conductance regulator gene directing SV40 t antigen expression induces malignant proliferation of ependymal cells in transgenic mice. *Oncogene* 1992, **7**: 993–997.

68. Danks RA, Orian JM, Gonzales MF, *et al.* Transformation of astrocytes in transgenic mice expressing SV40 t antigen under the transcriptional control of the glial fibrillary acidic protein promoter. *Cancer Res.* 1995, **55**: 4302–4310.

69. Uhrbom L, Hesselager G, Nistér M, Westermark B. Induction of brain tumors in mice using a recombinant platelet-derived growth factor B-chain retrovirus. *Cancer Res.* 1998, **58**: 5275–5279.

70. Holland EC, Hively WP, DePinho RA, Varmus HE. A constitutively active epidermal growth factor receptor cooperates with disruption of G_1 cell-cycle arrest pathways to induce glioma-like lesions in mice. *Genes Devel.* 1998, **12**: 3675–3685.

71. Holland EC, Hively WP, Gallo V, Varmus HE. Modeling mutations in the G_1 arrest pathway in human gliomas: overexpression of *cdk4* but not loss of *INK4a-ARF* induces hyperploidy in cultured mouse astrocytes. *Genes Devel.* 1998, **12**: 3644–3649.

72. Ding H, Roncari L, Shannon P, *et al.* Astrocyte-specific expression of activated *p21-ras* results in malignant astrocytoma formation in a transgenic mouse model of human gliomas. *Cancer Res.* 2001, **61**: 3826–3836.

73. Bajenaru ML, Hernandez MR, Perry A, *et al.* Optic nerve glioma in mice requires astrocyte *nf1* gene inactivation and *nf1* brain heterozygosity. *Cancer Res.* 2003, **63**: 8573–8577.

74. Holland EC, Celestino J, Dai CK, *et al*. Combined activation of *ras* and *akt* in neural progenitors induces glioblastoma formation in mice. *Nature Genet.* 2000, **25**: 55–57.
75. Jensen NA, Pedersen KM, Lihme F, *et al*. Astroglial *c-myc* overexpression predisposes mice to primary malignant gliomas. *J. Biol. Chem.* 2003, **278**: 8300–8308.
76. Weissenberger J, Steinbach JP, Malin G, *et al*. Development and malignant progression of astrocytomas in GFAP-v-*src* transgenic mice. *Oncogene* 1997, **14**: 2005–2013.
77. Reilly KM, Loisel DA, Bronson RT, McLaughlin ME, Jacks T. *Nf1/Trp53* mutant mice develop glioblastoma with evidence of strain-specific effects. *Nature Genet.* 2000, **26**: 109–113.
78. Weiss WA, Burns MJ, Hackett C, *et al*. Genetic determinants of malignancy in a mouse model for oligodendroglioma. *Cancer Res.* 2003, **63**: 1589–1595.
79. Ding H, Shannon P, Lau N, *et al*. Oligodendrogliomas result from the expression of an activated mutant epidermal growth factor receptor in a *ras* transgenic mouse astrocytoma model. *Cancer Res.* 2003, **63**: 1106–1113.
80. Dai C, Celestino J, Okada Y, *et al*. PDGF autocrine stimulation dedifferentiates cultured astrocytes and induces oligodendrogliomas and oligoastrocytomas from neural progenitors and astrocytes in vivo. *Genes Devel.* 2001, **15**: 1913–1925.
81. Weiner HL, Bakst R, Hurlbert MS, *et al*. Induction of medulloblastomas in mice by sonic hedgehog, independent of *glii. Cancer Res.* 2002, **62**: 6385–6389.
82. Tong WM, Ohgaki H, Huang H, *et al*. Null mutation of DNA strand break-binding molecule poly(ADP-ribose) polymerase causes medulloblastomas in *p53*(−/−) mice. *Am. J. Pathol.* 2003, **162**: 343–352.
83. Lee Y, McKinnon PJ. DNA ligase IV suppresses medulloblastoma formation. *Cancer Res.* 2002, **62**: 6395–6399.
84. Marino S, Vooijs M, van der Gulden H, Jonkers J, Berns A. Induction of medulloblastomas in *p53*-null mutant mice by somatic inactivation of Rb in the external granular layer cells of the cerebellum. *Genes Devel.* 2000, **14**: 994–1004.
85. Goodrich LV, Milenkovic L, Higgins KM, Scott MP. Altered neural cell fates and medulloblastoma in mouse patched mutants. *Science* 1997, **277**: 1109–1113.
86. Saylors RL, Sidransky D, Friedman HS, *et al*. Infrequent *p53* gene mutations in medulloblastomas. *Cancer Res.* 1991, **51**: 4721–4723.
87. Tada T, Wendland M, Watson N, *et al*. A head holder for magnetic resonance imaging that allows the stereotaxic alignment of spontaneously occurring intracranial mouse tumors. *J. Neurosci. Methods* 2002, **116**: 1–7.
88. Koutcher JA, Hu X, Xu S, *et al*. MRI of mouse models for gliomas shows similarities to humans and can be used to identify mice for preclinical studies. *Neoplasia* 2002, **4**: 480–485.
89. Culver KW, Ram Z, Wallbridge S, *et al*. In vivo gene transfer with retroviral vector-producer cells for treatment of experimental brain tumors. *Science* 1992, **256**: 1550–1552.
90. Xiao A, Wu H, Pandolfi PP, Louis DN, Van Dyke T. Astrocyte inactivation of the PRB pathway predisposes mice to malignant astrocytoma development that is accelerated by *PTEN* mutation. *Cancer Cell* 2002, **1**: 157–168.

23

Experimental models for demyelinating diseases

JASON M. LINK, RICHARD E. JONES, HALINA OFFNER,
AND ARTHUR A. VANDENBARK

23.1 Introduction

Multiple sclerosis (MS) is a demyelinating disease of the central nervous system (CNS) which manifests most commonly as weakness and sensory loss and is characterized by immune-mediated inflammation. Approximately 2.5 million individuals worldwide (400 000 in the USA) are afflicted with MS and among these, the disease is skewed toward Caucasians and females. The resultant economic burden caused by MS in the USA is approximately $20 billion. Superimposed on this cost is the personal burden of living with a debilitating condition for which there is no permanent cure and often no treatment of symptoms. MS is progressive in most patients and within 15 years of diagnosis, 70% of patients are unable to perform normal daily activities without assistance. The most frequently administered treatments (interferon (IFN)-β1a or IFN-β1b) for the most common disease course (relapsing–remitting MS) result in 30% fewer clinical exacerbations and can only delay onset of disability. Thus, researchers in autoimmunity and neurology are in pursuit of new treatments that can effectively and reliably halt or reverse progression of MS.

Establishing potential MS therapies requires an experimental animal model of the disease. The conventional animal model, experimental autoimmune encephalomyelitis (EAE), is a symptomatic and histologic recapitulation of MS based on a presumed etiology of autoimmune-mediated demyelination. In the earliest demonstrations of EAE, it was found that injections of brain or spinal cord extract could cause disease in primates[1] and that addition of an immunological adjuvant eliminated the requirement for repeated injections and decreased the number of days until onset of symptoms.[2] These studies revealed the immunological relevance of the demyelinating disease and this aspect was clearly confirmed when lymphocytes from diseased rats transferred disease.[3] Deductively, it was assumed that anti-self immune responses were

Handbook of Experimental Neurology, ed. Turgut Tatlisumak and Marc Fisher. Published by Cambridge University Press. © Cambridge University Press 2006.

sufficient for inflammation and demyelination in the CNS and could result in manifest neuropathy. Inductively, it was presumed that MS originated through a similar etiology and was mediated by aberrant anti-self responses. Thus, EAE has served as standard model for MS.

In EAE, autoimmunity leads to CNS inflammation that often yields demyelination of axons and results in a neurological condition that is histologically and symptomatically similar to MS. CNS damage in EAE is widely believed to be mediated by $CD4^+$ T cells as these cells are sufficient for the transfer of disease,[4] and eliminating $CD4^+$ populations prevents EAE.[5] Furthermore, dogma dictates that inflammation is mediated by a prevailing $CD4^+$ T helper (Th1) condition that is responsible for the initiation and continuation of EAE and possibly MS. However, this paradigm suffers from oversimplification as mice deficient for the hallmark Th1 cytokine, IFN-γ, are still susceptible to EAE (IFN-γ may even play a protective role)[6] and $CD4^+$ Th2 cells are sufficient for the transfer of disease in some immunocompromised EAE models.[7,8]

Many mammalian species are susceptible to EAE. And although rodent models are more phylogenetically distant from humans than are primates, rats and mice are the most commonly used EAE models. Since the first demonstration of EAE in mice,[9] rodent models have increased in popularity due to rapid breeding, ease of experimentation, available inbred strains, transgenic models, and gene knockout models (especially for mice). Moreover, there is a wealth of data exploring relationships between the encephalitogenicity of CNS-derived proteins and well-characterized mouse strains. This level of reductionism may reveal analogies between specific mouse strain/antigen combinations and particular courses or features of MS. Additionally, experimental mouse models with a well-documented etiology are well suited for testing MS therapies directed against specific causes of demyelination. In this chapter, we will outline the most commonly used models of rodent EAE, the procedures for inducing disease, and the expected outcomes.

The generic method for inducing EAE involves triggering a T cell response against whole spinal cord homogenate, myelin proteins, or synthetic peptides of myelin proteins. In rodents, the basic protocol for reliably inducing EAE involves subcutaneous injection of antigen plus adjuvant that has been homogenized as an oil/water emulsion. Earlier studies in rats and guinea pigs involved injection of the emulsion into the footpads, which produced very strong EAE but also granulomatous inflammation in the footpads. More recent preferred protocols in mice that avoid damage to the footpads involve multiple subcutaneous injections on the back near the base of the tail. The emulsion is a mixture of incomplete Freund's adjuvant (IFA) supplemented with 4 mg/ml heat-killed *Mycobacterium tuberculosis* or *M. butyricum* and the saline peptide solution. There is more than one standard procedure for homogenizing the injection material. Commonly, either a mechanical homogenizer is used or the material is mixed by drawing and withdrawing through a large-bore needle (18-gauge) and glass syringe until a stable emulsion is formed; i.e., a drop of the emulsion does not disperse when placed on an aqueous solution. The syringe extrusion method offers the advantage of homogenizing the oil/water emulsion in less time and is ideal for low volumes. However, it has been reported that lower force in the syringe extrusion method does not create the same type of vesicle/antigen complex. As a result, uptake by antigen-presenting cells at the site of injection may not be as efficient and slightly lower levels of disease incidence may result in some mouse strains.[10] Nonetheless, the syringe extrusion method produces a stable emulsion (does not disperse in an aqueous solution) and is a popular method. In approximately 10–12 days, animals begin to exhibit signs of neurological impairment that manifest first as loss of tail tonicity followed by hindlimb weakness and paralysis that progresses anteriorly. Additional symptoms include ataxia, weight loss, and incontinence.

The onset, severity, and disease course of EAE are quantitated by assigning a daily score to each mouse based on symptoms of paralysis. Scores for mice are usually based on a 5- or 6-point scale ranging from no symptoms (score of 0) to complete paralysis or a moribund condition (score of 6). The onset of disease is typically associated with a limp tail and/or mild hindlimb weakness demonstrated by an inability of the mouse to right itself after being turned on its back (score of 1). Generally within 1 or 2 days, the disease progresses to moderate hindlimb weakness (an awkward gait) and ataxia if present (score of 2), and then moderately severe hindlimb weakness (score of 3). Peak disease after active induction in wild-type animals is often maintained at a score of 3 or 4 (severe hindlimb weakness with legs beginning to drag behind and mild forelimb weakness). EAE can be relatively more severe (e.g., greater peak score, earlier onset) in mice with a progressive course of disease, following passive transfer of encephalitogenic T cell lines, in mice with transgenic T cell receptor (TCR), and in mice that lack regulatory components of the immune system. In these cases, mice might frequently exhibit paraplegia with moderate forelimb weakness (score of 5) or paraplegia with severe forelimb weakness or a moribund condition (score of 6). In addition to disease score, the level of disease can be qualified by histological examination of the spinal cord and/or brain. Even animal models with indistinguishable symptoms can exhibit different patterns of neurological damage, and a complete characterization of disease includes a description of the cause of the overt neurological impairment. Staining methods are available to identify leukocyte infiltration and inflammation, demyelination, and presence of axons.[11] Because histological consequences can be more severe in dorsal and sacral regions of the spinal cord, it is often informative to observe tissue sections procured from the rostral, middle, and caudal regions of spinal cords. And for the purpose of reliably reproducing results, multiple sections should be taken from each spinal cord region and spinal cords should be obtained from several mice.

Because variability in disease symptoms and course is beyond control even within a group of inbred mice receiving identical immunizations, it is important to use appropriate statistical measures when gauging treatment efficacies. For a typical EAE experiment in which one group of mice is given treatment and another is given only the vehicle, the type of statistical test to be used is dependent on the outcome being measured. If the values are based on a rating scale (e.g., EAE disease score) then the points on the scale are not equally spaced, and thus the scale is not an equal interval scale but rather it is an ordinal scale (similar to MS clinical scores measured by expanded disability status scale (EDSS) or ambulation index (AI)). Additionally, the distribution of data from disease scores is not reliably Gaussian; i.e., there is not a normal distribution of the data over an extended range, especially if data from one of the groups lies close to the bottom or top of the scale. Since parametric tests like the *t*-test require both an equal interval scale and a normal distribution, these tests are not appropriate for comparisons of disease scores between two groups; rather these types of analyses require tests for non-parametric data such as the Mann–Whitney or Kruskal–Wallis tests, used to compare mean daily or cumulative disease scores between two or more treatment groups, respectively. However, some features of disease course are measured on an equal interval scale and have a near-Gaussian distribution (e.g., day of onset and day of peak score) and comparisons of these features should be made using an unpaired *t*-test or multiple comparison tests such as the Bonferroni, Student–Neumann–Keuls, or Dunnetts. Categorical disease measurements such as disease incidence or death should be compared with the χ^2 or Fisher's exact test.

23.2 Models of disease

Although the general phenomenon of antigen-induced EAE is consistent across a range of experimental species, there is variation in the disease course that is dependent on which animal and which myelin antigen is used. Furthermore, there is inherent biological variation in EAE models that can result in a large standard deviation of clinical scores. Although this variation in

EAE helps to align it with the unpredictable and individual-specific course of MS, natural variation can make statistically significant demonstrations of treatment difficult. Thus, researchers should expect a range in severity of symptoms, time to onset, and incidence of disease despite the use of inbred strains. And the numbers of mice to be used for experimental and control groups should reflect this expected variation.

Because of the availability of inbred strains, rats and mice have served as by far the most popular model for EAE. And in most cases, there are more experimental advantages to using mice for which myriad gene deficient and transgenic strains are available. For both rats and mice, the most commonly used encephalitogenic myelin proteins are myelin basic protein (MBP), proteolipid protein (PLP), and myelin oligodendrocyte protein (MOG). Within these proteins, epitopes exist against which T cells can be stimulated to respond and subsequently elicit inflammatory reactions in the CNS. For these dominant epitopes T cell reactivity is either not eliminated during central tolerance in the thymus or peripheral tolerance mechanisms are overwhelmed by the immunization. In most cases, the dominant epitopes that alone are sufficient for disease induction are also the major reactive epitopes when animals are immunized with whole myelin protein. Table 23.1 and the following text list the most common rat and mouse models of EAE and indicate the inciting antigens and the expected disease course.

In rats, MBP was the first major encephalitogenic myelin protein identified[12–14] and both rat and guinea pig, but not bovine, MBP were found to be sufficient to induce disease in Lewis rats. Fractionation of MBP by limited pepsin cleavage demonstrated that the encephalitogenicity was limited to only finite regions of the protein[15] and the most encephalitogenic synthetic peptides in Lewis rats were found to be amino acids 68–86 and 87–99 for both Lewis and Buffalo rats.[16,17] The most commonly used mouse strains that are susceptible to MBP-induced EAE are B10.PL, PL/J, and SJL. However, the encephalitogenic peptides differ among these mouse strains due to differences in MHC II genes. B10.PL and PL/J are most susceptible to an acetylated N-terminal peptide (1–11), whereas SJL/J are susceptible to an encephalitogenic peptide in the mid region of MBP (i.e., 87–99).[18] The difference in response is due to which MBP peptides are capable of presentation by the endogenous major histocompatibility complex (MHC) class II molecules (B10.PL and PL/J mice bear $H-2^u$ and SJL/J mice bear $H-2^s$).[19]

Although early evidence indicated that PLP was a major CNS encephalitogenic protein of the CNS, well-purified PLP (in the absence of MBP contamination) was not demonstrated as an encephalitogen in Lewis rats until 1986 when 100 µg of purified protein + complete Freund's adjuvant (CFA) was

Table 23.1. *Major models for experimental autoimmune encephalomyelitis*

Mouse or rat strain	Encephalitogenic peptide	Method of disease induction and immunization[a]	Disease course	Requires pertussis toxin?
Lewis and Buffalo rats	MBP-68-86, MBP-87-99	Active, s.c., and passive	Monophasic	No
SJL/J	PLP-139-151, MOG-92-106	Active, s.c., and passive	Relapsing	No
SJL/J × C57Bl/6	MOG-35-55	Active, s.c., and passive	Relapsing	No
SJL/L × PL/J	PLP-139-151, PLP-43-64	Active, s.c., and passive	Relapsing	No
SJL/J × B10.PL	MBP-AC-1-11	Active, s.c., and passive	Relapsing	No
B10.PL	MBP-Ac-1-11	Active, s.c., and passive	Chronic	Yes
C57Bl/6	MOG-35-55	Active, s.c.; passive disease may require antibody transfer	Chronic	Yes
PL/J	MBP-Ac-1-11, PLP-43-64, MOG-35-55	Active, s.c., and passive	Relapsing (MOG-35-55)	Yes
MBP-85-99 TCR transgene (C57Bl/6)	MBP-85-99	No immunization required if mice are RAG-deficient	Chronic	No
MBP-1-11 TCR transgene (B10.PL)	MBP-1-11	No immunization required if mice are RAG-deficient and exposed to environmental antigens	Chronic	No
Lewis rats	MBP	High dose, i.v.	Tolerance to disease	No
MBP-1-11 TCR transgene	MBP-1-11 or spontaneous	Epicutaneous	Tolerance to disease	No
Lewis rats	MBP	Oral	Tolerance to disease	No

[a] i.v.,N intravenous; s.c., subcutaneous.

shown to induce a transient disease similar to MBP-induced EAE.[20] PLP is not readily water-soluble as it is a highly hydrophobic membrane protein and thus the use of encephalitogenic peptides is important in PLP-mediated disease. The major epitope in rats has been described as an N-terminal peptide from 217–240 but the peptide requires N-terminal acetylation in order to be encephalitogenic.[21] PLP was also shown to cause severe EAE in SJL mice, but PLP-induced disease was much less pronounced in other strains.[22] The major epitope[23] for the SJL model is PLP 139–151 and a commonly used variant contains a C140 S substitution to avoid disulfide bond formation.[24] Additionally, SJL mice can mount lymph node responses against other PLP peptides (e.g., PLP 103–116).[25] Currently, the most popular mouse models for actively induced disease involving PLP peptides are PLP 43–64 in PL/J mice and PLP 139–151 in SJL mice; F_1 mice (PLXSJL) are susceptible to both peptides.[26] Additionally, PLP epitopes clustering within three other regions of PLP (40–70, 100–119, and 178–209) have been described as encephalitogenic in mice of various MHC (I-A) haplotypes.[27]

MBP and PLP make up the majority of the mass of myelin (30% and 50%, respectively). Yet, responses against the MOG protein, only a fraction of the mass of myelin, are still sufficient to induce EAE and T cells specific for this protein are readily detectable in the peripheral blood of MS patients perhaps at even higher frequency than T cells specific for PLP and MBP.[28] Thus, the quantity of a myelin protein in the CNS is not directly, and may be inversely, proportional to its propensity to be targeted in MS and EAE. But, as it has been relatively recently identified, MOG responses have not been as comprehensively studied as those of PLP and MBP. Nonetheless, encephalitogenic responses against MOG protein and peptides have been demonstrated in rats and mice. Lewis rats exhibit a relapsing–remitting and demyelinating disease when immunized with either a peptide or recombinant protein of MOG,[24] thereby paralleling a common MS disease course. Interestingly, anti-MOG antibodies might play a major role in MOG-induced EAE and possibly MS since transfer of anti-MOG antibodies exacerbates EAE in Lewis rats.[29] MOG also causes both clinical and histological EAE in AB/H mice and SJL mice. In AB/H mice, several MOG epitopes are sufficient for disease (1–22, 43–57, and 134–148) whereas in SJL mice only one epitope is known to be encephalitogenic (92–106).[30] The MOG 35–55 peptide is encephalitogenic in PL/J mice and C57Bl/6 mice[28,31] and C57Bl/6 mice offer the advantage of a chronic, progressive form of EAE induced by MOG immunization and no reliance on antibodies for MOG-35–55 induced disease.[32]

23.3 Heterologous and homologous CNS proteins can both
induce disease

The requirements for immune-mediated demyelination require an anti-self
response targeted against myelin. Thus, immunization with a self protein is in
most cases the ideal method for generating such a response. However, the
major epitopes of myelin proteins that induce disease can be identical among
many species and thus synthetic peptides designed from several species
can induce equivalent disease. Moreover, epitopes from xenogeneic myelin
proteins, by chance, can be more adept at triggering T cell responses than
the autologous epitope, and due to cross-reactivity, the activated T cells
respond to the self epitope. For example, a form of hyperacute EAE is
induced in the Lewis rat by guinea pig (gp)MBP, whereas the self rat protein
results in a much less severe disease.[33] And in fact, gpMBP is highly encephalitogenic in many species including SJL mice.[34] Furthermore, rat, human,
and bovine MBP peptides have all been found to be encephalitogenic in
SJL mice.[8]

23.4 Relapsing models

Because of poorly traceable etiology there is no predictive test for MS and
diagnosis is dependent only on clinical observation of myriad disease courses
and magnetic resonance imaging (MRI) detection of new or active CNS
lesions. But since the EAE model can be adjusted to yield specific outcomes
(e.g., relapsing, chronic, etc.) researchers have the advantage of aligning causes
and matching treatments to a particular disease course.[35] The most popular
and reliable model for relapsing and remitting EAE (a common MS course)
results from PLP (or PLP 139–151) immunization of SJL mice or transfer of a
PLP 139–151 specific T cell line.[25,36] In this model, remission is defined as
a reduction from previous disease score for a period of at least 2 days and a
relapse is defined as an increase in clinical score (by at least a score of 1) for at
least 2 consecutive days following a remission period. Relapsing disease has
also been reliably produced in F_1 models, and these mixed-background mice
offer the advantage of retaining susceptibility to a desired myelin protein while
gaining the relapsing course. Relapsing models can be induced with both MBP
in SJL × PL/J mice[37] and with MOG in C57Bl/6 × SJL mice.[38] In rats, EAE is
typically acute and monophasic with onset at approximately days 10–14 and
recovery occurring after an additional 7–10 days.[39] However, a chronic,
relapsing disease has been induced in Lewis rats when they are given high
doses of gpMBP.[40]

23.5 Immunization site and adjuvants can modulate EAE

In addition to the specific myelin protein or peptide used as antigen, the outcomes of EAE are dependent on the makeup of the homogenized immunogen, in particular the adjuvant. The dose of myelin antigen does not play a major role in altering EAE and the standard dose of protein or peptide (100–200 μg) is likely greater than necessary, especially in rats where much lower doses (5–25 μg) are sufficient for disease induction and even lower doses of gpMBP can cause disease in rats and guinea pigs.[29,41] In contrast, the dose of heat-inactivated *Mycobacterium tuberculosis* (Mtb) in CFA is critically linked to disease outcome,[42] and doses of 400 μg of Mtb per animal are routinely administered. The requirements for CFA are the likely result of innate immune responses to pathogen associated molecular patterns (PAMPs) from the inactivated bacteria.[43] These innate responses are required to induce and guide specific adaptive immune responses. Surprisingly, pretreatment with CFA prevents future active induction of EAE[44] and additionally, immunization in the absence of innate immune signals from CFA can result in tolerance to the myelin antigen.[38,45] Thus, eliciting successive disease courses in the same animal presents a technical challenge.

Pertussis toxin (Ptx) from *Bordetella pertussis* was discovered as an adjuvant that augments the immune response to myelin proteins.[29,46] But evidence that Ptx increases vascular permeability of the blood–brain barrier provided an attractive explanation for the mechanism by which Ptx affects EAE; i.e., pathogenic, myelin-specific T cells can more readily engage the CNS.[47] This concept is still a popular rationale for the use of Ptx in EAE, but is contentious. More recent evidence indicates that the prominent role of Ptx in EAE is as it was originally used: as an adjuvant. In fact, most EAE models do not require Ptx in order to exhibit clinical disease, although time to onset may be longer and disease scores may be lower in the absence of Ptx.[48] Ptx is a G-protein inhibitor that directly alters leukocyte trafficking and can activate antigen-presenting cells. And as a result of its adjuvanticity, Ptx can substitute for CFA and elicit EAE of a typical severity and course. Moreover, Ptx can reverse the tolerance that is caused by injection of myelin antigens with IFA.[49] Despite the fact that EAE is not dependent on Ptx, making use of its adjuvanticity has become orthodox for many researchers and it is commonly included in EAE protocols especially in strains that are relatively resistant to disease. The exact protocol ranges from administering anywhere from 50 ng to 400 ng either given once or twice during or shortly after the immunization (e.g., 75 ng on the same day as immunization and 200 ng 2 days after immunization).

Ptx is effective when administered subcutaneously, intravenously, and intraperitoneally.

By far the most common route for immunization of myelin protein or peptides is subcutaneous. Mice and rats are usually immunized at more than one site (two to four) on the flank, or for rats, on the footpad (although footpad injections have raised serious animal welfare concerns and many institutions prohibit this method). Intramuscular injections are also sufficient for induction of EAE,[2] but many other routes can result in tolerance to the myelin antigen and protection from disease. Soluble myelin antigens can prevent or treat disease when administered either intravenously,[38] orally,[50] intraperitoneally,[51,52] or intrathymically.[53] Researchers should take caution with the subcutaneous route as epicutaneous injections[54] and high doses of antigen administered intravenously[38] have both been shown to tolerize animals against EAE.

23.6 Passive transfer of disease

In addition to inducing EAE by active immunization with myelin antigens and adjuvant, disease can be transferred by obtaining myelin specific T cells that have been appropriately stimulated, and transferring these cells to a susceptible, syngeneic recipient. In general, donor mice are immunized with whole spinal cord or a desired myelin antigen or peptide and at least 7 days later spleen or lymph node cells are restimulated in vitro and transferred to recipients. Passive (also termed adoptive) induction of EAE by cell transfer grants the researcher several advantages. Firstly, the time between induction and onset is shorter than active disease. Secondly, encephalitogenic T cell lines and clones can be expanded and preserved for future use ensuring that many recipients can be given nearly identical transfers and eliminating some of the variability inherent in active induction of disease. And thirdly, the effector functions of EAE can be studied in the absence of requirements for initiating pathogenic antigen specific cells in vivo (e.g., adjuvant).

The first transfers of disease in rats by either parabiosis[55] or injection of lymph node cells[3] resulted in relatively low incidence of disease. But this procedure was improved by eliminating suppression in recipients through irradiation,[56] and in vitro conditioning of T cells with the myelin antigen used in the donors and/or the T cell mitogen ConA. Importantly, passive transfer in Lewis rats produces transient EAE but the recovered rats, unlike in actively induced disease, are still susceptible to both active and passive EAE induction.[57] EAE is augmented and lower numbers of cells are required for disease when T cell lines are created through repeated stimulation with antigen and syngeneic antigen presenting cells.[58] In rats, potent T cell lines specific for gpMBP can transfer disease using as few as 0.1×10^6 cells and can transfer lethal disease with only 1×10^6 cells.[59] However, the number of transferred T cells required to induce EAE differs for each cell line generated and it is necessary for each researcher to titrate an appropriate dose after generating a new T cell line.

In mice, the antigens used to stimulate donor cells are typically the same antigens that can reliably induce active EAE, but occasionally modifications are made to the transfer protocol to produce more potent cell lines.[60] The specific outcome of EAE from passive transfer also matches that achieved by actively induced disease indicating that the discrete specificity for myelin controls the specific neurological impairment. For example, mice susceptible to actively induced relapsing–remitting disease also exhibit the disease course upon passive transfer.[61] However, there are exceptions in which EAE cannot be actively induced with a particular antigen, but T cells specific for the antigen can be generated and passively transfer disease, as is the case for MBP-specific cells in C57Bl/6 mice.[62] In contrast, there are also exceptions where passive transfer is not sufficient to elicit the same EAE symptoms that are induced with active immunization, such as with the dependency on B cells for MOG-induced disease in both rats and mice.[29,63]

23.7 Transgenic models

Different responses in mouse strains are often a function of different MHC backgrounds, and as an effect have differing abilities to process and present myelin peptides. It is well established that differences in myelin peptide encephalitogenicity and disease course are often a function of the MHC haplotype that is linked to the inbred strain.[25] And since variations in the manifestation of T cell-mediated disease in EAE depend largely on the genetic background, it is a reasonable expectation that individual disease patterns in MS patients would also vary accordingly. Thus, it is not surprising that the polygenic MHC combinations in an outbred human population yield a plethora of disease courses. But, investigating mouse models with transgenic MHC expression eliminates much of this variation, and mice expressing only human MHC (human leukocyte antigen, HLA) can be an excellent model for specific MS conditions. Moreover, mice expressing human MHC are optimal indicators of therapy that may successfully treat MS.

A number of genetic markers have been found to be associated with susceptibility to MS, including HLA alleles and TCR polymorphisms. Among these, the HLA–DR2 haplotype including the DRB1*1501 and DRB5*0101 alleles, confers the highest relative risk for Caucasian MS patients of Northern

European descent.[64] Mice expressing HLA-DR2 and no mouse MHC class II develop chronic symptoms of EAE and T cell infiltration into the CNS upon immunization with the myelin peptide MOG-35–55.[60] This disease course parallels the non-self-limiting MS disease process in HLA-DR2[+] MS patients. HLA transgenic mice are an excellent research tool for identifying MHC-binding epitopes of myelin proteins that may contribute to MS in humans as well as identifying therapies that can target T cells which bind these epitopes.

Although MHC is thought to play a major role in EAE, some differences in disease induction are dependent on the TCR repertoire. For instance, MBP does not induce disease in C57Bl/6 mice even when these mice express an MHC transgene known to present an encephalitogenic MBP epitope (85–99).[60,65] However, the insertion of a TCR transgene with specificity for the MBP-85–99 epitope allows susceptibility to EAE.[66,67] Thus, EAE is also dependent on the availability of appropriate genes in the TCR germline repertoire and it follows that mice expressing TCR transgenes with specificity for myelin encephalito-genic epitopes are excellent models for understanding pathology associated with different types of demyelination. In order to produce more etiologically simple models for disease and as proof of the principle that T cell specificity is a major factor in EAE, several groups have developed myelin peptide specific TCR transgenic mice.[67–70] Furthermore, by eliminating endogenous expression of TCR (and thus regulatory T cell populations) mouse models now exist wherein EAE develops spontaneously[67,68] (as it does with MS) and the factors that are causative of spontaneous EAE can now be investigated. In contrast to active and adoptive disease models that are used to study post-immunization disease etiology and pathophysiology, models of spontaneous disease (that do not require antigen sensitization) can be used to elucidate preimmunization mechanisms of disease.

In addition to spontaneous EAE in transgenic TCR mice, adoptive transfer methods utilizing transplanted hematopoietic cells and T cells in C.B-17 *scid/scid* mice[71] have revealed prepathogenic changes in the CNS associated with enhanced susceptibility to disease induction.[72,73] As an example, preinjection of activated T cells specific for non-myelin antigens into C.B-17 *scid/scid* mice results in their migration into the CNS where they promote recruitment of antigen-presenting cells from the circulation. Subsequent injection of myelin reactive T lymphocytes after such preconditioning causes more severe EAE, clearly implicating non-myelin-reactive T cells and antigen-presenting cells as important factors that control clinical severity and formation of new lesions at disease onset or during established disease.

The requirements for disease induction that are constant across strain and species barriers (providing a connection between EAE and MS) have been evaluated in allogeneic and xenogeneic transfers of T cells into C.B-17 *scid/scid* immunodeficient mice. In these types of experiments, transplanted hematopoietic cells are typically necessary to provide a source of syngeneic antigenpresenting cells in the CNS for presentation of antigen to transplanted allogeneic or xenogeneic T cells. Thus, SJL mouse (H-2^s) T cells and hematopoietic-derived cells induced EAE in allogeneic C.B-17 *scid/scid* (H-2^d) mice; and rat T cells and hematopoietic-derived cells (RT-1^l) were also capable of inducing disease in C.B-17 *scid/scid* mice.[74] Adoptive transfer of human cells from MS patients has been attempted with inconsistent results. Thus, it remains to be determined whether and under what conditions it might be possible to utilize adoptive transfers of human T cells in immunodeficient mice as an approach for examining pathogenic mechanisms mediated by human cells. If possible, such an in vivo experimental approach may be potentially valuable for testing treatments directed against disease-inducing human cells.

23.8 Summary

Over the last 80 years, EAE animal models have solidified the paradigm of autoimmunity as the principal cause of MS. In turn, these animal models have been used to investigate the etiology of autoimmunity and to test potential treatments. Currently, the most widely used treatments involve general immunosuppression. In addition to suboptimal efficacy, these treatments have myriad side effects including the attenuation of natural immune regulatory systems. However, the development of EAE models with more precise causation (e.g., inbred mouse strains, single myelin peptide reactivity, and designed TCR and MHC transgenes) have created highly relevant models in which to test disease component specific therapies. If successful, more specific therapies and perhaps therapies that can be tailored to individual patients will limit side effects and plausibly be of greater potency. Thus, the persistent investigation of well-refined animal models of EAE will allow further focus on and discovery of specific pathways and cell types that can be targeted for treatment of multiple sclerosis.

References

1. Rivers TM, Sprunt DH, Berry GP. Observations on attempts to produce acute disseminated encephalomyelitis in monkeys. *J. Exp. Med.* 1933, **58**: 39–53.
2. Kabat EA, Wolf A, Bezer AE. The rapid production of acute disseminated encephalomyelitis in rhesus monkeys by injection of heterologous and homologous brain tissue with adjuvants. *J. Exp. Med.* 1947, **85**: 117–130.

3. Paterson PY. Transfer of allergic encephalomyelitis in rats by means of lymph node cells. *J. Exp. Med.* 1960, **111**: 119–136.
4. Pettinelli CB, McFarlin DE. Adoptive transfer of experimental allergic encephalomyelitis in SJL/J mice after in vitro activation of lymph node cells by myelin basic protein: requirement for Lyt 1+ 2- T lymphocytes. *J. Immunol.* 1981, **127**: 1420–1423.
5. Waldor MK., *et al.* Reversal of experimental allergic encephalomyelitis with monoclonal antibody to a T-cell subset marker. *Science* 1985, **227**: 415–417.
6. Krakowski M, Owens T. Interferon-gamma confers resistance to experimental allergic encephalomyelitis. *Eur. J. Immunol.* 1996, **26**: 1641–1646.
7. Lafaille JJ, *et al.* Myelin basic protein-specific T helper 2 (Th2) cells cause experimental autoimmune encephalomyelitis in immunodeficient hosts rather than protect them from the disease. *J. Exp. Med.* 1997, **186**: 307–312.
8. Genain CP, *et al.* Late complications of immune deviation therapy in a nonhuman primate. *Science* 1996, **274**: 2054–2057.
9. Olitsky PK, Yager RH. Experimental disseminated encephalomyelitis in white mice. *J. Exp. Med.* 1949, **90**: 213–224.
10. Fillmore PD, *et al.* Genetic analysis of the influence of neuroantigen–complete Freund's adjuvant emulsion structures on the sexual dimorphism and susceptibility to experimental allergic encephalomyelitis. *Am. J. Pathol.* 2003, **163**: 1623–1632.
11. Dal Canto MC, *et al.* Two models of multiple sclerosis: experimental allergic encephalomyelitis (EAE) and Theiler's murine encephalomyelitis virus (TMEV) infection – a pathological and immunological comparison. *Microsc. Res. Tech.* 1995, **32**: 215–229.
12. Eylar EH, *et al.* Experimental allergic encephalomyelitis: an encephalitogenic basic protein from bovine myelin. *Arch. Biochem. Biophys.* 1969, **132**: 34–48.
13. Kies MW, Thompson EB, Alvord Jr EC. The relationship of myelin proteins to experimental allergic encephalomyelitis. *Ann. NY Acad. Sci.* 1965, **122**: 148–160.
14. Paterson PY ed. *Textbook of Immunopathology.* Experimental autoimmune (allergic) encephalomyelitis: induction, pathogenesis, and suppression. In Miescher PA, Muller-Eberhard HJ (eds.) *Textbook of Immunopathology,* vol. 1. New York: Gruene and Straton, 1976, pp. 179–213.
15. Martenson RE, Levine S, Sowindki R. The location of regions in guinea pig and bovine myelin basic proteins which induce experimental allergic encephalo- myelitis in Lewis rats. *J. Immunol.* 1975, **114**: 592–596.
16. Mannie MD, *et al.* Induction of experimental allergic encephalomyelitis in Lewis rats with purified synthetic peptides: delineation of antigenic determinants for encephalitogenicity, in vitro activation of cellular transfer, and proliferation of lymphocytes. *Proc. Natl Acad. Sci. USA* 1985, **82**: 5515–5519.
17. Jones RE, *et al.* The synthetic 87–99 peptide of myelin basic protein is encephalitogenic in Buffalo rats. *J. Neuroimmunol.* 1992, **37**: 203–212.
18. Kuchroo VK, *et al.* A single TCR antagonist peptide inhibits experimental allergic encephalomyelitis mediated by a diverse T cell repertoire. *J. Immunol.* 1994, **153**: 3326–3336.
19. Fritz RB, *et al.* Major histocompatibility complex-linked control of the murine immune response to myelin basic protein. *J. Immunol.* 1985, **134**: 2328–2332.
20. Yamamura T, *et al.* Experimental allergic encephalomyelitis induced by proteolipid apoprotein in Lewis rats. *J. Neuroimmunol.* 1986, **12**: 143–153.

21. Zhao W, *et al*. Identification of an N-terminally acetylated encephalitogenic epitope in myelin proteolipid apoprotein for the Lewis rat. *J. Immunol*. 1994, **153**: 901–909.

22. Tuohy VK, Sobel RA, Lees MB. Myelin proteolipid protein-induced experimental allergic encephalomyelitis: variations of disease expression in different strains of mice. *J. Immunol*. 1988, **140**: 1868–1873.

23. Tuohy VK, *et al*. Identification of an encephalitogenic determinant of myelin proteolipid protein for SJL mice. *J. Immunol*. 1989, **142**: 1523–1527.

24. Johns TG, *et al*. Myelin oligodendrocyte glycoprotein induces a demyelinating encephalomyelitis resembling multiple sclerosis. *J. Immunol*. 1995, **154**: 5536–5541.

25. Tuohy VK, *et al*. A synthetic peptide from myelin proteolipid protein induces experimental allergic encephalomyelitis. *J. Immunol*. 1988, **141**: 1126–1130.

26. Whitham RH, *et al*. Location of a new encephalitogenic epitope (residues 43 to 64) in proteolipid protein that induces relapsing experimental autoimmune encephalomyelitis in PL/J and (SJL × PL) F_1 mice. *J. Immunol*. 1991, **147**: 3803–3808.

27. Greer JM, *et al*. Immunogenic and encephalitogenic epitope clusters of myelin proteolipid protein. *J. Immunol*. 1996, **156**: 371–379.

28. Mendel I, Kerlero de Rosbo N, Ben-Nun A. A myelin oligodendrocyte glycoprotein peptide induces typical chronic experimental autoimmune encephalomyelitis in H-2b mice: fine specificity and T cell receptor V beta expression of encephalitogenic T cells. *Eur. J. Immunol*. 1995, **25**: 1951–1959.

29. Lennon VA, *et al*. Antigen, host and adjuvant requirements for induction of hyperacute experimental autoimmune encephalomyelitis. *Eur. J. Immunol*. 1976, **6**: 805–810.

30. Amor S, *et al*. Identification of epitopes of myelin oligodendrocyte glycoprotein for the induction of experimental allergic encephalomyelitis in SJL and Biozzi AB/H mice. *J. Immunol*. 1994, **153**: 4349–4356.

31. Kerlero de Rosbo N, Mendel I, Ben-Nun A. Chronic relapsing experimental autoimmune encephalomyelitis with a delayed onset and an atypical clinical course, induced in PL/J mice by myelin oligodendrocyte glycoprotein (MOG)-derived peptide: preliminary analysis of MOG T cell epitopes. *Eur. J. Immunol*. 1995, **25**: 985–993.

32. Zhang GX, *et al*. T cell and antibody responses in remitting–relapsing experimental autoimmune encephalomyelitis in (C57BL/6 × SJL) F_1 mice. *J. Neuroimmunol*. 2004, **148**: 1–10.

33. Skundric DS, *et al*. Distinct immune regulation of the response to H-2^b restricted epitope of MOG causes relapsing–remitting EAE in H-2$^{b/s}$ mice. *J. Neuroimmunol*. 2003, **136**: 34–45.

34. Pettinelli CB, *et al*. Encephalitogenic activity of guinea pig myelin basic protein in the SJL mouse. *J. Immunol*. 1982, **129**: 1209–1211.

35. Lublin FD. Relapsing experimental allergic encephalomyelitis: an autoimmune model of multiple sclerosis. *Springer Semin. Immunopathol*. 1985, **8**: 197–208.

36. Whitham RH, *et al*. Lymphocytes from SJL/J mice immunized with spinal cord respond selectively to a peptide of proteolipid protein and transfer relapsing demyelinating experimental autoimmune encephalomyelitis. *J. Immunol*. 1991, **146**: 101–107.

37. Fritz RB, Chou CH, McFarlin DE. Relapsing murine experimental allergic encephalomyelitis induced by myelin basic protein. *J. Immunol.* 1983, **130**: 1024–1026.

38. Swierkosz JE, Swanborg RH. Immunoregulation of experimental allergic encephalomyelitis: conditions for induction of suppressor cells and analysis of mechanism. *J. Immunol.* 1977, **119**: 1501–1506.

39. Paterson PY, *et al.* Immunologic determinants of experimental neurologic autoimmune disease and approaches to the multiple sclerosis problem. *Trans. Am. Clin. Climatol. Ass.* 1977, **89**: 109–118.

40. Feurer C, Prentice DE, Cammisuli S. Chronic relapsing experimental allergic encephalomyelitis in the Lewis rat. *J. Neuroimmunol.* 1985, **10**: 159–166.

41. McFarlin DE, *et al.* Experimental allergic encephalomyelitis in the rat: response to encephalitogenic proteins and peptides. *Science* 1973, **179**: 478–480.

42. Keith AB, McDermott JR. Optimum conditions for inducing chronic relapsing experimental allergic encephalomyelitis in guinea pigs. *J. Neurol. Sci.* 1980, **46**: 353–364.

43. Medzhitov R, Preston-Hurlburt P, Janeway Jr CA. A human homologue of the *Drosophila* Toll protein signals activation of adaptive immunity. *Nature* 1997, **388**: 394–397.

44. Hempel K, *et al.* Unresponsiveness to experimental allergic encephalomyelitis in Lewis rats pretreated with complete Freund's adjuvant. *Int. Arch. Allergy Appl. Immunol.* 1985, **76**: 193–199.

45. Heeger PS, *et al.* Revisiting tolerance induced by autoantigen in incomplete Freund's adjuvant. *J. Immunol.* 2000, **164**: 5771–5781.

46. Pitts OM, Varitek VA, Day ED. The antibody responses to myelin basic protein (BP) in Lewis rats: the effects of *Bordetella pertussis*. *J. Immunol.* 1975, **115**: 1114–1116.

47. Linthicum DS, Munoz JJ, Blaskett A. Acute experimental autoimmune encephalomyelitis in mice. I. Adjuvant action of *Bordetella pertussis* is due to vasoactive amine sensitization and increased vascular permeability of the central nervous system. *Cell Immunol.* 1982, **73**: 299–310.

48. Munoz JJ, Mackay IR. Adoptive transfer of experimental allergic encephalomyelitis in mice with the aid of pertussigen from *Bordetella pertussis*. *Cell Immunol.* 1984, **86**: 541–545.

49. Hofstetter HH, Shive CL, Forsthuber TG. Pertussis toxin modulates the immune response to neuroantigens injected in incomplete Freund's adjuvant: induction of Th1 cells and experimental autoimmune encephalomyelitis in the presence of high frequencies of Th2 cells. *J. Immunol.* 2002, **169**: 117–125.

50. Bitar DM, Whitacre CC. Suppression of experimental autoimmune encephalomyelitis by the oral administration of myelin basic protein. *Cell. Immunol.* 1988, **112**: 364–370.

51. Gaur A, *et al.* Amelioration of autoimmune encephalomyelitis by myelin basic protein synthetic peptide-induced anergy. *Science* 1992, **258**: 1491–1494.

52. Rivero VE, *et al.* Suppression of experimental autoimmune encephalomyelitis (EAE) by intraperitoneal administration of soluble myelin antigens in Wistar rats. *J. Neuroimmunol.* 1997, **72**: 3–10.

53. Goss JA, *et al.* Immunological tolerance to a defined myelin basic protein antigen administered intrathymically. *J. Immunol.* 1994, **153**: 3890–3898.

54. Bynoe MS, *et al*. Epicutaneous immunization with autoantigenic peptides induces T suppressor cells that prevent experimental allergic encephalomyelitis. *Immunity*. 2003, **19**: 317–328.

55. Lipton MMF, J., The transfer of experimental allergic encephalomyelitis in the rat by means of parabiosis. *J. Immunol*. 1953, **71**: 380–384.

56. Paterson PY, Richarson WP, Drobish DG. Cellular transfer of experimental allergic encephalomyelitis: altered disease pattern in irradiated recipient Lewis rats. *Cell Immunol*. 1975, **16**: 48–59.

57. Hinrichs DJ, Roberts CM, Waxman FJ. Regulation of paralytic experimental allergic encephalomyelitis in rats: susceptibility to active and passive disease reinduction. *J. Immunol*. 1981, **126**: 1857–1862.

58. Ben-Nun A, Wekerle H, Cohen IR. The rapid isolation of clonable antigen-specific T lymphocyte lines capable of mediating autoimmune encephalomyelitis. *Eur. J. Immunol*. 1981, **11**: 195–199.

59. Vandenbark AA, Gill T, Offner H. A myelin basic protein-specific T lymphocyte line that mediates experimental autoimmune encephalomyelitis. *J. Immunol*. 1985, **135**: 223–228.

60. Rich C, *et al*. Myelin oligodendrocyte glycoprotein-35–55 peptide induces severe chronic experimental autoimmune encephalomyelitis in HLA-DR2 transgenic mice. *Eur. J. Immunol*. 2004, **34**: 1251–1261.

61. Richert JR, *et al*. Myelin basic protein-specific T cell lines and clones derived from SJL/J mice with experimental allergic encephalomyelitis. *J. Neuroimmunol*. 1985, **8**: 129–139.

62. Shaw MK, *et al*. A combination of adoptive transfer and antigenic challenge induces consistent murine experimental autoimmune encephalomyelitis in C57BL/6 mice and other reputed resistant strains. *J. Neuroimmunol*. 1992, **39**: 139–149.

63. Trotter J, *et al*. Characterization of T cell lines and clones from SJL/J and (BALB/c × SJL/J)F1 mice specific for myelin basic protein. *J. Immunol*. 1985, **134**: 2322–2327.

64. Ghabanbasani MZ, *et al*. Importance of HLA-DRB1 and DQA1 genes and of the amino acid polymorphisms in the functional domain of DR beta 1 chain in multiple sclerosis. *J. Neuroimmunol*. 1995, **59**: 77–82.

65. Bernard CC. Experimental autoimmune encephalomyelitis in mice: genetic control of susceptibility. *J. Immunogenet*. 1976, **3**: 263–274.

66. Ellmerich S, *et al*. Disease-related epitope spread in a humanized T cell receptor transgenic model of multiple sclerosis. *Eur. J. Immunol*. 2004, **34**: 1839–1848.

67. Madsen LS, *et al*. A humanized model for multiple sclerosis using HLA-DR2 and a human T-cell receptor. *Nature Genet*. 1999, **23**: 343–347.

68. Lafaille JJ, *et al*. High incidence of spontaneous autoimmune encephalomyelitis in immunodeficient anti-myelin basic protein T cell receptor transgenic mice. *Cell* 1994, **78**: 399–408.

69. Kuchroo VK, *et al*. T cell receptor (TCR) usage determines disease susceptibility in experimental autoimmune encephalomyelitis: studies with TCR V beta 8.2 transgenic mice. *J. Exp. Med*. 1994, **179**: 1659–1664.

70. Goverman J, *et al*. Transgenic mice that express a myelin basic protein-specific T cell receptor develop spontaneous autoimmunity. *Cell* 1993, **72**: 551–560.

71. Schuler W, *et al*. Rearrangement of antigen receptor genes is defective in mice with severe combined immune deficiency. *Cell* 1986, **46**: 963–972.

72. Subramanian S, *et al*. T lymphocytes promote the development of bone marrow-derived APC in the central nervous system. *J. Immunol*. 2001, **166**: 370–376.

73. Jones RE, *et al*. Nonmyelin-specific T cells accelerate development of central nervous system APC and increase susceptibility to experimental autoimmune encephalomyelitis. *J. Immunol*. 2003, **170**: 831–837.
74. Jones RE, *et al*. Induction of experimental autoimmune encephalomyelitis in severe combined immunodeficient mice reconstituted with allogeneic or xenogeneic hematopoietic cells. *J. Immunol*. 1993, **150**: 4620–4629.

24

Animal models of Parkinson's disease

ANUMANTHA G. KANTHASAMY AND SIDDHARTH KAUL

24.1 Introduction

Parkinson's disease (PD) is a progressive neurodegenerative disorder characterized primarily by the gradual dopaminergic loss in the substantia nigra of the midbrain region. Development of PD can be sporadic or can be associated with genetic mutations and deficiencies, or may result from the combination of these two precipitating factors. The pathogenesis of PD has been studied in numerous experimental models developed to replicate the salient features of the disease in a controlled environment. Although no single model exists today that mimics all the neurological and neuropathological features of PD, each model presents a particular aspect of the disease process induced either by natural or artificial toxic agents or by genetically induced deficiencies in experimental animals. Epidemiological and laboratory results suggest that environmental factors play a predominant role in the induction and propagation of dopaminergic degeneration. However, numerous familial cases indicate that development of PD might be aggravated by pre-existing genetic deficiencies that act as predisposing factors. This chapter describes in detail the extensive research conducted using animal and tissue-culture models of Parkinson's disease induced by both toxins and genetic manipulation. Furthermore, salient experimental findings are thoroughly described with regard to current perspectives on neurotoxic mechanisms of genetic variations and environmental toxins.

24.2 6-Hydroxydopamine model of PD

6-Hydroxydopamine (6-OHDA) was first demonstrated to effectively replicate Parkinsonian neurotoxic pathology in rats by stereotaxic nigral injection in rats as early as 1975.[1] 6-OHDA selectively leads to the degeneration of neuronal cell bodies and the nerve terminals by exerting an inhibitory effect on the mitochondrial respiratory enzymes (complex I and IV).[2,3] Since 6-OHDA

Handbook of Experimental Neurology, ed. Turgut Tatlisumak and Marc Fisher. Published by Cambridge University Press. © Cambridge University Press 2006.

does not cross the blood–brain barrier, effective delivery can be achieved only by intracerebrally injecting the toxin directly into the substantia nigra or ventral tegmental areas by stereotactic techniques. Furthermore, 6-OHDA is not only taken up by the dopaminergic neurons but also by the noradrenergic neurons due to which selectivity of action might be compromised. To address this, relative selectivity is usually ensured by preinjecting the animals with a noradrenalin neurotransmitter blocking agent like des-methylimipramine, and by stereotaxic injections of the toxin directly in the desired area of the midbrain.

The most commonly used 6-OHDA paradigm is the unilateral intracerebral injection into the medial forebrain bundle (MFB) of the rat brain. This model is popular due to several factors: firstly, the rat is a very responsive animal model to 6-OHDA and cost-effective; secondly, unilateral lesioning allows comparison of the normal and the lesioned sides of the same animal which is relevant to the disease; lastly, bilateral treatment with the toxin can induce systemic effects like aphagia (inability to swallow food) which necessitates the use of additional life and nutritional support thus confounding the process of data collection[4] though one study does advocate the concurrent analysis of a unilateral and bilateral lesioning in the rat model[5] as the most effective method of developing an effective PD model. A characteristic test to determine nigral damage in rats lesioned with 6-OHDA is the rotational movement analysis via injection of the dopamine releasing drugs D-amphetamine (DA) or apomorphine systemically in the animals. Lesions formed less than 1 week prior cause an ipsilateral rotation in animals upon administration of DA due to its release from the damaged dopaminergic system. Alternately, contralateral rotation of the animal occurs upon administration of DA when lesions are formed more than 1 week prior, since DA is depleted from the lesioned side and is now released from the non-lesioned dopaminergic neurons causing a contralateral rotation of the animal.[4] Apomorphine is generally considered the best alternative to DA since it can determine the extent of the dopaminergic lesion as it involves modulation of dopamine release from the axons of the neurons. A TH-positive neuronal loss of approximately 85%–90% is required to elicit a rotational response to apomorphine, since it was observed that rats exhibiting a loss of less than 75% neuronal loss do not exhibit any drug-induced response.[6] In addition to nigral lesion, injection of small doses of 6-OHDA in the striatum also have been demonstrated to induce damage in the nerve terminal as well as in the cell body.[7]

The major criticism of the 6-OHDA model is that it depicts an acute model of dopaminergic degeneration which does not mimic the slow progressive nature of PD in human patients. Furthermore, the 6-OHDA model does not affect multiple midbrain areas, such as the locus coeruleus, as documented in human PD pathology. Indeed when the dopaminergic nerve terminal damage induced in a 6-OHDA animal model of PD was combined with noradrenaline depletion from the locus coeruleus, a potentiation in the loss of dopamine was almost twofold greater.[8] In addition, some investigators use a bilateral lesion model as compared to the unilateral MFB model, indicating that the former may not always produce exclusively ipsilateral motor manifestations of the toxicity, and results obtained from rotational measurements may not reflect actual central nervous system(CNS) pathology.[9] Regardless of the benefits or drawbacks, the 6-OHDA model has been used extensively to study and demonstrate the effectiveness of various therapeutic measures like genetic implantation of growth factors,[10,11] possible development of surgical therapies like ablation of the subthalamic nucleus,[12] use of experimental drugs like anti-inflammatory agents (aspirin),[13] and antioxidants like cabergoline or melatonin.[14]

24.3 MPTP-induced model of PD

The neurotoxic effects of MPTP (1-methyl-4-phenyl-1, 2, 3, 6-tetrahydropyridine) were discovered when some drug addicts in California accidentally self-administered a contaminant of the then widely prevalent "synthetic heroin" MPPP (1-methyl-4-phenyl-propion-oxypiperidine) and developed neurological symptoms resembling Parkinson's disease which were completely reversed by the administration of L-dopa.[15,16] The clinical symptomatology and biochemical changes observed in these patients were remarkably similar to those observed in PD patients except for the characteristic presence of the Lewy bodies.[17] MPTP initiates cellular toxicity via a two-step transformation to its ionic form MPP^+ due to the action of the glial enzyme monoamine oxidase B (MAO-B) which includes the formation of an unstable charged intermediate $(MPDP^+)$.[18]

A variety of animal species has been studied with respect to the development of an effective laboratory model of PD using the neurotoxic effects of MPTP. Rats have been shown to be insensitive to MPTP-induced neurotoxicity even though they tend to accumulate MPP^+ in the nigrostriatal dopaminergic terminals.[19] Although recent studies with the MPTP-induced model in rats have garnered some popular interest as a model to study the induction of memory deficits seen in Parkinson's disease,[20,21] they are not traditionally a well-accepted model of PD. Mice have been the preferred species to develop MPTP-induced model of dopaminergic toxicity[22] (Table 24.1) and the C57/Bl strain is shown to be more susceptible to the toxic effects of MPTP than other

Table 24.1. *Summary of MPTP-induced C57/Bl mouse models of PD*

MPTP dose[a]	Biochemical finding	References
30 mg/kg/d 5 d (150 mg)	Dopaminergic neuronal degeneration involves apoptotic cell death	50
	Caspase-3 and caspase-8 play important role in dopaminergic apoptotic process	42, 51
	Bax plays an important role in dopaminergic neurotoxicity	33, 38
20 mg/kg/2 hr 4 i.p. (80 mg)	p53 inhibition protects dopaminergic neurons	52
	PARP activation in dopaminergic neuronal apoptosis (PARP−/− knockout mice)	47, 53
15 mg/kg/2 hr 4 i.p. (60 mg)	Caspase-9 activates caspase-8 and bid cleavage	44
20–40 mg/kg single dose i.p.	c-JNK inhibition protects dopaminergic neurons from apoptosis	54, 55
	Rapid upregulation of c-Jun, c-fos, and Bax in all brain regions	56
10 mg/kg 4 i.p. 24-hr interval (40 mg)	Bcl-2 overexpression protects dopaminergic neurons from apoptotic degeneration	57

[a] i.p., intraperitoneally.

strains like the BALB/c mice.[23] Primates are perhaps the most relevant, widely used animal species in the development of PD models and possibly the most sensitive to neurotoxic effects of MPTP (Table 24.2).[24] Following sections will attempt to outline concisely the tremendous amount of data that has been collected regarding what is known about the cellular mechanisms of MPTP-induced dopaminergic cell death and it relevance to the development of PD.

MPTP, once processed by the glial cells to its ionic form MPP^+, is selectively concentrated in the dopaminergic neurons, via the cell-membrane-bound dopamine transporter $(DAT)^{25}$ where it can have numerous intraneuronal fates. MPP^+ accumulates in the mitochondrion of the dopaminergic neurons and acts to inhibit complex I of the respiratory chain thus precipitating a significant depletion of the essential energy molecule ATP.[26] ATP depletion not only results is an energy crisis but also affects downstream biochemical processes that require ATP as a cofactor for proper function like the nuclear DNA repair enzyme PARP (poly-ADP-ribose polymerase, which adds ADP ribose groups from NAD to DNA) which compromises cellular function to a great extent.[27] The block in the electron transport chain prevents the enzymes

Table 24.2. *Summary of MPTP-induced primate models of PD*[a]

MPTP dose[b]	Pathophysiological finding	References
2.5 mg/kg single s.c.	Neurodegenerative findings within 24 hr of toxin administration (squirrel monkey)	58
2 mg/kg repeated i.p.	Selective neuronal loss in substantia nigra pars compacta (squirrel monkey)	59
4 mg intracaudate	Parkinsonian symptoms at 1 week: hypokinesia and curved posture (common marmoset)	60
15 doses (0.5–4.5 mg/kg i.p.) 25 mg total dose, 29 days	16 days: rigid posture, profound hypokinesia, and abnormal motor behavior (common marmoset)	61
1 mg/kg i.p. bi-weekly 4 mths	2 groups: 1 studied after 4 months and other 8 mths after end of dosage (common marmoset)	62
2 mg/kg i.p.	Calcium channel blocker nimodipine blocks MPTP-induced substantia nigra TH$^+$ neuronal loss (common marmoset)	63
2 mg/kg s.c./day for 5 days	Dopamine uptake but not serotonin inhibits MPTP-induced toxicity (common marmoset)	64
	Development of a new global dyskinesia rating scale (GDRS) for squirrel monkey dyskinesias in response to MPTP toxicity	65

[a] For review of contribution of MPTP primate model to PD see reference 66.
[b] s.c., subcutaneously.

from harnessing the free molecular oxygen which in turn results in the generation of large quantities of reactive superoxide radicals and oxidative damage.[28] We have also shown that MPP$^+$ induces significant generation of reactive oxygen species in dopaminergic neurons within a period of 10 min.[29]

Further oxidative stress can result when MPP$^+$ causes rapid efflux of the neurotransmitter dopamine from the postsynaptic vesicles resulting in oxidation and generation of hydroxyl radicals.[30] MPP$^+$ also leads to a selective mitochondrial DNA (mtDNA) damage by inhibiting the incorporation of 5-bromo-2′deoxyuridine into the mtDNA but not into the nuclear DNA.[31] MPP$^+$ toxicity induces translocation of the proapoptotic protein Bax to the mitochondrial membrane that upon oligomerization of Bax with BH3 cell death domains like t-bid, the mitochondrial membrane permeabilizes and cytochrome c is released from the intermembrane space into the cytosol.[32–34]

Cytochrome *c* release from the mitochondrial inner membrane is closely regulated by cytoplasmic and mitochondrial proteins like Bcl-2, Bax, and Bad.[35] Overexpression of Bcl-2 can induce significant protection against apoptosis in cells lines exposed to MPP^+ either via interaction with proapoptotic proteins like Bad and Bax or via the inactivation of cellular proteases like caspase-3 and calpains,[36,37] and Bax, a well-known Bcl-2 family proapoptotic protein, is significantly upregulated in MPTP-treated mice exhibiting neurodegenerative processes.[38] Upon release from the inner mitochondrial membrane, cytochrome *c* acts as an essential cofactor for the activation of a *ced-4* homologous apoptotic factor Apaf-1 in the cytosol, which in turn is responsible for cleaving the pro-caspase-9 to the active caspase-9 enzyme.[39] Caspase-9 activation is a premonitory step in the development and propagation of the apoptotic cascade in the cellular environment. Activated caspase-9 cleaves pro-caspase-3 to its active enzymatic form. MPP^+-induced caspase-3 activity was first demonstrated in cerebellar granule neuronal cultures at concentrations of 10–100 μM.[40] Indeed a meticulous study of human brain samples also indicated significantly depleted numbers of caspase-3 positive neurons in the substantia nigra of PD patients than in time-matched normal brains, suggesting caspase-3-expressing neurons were more susceptible to neurodegenerative pathology than those not expressing the active enzyme.[41] In addition other studies have shown that activation of caspase-9 is essential along with the activation of the effector caspase-3 for the apoptotic process involved in both MPTP-induced[42] and MPP^+-induced[29,43,44] neurotoxicity in various models of PD.

Caspase-3 is a cysteine protease that is known to act on various cytoplasmic and nuclear downstream substrates to advance the process of programmed cell death.[41] In the cytoplasmic compartment, active caspase-3 can proteolytically activate the pro-apoptotic protein kinase C-delta (PKCδ) to induce cellular apoptosis.[29] Caspase-3 also redistributes to the nuclear compartment and proteolytically cleaves numerous putative nuclear substrates like PARP and DNA-dependent protein kinase (DNA-PK) to precipitate nuclear chromatin degradation and apoptosis.[45,46] PARP is substrate target in MPTP-induced neuronal apoptosis and its proteolytic cleavage results in an inactive enzyme precipitating DNA fragmentation and apoptosis.[47,48] DNA-PK, a serine-threonine kinase that is responsible for DNA double-strand repair, is also inactivated by proteolytic action of caspase-3 in the nucleus.[49]

Though the MPTP-induced neurotoxicity model has remained the most popular PD model and has yielded an enormous amount of information regarding the cellular and pathological changes occurring during dopaminergic degeneration, the exact mechanism of cell death still remains to be completely understood. Further research continues with this model of PD in the quest to completely elucidate the mechanisms of selective dopaminergic cell death in PD.

24.4 Paraquat-induced model of neurodegeneration

Paraquat (1, 1'-dimethyl-4, 4'-bipyridinium) (Fig. 24.1) is a widely used herbicide that structurally resembles MPP[+] and was implicated as a principal toxic agent responsible for neurological disorders in a subset of a Taiwanese farming community.[67] Cerebral poisoning was first reported in 1980 when four patients died of paraquat exposure and exhibited cerebral hemorrhages, glial reactions, and edema.[68] Later a comparative study found the pathological changes induced by paraquat were like those induced by the Parkinsonian toxin MPTP in a species of frog[69] as well as in isolated rat hepatocytes[70] and the concept of a link between pesticide toxicity and Parkinson's disease was born.[71–73] Independent epidemiological studies showed a distinct relationship between exposure to paraquat in the environment and increased risk for developing Parkinson's disease[67,74,75] especially in the developing nations.[76]

Although some earlier investigative reports might have suggested that paraquat may not specifically cause dopaminergic toxicity as effectively as MPTP,[71,77] overwhelming evidence to the contrary has demonstrated the usefulness of paraquat for studying the cellular mechanisms involved in the development of PD. Recent investigations have shown that paraquat toxicity can lead to significant and specific dopaminergic degenerative changes in cellular PD models[78] and in C57/Bl mouse models of PD.[79,80] Chun *et al.* showed a very close correlation between the toxicant action of the known Parkinsonian ionic compound MPP[+] and various environmental contaminants like paraquat, dieldrin, and manganese[81] in a nigral dopaminergic cell line, further underscoring the role

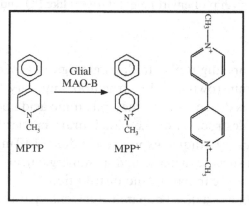

Figure 24.1. Structure of paraquat.

Table 24.3. *Summary of findings in the paraquat-induced model of PD*[a]

Paraquat (PQ) dose	Model	Conclusions	References
PQ	C57/Bl mice	Characterization of PQ as a useful model to study neurological disease pathology	90
Intranigral PQ 10 µg injection	Male Wistar rats	Intranigral PQ injection induces significant dopaminergic degeneration	91
5–10 mg/kg i.p. 1 week/3 weeks	C57/Bl mice	Selective age-dependent dopaminergic toxicity	83
10 µM PQ	PC12 dopaminergic cells	Activation of transcription factor AP-1 and apoptosis	78
10 mg PQ + 30 mg/kg maneb 2 weeks/ 6 weeks	C57/Bl mice	PQ + maneb combination induced selective nigrostriatal degeneration	79
10 mg/kg i.p.	C57/Bl mice	PQ can be absorbed across the blood–brain barrier and lead to dopaminergic neuronal degeneration	80
50 µM PQ or 10 µM PQ + 1 µM MPP$^+$	Organotypic midbrain cultures	Low dose exposure of midbrain neurons to PQ increases vulnerability by excitotoxic mechanisms	85
7 mg/kg 1 dose/2 days 10 doses	C57/Bl mice	JNK signaling cascade is a direct mediator of PQ-mediated dopaminergic toxicity	92

[a] For review of relationship of environmental toxins like PQ and rotenone to PD see reference 75.

environmental factors might play in dopaminergic degeneration. Paraquat is taken up in the brain (owing to its structural similarity to MPP$^+$) but the specific absorption is dependent on a neutral amino acid uptake carrier system and not the direct destruction of the blood–brain barrier by paraquat or its essential metabolites.[82] Paraquat exposure at a dose of 10 mg/kg can lead to an age-dependent and specific increase in dopaminergic neuronal cell loss which was significantly specific in nature and distribution.[79,83]

In addition to acting as a direct dopaminergic toxin, paraquat can also act as a potentiation factor for other forms of neuronal toxins like the manganese-based fungicide maneb (manganese ethylene-bis-dithiocarbamate)[79,84] in mice and MPP[+] in organotypic midbrain cultures.[85] Furthermore paraquat can synergize with chronic iron exposure induced dopaminergic abnormalities seen in PD.[86] Such synergistic activities of pesticides in the environment may indicate a direct link between the environmental exposure and development of neurodegenerative disorders since the real-time exposure of humans to toxicants is rarely unique to one agent but a combination of organic exposures. To support this hypothesis more recent studies point to the possibility of the development of an age-dependent dopaminergic pathology upon exposure to paraquat along with maneb in C57/Bl mice which mimics the gradual progressive nature of the disease in humans.[87]

Accelerated aggregation of amyloidal proteins like α-synuclein could be an additional signaling mechanisms that can be precipitated by paraquat toxicity and in this respect it mimics many other allied environmental organic compounds like dieldrin and manganese.[88,89] Dosage regimens and the significant findings that have been described in the paraquat model of PD are outlined in Table 24.3.

24.5 Rotenone-induced PD model

Rotenone, a highly lipophilic ketone complex (Fig. 24.2), has been widely used as a garden pesticide due to its short biodegradation time and effective toxicity in insects. It is a mitochondrial toxin which can interfere with the electron transport process by inhibition of the enzyme complex I in the mitochondrial cristae.[93,94] and induce damage to dopaminergic neurons. Complex I inhibition leads to metabolic effects like the acute reduction in ATP levels that

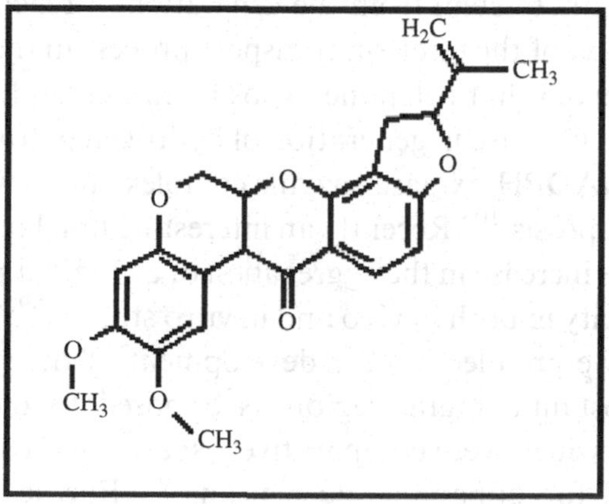

Figure 24.2. Structure of rotenone.

induces depolarization-associated Ca^{2+} influx into the neurons via the NMDA receptors; Ca^{2+} influx further aggravates mitochondrial damage thus precipitating a cycle of oxidative stress and apoptotic events.[95] These effects are strikingly similar to the action of the dopaminergic toxin MPP^+ in various cellular and animal models, which validates the use of rotenone as a viable tool to study the pathogenic mechanisms involved in PD. Although ATP depletion would not result in the preferential targeting of the dopaminergic system, some investigators have suggested oxidative stress as a plausible cause of neuronal cell death and argue the heightened susceptibility of dopamine-producing neurons to oxidation damage results in the specific neuronal damage.[96]

Recent studies have identified rotenone exposure as a putative environmental causative agent for development of amyloidal-based neurodegenerative disorders like Lewy body dementia and P3D.[97,98] Although systemic administration of rotenone was initially established to produce dopaminergic toxicity similar to that observed with the Parkinsonian toxin MPP^+,[99] subsequent studies also demonstrated a lack of a specific relationship between rotenone toxicity, neurological deficits, and the dopaminergic system even though dopamine levels and striatal neurons were altered drastically.[100,101] A later study showed that upon chronic intrajugular transfusion of rotenone at an optimal dose of 2–3 mg/kg clearly replicated the behavioral, neuropathological, and chemical changes characteristic of PD in the substantia nigra of Lewis rats.[102,103]

Rotenone exposure in an in vitro model of neuronal apoptosis revealed systemic activation of apoptotic signaling beginning with oxidative stress and cytochrome c release, culminating in caspase-3-mediated cell death.[94] In vivo data reveal that 1.5–2.5 mg/kg intraperitoneal exposure to rotenone over an extended period of time results in an increased dopaminergic neuronal loss and expression of Parkinsonian symptoms in rats.[104] The mechanism of rotenone neurotoxicity appears to stem from the generation of reactive oxygen species due to the disruption of the electron transport process in the mitochondria.[105] Indeed it was observed that rotenone exposure in human leukemic cells (HL-60) induced a rapid increase in generation of hydrogen peroxide (H_2O_2) via the activation of the NADPH oxidase enzyme complex, along with mitochondrial disruption and apoptosis.[106] Recently an interesting link has also been demonstrated between the increase in the aggregation of amyloidal protein α-synuclein and rotenone toxicity in both in vivo and in vitro studies.[89,107] The studies also indicated a selective predilection for development of the synuclein inclusion bodies in the substantia nigral region as opposed to the striatal and the thalamic neurons, which were comparatively spared, indicating the specificity of this PD model for dopaminergic neurons.[107] Furthermore, in a breakthrough study done recently, significant neurobehavioral changes induced by the bilateral administration of rotenone to the median forebrain bundle of rats were reversed by treatment with the anti-Parkinsonian drug L-dopa (5–10 mg/kg + Benserazide, a clinically utilized Parkinsonian drug).[108] The above data establish rotenone as a primary candidate for studying the effects of Parkinsonian pathology and treatment. However, a caution should be noted regarding the high mortality associated with rotenone model mainly due to systematic toxicity.

Current research demonstrates that rotenone has indeed proven to be a vital tool in the study of neurodegenerative disorders, as it induces Lewy-body-like inclusions in treated animal models, unlike most currently used Parkinsonian toxins.[102,103] The rotenone model has also further strengthened the existing hypothesis that mitochondrial complex I inhibition may be critical to the nigral dopaminergic neuronal loss,[109] even though the same investigation raised a query on the selectivity of the rotenone toxicity to target dopaminergic neurons by showing damage to striatal non-dopaminergic neurons at the same levels used to develop the nigral pathology.

24.6 Proteosomal inhibitor-induced PD model

Inclusion bodies found in various regions of the brain including the substantia nigra pars compacta, locus coeruleus, and the nucleus basalis of Meynert, known as Lewy bodies, are a pathological hallmark of Parkinson's disease.[110,111] The ubiquitin–proteosome system (UPS) is a molecular pathway in cells involved in the tagging, transport, and degradation of excessive protein structures. Impaired function of this system induces the development of intracellular protein aggregosomes as well as dopaminergic apoptosis, resulting in a model which replicates the pathological features of PD.[112–115] Furthermore, proteosome function was severely affected in the substantia nigra of PD patients as compared to age-matched unaffected control brain samples.[115]

The development of a novel PD model has been recently described based on the utilization of both naturally occurring and synthetic inhibitors of the proteosome pathway epoxomicin and PSI (Z-Ile-Glu(OtBu)-Ala-Leu-al), respectively.[116] The model was developed as follows: male Sprague-Dawley rats were treated with 3–6 mg/kg PSI or 1.5 mg/kg epoxomicin over a period of 2 weeks via six injections. The animals were then monitored for a period of 21 weeks bi-weekly for changes in behavioral patterns and development of motor changes. Morbidity was not increased and appetite and health of the rats were not decreased during the subsequent weeks; however, all treated animals developed mild bradykinesia 1–2 weeks after the end of treatment, which progressively worsened by the 6th week to frank rigidity and severe bradykinesia.

These symptoms were significantly attenuated by the administration of both apomorphine and L-dopa. Pathological analysis revealed a compensatory increase in proteosomal activity in all parts of the brain, which was dramatically reduced by the 4th week post-treatment in the ventral midbrain and the lower brain stem regions. Tyrosine hydroxylase and eosin staining revealed fairly specific neuronal loss, mostly due to apoptotic cell death, in the substantia nigra pars compacta, while the substantia nigra pars reticularis and the adjacent areas were relatively unchanged. Furthermore, in addition to the substantia nigra pars compacta lesions, selective lesions affecting the locus coeruleus, dorsal motor nucleus of vagus, and nucleus basalis of Meynert were observed; these lesions closely mimic PD pathogenesis and are often absent in conventional toxin-induced PD models. Finally, densely staining inclusion bodies immunoreactive to α-synuclein, synphilin, and γ-tubulin (but not to β-synuclein) were observed in the substantia nigra pars compacta, locus coeruleus, and the nucleus basalis of Meynert brain regions of the treated animals. This model was first to effectively replicate the many specific and regional salient clinical and pathological features of Parkinson's disease.

24.7 Genetic models of PD

Most PD cases occur sporadically in the majority of the affected population yet various studies conducted over the last couple of decades have indicated the fact that the occurrence of the disease may actually be multifactorial in origin with numerous genetic factors playing a major role as well.[117] Epidemiological studies have further shown that the affected individuals with genetically acquired PD have an onset age of at least a decade younger than those with the sporadic form of the disease.[118,119]

Alpha-synuclein is a highly expressed brain protein that has been primarily associated with the development of the characteristic Parkinsonian inclusion Lewy bodies. Two PARK1 (α-synuclein) mutations, A30P (G88 C on gene) and A53T (G209 A on gene), located on chromosome 4 (p21–22), were the first loci associated with the development of familial PD in a Greek kindred family. Studies showed that these individuals had an early mean age of onset (~45 years) and relatively rapid disease progression.[118,120,121] Subsequent studies have disputed the significance of the synuclein mutation by demonstrating that this phenomenon is extremely rare,[122,123] and that no other mutated loci have been determine despite extensive epidemiological studies of affected families. Yet, significant findings regarding the pathogenesis of synuclein mutations have been discovered in the last 5 years. The localization of α-synuclein protein was shown in the brain samples of the Contursi kindred, which seemed to be in the caudate nucleus while being absent from the control brains and the frontal cortex of the affected individuals.[124] Furthermore α-synuclein mutant forms promote early aggregation of the protein in the neuronal systems,[125] which was described as the propensity of the mutant forms to oligomerize readily instead of forming protofibrils,[126,127] and that this property was shared by both the known synuclein mutant forms A30P and A53T. The spontaneous preponderance of the mutant forms to aggregate in vitro was determined to be related to the ready self-aggregation of the partially folded intermediates rather than a change in the native monomeric species of the synuclein protein.[128] Transgenic mice overexpressing the mutant synuclein form A53T developed marked increases in Lewy body pathology, neuronal degeneration, and motor defects.[129,130]

Studies further determined that the A53T mutant form of synuclein induces more significant neurodegenerative changes and protein aggregation in overexpressing transgenic mice than the A30P mutant form of the protein.[131] Human patients afflicted with the familial form of PD due to the A53T mutation have numerous ubiquitously present α-synuclein aggregative formations, implicating this process either in the induction of or in the course of disease development.[132]

Interestingly, the lipid bilayer interaction with the synuclein protein might play an important role in the development of the intracellular aggregated forms.[133–135] Free α-synuclein usually exists in an unfolded state, but when this protein interacts with membrane lipid molecules via the N-terminal, it adopts varied helical conformations[136] which are not altered by the mutant form A53T.[137] The reduced aggregative activity of the A30P mutant as compared to the A53T mutant could be explained partly by the fact that the A30P mutant loses its ability to interact with the membranes while the A53T mutant and the native protein interact normally.[138] Though the role of lipid interactions in the development of amyloid aggregation is still not well outlined, some results indicate that the initial aggregative process occurs in lipid droplets, and micelles in the cell membrane subsequently become aggravated by disease-causing processes.[138] Beta-synuclein, another synuclein protein family member, has thus far not been associated with the pathogenesis of PD, but recent studies have highlighted neuroprotective modulation associated with this protein form. Beta-synuclein can inhibit the formation of α-synuclein protofibrils[139] or act as an anti-aggregative protein,[140] but can also be neuroprotective by modulating signaling mechanisms like the Akt[141] and the p53 pathways[142] to reduce cellular toxicity.

The native form of the α-synuclein protein has recently been investigated with regard to development of neuroprotective mechanisms in PD. Alpha-synuclein mRNA levels were greatly reduced in PD patient brains as compared to normal controls,[143] and rats exposed to 6-OHDA had reduced levels of α-synuclein protein in the substantia nigra,[144] indicating that the native form of the protein did indeed play a role in dopaminergic survival. Additionally, transcription levels of synuclein protein were markedly reduced in adult and old mice after a significant burst during the developmental stages, which might explain the occurrence of PD in the later stages of life and the absence in the early formative years.[145] Recent studies have also shown that overexpression of the native form of α-synuclein can protect dopaminergic neurons from toxicity by either reducing oxidative stress[146–148] or by transcriptional regulation of proteins,[149] by counteracting the effects of neurotoxins by as yet unknown mechanisms,[150] or by direct modulation of apoptotic signaling molecules like Bcl-2.[151] Taken together, the mutant form of α-synuclein is toxic towards the dopaminergic system and this toxicity does not yet explain completely the sporadic nature of the disease. Also, the neurophysiological role of an abundantly expressed protein must be explored further as a possible neuroprotectant against development of neurodegenerative processes like PD.

Parkin (PARK 2) is another locus (chromosome 6q25.2–27) identified in the autosomal recessive juvenile form of PD (AR-JP) demonstrated to induce early onset of disease pathology.[152,153] Although preliminary reports cite that parkin mutations are relatively rare even among autosomal recessive PD patients, as many as 60 different mutations have been identified so far.[154] A mutation in the codon 167 of the parkin gene[155] as well as a homozygous exon 4 deletion have been implicated in early-onset AR-JP disease.[156] Interestingly, studies in PD patients with parkin mutations have shown inconsistent involvement of the dopaminergic system and the development of the cardinal pathological finding of Lewy bodies in the nigral system,[157,158] prompting a debate as to whether ubiquitination actually precedes the development of Lewy bodies.

Parkin is a type of E3 ubiquitin ligase responsible for tagging proteins within cells with ubiquitin (ubiquitination) for subsequent proteosomal degradation. Mutations in the parkin protein have been associated with the development of protein aggregates within neurons.[159,160] This may explain why ubiquitin and α-synuclein are the major components of Lewy bodies,[161] which represent the failure of the ubiquitination system in PD patients. Parkin co-localized with α-synuclein in the Lewy bodies of patients with four allied neurodegenerative disorders, indicating that the protein was absolutely involved in some process during the formation of the inclusion structures.[162,163] In addition, brains of AR-JP patients with an inherently mutated form of the parkin protein are conspicuously missing Lewy bodies because these patients have a non-functioning form of the protein.[164] Some of the other defined substrates of parkin are Pael-R (parkin-associated endothelin receptor-like receptor),[165] which accumulates in brains of AR-JP patients, glycosylated α-synuclein, CDCrel-1 (a synaptic vesicle related protein),[166] and another as yet uncharacterized protein (30 kDa).[167]

During recent years, parkin has emerged as an important molecule in the development of neuroprotective strategies in PD. The neurotoxic effects of dopamine and 6-OHDA, but not those of hydrogen peroxide and rotenone, were significantly attenuated by the expression of parkin protein as compared with the mutant expression form which aggravated the toxic effects.[168] Parkin rescues catecholaminergic neurons from neurotoxic effects of mutant forms of synuclein by reducing the sensitivity of the proteosome pathway to the adverse effects of proteosome inhibitors and the mutant synuclein.[169] Interestingly, following endoplasmic reticulum stress, the expression of wild-type parkin protein in astrocytes was increased as compared to neuronal cells, indicating that parkin may attenuate oxidative stress.[170] Induction of transient focal ischemia led to a significant reduction in levels of parkin in C57/Bl mice, suggesting involvement of the protein in development of PD due to recurrent ischemic episodes.[171] Parkin also acts in a neuroprotective manner in manganese-induced neurotoxicity,[172] cellular death induced by Pael-R,[173] and α-synuclein-induced cytotoxicity,[174] and it prevents cytochrome *c* release and caspase-3 activation in ceramide-induced cellular apoptosis.[175]

Another genetic candidate investigated in relation to PD pathogenesis development is UCH-L1 (PARK5), a gene that encodes ubiquitin C-hydrolase-L1, first identified in a family that exhibited dominant inheritance of PD.[176] UCH-L1 is almost as highly expressed in the brain (1% of total protein) as the presynaptic protein synuclein and is believed to be involved in the ubiquitination and proteosome-induced degradation of intracellular proteins. UCH-L1 has either a beneficial hydrolase activity or a damaging activity involving ligase, depending on cell type as well as the type of insult.[177] PARK6, on chromosome 1p35–36, and PARK 7, on chromosome 1p36, are commonly associated with AR-JP.[178,179]

24.8 Knockout mouse models of PD

Dopamine is the major neurotransmitter of the dopaminergic neurons that is selectively degenerated in diseases like PD, and the functional aspects of dopaminergic homeostasis are being studied in an effort to elucidate the mechanism of pathogenesis. Genetic mutations to induce the absence of dopamine (D2) receptors in inbred C57/Bl mice caused dyskinesias and locomotor deficiencies akin to those seen in dopaminergic deficits.[180,181] Knockout mouse models deficient in the production of the dopamine transporter demonstrated significant defects in dopamine metabolism, indicating that the transporter is important in neurotransmitter homeostasis in the substantia nigra.[182]

Oxidative stress has long been implicated as one of the more plausible etiological conditions precipitating neurodegenerative disorders. Nitric oxide synthase knockout mice exhibit increased neuroprotection towards Parkinsonian toxins.[183] Furthermore, mice genetically deficient in superoxide dismutase isoforms, an endogenous antioxidant system, show increased susceptibility to mitochondrial toxicity; many known toxins induce neuronal apoptosis via mitochondrial toxicity.[184,185] More recently, the membrane-bound enzyme complex NADPH oxidase has been increasingly studied as a possible source of generation of oxidative stress not only in the neuroglial environment but also in neuronal cells.[186,187]

Knockout mouse models have recently been used to demonstrate the involvement of various molecules in the development of pathogenesis in PD. Mice deficient in tumor necrosis factor (TNF) (death domain) receptors exhibit reduced susceptibility to neurotoxic stimuli.[188] Alpha-synuclein-null mice were more susceptible to toxicity after administration of MPTP than wild-type mice, indicating that synuclein protein might play an important role in the neuroprotection of dopaminergic cells.[189] Glial-derived neurotrophic factor (GDNF) is responsible for neuroprotective effects in the midbrain, and knockout studies in mice validate this hypothesis; these mice showed impaired locomotor activity as well as dopaminergic deficits.[190] Caffeine and adenosine receptor inactivation also protect the dopaminergic system in knockout models of PD.[191] Nurr-1 is an important genetic determinant of dopamine synthesis in the brain. Development of the dopaminergic system was not impaired in knockout mice deficient in Nurr-1, but terminal differentiation of the dopaminergic neurons was impaired and effective synaptic dopaminergic connections were not formed.[192]

Acknowledgments

This work was supported by the National Institutes of Health grants NS 38644, ES 10586, and NS 45133.

References

1. Mendez JS, Finn BW. Use of 6-hydroxydopamine to create lesions in catecholamine neurons in rats. *J. Neurosurg.* 1975, **42**: 166–173.
2. Glinka Y, Gassen M, Youdim MB. Mechanism of 6-hydroxydopamine neurotoxicity. *J. Neural Transm. (Suppl.)* 1997, **50**: 55–66.

3. Ungerstedt U. 6-Hydroxydopamine induced degeneration of central monoamine neurons. *Eur. J. Pharmacol.* 1968, **5**: 107–110.

4. Ungerstedt U. Adipsia and aphagia after 6-hydroxydopamine-induced degeneration of the nigro-striatal dopamine system. *Acta Physiol. Scand. (Suppl.)* 1971, **367**: 95–122.

5. Roedter A, Winkler C, Samii M, *et al.* Comparison of unilateral and bilateral intrastriatal 6-hydroxydopamine-induced axon terminal lesions: evidence for interhemispheric functional coupling of the two nigrostriatal pathways. *J. Comp. Neurol.* 2001, **432**: 217–229.

6. Hefti F, Melamed E, Wurtman RJ. Partial lesions of the dopaminergic nigrostriatal system in rat brain: biochemical characterization. *Brain Res.* 1980, **195**: 123–137.

7. Przedborski S, Levivier M, Jiang H, *et al.* Dose-dependent lesions of the dopaminergic nigrostriatal pathway induced by intrastriatal injection of 6-hydroxydopamine. *Neuroscience* 1995, **67**: 631–647.

8. Srinivasan J, Schmidt WJ. Potentiation of Parkinsonian symptoms by depletion of locus coeruleus noradrenaline in 6-hydroxydopamine-induced partial degeneration of substantia nigra in rats. *Eur. J. Neurosci.* 2003, **17**: 2586–2592.

9. Whishaw IQ, Pellis SM, Gorny BP. Skilled reaching in rats and humans: evidence for parallel development or homology. *Behav. Brain Res.* 1992, **47**: 59–70.

10. Kirik D, Georgievska B, Rosenblad C, Bjorklund A. Delayed infusion of GDNF promotes recovery of motor function in the partial lesion model of Parkinson's disease. *Eur. J. Neurosci.* 2001, **13**: 1589–1599.

11. Akerud P, Canals JM, Snyder EY, Arenas E. Neuroprotection through delivery of glial cell line-derived neurotrophic factor by neural stem cells in a mouse model of Parkinson's disease. *J. Neurosci.* 2001, **21**: 8108–8118.

12. Paul G, Meissner W, Rein S, *et al.* Ablation of the subthalamic nucleus protects dopaminergic phenotype but not cell survival in a rat model of Parkinson's disease. *Exp. Neurol.* 2004, **185**: 272–280.

13. Carrasco E, Werner P. Selective destruction of dopaminergic neurons by low concentrations of 6-OHDA and MPP$^+$: protection by acetylsalicylic acid aspirin. *Parkinsonism Relat. Disord.* 2002, **8**: 407–411.

14. Yoshioka M, Tanaka K, Miyazaki I, *et al.* The dopamine agonist cabergoline provides neuroprotection by activation of the glutathione system and scavenging free radicals. *Neurosci. Res.* 2002, **43**: 259–267.

15. Langston JW. Mechanisms underlying neuronal degeneration in Parkinson's disease: an experimental and theoretical treatise. *Mov. Disord.* 1989, **4**(Suppl. 1): S15–S25.

16. Bradbury AJ, Costall B, Domeney AM, *et al.* 1-methyl-4-phenylpyridine is neurotoxic to the nigrostriatal dopamine pathway. *Nature* 1986, **319**: 56–57.

17. Langston JW, Ballard P, Tetrud JW, Irwin I. Chronic Parkinsonism in humans due to a product of meperidine-analog synthesis. *Science* 1983, **219**: 979–980.

18. Chiba K, Trevor A, Castagnoli Jr N. Metabolism of the neurotoxic tertiary amine, MPTP, by brain monoamine oxidase. *Biochem. Biophys. Res. Commun.* 1984, **120**: 574–578.

19. Zuddas A, Fascetti F, Corsini GU, Piccardi MP. In brown Norway rats, MPP$^+$ is accumulated in the nigrostriatal dopaminergic terminals but it is not neurotoxic: a model of natural resistance to MPTP toxicity. *Exp. Neurol.* 1994, **127**: 54–61.

20. Da Cunha C, Gevaerd MS, Vital MA, *et al.* Memory disruption in rats with nigral lesions induced by MPTP: a model for early Parkinson's disease amnesia. *Behav. Brain Res.* 2001, **124**: 9–18.

428 *Anumantha G. Kanthasamy and Siddharth Kaul*

21. Miyoshi E, Wietzikoski S, Camplessei M, *et al.* Impaired learning in a spatial working memory version and in a cued version of the water maze in rats with MPTP-induced mesencephalic dopaminergic lesions. *Brain Res. Bull.* 2002, **58**: 41–47.
22. Lau YS, Meredith GE. From drugs of abuse to Parkinsonism: the MPTP mouse model of Parkinson's disease. *Methods Mol. Med.* 2003, **79**: 103–116.
23. Sedelis M, Hofele K, Auburger GW, *et al.* MPTP susceptibility in the mouse: behavioral, neurochemical, and histological analysis of gender and strain differences. *Behav. Genet.* 2000, **30**: 171–182.
24. Langston JW, Langston EB, Irwin I. MPTP-induced Parkinsonism in human and non-human primates: clinical and experimental aspects. *Acta Neurol. Scand. (Suppl.)* 1984, **100**: 49–54.
25. Bezard E, Gross CE, Fournier MC, *et al.* Absence of MPTP-induced neuronal death in mice lacking the dopamine transporter. *Exp. Neurol.* 1999, **155**: 268–273.
26. Przedborski S, Jackson-Lewis V. Mechanisms of MPTP toxicity. *Mov. Disord.* 1998, **13** (Suppl. 1): 35–38.
27. Cosi C, Marien M. Implication of poly (ADP-ribose) polymerase (PARP) in neurodegeneration and brain energy metabolism: decreases in mouse brain NAD^+ and ATP caused by MPTP are prevented by the PARP inhibitor benzamide. *Ann. NY Acad. Sci.* 1999, **890**: 227–239.
28. Cleeter MW, Cooper JM, Schapira AH. Irreversible inhibition of mitochondrial complex I by 1-methyl-4-phenylpyridinium: evidence for free radical involvement. *J. Neurochem.* 1992, **58**: 786–789.
29. Kaul S, Kanthasamy A, Kitazawa M, Anantharam V, Kanthasamy AG. Caspase-3 dependent proteolytic activation of protein kinase Cdelta mediates and regulates 1-methyl-4-phenylpyridinium (MPP^+)-induced apoptotic cell death in dopaminergic cells: relevance to oxidative stress in dopaminergic degeneration. *Eur. J. Neurosci.* 2003, **18**: 1387–1401.
30. Obata T, Yamanaka Y, Kinemuchi H, Oreland L. Release of dopamine by perfusion with 1-methyl-4-phenylpyridinium ion (MPP^+) into the striatum is associated with hydroxyl free radical generation. *Brain Res.* 2001, **906**: 170–175.
31. Miyako K, Irie T, Muta T, *et al.* 1-Methyl-4-phenylpyridinium ion (MPP^+) selectively inhibits the replication of mitochondrial DNA. *Eur. J. Biochem.* 1999, **259**: 412–418.
32. Fiskum G, Starkov A, Polster BM, Chinopoulos C. Mitochondrial mechanisms of neural cell death and neuroprotective interventions in Parkinson's disease. *Ann. NY Acad. Sci.* 2003, **991**: 111–119.
33. Vila M, Jackson-Lewis V, Vukosavic S, *et al.* Bax ablation prevents dopaminergic neurodegeneration in the 1-methyl-4-phenyl-1,2,3,6-tetrahydropyridine mouse model of Parkinson's disease. *Proc. Natl Acad. Sci. USA* 2001, **98**: 2837–2842.
34. Cassarino DS, Parks JK, Parker Jr WD, Bennett Jr JP. The Parkinsonian neurotoxin MPP^+ opens the mitochondrial permeability transition pore and releases cytochrome *c* in isolated mitochondria via an oxidative mechanism. *Biochim. Biophys. Acta* 1999, **1453**: 49–62.
35. Cheng EH, Wei MC, Weiler S, *et al.* BCL-2, BCL-X(L) sequester BH3 domain-only molecules preventing BAX- and BAK-mediated mitochondrial apoptosis. *Mol. Cell* 2001, **8**: 705–711.
36. Choi WS, Lee EH, Chung CW, *et al.* Cleavage of Bax is mediated by caspase-dependent or -independent calpain activation in dopaminergic neuronal cells: protective role of Bcl-2. *J. Neurochem.* 2001, **77**: 1531–1541.

37. Oh YJ, Wong SC, Moffat M, O'Malley KL. Overexpression of Bcl-2 attenuates MPP$^+$, but not 6-ODHA, induced cell death in a dopaminergic neuronal cell line. *Neurobiol. Dis.* 1995, **2**: 157–167.

38. Hassouna I, Wickert H, Zimmermann M, Gillardon F. Increase in bax expression in substantia nigra following 1-methyl-4-phenyl-1,2,3,6-tetrahydropyridine (MPTP) treatment of mice. *Neurosci. Lett.* 1996, **204**: 85–88.

39. Zou H, Li Y, Liu X, Wang X. An APAF-1 cytochrome *c* multimeric complex is a functional apoptosome that activates procaspase-9. *J. Biol. Chem.* 1999, **274**: 11549–11556.

40. Du Y, Dodel RC, Bales KR, *et al.* Involvement of a caspase-3-like cysteine protease in 1-methyl-4-phenylpyridinium-mediated apoptosis of cultured cerebellar granule neurons. *J. Neurochem.* 1997, **69**: 1382–1388.

41. Hartmann A, Hunot S, Michel PP, *et al.* Caspase-3: a vulnerability factor and final effector in apoptotic death of dopaminergic neurons in Parkinson's disease. *Proc. Natl Acad. Sci. USA.* 2000, **97**: 2875–2880.

42. Turmel H, Hartmann A, Parain K, *et al.* Caspase-3 activation in 1-methyl-4-phenyl-1,2,3,6-tetrahydropyridine (MPTP)-treated mice. *Mov. Disord.* 2001, **16**: 185–189.

43. Dodel RC, Du Y, Bales KR, *et al.* Peptide inhibitors of caspase-3-like proteases attenuate 1-methyl-4-phenylpyridinum-induced toxicity of cultured fetal rat mesencephalic dopamine neurons. *Neuroscience* 1998, **86**: 701–707.

44. Viswanath V, Wu Y, Boonplueang R, *et al.* Caspase-9 activation results in downstream caspase-8 activation and bid cleavage in 1-methyl-4-phenyl-1,2,3,6-tetrahydropyridine-induced Parkinson's disease. *J. Neurosci.* 2001, **21**: 9519–9528.

45. Mandal M, Adam L, Kumar R. Redistribution of activated caspase-3 to the nucleus during butyric acid-induced apoptosis. *Biochem. Biophys. Res. Commun.* 1999, **260**: 775–780.

46. Casciola-Rosen L, Nicholson DW, Chong T, *et al.* Apopain/CPP32 cleaves proteins that are essential for cellular repair: a fundamental principle of apoptotic death. *J. Exp. Med.* 1996, **183**: 1957–1964.

47. Mandir AS, Przedborski S, Jackson-Lewis V, *et al.* Poly(ADP-ribose) polymerase activation mediates 1-methyl-4-phenyl-1, 2,3,6-tetrahydropyridine (MPTP)-induced Parkinsonism. *Proc. Natl Acad. Sci. USA* 1999, **96**: 5774–5779.

48. Cosi C, Colpaert F, Koek W, Degryse A, Marien M. Poly(ADP-ribose) polymerase inhibitors protect against MPTP-induced depletions of striatal dopamine and cortical noradrenaline in C57B1/6 mice. *Brain Res.* 1996, **729**: 264–269.

49. Han Z, Malik N, Carter T, *et al.* DNA-dependent protein kinase is a target for a CPP32-like apoptotic protease. *J. Biol. Chem.* 1996, **271**: 25035–25040.

50. Tatton NA, Kish SJ. In situ detection of apoptotic nuclei in the substantia nigra compacta of 1-methyl-4-phenyl-1,2,3,6-tetrahydropyridine-treated mice using terminal deoxynucleotidyl transferase labelling and acridine orange staining. *Neuroscience* 1997, **77**: 1037–1048.

51. Hartmann A, Troadec JD, Hunot S, *et al.* Caspase-8 is an effector in apoptotic death of dopaminergic neurons in Parkinson's disease, but pathway inhibition results in neuronal necrosis. *J. Neurosci.* 2001, **21**: 2247–2255.

52. Duan W, Zhu X, Ladenheim B, *et al.* p53 inhibitors preserve dopamine neurons and motor function in experimental parkinsonism. *Ann. Neurol.* 2002, **52**: 597–606.

53. Wang H, Shimoji M, Yu SW, Dawson TM, Dawson VL. Apoptosis inducing factor and PARP-mediated injury in the MPTP mouse model of Parkinson's disease. *Ann. NY Acad. Sci.* 2003, **991**: 132–139.

54. Saporito MS, Brown EM, Miller MS, Carswell S. CEP-1347/KT-7515, an inhibitor of c-jun N-terminal kinase activation, attenuates the 1-methyl-4-phenyl tetrahydropyridine-mediated loss of nigrostriatal dopaminergic neurons in vivo. *J. Pharmacol. Exp. Ther.* 1999, **288**: 421–427.

55. Saporito MS, Thomas BA, Scott RW. MPTP activates c-Jun NH(2)-terminal kinase (JNK) and its upstream regulatory kinase MKK4 in nigrostriatal neurons in vivo. *J. Neurochem.* 2000, **75**: 1200–1208.

56. Chen JY, Hsu PC, Hsu IL, Yeh GC. Sequential up-regulation of the *c-fos*, *c-jun* and *bax* genes in the cortex, striatum and cerebellum induced by a single injection of a low dose of 1-methyl-4-phenyl-1,2,3,6-tetrahydropyridine (MPTP) in C57Bl/6 mice. *Neurosci. Lett.* 2001, **314**: 49–52.

57. Offen D, Beart PM, Cheung NS, *et al.* Transgenic mice expressing human Bcl-2 in their neurons are resistant to 6-hydroxydopamine and 1-methyl-4-phenyl-1,2,3,6-tetrahydropyridine neurotoxicity. *Proc. Natl Acad. Sci. USA* 1998, **95**: 5789–5794.

58. Forno LS, DeLanney LE, Irwin I, Langston JW. Evolution of nerve fiber degeneration in the striatum in the MPTP-treated squirrel monkey. *Mol. Neurobiol.* 1994, **9**: 163–170.

59. Langston JW, Forno LS, Rebert CS, Irwin I. Selective nigral toxicity after systemic administration of 1-methyl-4- phenyl-1,2,5,6-tetrahydropyrine (MPTP) in the squirrel monkey. *Brain Res.* 1984, **292**: 390–394.

60. Imai H, Nakamura T, Endo K, Narabayashi H. Hemiparkinsonism in monkeys after unilateral caudate nucleus infusion of 1-methyl-4-phenyl-1,2,3,6-tetrahydropyridine (MPTP): behavior and histology. *Brain Res.* 1988, **474**: 327–332.

61. Russ H, Mihatsch W, Gerlach M, Riederer P, Przuntek H. Neurochemical and behavioural features induced by chronic low dose treatment with 1-methyl-4-phenyl-1,2,3,6-tetrahydropyridine (MPTP) in the common marmoset: implications for Parkinson's disease? *Neurosci. Lett.* 1991, **123**: 115–118.

62. Albanese A, Granata R, Gregori B, *et al.* Chronic administration of 1-methyl-4-phenyl-1,2,3,6-tetrahydropyridine to monkeys: behavioural, morphological and biochemical correlates. *Neuroscience* 1993, **55**: 823–832.

63. Kupsch A, Sautter J, Schwarz J, *et al.* 1-Methyl-4-phenyl-1,2,3,6-tetrahydropyridine-induced neurotoxicity in non-human primates is antagonized by pretreatment with nimodipine at the nigral, but not at the striatal level. *Brain Res.* 1996, **741**: 185–196.

64. Hansard MJ, Smith LA, Jackson MJ, Cheetham SC, Jenner P. Dopamine, but not norepinephrine or serotonin, reuptake inhibition reverses motor deficits in 1-methyl-4-phenyl-1,2,3,6-tetrahydropyridine-treated primates. *J. Pharmacol. Exp. Ther.* 2002, **303**: 952–958.

65. Jakowec MW, Donaldson DM, Barba J, Petzinger GM. Postnatal expression of alpha-synuclein protein in the rodent substantia nigra and striatum. *Devel. Neurosci.* 2001, **23**: 91–99.

66. Jenner P. The contribution of the MPTP-treated primate model to the development of new treatment strategies for Parkinson's disease. *Parkinsonism Relat. Disord.* 2003, **9**: 131–137.

67. Liou HH, Tsai MC, Chen CJ, *et al.* Environmental risk factors and Parkinson's disease: a case-control study in Taiwan. *Neurology* 1997, **48**: 1583–1588.

68. Grant H, Lantos PL, Parkinson C. Cerebral damage in paraquat poisoning. *Histopathology* 1980, **4**: 185–195.

69. Barbeau A, Dallaire L, Buu NT, *et al.* New amphibian models for the study of 1-methyl-4-phenyl-1,2,3,6- tetrahydropyridine (MPTP). *Life Sci.* 1985, **36**: 1125–1134.

70. Di Monte D, Sandy MS, Ekstrom G, Smith MT. Comparative studies on the mechanisms of paraquat and 1-methyl-4-phenylpyridine (MPP^+) cytotoxicity. *Biochem. Biophys. Res. Commun.* 1986, **137**: 303–309.

71. Koller WC. Paraquat and Parkinson's disease. *Neurology* 1986, **36**: 1147.

72. Rajput AH, Uitti RJ. Paraquat and Parkinson's disease. *Neurology* 1987, **37**: 1820–1821.

73. Sanchez-Ramos JR, Hefti F, Weiner WJ. Paraquat and Parkinson's disease. *Neurology* 1987, **37**: 728.

74. Tanner CM, Ottman R, Goldman SM, *et al.* Parkinson disease in twins: an etiologic study. *J. Am. Med. Ass.* 1999, **281**: 341–346.

75. Di Monte DA. The environment and Parkinson's disease: is the nigrostriatal system preferentially targeted by neurotoxins? *Lancet Neurol.* 2003, **2**: 531–538.

76. Wesseling C, van Wendel de Joode B, Ruepert C, *et al.* Paraquat in developing countries. *Int. J. Occup. Environ. Health* 2001, **7**: 275–286.

77. Markey SP, Weisz A, Bacon JP. Reduced paraquat does not exhibit MPTP-like neurotoxicity. *J. Anal. Toxicol.* 1986, **10**: 257.

78. Li X, Sun AY. Paraquat induced activation of transcription factor AP-1 and apoptosis in PC12 cells. *J. Neural Transm.* 1999, **106**: 1–21.

79. Thiruchelvam M, Brockel BJ, Richfield EK, Baggs RB, Cory-Slechta DA. Potentiated and preferential effects of combined paraquat and maneb on nigrostriatal dopamine systems: environmental risk factors for Parkinson's disease? *Brain Res.* 2000, **873**: 225–234.

80. Brooks AI, Chadwick CA, Gelbard HA, Cory-Slechta DA, Federoff HJ. Paraquat-elicited neurobehavioral syndrome caused by dopaminergic neuron loss. *Brain Res.* 1999, **823**: 1–10.

81. Chun HS, Gibson GE, DeGiorgio LA, *et al.* Dopaminergic cell death induced by MPP(+), oxidant and specific neurotoxicants shares the common molecular mechanism. *J. Neurochem.* 2001, **76**: 1010–1021.

82. Shimizu K, Ohtaki K, Matsubara K, *et al.* Carrier-mediated processes in blood–brain barrier penetration and neural uptake of paraquat. *Brain Res.* 2001, **906**: 135–142.

83. McCormack AL, Thiruchelvam M, Manning-Bog AB, *et al.* Environmental risk factors and Parkinson's disease: selective degeneration of nigral dopaminergic neurons caused by the herbicide paraquat. *Neurobiol. Dis.* 2002, **10**: 119–127.

84. Thiruchelvam M, Richfield EK, Goodman BM, Baggs RB, Cory-Slechta DA. Developmental exposure to the pesticides paraquat and maneb and the Parkinson's disease phenotype. *Neurotoxicology* 2002, **23**: 621–633.

85. Shimizu K, Matsubara K, Ohtaki K, Shiono H. Paraquat leads to dopaminergic neural vulnerability in organotypic midbrain culture. *Neurosci. Res.* 2003, **46**: 523–532.

86. Andersen JK. Paraquat and iron exposure as possible synergistic environmental risk factors in Parkinson's disease. *Neurotox. Res.* 2003, **5**: 307–313.

87. Thiruchelvam M, Richfield EK, Baggs RB, Tank AW, Cory-Slechta DA. The nigrostriatal dopaminergic system as a preferential target of repeated exposures to combined paraquat and maneb: implications for Parkinson's disease. *J. Neurosci.* 2000, **20**: 9207–9214.

88. Uversky VN, Li J, Fink AL. Metal-triggered structural transformations, aggregation, and fibrillation of human alpha-synuclein: a possible molecular NK between Parkinson's disease and heavy metal exposure. *J. Biol. Chem.* 2001, **276**: 44284–44296.

89. Uversky VN, Li J, Fink AL. Pesticides directly accelerate the rate of alpha-synuclein fibril formation: a possible factor in Parkinson's disease. *FEBS Lett.* 2001, **500**: 105–108.

90. Corasaniti MT, Strongoli MC, Rotiroti D, Bagetta G, Nistico G. Paraquat: a useful tool for the in vivo study of mechanisms of neuronal cell death. *Pharmacol. Toxicol.* 1998, **83**: 1–7.

91. Liou HH, Chen RC, Tsai YF, *et al.* Effects of Paraquat on the substantia nigra of the Wistar rats: neurochemical, histological, and behavioral studies. *Toxicol. Appl. Pharmacol.* 1996, **137**: 34–41.

92. Peng J, Mao XO, Stevenson FF, Hsu M, Andersen JK. The herbicide Paraquat induces dopaminergic nigral apoptosis through sustained activation of the JNK pathway. *J. Biol. Chem.* 2004.

93. Schuler F, Casida JE. Functional coupling of PSST and ND1 subunits in NADH: ubiquinone oxidoreductase established by photoaffinity labeling. *Biochim. Biophys. Acta* 2001, **1506**: 79–87.

94. Greenamyre JT, Sherer TB, Betarbet R, Panov AV. Complex I and Parkinson's disease. *IUBMB Life* 2001, **52**: 135–141.

95. Greenamyre JT, MacKenzie G, Peng TI, Stephans SE. Mitochondrial dysfunction in Parkinson's disease. *Biochem. Soc. Symp.* 1999, **66**: 85–97.

96. Giasson BI, Duda JE, Murray IV, *et al.* Oxidative damage linked to neurodegeneration by selective alpha-synuclein nitration in synucleinopathy lesions. *Science* 2000, **290**: 985–989.

97. Trojanowski JQ. Rotenone neurotoxicity: a new window on environmental causes of Parkinson's disease and related brain amyloidoses. *Exp. Neurol.* 2003, **179**: 6–8.

98. Orth M, Tabrizi SJ. Models of Parkinson's disease. *Mov. Disord.* 2003, **18**: 729–737.

99. Heikkila RE, Nicklas WJ, Vyas I, Duvoisin RC. Dopaminergic toxicity of rotenone and the 1-methyl-4-phenylpyridinium ion after their stereotaxic administration to rats: implication for the mechanism of 1-methyl-4-phenyl-1,2,3,6-tetrahydropyridine toxicity. *Neurosci. Lett.* 1985, **62**: 389–394.

100. Ferrante RJ, Schulz JB, Kowall NW, Beal MF. Systemic administration of rotenone produces selective damage in the striatum and globus pallidus, but not in the substantia nigra. *Brain Res.* 1997, **753**: 157–162.

101. Thiffault C, Langston JW, Di Monte DA. Increased striatal dopamine turnover following acute administration of rotenone to mice. *Brain Res.* 2000, **885**: 283–288.

102. Betarbet R, Sherer TB, MacKenzie G, *et al.* Chronic systemic pesticide exposure reproduces features of Parkinson's disease. *Nature Neurosci.* 2000, **3**: 1301–1306.

103. Sherer TB, Betarbet R, Stout AK, *et al.* An in vitro model of Parkinson's disease: linking mitochondrial impairment to altered alpha-synuclein metabolism and oxidative damage. *J. Neurosci.* 2002, **22**: 7006–7015.

104. Alam M, Schmidt WJ. Rotenone destroys dopaminergic neurons and induces Parkinsonian symptoms in rats. *Behav. Brain Res.* 2002, **136**: 317–324.

105. Betarbet R, Sherer TB, Di Monte DA, Greenamyre JT. Mechanistic approaches to Parkinson's disease pathogenesis. *Brain Pathol.* 2002, **12**: 499–510.

106. Tada-Oikawa S, Hiraku Y, Kawanishi M, Kawanishi S. Mechanism for generation of hydrogen peroxide and change of mitochondrial membrane potential during rotenone-induced apoptosis. *Life Sci.* 2003, **73**: 3277–3288.

107. Sherer TB, Kim JH, Betarbet R, Greenamyre JT. Subcutaneous rotenone exposure causes highly selective dopaminergic degeneration and alpha-synuclein aggregation. *Exp. Neurol.* 2003, **179**: 9–16.

108. Alam M, Mayerhofer A, Schmidt WJ. The neurobehavioral changes induced by bilateral rotenone lesion in medial forebrain bundle of rats are reversed by L-DOPA. *Behav. Brain Res.* 2004, **151**: 117–124.

109. Hoglinger GU, Feger J, Prigent A, *et al.* Chronic systemic complex I inhibition induces a hypokinetic multisystem degeneration in rats. *J. Neurochem.* 2003, **84**: 491–502.

110. Braak H, Del Tredici K, Bratzke H, *et al.* Staging of the intracerebral inclusion body pathology associated with idiopathic Parkinson's disease (preclinical and clinical stages). *J. Neurol.* 2002, **249** (Suppl. 3): III/1–5.

111. Forno LS. Neuropathology of Parkinson's disease. *J. Neuropathol. Exp. Neurol.* 1996, **55**: 259–272.

112. Lang-Rollin I, Vekrellis K, Wang Q, Rideout HJ, Stefanis L. Application of proteasomal inhibitors to mouse sympathetic neurons activates the intrinsic apoptotic pathway. *J. Neurochem.* 2004, **90**: 1511–1520.

113. Ardley HC, Scott GB, Rose SA, Tan NG, Robinson PA. UCH-L1 aggresome formation in response to proteasome impairment indicates a role in inclusion formation in Parkinson's disease. *J. Neurochem.* 2004, **90**: 379–391.

114. McNaught KS, Bjorklund LM, Belizaire R, *et al.* Proteasome inhibition causes nigral degeneration with inclusion bodies in rats. *NeuroReport* 2002, **13**: 1437–1441.

115. McNaught KS, Jenner P. Proteasomal function is impaired in substantia nigra in Parkinson's disease. *Neurosci. Lett.* 2001, **297**: 191–194.

116. McNaught KS, Perl DP, Brownell AL, Olanow CW. Systemic exposure to proteasome inhibitors causes a progressive model of Parkinson's disease. *Ann. Neurol.* 2004, **56**: 149–162.

117. Moilanen JS, Autere JM, Myllyla VV, Majamaa K. Complex segregation analysis of Parkinson's disease in the Finnish population. *Hum. Genet.* 2001, **108**: 184–189.

118. Polymeropoulos MH, Lavedan C, Leroy E, *et al.* Mutation in the alpha-synuclein gene identified in families with Parkinson's disease. *Science* 1997, **276**: 2045–2047.

119. Marder K, Logroscino G, Alfaro B, *et al.* Environmental risk factors for Parkinson's disease in an urban multiethnic community. *Neurology* 1998, **50**: 279–281.

120. Athanassiadou A, Voutsinas G, Psiouri L, *et al.* Genetic analysis of families with Parkinson disease that carry the Ala53Thr mutation in the gene encoding alpha-synuclein. *Am. J. Hum. Genet.* 1999, **65**: 555–558.

121. Papapetropoulos S, Paschalis C, Athanassiadou A, *et al.* Clinical phenotype in patients with alpha-synuclein Parkinson's disease living in Greece in comparison with patients with sporadic Parkinson's disease. *J. Neurol. Neurosurg. Psychiat.* 2001, **70**: 662–665.

122. Farrer M, Wavrant-De Vrieze F, Crook R, *et al.* Low frequency of alpha-synuclein mutations in familial Parkinson's disease. *Ann. Neurol.* 1998, **43**: 394–397.

123. Vaughan JR, Farrer MJ, Wszolek ZK, *et al.* Sequencing of the alpha-synuclein gene in a large series of cases of familial Parkinson's disease fails to reveal any further mutations: the European Consortium on Genetic Susceptibility in Parkinson's Disease (GSPD). *Hum. Mol. Genet.* 1998, **7**: 751–753.

124. Langston JW, Sastry S, Chan P, *et al.* Novel alpha-synuclein-immunoreactive proteins in brain samples from the Contursi kindred, Parkinson's, and Alzheimer's disease. *Exp. Neurol.* 1998, **154**: 684–690.

125. Narhi L, Wood SJ, Stevenson S, *et al.* Both familial Parkinson's disease mutations accelerate alpha-synuclein aggregation. *J. Biol. Chem.* 1999, **274**: 9843–9846.

126. Conway KA, Harper JD, Lansbury Jr PT. Fibrils formed in vitro from alpha-synuclein and two mutant forms linked to Parkinson's disease are typical amyloid. *Biochemistry* 2000, **39**: 2552–2563.

127. Conway KA, Lee SJ, Rochet JC, *et al.* Accelerated oligomerization by Parkinson's disease linked alpha-synuclein mutants. *Ann. NY Acad. Sci.* 2000, **920**: 42–45.

128. Li J, Uversky VN, Fink AL. Effect of familial Parkinson's disease point mutations A30P and A53T on the structural properties, aggregation, and fibrillation of human alpha-synuclein. *Biochemistry* 2001, **40**: 11604–11613.

129. Sommer B, Barbieri S, Hofele K, *et al.* Mouse models of alpha-synucleinopathy and Lewy pathology. *Exp. Gerontol.* 2000, **35**: 1389–1403.

130. Lo Bianco C, Ridet JL, Schneider BL, Deglon N, Aebischer P. Alpha-synucleinopathy and selective dopaminergic neuron loss in a rat lentiviral-based model of Parkinson's disease. *Proc. Natl Acad. Sci. USA* 2002, **99**: 10813–10818.

131. Lee MK, Stirling W, Xu Y, *et al.* Human alpha-synuclein-harboring familial Parkinson's disease-linked Ala-53 → Thr mutation causes neurodegenerative disease with alpha-synuclein aggregation in transgenic mice. *Proc. Natl Acad. Sci. USA* 2002, **99**: 8968–8973.

132. Kotzbauer PT, Trojanowsk JQ, Lee VM. Lewy body pathology in Alzheimer's disease. *J. Mol. Neurosci.* 2001, **17**: 225–232.

133. Jo E, McLaurin J, Yip CM, St George-Hyslop P, Fraser PE. Alpha-synuclein membrane interactions and lipid specificity. *J. Biol. Chem.* 2000, **275**: 34328–34334.

134. Davidson WS, Jonas A, Clayton DF, George JM. Stabilization of alpha-synuclein secondary structure upon binding to synthetic membranes. *J. Biol. Chem.* 1998, **273**: 9443–9449.

135. Zhu M, Li J, Fink AL. The association of alpha-synuclein with membranes affects bilayer structure, stability and fibril formation. *J. Biol. Chem.* 2003.

136. Bussell Jr R, Eliezer D. Residual structure and dynamics in Parkinson's disease-associated mutants of alpha-synuclein. *J. Biol. Chem.* 2001, **276**: 45996–46003.

137. Perrin RJ, Woods WS, Clayton DF, George JM. Interaction of human alpha-synuclein and Parkinson's disease variants with phospholipids: structural analysis using site-directed mutagenesis. *J. Biol. Chem.* 2000, **275**: 34393–34398.

138. Cole NB, Murphy DD. The cell biology of alpha-synuclein: a sticky problem? *Neuromol. Med.* 2002, **1**: 95–109.

139. Park JY, Lansbury Jr PT. Beta-synuclein inhibits formation of alpha-synuclein protofibrils: a possible therapeutic strategy against Parkinson's disease. *Biochemistry* 2003, **42**: 3696–3700.

140. Windisch M, Hutter-Paier B, Rockenstein E, *et al.* Development of a new treatment for Alzheimer's disease and Parkinson's disease using anti-aggregatory beta-synuclein-derived peptides. *J. Mol. Neurosci.* 2002, **19**: 63–69.

141. Hashimoto M, Bar-On P, Ho G, *et al.* Beta-synuclein regulates Akt activity in neuronal cells: a possible mechanism for neuroprotection in Parkinson's disease. *J. Biol. Chem.* 2004, **279**: 23622–23629.

142. da Costa CA, Masliah E, Checler F. Beta-synuclein displays an antiapoptotic p53-dependent phenotype and protects neurons from 6-hydroxydopamine-induced caspase 3 activation: cross-talk with alpha-synuclein and implication for Parkinson's disease. *J. Biol. Chem.* 2003, **278**: 37330–37335.

143. Neystat M, Lynch T, Przedborski S, *et al.* Alpha-synuclein expression in substantia nigra and cortex in Parkinson's disease. *Mov. Disord.* 1999, **14**: 417–422.

144. Kholodilov NG, Oo TF, Burke RE. Synuclein expression is decreased in rat substantia nigra following induction of apoptosis by intrastriatal 6-hydroxydopamine. *Neurosci. Lett.* 1999, **275**: 105–108.

145. Petersen K, Olesen OF, Mikkelsen JD. Developmental expression of alpha-synuclein in rat hippocampus and cerebral cortex. *Neuroscience* 1999, **91**: 651–659.

146. Orth M, Tabrizi SJ, Tomlinson C, *et al.* G209A mutant alpha synuclein expression specifically enhances dopamine induced oxidative damage. *Neurochem. Int.* 2004, **45**: 669–676.

147. Wersinger C, Sidhu A. Attenuation of dopamine transporter activity by alpha-synuclein. *Neurosci. Lett.* 2003, **340**: 189–192.

148. Hashimoto M, Hsu LJ, Rockenstein E, *et al.* Alpha-synuclein protects against oxidative stress via inactivation of the *c-Jun* N-terminal kinase stress-signaling pathway in neuronal cells. *J. Biol. Chem.* 2002, **277**: 11465–11472.

149. Baptista MJ, O'Farrell C, Daya S, *et al.* Co-ordinate transcriptional regulation of dopamine synthesis genes by alpha-synuclein in human neuroblastoma cell lines. *J. Neurochem.* 2003, **85**: 957–968.

150. Manning-Bog AB, McCormack AL, Purisai MG, Bolin LM, Di Monte DA. Alpha-synuclein overexpression protects against paraquat-induced neurodegeneration. *J. Neurosci.* 2003, **23**: 3095–3099.

151. Seo JH, Rah JC, Choi SH, *et al.* Alpha-synuclein regulates neuronal survival via Bcl-2 family expression and PI3/Akt kinase pathway. *FASEB J.* 2002, **16**: 1826–1828.

152. Hattori N, Kitada T, Matsumine H, *et al.* Molecular genetic analysis of a novel *Parkin* gene in Japanese families with autosomal recessive juvenile Parkinsonism: evidence for variable homozygous deletions in the *Parkin* gene in affected individuals. *Ann. Neurol.* 1998, **44**: 935–941.

153. Leroy E, Anastasopoulos D, Konitsiotis S, Lavedan C, Polymeropoulos MH. Deletions in the *Parkin* gene and genetic heterogeneity in a Greek family with early onset Parkinson's disease. *Hum. Genet.* 1998, **103**: 424–427.

154. Abbas N, Lucking CB, Ricard S, *et al.* A wide variety of mutations in the parkin gene are responsible for autosomal recessive parkinsonism in Europe: French Parkinson's Disease Genetics Study Group and the European Consortium on Genetic Susceptibility in Parkinson's Disease. *Hum. Mol. Genet.* 1999, **8**: 567–574.

155. Satoh J, Kuroda Y. Association of codon 167 Ser/Asn heterozygosity in the *Parkin* gene with sporadic Parkinson's disease. *NeuroReport* 1999, **10**: 2735–2739.

156. Hayashi S, Wakabayashi K, Ishikawa A, *et al.* An autopsy case of autosomal-recessive juvenile Parkinsonism with a homozygous exon 4 deletion in the parkin gene. *Mov. Disord.* 2000, **15**: 884–888.

157. van de Warrenburg BP, Lammens M, Lucking CB, *et al*. Clinical and pathologic abnormalities in a family with parkinsonism and *Parkin* gene mutations. *Neurology* 2001, **56**: 555–557.
158. Farrer M, Chan P, Chen R, *et al*. Lewy bodies and Parkinsonism in families with *Parkin* mutations. *Ann. Neurol.* 2001, **50**: 293–300.
159. Dawson TM, Dawson VL. Rare genetic mutations shed light on the pathogenesis of Parkinson disease. *J. Clin. Invest.* 2003, **111**: 145–151.
160. Forloni G, Terreni L, Bertani I, *et al*. Protein misfolding in Alzheimer's and Parkinson's disease: genetics and molecular mechanisms. *Neurobiol. Aging.* 2002, **23**: 957–976.
161. Takahashi H. [Juvenile parkinsonism: its neuropathological aspects.] *No To Shinkei.* 1994, **46**: 523–529. (In Japanese)
162. Schlossmacher MG, Frosch MP, Gai WP, *et al*. Parkin localizes to the Lewy bodies of Parkinson disease and dementia with Lewy bodies. *Am. J. Pathol.* 2002, **160**: 1655–1667.
163. Shimura H, Schlossmacher MG, Hattori N, *et al*. Ubiquitination of a new form of alpha-synuclein by *Parkin* from human brain: implications for Parkinson's disease. *Science* 2001, **293**: 263–269.
164. Kahle PJ, Neumann M, Ozmen L, *et al*. Subcellular localization of wild-type and Parkinson's disease-associated mutant alpha-synuclein in human and transgenic mouse brain. *J. Neurosci.* 2000, **20**: 6365–6373.
165. Imai Y, Soda M, Murakami T, *et al*. A product of the human gene adjacent to parkin is a component of Lewy bodies and suppresses Pael receptor-induced cell death. *J. Biol. Chem.* 2003, **278**: 51901–51910.
166. Zhang Y, Gao J, Chung KK, *et al*. Parkin functions as an E2-dependent ubiquitin-protein ligase and promotes the degradation of the synaptic vesicle-associated protein, CDCrel-1. *Proc. Natl Acad. Sci. USA* 2000, **97**: 13354–13359.
167. Shimura H, Hattori N, Kubo S, *et al*. Familial Parkinson disease gene product, parkin, is a ubiquitin-protein ligase. *Nature Genet.* 2000, **25**: 302–305.
168. Jiang H, Ren Y, Zhao J, Feng J. *Parkin* protects human dopaminergic neuroblastoma cells against dopamine-induced apoptosis. *Hum. Mol. Genet.* 2004, **13**: 1745–1754.
169. Petrucelli L, O'Farrell C, Lockhart PJ, *et al*. *Parkin* protects against the toxicity associated with mutant alpha-synuclein: proteasome dysfunction selectively affects catecholaminergic neurons. *Neuron* 2002, **36**: 1007–1019.
170. Ledesma MD, Galvan C, Hellias B, Dotti C, Jensen PH. Astrocytic but not neuronal increased expression and redistribution of parkin during unfolded protein stress. *J. Neurochem.* 2002, **83**: 1431–1440.
171. Mengesdorf T, Jensen PH, Mies G, Aufenberg C, Paschen W. Down-regulation of parkin protein in transient focal cerebral ischemia: a link between stroke and degenerative disease? *Proc. Natl Acad. Sci. USA* 2002, **99**: 15042–15047.
172. Higashi Y, Asanuma M, Miyazaki I, *et al*. Parkin attenuates manganese-induced dopaminergic cell death. *J. Neurochem.* 2004, **89**: 1490–1497.
173. Takahashi R, Imai Y. Pael receptor, endoplasmic reticulum stress, and Parkinson's disease. *J. Neurol.* 2003, **250** (Suppl. 3): III25–9.
174. Baptista MJ, Cookson MR, Miller DW. Parkin and alpha-synuclein: opponent actions in the pathogenesis of Parkinson's disease. *Neuroscientist* 2004, **10**: 63–72.
175. Darios F, Corti O, Lucking CB, *et al*. *Parkin* prevents mitochondrial swelling and cytochrome c release in mitochondria-dependent cell death. *Hum. Mol. Genet.* 2003, **12**: 517–526.

176. Briggs MD, Mortier GR, Cole WG, *et al*. Diverse mutations in the gene for cartilage oligomeric matrix protein in the pseudoachondroplasia–multiple epiphyseal dysplasia disease spectrum. *Am. J. Hum. Genet.* 1998, **62**: 311–319.

177. Liu Y, Fallon L, Lashuel HA, Liu Z, Lansbury Jr PT. The UCH-L1 gene encodes two opposing enzymatic activities that affect alpha-synuclein degradation and Parkinson's disease susceptibility. *Cell* 2002, **111**: 209–218.

178. Valente EM, Bentivoglio AR, Dixon PH, *et al*. Localization of a novel locus for autosomal recessive early-onset parkinsonism, PARK6, on human chromosome 1p35–p36. *Am. J. Hum. Genet.* 2001, **68**: 895–900.

179. Bonifati V, Dekker MC, Vanacore N, *et al*. Autosomal recessive early-onset Parkinsonism is linked to three loci: PARK2, PARK6, and PARK7. *Neurol. Sci.* 2002, **23** (Suppl. 2): S59–S60.

180. Baik JH, Picetti R, Saiardi A, *et al*. Parkinsonian-like locomotor impairment in mice lacking dopamine D2 receptors. *Nature* 1995, **377**: 424–428.

181. Dracheva S, Haroutunian V. Locomotor behavior of dopamine D1 receptor transgenic/D2 receptor deficient hybrid mice. *Brain Res.* 2001, **905**: 142–151.

182. Jaber M, Jones S, Giros B, Caron MG. The dopamine transporter: a crucial component regulating dopamine transmission. *Mov. Disord.* 1997, **12**: 629–633.

183. Grunewald T, Beal MF. NOS knockouts and neuroprotection. *Nature Med.* 1999, **5**: 1354–1355.

184. Andreassen OA, Ferrante RJ, Dedeoglu A, *et al*. Mice with a partial deficiency of manganese superoxide dismutase show increased vulnerability to the mitochondrial toxins malonate, 3- nitropropionic acid, and MPTP. *Exp. Neurol.* 2001, **167**: 189–195.

185. Maier CM, Chan PH. Role of superoxide dismutases in oxidative damage and neurodegenerative disorders. *Neuroscientist* 2002, **8**: 323–334.

186. Wu DC, Teismann P, Tieu K, *et al*. NADPH oxidase mediates oxidative stress in the 1-methyl-4-phenyl-1,2,3,6-tetrahydropyridine model of Parkinson's disease. *Proc. Natl Acad. Sci. USA*. 2003, **100**: 6145–6150.

187. Gao HM, Liu B, Hong JS. Critical role for microglial NADPH oxidase in rotenone-induced degeneration of dopaminergic neurons. *J. Neurosci.* 2003, **23**: 6181–6187.

188. Sriram K, Matheson JM, Benkovic SA, *et al*. Mice deficient in TNF receptors are protected against dopaminergic neurotoxicity: implications for Parkinson's disease. *FASEB J.* 2002, **16**: 1474–1476.

189. Dauer W, Kholodilov N, Vila M, *et al*. Resistance of alpha-synuclein null mice to the Parkinsonian neurotoxin MPTP. *Proc. Natl Acad. Sci. USA* 2002, **99**: 14524–14529.

190. Gerlai R, McNamara A, Choi-Lundberg DL, *et al*. Impaired water maze learning performance without altered dopaminergic function in mice heterozygous for the GDNF mutation. *Eur. J. Neurosci.* 2001, **14**: 1153–1163.

191. Chen JF, Xu K, Petzer JP, *et al*. Neuroprotection by caffeine and A(2A) adenosine receptor inactivation in a model of Parkinson's disease. *J. Neurosci.* 2001, **21**: RC143.

192. Witta J, Baffi JS, Palkovits M, *et al*. Nigrostriatal innervation is preserved in Nurr1-null mice, although dopaminergic neuron precursors are arrested from terminal differentiation. *Brain Res. Mol. Brain Res.* 2000, **84**: 67–78.

25

Animal models of epilepsy

RICARDO M. ARIDA, ALEXANDRE V. SILVA, MARGARETH R. PRIEL,
AND ESPER A. CAVALHEIRO

25.1 Introduction

Epilepsy is a common disorder of the brain affecting approximately 1–3% of people worldwide. Clinically, the epilepsies are characterized by spontaneous, recurrent epileptic seizures, either convulsive or non-convulsive, which are caused by partial or generalized discharges in the brain. Important advances have been made in the diagnosis and treatment of seizures disorders. Although many antiepileptic drugs (AEDs) have been introduced, approximately 30% of patients remain pharmacoresistant.[1]

Animal models of seizures and epilepsy have played a fundamental role in the understanding of the physiological and behavioral changes associated with human epilepsy. They allow us to determine the nature of injuries that might contribute to the development of epilepsy, to observe and intercede in the disease process subsequent to an injury preceding the onset of spontaneous seizures, and also to study the chronically epileptic brain in detail, using physiological, pharmacological, molecular, and anatomical techniques.

Some criteria for a good animal model should be satisfied before the model could be considered useful for a particular human seizure or epilepsy condition. As the pattern of electroencephalograph (EEG) activity is a hallmark of seizures and epilepsy, the animal model should exhibit similar electrophysiological patterns to those observed in the human condition. The animal model should display similar pathological changes to those found in humans, it should respond to AEDs with similar mechanisms of action, and behavioral characteristics should in some way reflect the behavioral manifestations observed in humans. This chapter briefly reviews those models that most closely approximate human epilepsy.

25.2 Experimental models of temporal lobe epilepsy

Epidemiological data have shown that the most frequent type of seizures in humans are complex partial seizures with or without generalization, which

Handbook of Experimental Neurology, ed. Turgut Tatlisumak and Marc Fisher. Published by Cambridge University Press. © Cambridge University Press 2006.

occur in about 40–50% of all patients with epilepsy.[2] The majority (70–80%) of complex partial seizures originate in the temporal lobes, particularly in the hippocampus and amygdala, and the term temporal lobe epilepsy (TLE) is used in this regard. Animal models constitute one of our most valuable tools to better understand the pathophysiology of TLE.

Based on factors that contribute to the development of TLE, some characteristics of the ideal animal model can be suggested. For instance, the ideal animal model of TLE would be expected to display spontaneous seizures some time after an initiating insult, i.e., the latent period. The latent period between the initial insult and the occurrence of a behavioral seizure would be expected to be days to weeks in duration and should reflect a period in which the animal does not display behavioral seizures. The latent period also is considered the phase in which functional and structural reorganization is occurring as a consequence of a specific series of pathologic events. Therefore, the functional and structural reorganization that contributes to the expression of spontaneous seizures should also be consistent with that observed in human tissue.

The ideal model of human TLE may also be characterized by additional neuroplastic changes that manifest as pharmacologic resistance to existing AEDs or cognitive impairment. There are several animal models of epileptogenesis that share many similarities with TLE and have been used to study the molecular biology of the epileptogenic process. These animal models involve experimental manipulations in which the epileptic condition results in brain damage induced by an acute episode of status epilepticus. This event can be triggered through two mechanisms: administration of a chemical convulsant, such as pilocarpine or kainic acid (KA), or electrical stimulation (amygdala, perforant path, or hippocampus) (for review see reference 3). Induction of status epilepticus allows the animals to have persistent seizures for more than 1 hr. Unlike kindling and other models of acquired epilepsy, an extremely high proportion of animals that survive the initial status epilepticus episode develop spontaneous seizures after a latent period of days to weeks. The presence of a latent period between the initiating insult and the first spontaneous seizure satisfies an important criterion for a model of acquired epilepsy. Among many animal models of TLE, this review focuses on three specific models of epileptogenesis: the kindling model, the pilocarpine model, and KA model (for review see reference 4).

25.2.1 Kindling model

Since its introduction in 1969, kindling has become one of the most widely used animal models of epilepsy.[5] Kindling can be induced by the repeated administration of a subconvulsive stimulus administered through a bipolar electrode implanted into a limbic structure such as the amygdala, hippocampus, entorhinal cortex, or other brain areas. Over a period of several stimulation days, the animal displays both behavioral and electrographic seizures that spread to become secondarily generalized. In rats stimulated in the amygdala, the initial stimulus often elicits focal paroxysmal activity (i.e., so-called "after-discharges") without apparent clinical seizure activity. Subsequent stimulations induce the progressive development of seizures, generally evolving through the following stages: (1) immobility, facial clonus, eye closure, twitching of the vibrissae, (2) head nodding, (3) unilateral forelimb clonus, (4) rearing, and (5) rearing and falling accompanied by secondary generalized clonic seizure.[6] The behavior observed in stages 1 and 2 mimics that found in human complex partial (limbic or temporal lobe) seizures; the behavior in the latter three stages would be consistent with complex partial seizures evolving to generalized motor seizures. Furthermore, the electrical threshold for induction of after-discharges significantly decreases during kindling development. An animal is usually considered being fully kindled after it displays several (e.g., at least three) stage 5 seizures and a stable duration of electrographic after-discharge (typically 60–80 s in duration).

The increased convulsive sensitivity persists for at least several months after kindling has been established and does appear to reflect permanent changes in brain function.[5] If kindling stimulation is continued, animals develop spontaneous seizures demonstrating that kindling has resulted in epileptogenesis. Pinel *et al.* first described these spontaneous seizures in kindled rats.[7] However, before the spontaneous seizures appeared, it was demonstrated that kindling progressed beyond stage 5 seizure levels and involved more severe events characterized by brainstem evoked seizures (labeled as stages 6–8).[8]

Although it is not routinely observed, different species of kindled animals can develop spontaneous recurrent seizures, reinforcing the concept that brain networks become permanently hyperexcitable after repeated partial seizures.[9] All animal species examined are susceptible to kindling including frog, reptile, rat, mouse, rabbit, dog, cat, rhesus monkey, and baboon.[9]

Unlike the status epilepticus models discussed below, seizures in the kindling models are usually evoked rather than spontaneous. However, with repeated stimulation the kindled rat eventually displays spontaneous seizures. Because the seizures are evoked rather than spontaneous, the kindled rat does not display a "latent" period. Nevertheless, the changes that take place with each stimulation lead to changes in plasticity that contribute to a permanent state of hyperexcitability. In this regard, the development of a stage 5 seizure can be viewed as epileptogenesis. The pathophysiology of kindling is very similar to that of human mesial TLE. For example, kindling leads to structural and functional changes characterized by neuronal cell loss, gliosis, neurogenesis, and mossy fiber sprouting. In some animals, the plasticity changes associated with repeated kindled seizures may also lead to cognitive impairment.[10] Because the kindled seizure is evoked rather than spontaneous and lacks a definable latent period, it is not necessarily considered to be an ideal model of epileptogenesis. Nevertheless, the kindling model has been used extensively in the search for novel AEDs for the treatment of partial seizures. For these studies, the drug is tested in the fully kindled rat to determine whether it prevents the expression of the evoked kindled seizure. The kindling model has also been used to assess whether a drug administered during the kindling process will prevent or delay the development of kindling.[11]

25.2.2 *Pilocarpine model*

The pilocarpine model of epilepsy reproduces the main features of human TLE in rats and mice. The pilocarpine model as well as the KA model are probably the most commonly studied chemical-inductive models for TLE. The first evidence that rats with brain damage induced by pilocarpine-triggered status epilepticus could develop spontaneous recurrent seizures (SRSs) in the long run occurred in 1983.[12] The pilocarpine model was fully characterized in rats in the following years.[13,14]

As extensively described by Turski *et al.* a single high dose of pilocarpine (300–380 mg/kg intraperitoneally (i.p.)), a potent muscarinic cholinergic agonist originally isolated from the leaves of a South American shrub, acutely induces sequential behavioral and electrographic changes indicative of sustained epileptic activity, resulting in widespread damage to the forebrain in both rats and mice.[15] The initial alterations comprise akinesia, ataxia, facial automatisms, and head tremor. After 15–25 min those changes evolve to motor limbic seizures with rearing, forelimb clonus, salivation, intense masticatory movements, and falling. Such fits recur every 2–8 min and lead to status epilepticus within 50–60 min after pilocarpine administration that lasts for up 12 hr, rendering the animals prostrate or critically ill. The first 24 hr taken by those manifestations, when the lethality rate reaches 30%, was called the acute period.

Electrographic changes immediately after pilocarpine injection includes a significant theta rhythm superceding the background activity in the hippocampus and low voltage fast activity in the cortex. This progresses to high voltage fast activity with spikes in the hippocampus. Sequentially, spiking activity spreads to the cortex and evolves into electrographic seizures that

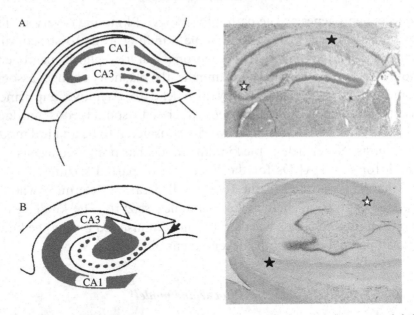

Figure 25.1. Hippocampal damage in human and animal temporal lobe epilepsy. On the left, anatomical diagrams of (A) rat and (B) human hippocampal formation. On the right, histological pattern of (A) rat and (B) human hippocampal damage. Arrows in A and B point to the hippocampal fissure. Note the typical neuronal cell loss in CA1 (black stars) and CA3 (white stars).

recur every 2–8 min and finally become continuous within 50–60 min after pilocarpine administration. This pattern of electrographic activity is sustained for 6–12 hr and then gradually abates during the next 12–24 hr. Morphological analysis of the brains by the end of this period shows characteristic damage preferentially distributed in the hippocampus, thalamus, amygdaloid complex, pyriform and entorhynal cortex, neocortex, and substantia nigra.[15] After a silent period (seizure-free phase) that varies from 4 to 44 days (mean 14.8 ± 3.0 days) all surviving animals start exhibiting the SRSs which characterize the chronic period, varying from 2 to 15 seizure episodes per month (mean of 2–3 seizures per week). Behaviorally, a spontaneous seizure is characterized by facial automatisms, head nodding, forelimb clonus, rearing, and falling, and electrographically by paroxysmal hippocampal discharges that rapidly spread to cortical regions.[13,14] The behavioral analysis of this model has been reviewed in detail.[16]

Morphological analysis of the brain after pilocarpine-induced status epilepticus demonstrates cell loss in the hippocampal subfields CA1 and CA3 (Fig. 25.1) and in the hilus of dentate gyrus, in the septum, olfactory tubercle, amygdala, piriform cortex, neocortex, and thalamic nuclei.[12,17]

Supragranular sprouting of the mossy fibers is also observed, starting as early as 4 days after status epilepticus and increases with time reaching a plateau by 100-day survival.[18]

Pretreatment with lithium chloride 24 hr prior to pilocarpine injection, at a dose of 3 mEq/kg, i.p., potentiates the epileptogenic action of pilocarpine and the amount of the drug can be reduced by a factor of 10. Behavioral manifestations and the pattern of seizure-induced brain damage after high doses of pilocarpine and lithium/pilocarpine models are very similar. It seems that the lithium–pilocarpine protocol reduces mortality, and avoids many of the peripheral cholinomimetic side effects of high doses of pilocarpine.[19]

In addition to the systemic injection of pilocarpine, local administration of pilocarpine delivered either intracerebroventricularly or directly into the hippocampus has been used in studies assessing seizure-induced changes in amino acid levels and the effectiveness of some antiepileptic agents.[20,21]

25.2.3 Kainic acid model

In addition to the pilocarpine model, seizures induced by the excitotoxic glutamate analogue kainite (KA) have increasingly been used as a model of TLE. KA (in Japanese literally "the ghost of the sea") was isolated some decades ago from the seaweed *Digenea simplex*[22] which had been extensively used in post-war Japan to eradicate ascariasis. It was originally suggested by Olney *et al.* that KA and other analogs of glutamate are toxic since they activate glutamate receptors on neuronal surfaces resulting in prolonged depolarization, neuronal swelling, and death.[23]

KA can be systemically or intracerebrally injected into an animal and rapidly produce acute seizures.[24] In rodents, large doses of the drug induce severe acute seizures with subsequent status epilepticus, which is followed by a quiescent period of usually several weeks.[25] This latent period is followed by the development of spontaneous recurrent seizures. A convulsant dose of KA induces a variety of behavioral manifestations which mimic some automatisms observed in human TLE. Administration of KA to the rat elicits behavioral changes dependent on the dose and route of administration. Systemic administration (and injections into the amygdala) induces wet-dog shakes, sniffing, and masticatory movements followed by repetitive head nodding, rearing, forelimbs clonus, and sudden loss of upright posture. Between 1 and 2 hr after KA injection, the animal displays full status epilepticus. Injections into the rat hippocampal formation produce wet-dog shakes, forelimb clonus, and episodes of hyperactivity characterized by circling away from the injected side. In the course of the seizure, intermittent tonic–clonic convulsions may occur.

In summary, by whatever route it is administrated, KA initiates convulsive behavior that persists for hours (12–24 hr) after a single injection.

Electrographic recordings from cortical and subcortical structures have confirmed that the main three phases of behavioral abnormalities (staring, individual limbic seizures, status epilepticus) correspond respectively to: (1) a localized paroxysmal discharges in the hippocampus (2) involvement of other limbic structures (amygdala), and then (3) generalization to a number of other non-limbic structures. The hippocampus has a particular low threshold to parenteral KA.[26] Seizure activity is observed very soon after KA injection by various routes, usually within 5 min. When injections of KA are made into a localized region of the limbic system, seizure activity originates in that region.[25,27] After parenteral administration of KA, seizures appear first in the hippocampal area or amygdaloid complex.[28] Electrographic seizures quickly propagate throughout the limbic circuit.

The excitotoxic damage caused directly by KA is not selective if injected into any part of the brain,[23] i.e., practically all cell types present within the effective injection site will undergo edematous changes and degeneration. However, following intracerebroventricular or intraperitoneal injections some degree of selectivity appears; areas containing a high concentration of kainate receptors will be preferentially destroyed. The most extensively damaged area is the CA3 region of the hippocampus.[29] In addition to local effects, KA injections will also result in damage in distant brain regions which receive excitatory input from the injected area.[30,31] Injections of KA were shown to lead to cell death in the hippocampus, amygdala, entorhinal cortex, and medial thalamic nuclei.[27,28] The so-called "distant damage" is likely to be caused by hyperactivity in afferent excitatory pathways rather than by the direct action of kainate on its receptor.

Several well-characterized models have been described in the last decades and in many ways mimic complex partial seizures observed in patients with TLE. The three models discussed in this review are certainly the most commonly studied models for TLE and the recognition of these models is attributed to the satisfaction of many criteria necessary for a good animal model described above.

25.3 Experimental models of epilepsy in the developing brain

Epileptic seizures are frequently observed in the nursery and neonatal intensive care and may have different follow-up patterns, from complete recovery to permanent cognitive deficits or death. Clinical evidence suggests that the occurrence of seizures in the developing brain present two important aspects: (1) the immature brain has a lower threshold for seizures and (2) seizures during development show clinical manifestations different from those observed in adults. Moreover, some seizures are able to modify the maturational process and lead to chronic epilepsy and/or cognitive deficits.[32]

The immature brain has higher levels of excitability and hypersynchronicity among groups of neurons.[33] That hypersynchronicity can be related to an increased number of synapses in the developing brain, a higher number of gap junctions, or to the transient increased expression of some receptors for the excitatory amino acids. In fact, in the early postnatal period there is a preponderance of excitability over inhibition.[34]

Although gamma-aminobutyric acid (GABA)a receptors are expressed beginning in the embryonic period, their stimulation by specific agonists during the early phases of development results in an excitatory effect.[35] The activation of GABAa depolarizes the immature neuroblasts and neurons in all the regions of the central nervous system. This depolarization is derived from the increase of intracellular chloride concentration. When GABAergic and glutamatergic synapses are co-activated during physiological activity, GABAa receptors can facilitate the activation of the N-methyl-D-aspartate (NMDA) glutamatergic receptors playing a similar role to the AMPA (amino-3-hydroxy-5-methyl-4-isoxazol proprionic acid) receptor that will appear later.[36] Moreover, in the initial phases of the developmental process, some excitatory amino acid receptors have a transient increased expression. This increased expression of NMDA and AMPA receptors in the early periods of the postnatal life coincides with rapid growth and cerebral differentiation,[37] representing a window of increased synaptic plasticity.[38]

The developmental process of the nervous system is characterized by the sequential occurrence of characteristic stages in each structure or area. Insults that occur in developing brain result in the transitory interruption of the normal maturational process and are followed by an intrinsic attempt at compensation. Studies suggest that large regions of cerebral injury in animals and humans during the early phases of development can result in a relatively small functional deficit. Among the factors that contribute to this recovery one should consider the greater propensity for brain plasticity during development. This plasticity is characterized by the occurrence of reversible (functional plasticity) and of long-term changes. Natural or artificial, internal or external stimulations can start this phenomenon resulting in positive or negative changes and its mechanisms are based on the modulation of the synaptic transmission.[39] In fact, the brain has plasticity mechanisms during the entire developmental period showing changes in the synaptic pattern, until it reaches the "adult brain" pattern. Therefore, developing brain exhibits a dynamic process of modifications and the possibility of different responses according to the age, intensity, and type of insult suffered.

Although important contributions have been made by different experimental studies of seizures in developing rats the clear relationship between seizures and definitive deficits later in life has not been completely elucidated. Here we describe several epilepsy models used in developing rats.

25.3.1 Partial epilepsy models

The occurrence of status epilepticus or prolonged febrile seizures during childhood as well as trauma or meningitis has been related to the late appearance of TLE. This hypothesis suggests that TLE could be a consequence of an initial precipitating injury leading to damage of selective hippocampal neuronal groups,[40] and resulting in hippocampal excitatory and inhibitory circuitry reorganization and mossy fiber sprouting.

Pilocarpine model

The pilocarpine model[14] has been used as a model of human TLE. As mentioned, this muscarinic cholinergic agonist, in adult rats, induces a rapid onset of limbic seizures culminating in status epilepticus and after a symptom-free period recurrent spontaneous seizures can be observed. In developing rats, the doses of pilocarpine needed to induce status epilepticus change according to age, and the youngest animals need the highest intraperitoneal dose.[41] Chronic seizures and brain damage following pilocarpine-induced status epilepticus can be observed only if status epilepticus is induced after the 18th day of life. The latent period to the chronic phase is longer in developing animals when compared to adult rats. Younger rats (less than 18 days old) do not develop spontaneous seizures as late consequence of pilocarpine-induced status epilepticus.[41] In addition, animals suffering multiple pilocarpine-induced status epilepticus at postnatal days 7–9 demonstrated several EEG changes, including frequent spiking activity and ictal discharges, and cognitive deficits but rare convulsive seizures that are not accompanied by evident neuronal loss in limbic or neocortical structures.[45] Moreover, animals exhibit chronic hippocampal hyperexcitability in the CA1 area and persistent latent epileptogenesis can be observed.[42]

Kainic acid model

Kainic acid doses and features are age dependent. Seven-day-old rats (P7) need a lower dose (2 mg/kg) while 10 mg/kg or more is required to induce status epilepticus in adult rats.[43] Even the manifestations are different: young animals show more scratching than wet-dog shakes, tonic–clonic seizures can be observed after postnatal day 7, and clonic seizures are present only if status epilepticus is induced after the 3rd week of life. Developing rats submitted to status epilepticus induced by KA before 30 days of life do not present hippo-campal neuronal loss, synaptic reorganization, or late recurrent spontaneous seizures[44,45] as observed in adult rats. Furthermore cognitive deficits have also been described in animals submitted to KA-induced status epilepticus at P20, P30, and P60. However behavioral deficits are absent in animals submitted to status epilepticus at P5 and P10.[46] Studies with multiple KA-induced status epilepticus in immature rats (P20–26) did not induce hippocampal damage.[47]

Kindling model

In immature rats the typical kindling paradigm used has been 1s, 60 Hz stimulations using interstimulus intervals of 15 min to 24 hr.[48] However, the threshold to after-discharge and the number of stimulus to reach the kindled state vary according to age. Fifteen-day-old rats have a higher amygdala after-discharge threshold than adult rats. The after-discharge threshold of animals submitted to amygdala kindling during the 3rd or 4th weeks is lower than that observed in younger or older animals. These animals also need a greater number of stimuli to reach the kindled state.[49]

25.3.2 Generalized epilepsy models

Generalized seizures can be frequently observed during development and the increased susceptibility to these seizures probably involves several brain struc-tures.[34] The following models are currently used in several laboratories, but do not strictly represent epilepsy models since they fail to reproduce the hallmark of the human syndrome that is the occurrence of spontaneous seizures. They should be more appropriately considered as models of seizures or convulsions.

Pentylenetetrazol (PTZ) model

Pentylenetetrazol (PTZ) has been used as an epilepsy model in developing brain since the late 1960s. Although it is known that PTZ is a GABA antagonist, its mechanism of action is not fully understood. The features of seizures induced by the systemic application of PTZ to immature rats are age-dependent. Tonic–clonic seizures are similar to those observed in adult rats but the clonic pattern is not fully present until the age of 21 days.[43] EEG recordings show spike-wave activity during clonic and tonic–clonic seizures that usually start in one hemisphere with posterior involvement of both hemispheres but without synchronization. On the other hand, repetitive seizures induced in developing rats by PTZ at P10 to P14 result in recurrent seizures and cognitive deficits without morphologic changes.[50]

Flurothyl model

Flurothyl ether (bis-2,2,2-triflurothyl ether) is a volatile convulsant gas with a fast action largely used to measure the threshold to generalized seizures. Its mechanism of action remains unclear but some studies have suggested that flurothyl could induce increased presynaptic transmission or postsynaptic conductance. Other putative mechanism is the inhibition of GABA synthesis.[51] It has been demonstrated that the mortality of 2-week-old rats submitted to fluorothyl-induced seizures is lower when compared to that observed in adult rats.[52] Behavioral manifestations are accompanied by EEG correlates characterized by high-frequency discharges (4–7 Hz) followed by continuous rhythmic spiking in cortex and hippocampus. However, hippocampal neuronal loss or aberrant sprouting was not observed.

25.4 Models of malformations of cortical development

Malformations of cortical development (MCD) are a heterogeneous group of anatomical derangements of the cortical mantle whose pathological features depend largely on the timing of the defect in the developmental process and to a lesser extent on its cause.[53] MCD range in severity from minor displacements of a few neurons to massive rearrangements of cortical structure. MCD are associated with neurological deficits and particularly epilepsy. In fact, 8–12% of cases of intractable epilepsy are associated with MCD, while 14–26% of surgically treated cases of pediatric epilepsy have MCD.[54]

There is a controversy about whether a malformation by itself or the adjacent abnormal cortex is the generator of epileptic activity. It is also not clear why some malformations are so refractory to AEDs. Recent progress in human molecular genetics has allowed the identification of several genes whose mutations lead to both malformations and epilepsy. In parallel, several genetic and non-genetic rodent models of MCD have been shown to be associated with either spontaneous seizures or hyperexcitability. Animals with induced MCD have a low seizure threshold and morphological changes similar to those found in human dysgenic brains.

Before describing animal models of MCD, it is important to distinguish between diffuse malformations that affect all neocortical structures and focal malformations that primarily target restricted cortical regions. Examples of diffuse malformations include the lissencephalies and the band heterotopias, whereas focal malformations comprise focal polymicrogyria and focal cortical dysplasia.[53] The important point to remember is that, in humans, any cortical malformation (diffuse or focal) can result in epilepsy.

25.4.1 Non-genetic models of MCD

Several teratogenic agents are known to cross the placenta and cause cortical malformations in the offspring. Generally, teratogenic treatments interfere with neurogenesis and neuronal migration, and thus cause microcephaly and disorganized cortical cytoarchitecture. Two models have been largely used to study the mechanisms and consequences of MCD by producing severe and reliably reproducible malformations. These models involve prenatal exposure to the DNA alkylating agent methylazoxymethanol (MAM) or gamma or X irradiation. Both treatments are more effective when applied around embryonic days 14–16 in rats. MAM[55] and irradiation[56] are basically antimitotic treatments that selectively kill dividing cells in the proliferative epithelium. MAM- or irradiation-exposed animals are invariably microcephalic and have partial corpus callosum agenesis with ventricular enlargement. In addition, they develop subcortical and intracortical heterotopias[57,58] formed by neurons that fail to migrate correctly, together with distinct disorganized laminar arrangements in both neocortical and hippocampal structures.[59]

In vivo EEG studies in irradiated animals showed an increased propensity for electrographic seizures in the presence of the sedating agents aceleromazine and xylazine.[60] Moreover, in vitro neocortical slices containing dysplastic cortex present enhanced excitability as compared to control neocortex when GABAergic inhibition is blocked with bicuculline methiodide.[61] The irradiated cortex is characterized by reduction in size, volume, and number of neurons and fibers,[62] reflecting the original lethal injury to neuronal precursors. Consequently, only neurons that survived this injury were able to continue their, albeit altered, development. The result is altered corticogenesis characterized by significant changes in neurons, fiber circuitry, and microvascularization.

Prenatal exposure to MAM in rats is able to induce neuronal heterotopias[57] that share striking similarities with those observed in human periventricular nodular heterotopia, a cerebral dysgenesis frequently associated with drug-resistant focal seizures. MAM exerts its effect by methylating pyrimidine bases in a time window of 2–24 hr, with maximal activity at 12 hr after administration.[55] A single MAM exposure on embryonic day 15 (E15), corresponding in rodents to the neurogenic peak at the neocortex, produce hippocampal heterotopias primarily involving the CA1 and CA2 subfields, reduction of cortical thickness, and subcortical neuronal heterotopia. Hippocampal neurons in

MAM rats are hyperexcitable in vitro[63] and animals show increased suscept-ibility to flurothyl- and hyperthermia-induced seizures in vivo.[64,65]

Besides MAM and irradiation models, there is another widely used non-genetic model of MCD that was described by Dvorak and colleagues in 1978.[66] Through freeze-induced lesions to the neonatal rat (postnatal days 0–2) cor-tical plate, these authors subsequently observed a focal four-layered cortex composed of a molecular layer, two external layers, and a deep layer.[66] This cortical malformation mimics human layered microgyria[67] and was inter-preted as a consequence of the migration of external layers through lesioned infragranular layers that were postmigratory at the time of the lesion.[68] A similar effect can be obtained by neonatal cortical injections of the glutamate agonist ibotenate in mice.[69] The "freezing model" of MCD has been exten-sively used to characterize the mechanisms of epileptogenicity associated with focal malformations. An epileptiform response to subconvulsive stimulation of the white matter was observed in cortical regions adjacent to the micro-gyrus.[70] The microgyrus itself, however, was never found to be the focus for abnormal seizure discharges. In fact, hyperexcitability is even conserved when the microgyrus is dissected out of the slice.[71]

25.4.2 Genetic models of MCD

Recent progress in human molecular genetics has allowed the identification of several genes whose mutations lead to both malformations and epilepsy. In parallel, several genetic rodent models of MCD have been shown to be associated with either spontaneous seizures or hyperexcitability. It is impor-tant to note that, as in other models of chronic epileptogenesis, it seems likely that more than one underlying pathophysiologic mechanism will turn out to be present in each genetic model.

More than 40 years ago, an autosomal mutation causing neurologic disorders associated with an abnormal pattern of lamination in all cortical structures (e.g., neocortex, hippocampus, and cerebellum) was identified in mice.[72,73] The so-called "reeler mouse" has been described as having a reversed cortex, with the deeper layers assuming an external position.[74] Reelin, the affected protein in reeler mice, is an extracellular serine protease that binds to several receptors in the migrating neurons.[75] During normal corticogenesis, reelin detaches the neuron from the radial glia arresting migration. Mutant mice with reduced reelin expression develop cortical malformations, with inverted outside-in lamination, and epileptic seizures. Similar phenotypes were recently reported in other mutant mice such as the *scrambler* mouse[76] and mice with engineered mutation (knockout) on the cyclin-dependant kinase cdk5 and its activator p35.[77,78]

Another mutant rodent, the *tish* rat, has been used to study a particular subtype of MCD: the subcortical band heterotopia, also called "double cortex." Subcortical band heterotopia is characterized by a large collection of heterotopic neurons located in the white matter below a normal-appearing cortex.[79] Similarly, mutant rats display a telencephalic internal structural heterotopia (TISH), characterized as a distinct band of heterotopic neocortex extending dorsally from the frontal to the dorsoparietal neocortex.[80] The heterotopia is present bilaterally, contains neurons with neocortical appearance, and displays near-normal connections with subcortical targets.[81] The affected animals typically exhibited partial seizures with variable secondary generalization.[80]

In recent years, it has been shown that animal models of cortical malformations can exhibit cortical hyperexcitability, with the exception of the reeler mouse that has various neurologic deficits but not epilepsy. Although malformed cortex can cause intrinsic hyperexcitability both in humans and in experimental models, some rodents with experimentally induced MCD do not have spontaneous seizures. Therefore, it is clear that the presence of a cortical malformation (although it can result in a significant hyperexcitability) does not necessarily result in a spontaneous epileptic phenotype.

Conclusion

This chapter represents only the beginning of what should be known about the most commonly used experimental models of epilepsy. There is an overwhelming need to develop new models and to investigate existing models for incorporation into the process of therapy discovery for epileptogenesis. Models that are age appropriate (for the developing, mature, and elderly brain) must be developed and the identification of genetic models with close parallels to human conditions is necessary. Models of chronic epilepsy with spontaneous seizures may be the best suited for the development of new therapies.

References

1. Schachter SC. Epilepsy. *Neurol. Clin.* 2001, **19**: 57–78.
2. Loscher W, Schmidt D. Strategies in antiepileptic drug development: is rational drug design superior to random screening and structural variation? *Epilepsy Res.* 1994, **17**: 95–134.
3. Walker MC, White HS, Sander JW. Disease modification in partial epilepsy. *Brain* 2002, **125**: 1937–1950.
4. Goodman JH. Experimental models of status epilepticus. In Peterson SL, Albertson TE (eds.) *Neuropharmacological Methods in Epilepsy Research.* Boca Raton, FL: CRC Press, 1998, pp. 95–125.

5. Sato M, Racine RJ, McIntyre DC. Kindling: basic mechanisms and clinical validity. *Electroenceph. Clin. Neurophysiol.* 1990, **76**: 459–472.

6. Racine RJ. Modification of seizure activity by electrical stimulation. II. Motor seizure. *Electroenceph. Clin. Neurophysiol.* 1972, **32**: 281–294.

7. Pinel JP, Mucha J, Phillips RF, *et al.* Spontaneous seizures generated in rats by kindling: a preliminary report. *Physiol. Psychol.* 1975, **3**: 127–129.

8. Pinel JP, Rovner JLI. Experimental epileptogenesis: kindling-induced epilepsy in rats. *Exp. Neurol.* 1978, **58**: 190–202.

9. McNamara JO, Wada JA. Kindling model. In Engel J, Pedley T (eds.) *Epilepsy: A Comprehensive Textbook*. Philadelphia, PA: Lippincott-Raven, 1997, pp. 419–425.

10. Pitkanen A, Sutula TP. Is epilepsy a progressive disorder? Prospects for new therapeutic approaches in temporal lobe epilepsy. *Lancet Neurol.* 2002, **1**: 173–181.

11. White HS. Animal models of epileptogenesis. *Neurology* 2002, **59**(Suppl. 5): S7–S14.

12. Turski WA, Czuczwar SJ, Cavalheiro EA, Turski L, Kleinrok Z. Acute and long-term effects of systemic pilocarpine in rats: spontaneous recurrent seizures as a possible model of temporal lobe epilepsy. *Naunyn-Schmiedebergs Arch. Pharmacol.* 1983, **324**: 25R.

13. Leite JP, Bortolotto ZA, Cavalheiro EA. Spontaneous recurrent seizures in rats: an experimental model of partial epilepsy. *Neurosci. Biobehav. Rev.* 1990, **14**: 511–517.

14. Cavalheiro EA, Leite JP, Bortolotto ZA, *et al.* Long-term effects of pilocarpine in rats: structural damage of the brain triggers kindling and spontaneous recurrent seizures. *Epilepsia* 1991, **32**: 778–782.

15. Turski WA, Cavalheiro EA, Schwarz M, *et al.* Limbic seizures produced by pilocarpine in rats: behavioural, electroencephalographic and neuropathological study. *Behav. Brain Res.* 1983, **9**: 315–335.

16. Arida RM, Scorza FA, Peres CA, Cavalheiro EA. The course of untreated seizures in the pilocarpine model of epilepsy. *Epilepsy Res.* 1999, **34**: 99–107.

17. Turski L, Cavalheiro EA, Sieklucka-Dziuba M, *et al.* Seizures produced by pilocarpine: neurophatological sequelae and activity of glutamate decarboxylase in the forebrain. *Brain Res.* 1986, **398**: 37–48.

18. Mello LEAM, Cavalheiro EA, Tan AM, *et al.* Circuit mechanisms of seizures in the pilocarpine model of chronic epilepsy: cell loss and mossy fiber sprouting. *Epilepsia* 1993, **34**: 985–995.

19. Clifford DB, Olney JW, Maniotis A, Collins RC, Zorumski CF. The functional anatomy and pathology of lithium/pilocarpine and high-dose pilocarpine seizures. *Neuroscience* 1987, **23**: 953–968.

20. Millan MH, Chapman AG, Meldrum BS. Extra-cellular amino acid levels in hippocampus during pilocarpine-induced seizures. *Epilepsy Res.* 1993, **14**: 139–148.

21. Smolders I, Khan GM, Lindekens H, *et al.* Effectiveness of vigabatrin against focally evoked pilocarpine-induced seizures and concomitant changes in extracellular hippocampal and cerebellar glutamate, γ-aminobutyric acid and dopamine levels, a microdialysis–electrocorticography study in freely moving rats. *J. Pharmacol. Exp. Ther.* 1997, **283**: 1239–1248.

22. Takemoto T. Isolation and structural identification of naturally occurring excitatory amino acids. In McGeer EG, Olney JW, McGeer P (eds.) *Kainic Acid as a Tool in Neurobiology*. New York: Raven Press, 1978, pp. 1–15.

23. Olney JW. Neurotoxicity of excitatory amino acids. In McGeer EG, Olney JW, McGeer P (eds.) *Kainic Acid as a Tool in Neurobiology*. New York: Raven Press, 1978, pp. 95–121.
24. Nadler V. Kainic acid as a tool for the study of temporal lobe epilepsy. *Life Sci.* 1981, **29**: 2031–2042.
25. Cavalheiro EA, Riche DA, Le Gal La Salle G. Long-term effects of intrahippocampal kainic acid injection in rats: a method for inducing spontaneous recurrent seizures. *Electroenceph. Clin. Neurophysiol.* 1982, **53**: 581–589.
26. Ben-Ari Y, Tremblay E, Riche D, Ghilini G, Naquet R. Electrographic, clinical and pathological alterations following systemic alterations of kainic acid, bicuculine and pentetrazole: metabolic mapping using the deoxyglucose method with special reference to the pathology of epilepsy. *Neuroscience* 1981, **6**: 1361–1391.
27. Ben-Ari Y, Tremblay E, Ottersen OP. Injections of kainic acid into the amygdaloid complex of the rat: an electrographic, clinical and histological study in relation to the pathology of epilepsy. *Neuroscience* 1980, **5**: 515–528.
28. Ben-Ari Y, Tremblay E, Ottersen OP, Meldrum BS. The role of epileptic activity in hippocampal and "remote" cerebral lesions induced by kainic acid. *Brain Res.* 1980, **191**: 79–97.
29. Nadler JV, Perry BW, Cotman CW. Intraventricular kainic acid preferentially destroys hippocampal pyramidal cells. *Nature* 1978, **271**: 676–677.
30. Ben-Ari Y, Tremblay E, Ottersen OP, Naquet R. Evidence suggesting secondary epileptogenic lesions after kainic acid: pretreatment with diazepam reduces distant but not local brain damage. *Brain Res.* 1979, **165**: 362–365.
31. Nadler JV, Perry BW, Gentry C, Cotman CW. Degeneration of hippocampal CA3 pyramidal cells induced by intraventricular kainic acid. *J. Comp. Neurol.* 1980, **192**: 333–359.
32. Jensen FE. Acute and chronic effects of seizures in the developing brain: experimental models. *Epilepsia* 1999, **40**(Suppl. 1): S51–S58.
33. Schwartzkroin PA. Basic mechanisms of epileptogenesis. In Wyllie E (ed.) *The Treatment of Epilepsy: Principles and Practice*. Baltimore, MD: Williams & Wilkins, 1993, pp. 83–98.
34. Moshé SL, Koszer S, Wolf SM, Cornblath M. Developmental aspects of epileptogenesis. In Wyllie E (ed.) *The Treatment of Epilepsy: Principles and Practice*. Baltimore, MD: Williams & Wilkins, 1993, pp. 139–150.
35. Cherubini E, Rovira C, Gaiarsa JL, Corradetti R, Ben-Ari Y. GABA mediated excitation in immature rat CA3 hippocampal neurons. *Int. J. Devel. Neurosci.* 1990, **8**: 481–490.
36. Ben-Ari Y, Khazipov R, Leinekugel X, Caillard O, Gaiarsa JL. GABAA, NMDA and AMPA receptors: a developmentally regulated 'ménage à trois'. *Trends Neurosci.* 1997, **20**: 523–529.
37. McDonald JW, Johnston MV. Excitatory amino acid neurotoxicity in the developing brain. *NIDA Res. Monogr.* 1993, **133**: 185–205.
38. Swann JW, Smith KL, Brady RJ. Neural networks and synaptic transmission in immature hippocampus. *Adv. Exp. Med. Biol.* 1990, **268**: 161–171.
39. Trojan S, Pokorny J. Theoretical aspects of neuroplasticity. *Physiol. Res.* 1999, **48**: 87–97.
40. Mathern GW, Price G, Rosales C, *et al*. Anoxia during kainate status epilepticus shortens behavioral convulsions but generates hippocampal neuron loss and supragranular mossy fiber sprouting. *Epilepsy Res.* 1998, **30**: 133–151.

41. Priel MR, Santos NF, Cavalheiro EA. Developmental aspects of the pilocarpine model of epilepsy. *Epilepsy Res.* 1996, **26**: 115–121.
42. Santos NF, Marques RH, Correia L, *et al.* Multiple pilocarpine-induced status epilepticus in developing rats: a long-term behavioral and electrophysiological study. *Epilepsia* 2000, **41**(Suppl. 6): S57–S63.
43. Velisek L, Veliskova J, Moshe SL. Developmental seizure models. *Ital. J. Neurol. Sci.* 1995, **16**: 127–133.
44. Stafstrom CE, Thompson JL, Holmes GL. Kainic acid seizures in the developing brain: status epilepticus and spontaneous recurrent seizures. *Devel. Brain Res.* 1992, **65**: 227–236.
45. Sperber EF, Haas KZ, Stanton PK, Moshé SL. Resistance of the immature hippocampus to seizure-induced synaptic reorganization. *Devel. Brain Res.* 1991, **60**: 88–93.
46. Stafstrom CE, Holmes GL, Chronopoulos A, Thurber S, Thompson JL. Age-dependent cognitive and behavioral deficits following kainic acid-induced seizures. *Epilepsia* 1993, **34**: 420–432.
47. Sarkisian MR, Tandon P, Liu Z, *et al.* Multiple kainic acid seizures in the immature and adult brain: ictal manifestations and long-term effects on learning and memory. *Epilepsia* 1997, **38**: 1157–1166.
48. Holmes GL, Thompson JL. Rapid kindling in the prepubescent rat. *Brain Res.* 1987, **433**: 281–284.
49. Moshe SL, Sharpless NS, Kaplan J. Kindling in developing rats: variability of afterdischarge thresholds with age. *Brain Res.* 1981, **211**: 190–195.
50. Holmes GL, Sarkisian M, Ben-Ari Y, Chevassus-au-Louis N. Mossy fiber sprouting after recurrent seizures during early development in rats. *J. Comp. Neurol.* 1999, **404**: 537–553.
51. Green AR, Metz A, Minchin MC, Vincent ND. Inhibition of the rate of GABA synthesis in regions of rat brain following a convulsion. *Br. J. Pharmacol.* 1987, **92**: 5–11.
52. Sperber EF, Haas KZ, Romero MT, Stanton PK. Flurothyl status epilepticus in developing rats: behavioral, electrographic histological and electrophysiological studies. *Devel. Brain Res.* 1999, **116**: 59–68.
53. Barkovich AJ, Kusniecky RI, Dobyns WB, *et al.* A classification scheme for malformations of cortical development. *Neuropediatrics* 1996, **27**: 59–63.
54. Polkey CE. Cortical dysplasia: resective surgery in children. In Guerrini R, Andermann F, Canapicchi R, *et al.* (eds.) *Dysplasias of Cerebral Cortex and Epilepsy.* Philadelphia, PA: Lippincott-Raven, 1996, pp. 435–439.
55. Cattaneo E, Reinach B, Caputi A, Cattabeni F, Di Luca M. Selective in vitro blockade of neuroepithelial cells proliferation by methylazoxymethanol acetate, a molecule capable of inducing long lasting functional impairments. *J. Neurosci. Res.* 1995, **41**: 640–647.
56. Hicks SP, D'Amato CJ, Lowe MJ. The development of the mammalian nervous system. I. Malformation of the brain, especially the cerebral cortex, induced in rats by radiation. II. Some mechanisms of the malformations of the cortex. *J. Comp. Neurol.* 1959, **113**: 435–69.
57. Collier PA, Ashwell KW. Distribution of neuronal heterotopiae following prenatal exposure to methylazoxymethanol. *Neurotoxicol. Teratol.* 1993, **15**: 439–444.
58. Chevassus-au-Louis N, Rafiki A, Jorquera I, Ben-Ari Y, Represa A. Neocortex in the hippocampus: morpho-functional analysis of CA1 heterotopias after prenatal

treatment with methylazoxymethanol in rats. *J. Comp. Neurol.* 1998, **394**: 520–536.

59. Ferrer I, Alcantara S, Zujer MI, Cinos C. Structure and pathogenesis of cortical nodules induced by prenatal X-irradiation in the rat. *Acta Neuropathol.* 1993, **85**: 205–212.

60. Roper SN, Gilmore RL, Houser CR. Experimentally induced disorders of neuronal migration produce an increased propensity for electrographic seizures in rats. *Epilepsy Res.* 1995, **21**: 205–219.

61. Roper SN, Abraham LA, Streit WJ. Exposure to in utero irradiation produces disruption of radial glia in rats. *Devel. Neurosci.* 1997, **19**: 521–528.

62. Marin-Padilla M, Tsai RJ, King MA, Roper SN. Altered corticogenesis and neuronal morphology in irradiation-induced cortical dysplasia: a Golgi–Cox study. *J. Neuropathol. Exp. Neurol.* 2003, **62**: 1129–1143.

63. Baraban SC, Schwartzkroin PA. Electrophysiology of CA1 pyramidal neurons in an animal model of neuronal migration disorders: prenatal methylazoxymethanol treatment. *Epilepsy Res.* 1995, **22**: 145–156.

64. Baraban SC, Schwartzkroin PA. Flurothyl seizure susceptibility in rats following prenatal methylazoxymethanol treatment. *Epilepsy Res.* 1996, **23**: 189–194.

65. Germano IM, Zhang YF, Sperber EF, Moshe SL. Neuronal migration disorders increase susceptibility to hyperthermia-induced seizures in developing rats. *Epilepsia* 1996, **37**: 902–910.

66. Dvorak K, Feit J, Jurankova Z. Experimentally induced focal microgyria and status verrucosus deformis in rats: pathogenesis and interrelation – histological and autoradiographical study. *Acta Neuropathol.* 1978, **44**: 121–129.

67. MacBride M, Temper T. Pathogenesis of four-layered microgyric cortex in man. *Acta Neuropathol.* 1982, **57**: 93–98.

68. Rosen GD, Sherman GF, Galaburda AM. Birthdates of neurons in induced microgyria. *Brain Res.* 1996, **727**: 71–8.

69. Marret S, Mukendi R, Gadisseux J-F, Gressens P, Evrard P. Effect of ibotenate on brain development: an excitotoxic mouse model of microgyria and posthypoxic-like lesions. *J. Neuropathol. Exp. Neurol.* 1995, **54**: 358–370.

70. Jacobs KM, Gutnick MJ, Prince DA. Hyperexcitability in a model of cortical maldevelopment. *Cereb. Cortex* 1996, **6**: 514–523.

71. Jacobs KM, Prince DA. Chronic focal neocortical epileptogenesis: does disinhibition play a role? *Can. J. Physiol. Pharmacol.* 1997, **75**: 500–507.

72. Falconer D. Two new mutants, *scrambler* and *reeler*, with neurological actions in the house mouse. *J. Genet.* 1951, **50**: 192–201.

73. Caviness Jr VS. Patterns of cell and fiber distribution in the neocortex of the reeler mutant mice. *J. Comp. Neurol.* 1976, **170**: 435–448.

74. Caviness Jr VS, Sidman RL. Time of origin of corresponding cell classes in the cerebral cortex of normal and reeler mutant mice: an autoradiographic analysis. *J. Comp. Neurol.* 1973, **148**: 141–151.

75. Jossin Y, Bar I, Ignatova N, *et al.* The reelin signaling pathway: some recent developments. *Cereb. Cortex* 2003, **13**: 627–633.

76. Sweet HO, Bronson RT, Johnson KR, Cook SA, Davisson MT. *Scrambler*, a new neurological mutation of the mouse with abnormalities of neuronal migration. *Mamm. Genome* 1996, **7**: 798–802.

77. Chae T, Kwon YT, Bronson R, *et al.* Mice lacking p35, a neuronal specific activator of cdk5, display cortical lamination defects, seizures, and adult lethality. *Neuron* 1997, **18**: 29–42.

78. Pearlman AL, Faust PL, Hatten ME, Brunstrom JE. New directions for neuronal migration. *Curr. Opin. Neurobiol.* 1998, **8**: 45–54.
79. Barkovich AJ, Kjos BO. Gray matter heterotopias: MR characteristics and correlation with developmental and neurologic manifestations. *Radiology* 1992, **182**: 493–499.
80. Lee KS, Schottler F, Collins JL, *et al.* A genetic model of human neocortical heterotopia associated with seizures. *J. Neurosci.* 1997, **17**: 6236–6242.
81. Schotter F, Couture D, Rao A, Kahn H, Lee KS. Subcortical connections of normotopic and heterotopic neurons in sensory and motor cortices of the tish mutant rat. *J. Comp. Neurol.* 1998, **25**: 29–42.

26

Experimental models of hydrocephalus

OSAAMA H. KHAN AND MARC R. DEL BIGIO

26.1 Introduction

Hydrocephalus is a common neurological condition characterized by impairment of cerebrospinal fluid (CSF) flow with subsequent enlargement of CSF-containing ventricular cavities in the brain. CSF absorption occurs through arachnoid villi into venous sinuses and along cranial and spinal nerves into lymphatics.[1] Enlarging ventricles damage the surrounding brain tissue. In children, hydrocephalus is associated with mental retardation, physical disability, and impaired growth. The pathogenesis of brain dysfunction includes alterations in the chemical environment of brain, chronic ischemia in white matter, and physical damage to axons with ultimate disconnection of neurons.[2–4] Hydrocephalus is the second most frequent congenital malformation (after spina bifida) of the nervous system, occurring in 5–6 per 10 000 live births.[5] It also develops in 80% of patients with spina bifida,[6] and 15% of premature (<30 weeks) infants following intraventricular hemorrhage.[7] Hydrocephalus can develop later in childhood or adulthood as a consequence of brain tumors, meningitis, brain injury, or subarachnoid hemorrhage.

For detailed discussions of the pathology of hydrocephalus see previous reviews (references 2 and 3). Briefly summarized, the ependyma lining the ventricles is damaged. In the subependymal layer, reactive gliosis is almost always observed and mitotic activity occurs among subependymal cells.[8] Hydrocephalus can cause reduction in cerebral blood flow and alterations in oxidative metabolism in subcortical regions[9,10] where white-matter axons and myelin are the main target of damage in hydrocephalus.[11,12] Imaging studies indicate that the brain is edematous in the periventricular region.[13] Severe hydrocephalus can cause thinning of the cerebral cortex and atrophy of the basal ganglia.[2] Age of the animal and mode of induction of hydrocephalus are important factors in determining the pathology.[14]

Handbook of Experimental Neurology, ed. Turgut Tatlisumak and Marc Fisher. Published by Cambridge University Press. © Cambridge University Press 2006.

26.2 Animal models

Hochwald categorized methods for inducing hydrocephalus:[15] (1) obstruction to CSF flow through the aqueduct of Sylvius and foramen of Monro, or the basilar cisterns and the cisterna magna, (2) interference with the flow of blood through the great vein of Galen, and (3) creation of primary congenital malformations of the neural tube or neurological anomalies secondary to axial skeletal dysraphic states caused by exogenous insults with teratogens directed at pregnant mammals. To study the pathophysiology of hydrocephalic brain damage (in contrast to the causes of hydrocephalus), the method of induction should cause the ventricles to enlarge but should not directly affect the brain, which chemical, radiation, and viral induction methods can do. The range of species used includes mouse, rat, guinea pig, rabbit, cat, dog, pig,[16] fetal lamb,[17] and primates such as *Macaca mulatta*[18] and Rhesus monkey.[19]

When choosing a model, several factors need to be addressed such as animal availability, the pathological aspects one wishes to explore, age, time course of hydrocephalus, and methods for assessing physical, behavioral, and/or biochemical changes.[14,20] Unlike humans, rodents have only narrow layers of periventricular white matter and their brains are lissencephalic (i.e., no gyri), therefore there are limitations in the applicability.

26.2.1 Hereditary models of hydrocephalus

hy3 mouse

The spontaneous hydrocephalus murine mutant model (*hy3*) was identified in 1943.[21] Perinatal onset is associated with alterations in periventricular tissues and eventually the cerebral cortex.[22] The underlying pathological mechanisms are not completely understood. It is an autosomal recessive trait.[23] More recently a random transgenic insertion on chromosome 8 led unexpectedly to hydrocephalus in mice and genetic crosses between hemizygous OVE459 mice and mice heterozygous for *hy3* produced hydrocephalic offspring with a frequency of 22%, demonstrating that these two mutations are allelic.[24–26]

hyh mouse

A lethal recessive mutation in the C57/Bl/10 J mouse strain was labeled hydrocephalus with hop gait (*hyh*). Morphological changes are evident between 4 and 10 weeks of age with enlargement of lateral and third ventricles, and narrowing of the cerebral aqueduct. The *hyh* locus has been mapped to the proximal end of chromosome 7.[27] The soluble *N*-ethylmalemide-sensitive factor (NSF) attachment protein alpha-*S*-nitroso-*N*-acetylpenicillamine (alpha-SNAP) has been identified as the only mutated protein.[28,29] The mutation causes a smaller cerebral cortex due to reduced progenitor pool of late-born upper-layer cortical neurons.[30] Obliteration of distal end of aqueduct and severe hydrocephalus has been observed.[31]

L1 cell adhesion molecule

L1 cell adhesion molecule (L1 CAM) is a member of the superfamily of immunoglobulin (Ig)-related cell adhesion molecules. It plays a pivotal role in growth and guidance of particular axon tracts in the developing nervous system.[32] In humans, mutations in L1 are associated with a neurological syndrome termed CRASH, which includes corpus callosum agenesis, mental retardation, adducted thumbs, spasticity, and X-linked hydrocephalus.[33,34] The L1 CAM gene is located at Xq28 in humans[35] and pathological human mutations are believed to eliminate exon 2.[36] In the mouse model, the size of the corticospinal tract corpus callosum is reduced and, depending on genetic background, the lateral ventricles are often enlarged. In vitro, neurite outgrowth is impaired[37] and surface ligand interactions are altered.[38] In the cerebral cortex, many pyramidal neurons in layer V exhibit undulating apical dendrites that do not reach layer I. The hippocampus is small, with fewer pyramidal and granule cells.[39]

Transforming growth factor-1

Mice that overexpress transforming growth factor-1 (TGF-1) were generated in an attempt to study astrocytic response to injury. The unexpected result was severe ventricle enlargement, spasticity, limb tremors, and ataxia with death by 3 weeks of age.[40–42] Injection of human TGF-1 into the subarachnoid space of 10-day-old mice results in hydrocephalus.[43] In all cases, the cause appears to be obliteration of CSF pathways in the subarachnoid space. This cytokine may play a role in post-meningitis and subarachnoid hemorrhage meningeal scarring.

H-Tx rat

The Hydrocephalus Texas (H-Tx) rat has been extremely well studied. H-Tx was described in 1981[44] and probably arose from the Lewis strain of Sprague-Dawley rats.[45] The H-Tx rat is a homozygous carrier of an autosomal recessive gene with incomplete penetrance.[46–50] There is an epigenetic factor that increases in fetuses if suckling pups are present during gestation.[51] Strong linkages to the trait are on loci of chromosomes 10, 11, and 17 with weaker linkages on 4, 9, and 19.[47] Jones's group and others have published morphological,[45,52,53] metabolic,[54] and behavioral[55] descriptions. The rats have fetal-onset associated with the closure of the cerebral aqueduct. The precise mechanisms through which narrowing occurs is not clear. Even non-hydrocephalic H-Tx rats have abnormal behavior.[56]

LEW/Jms rat

The LEW/Jms rat strain, described in 1983,[57] was derived from an inbred strain of Wistar–Lewis rats at the University of Tokyo. In most respects, the phenotype for LEW/Jms is similar in onset and pathophysiology to that of H-Tx.[58]

26.2.2 Mechanical models of hydrocephalus

Injections into the cisterna magna

Dandy and Blackfan described induction of hydrocephalus by injecting lampblack (i.e., charcoal soot) into the cisterna magna of dogs.[59] Injections of many substances can be done percutaneously or with surgical exposure of the skull base. CSF of an equal volume may be withdrawn, but this is not always necessary because spontaneous leakage of CSF around the needle tends to occur. A sufficiently small needle must be used to avoid reflux (e.g., 28-gauge in the rat). Proper flexion of the neck (Fig. 26.1) is necessary so that the substance is delivered into the foramen magnum and/or fourth ventricle while avoiding injury to the brainstem. In the case of the rodent, this flexion can be achieved by placing the chest on a sponge support with application of gentle pressure on the snout and mid-back. Larger animals (rabbits, dogs, etc.) usually require more rigid fixation, for example with a maxillary clamp. In rodents the foramen magnum can be palpated after the neck is shaved and cleansed with iodine or 70% ethanol. The needle should enter the dorsal foramen magnum, and be almost parallel to the cervical spine. In mature rodents and larger animals, as the needle passes through the dura a sudden loss of resistance is felt. In small animals the needle should be advanced no more than 1–2 mm beyond this point. If the foramen magnum is surgically exposed through a midline suboccipital/cervical incision, a pad of surgical

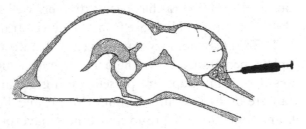

Figure 26.1. Diagram showing position of needle entry for cisternal injection in rodents.

hemostasis material (e.g., Gelfoam) can be placed over the puncture site. A retention suture can be used to approximate the cervical muscles in the midline to help retain this material.

We have used many types of anesthesia including cooling for neonatal rodents, ketamine–xylazine delivered parenterally, and inhalation of halothane or isofluorane by nose cone. The latter has the advantage of rapid recovery, but it is sometimes difficult to keep the nose cone in place during neck flexion. After recovery, the animal should be closely observed for head tilt, leaning to one side, circling, or hemiparesis, which indicate injury to brainstem or spinal cord. Some recovery of head tilt may occur but paretic animals should be euthanized. Seizures, presumably the result of a more general irritative phenomenon, may occasionally occur. Most animals exhibit signs of lethargy, weakness, and ataxia for a few days post-induction. Delayed gain of weight is often the earliest indicator of successful induction of hydrocephalus.

Kaolin

Kaolin-induced subarachnoid space occlusion is among the most commonly used models.[60] Kaolin is a whitish, clay-like substance (aluminum silicate) that is placed in suspension (250 mg/ml kaolin in 0.9% saline) before injection. It mimics post-meningitis or post-subarachnoid hemorrhage hydrocephalus with scarring in the subarachnoid space. It is simple, reproducible, and inexpensive, and is not species dependent. The optimum volume depends on size of the animal. The severity can be titrated according to dose. Neonatal (less than 1 week old) rats receive 0.02 ml, while 0.05 ml is given to young and adult rats.[61] Only recently has kaolin use been reported in mice (Hatta 2006).[62] However, we have had only a low success rate in our laboratory, probably due to the small size of the cisterna magna and the fact that the ventricle walls in mice have extensive sites of ependymal fusion and therefore do not dilate readily. During injection into neonatal rodents, kaolin can be seen spreading beneath the translucent occipital bone. Other authors report effectiveness of 0.2–0.5 ml in young rabbits[63] and 3 ml in adult dogs.[64] Kaolin spreads with CSF flow and following sacrifice it can be identified on the ventral surface of the brainstem and as far as the olfactory tracts or middle cerebral arteries (Fig. 26.2). In addition to ventricle enlargement, syrinx formation can occur in the cervical and thoracic spinal cord. Microscopically, kaolin engulfed by macrophages can be identified as small black refractive granules. The inflammatory cells are embedded in a delicate collagen web in the subarachnoid space. Although we have observed no astroglial or microglial reaction in adjacent brain matter,[8] T lymphocytes have been reported to appear early in the subarachnoid compartment and adjacent to brain tissue following kaolin injections.[65]

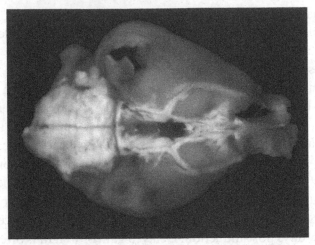

Figure 26.2. Photograph showing base of adult rat brain with severe hydrocephalus, 9 months after kaolin injection into the cisterna magna. The kaolin appears as a white layer on the surface of the brainstem, around the hypothalamus, and along the middle cerebral arteries.

Fibroblast growth factor

Fibroblast growth factor (FGF-2) or basic FGF can induce proliferation of fibroblasts, endothelial cells, smooth muscle cells, as well as other cells.[66] Hydrocephalus was induced in adult Sprague-Dawley rats by infusing recombinant FGF-2 at 1 μg/day into the lateral ventricle for 2–12 days.[67] High doses of FGF in mice resulted in enlargement of the ventricles and thinning of the cortex.[68] Exogenous FGF can affect brain cell survival and differentiation directly without causing hydrocephalus.[69]

Silastic oil

Silastic oil injected into the cisterna magna produces a pure mechanical obstruction without inflammatory changes in the subarachnoid compartment.[70–72] This transparent substance is available in different viscosities; typically a viscosity of 5000–10 000 centistokes is optimal. The oil sits in the fourth ventricle and subarachnoid space. The injection method is essentially the same as for kaolin; however, because the viscosity is greater a larger needle (>23-gauge) must be used. Severe ventriculomegaly and high pressures are not possible. In an attempt to increase the success rate, 5 ml of silastic elastomer solution, which hardens after injection, has been used in dogs.[73,74]

Cyanoacrylic gel

Luciano and coworkers described a model applicable to large animals.[75,76] Cyanoacrylic gel glue is injected into adult dogs to create surgical occlusion of the fourth ventricle. The large size of the canine brain enables implementation and testing of novel diagnostic and treatment modalities. Surgeries are performed with the dog in the prone position in a stereotaxic head frame. A suboccipital craniectomy exposes the fourth ventricle floor. Obstructions are produced by placing flexible silicone tubing (outer diameter 1.5 mm) connected to an 18-gauge catheter in the fourth ventricle. Through this catheter 0.25–0.35 ml of surgical grade cyanoacrylic gel glue (Loctite Corp., Newington, CT) is delivered. The rapidly curing glue does not significantly compress or deform surrounding tissues, while it adheres to the ependymal and pial membranes of the brainstem and cerebellum. Therefore potential for CSF leakage is minimal. The catheter remains in place. Postoperatively, animals receive anti-inflammatory, antibiotic, and analgesic drugs. Histologically, multinucleate foreign body giant cells can be seen at sites of contact between glue and tissue.

Plugs

Dandy and Blackfan used a piece of cotton to surgically occlude the aqueduct of Sylvius via the fourth ventricle.[59] Cellophane cylinders have also been used with a success rate of 75% in dogs.[77] The major disadvantage of this model is that it is a major surgical procedure with a high likelihood of damage to brainstem structures. Therefore, this model should probably be only used for acute experiments. Small (~0.5 ml volume) ballons have been inflated in the cisterna magna of adult rats with some success (Kim 1999).[78]

Venous occlusion

Dandy also described ligation of the vena magna galeni or sinus rectus as a way of creating hydrocephalus in dogs.[79] The rationale is that some CSF is absorbed through the venous system. Hydrocephalus due to elevated venous pressure certainly occurs in human infants,[80,81] but seldom in older children or adults.[82] Obliteration of the internal and external jugular veins at the base of the skull of adult dogs results in moderate hydrocephalus.[83] A similar result can be achieved in adult rabbits.[84]

26.3 Methods of assessment

26.3.1 Behavior

Hydrocephalus in immature animals whose skull sutures are not fused is associated with a dome-shaped head and/or persistent fontanel (Fig. 26.3). However, the correlation between head width and ventricle size is not accurate. In mature animals the head does not enlarge and the degree of lethargy or retardation of weight gain may be more valid indicators. We and others have used behavioral

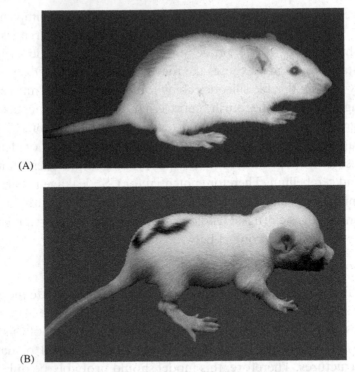

Figure 26.3. Photographs showing (A) a normal 17-day-old rat and (B) a hydrocephalic rat of the same age that received kaolin injection on day 1. The body is smaller, the head is domed, and the legs are positioned abnormally.

methods to study hydrocephalic rats. In neonatal rats we have observed that acquisition of early motor behaviors such as righting reflex, pivoting, negative geotaxis, and wire-hanging are delayed.[85] In young and adult rats, deficits in memory can be assessed using a water maze[55,56] or radial arm maze.[86] Posture, movement, and gait can be assessed using treadmills, rotorods, automated activity monitoring, and open field test to assess lethargy.[12,87]

26.3.2 Imaging

There is inherent variability in the models; therefore it is important to image the brain in vivo. Barkovich has compared the range of imaging techniques used on humans;[13] similar methods can be used in animals. Ultrasonography has been used for kittens,[88] dogs,[73] and piglets.[16] However, it cannot be used when the skull sutures are fused because ultrasound does not penetrate bone. Furthermore, the resolution is not very good. Computerized tomography (CT) scanning has been used to image hydrocephalic cats, dogs, etc.[89,90] A new bench-top CT (SkyScan, Aartselaar, Belgium) could be conveniently used for

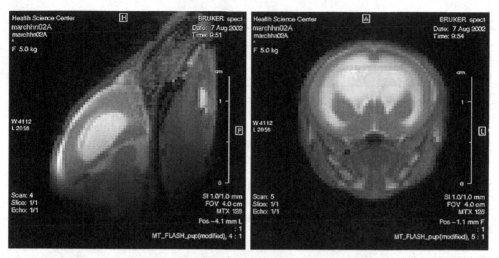

Figure 26.4. T2-weighted magnetic resonance images showing (left) sagittal and (right) coronal views of brain of 7-day-old hydrocephalic rat that received kaolin injection on day 1. The ventricles are enlarged and the external capsule white matter is edematous (bright signal).

rodents. Many laboratories now use magnetic resonance (MR) imaging which provides superb anatomical resolution as well as metabolic imaging capability in any species (Fig. 26.4).[53,87,91,92] Ventricle size can be measured quickly with Evans ratios (ventricle width/brain width) or complete image sets can be assessed by planimetry to calculate the brain and ventricle volumes.[12]

26.3.3 Histology

After sacrifice and opening of the skull, the expansion and thinning of the cerebrum can be assessed. If the brain is very thin, it will tend to collapse as CSF leaks out. Fixed brains are slightly more rigid. If sectioned in the coronal plane, the ventricle width or area can be determined in the fresh state or after sectioning for histologic preparation. In vivo imaging, however, is inherently more accurate.

26.4 Summary

Many animal models are available for studies of hydrocephalus (Table 26.1). Genetic models might have associated brain changes not directly due to hydrocephalus, but they are predictable and they mimic some types of human fetal-onset hydrocephalus. Artificial induction models vary in the invasiveness, expense, and the extent to which they mimic human situations. The investigator must choose the model that will allow proper study of the

Table 26.1. *Summary of animal models of hydrocephalus*

Experimental model	Advantages	Disadvantages
Mouse mutant models	Resurgence of interest because genetic exploration/ understanding feasible; relatively inexpensive, reproducible	Cost of maintaining breeding colony; applicability awaits understanding of underlying cause of hydrocephalus; too small for surgical interventions
Rat mutant models	Spontaneous neonatal hydrocephalus; predictable; surgical intervention possible	Genetic explanation unknown; possible brain abnormalities in unaffected animals of same strain; cost of maintaining breeding colony
Kaolin injection into cisterna magna	Easy; inexpensive; titratable severity; any age and any animal possible	Possible broader effect of inflammation
Silicone oil injection into cisterna magna	Easy; inexpensive; pure mechanical obstruction	Severe ventriculomegaly and high pressures not possible
Cyanoacrylate glue injection into cisterna magna of dogs	Large animal therefore modeling of complex surgical systems possible	Technically complicated and expensive
Fibroblast growth factor injection into cisterna magna	Easy; fibrotic obstruction in subarachnoid space	Expensive; fibroblast growth factor might affect brain cells directly

topic in question. Imaging of animals is expensive but critical for linking animal studies to the human disorder, for studying the dynamics of ventricle enlargement, and for neuroprotective studies which require assignment to treatment groups prior to sacrifice. Recognizing the applicability and limitations of these models is critical to understanding human hydrocephalus.

References

1. Papaiconomou C, Bozanovic-Sosic R, Zakharov A, Johnston M. Does neonatal cerebrospinal fluid absorption occur via arachnoid projections or extracranial lymphatics? *Am. J. Physiol. Regul. Integr. Comp. Physiol.* 2002, **283**: R869–R876.
2. Del Bigio MR. Neuropathological changes caused by hydrocephalus. *Acta Neuropathol. (Berlin)* 1993, **85**: 573–585.
3. Del Bigio MR. Pathophysiologic consequences of hydrocephalus. *Neurosurg. Clin. N. Am.* 2001, **12**: 639–649.

4. Del Bigio MR, McAllister JP II. Hydrocephalus: pathology. In Choux M, Di Rocco C, Hockley AD, Walker ML (eds.) *Pediatric Neurosurgery*. London: Churchill Livingstone, 1999, pp. 217–236.

5. Wiswell TE, Tuttle DJ, Northam RS, Simonds GR. Major congenital neurologic malformations: a 17-year survey. *Am. J. Dis. Child.* 1990, **144**: 61–67.

6. Stein SC, Schut L. Hydrocephalus in myelomeningocele. *Child's Brain* 1979, **5**: 413–419.

7. Holt PJ, Allan WC. The natural history of ventricular dilatation in neonatal intraventricular hemorrhage and its therapeutic implications. *Ann. Neurol.* 1981, **10**: 293–294.

8. Del Bigio MR, Zhang YW. Cell death, axonal damage, and cell birth in the immature rat brain following induction of hydrocephalus. *Exp. Neurol.* 1998, **154**: 157–169.

9. Hochwald GM, Boal RD, Marlin AE, Kumar AJ. Changes in regional blood-flow and water content of brain and spinal cord in acute and chronic experimental hydrocephalus. *Devel. Med. Child Neurol. (Suppl.)* 1975, **35**: 42–50.

10. Chumas PD, Drake JM, Del Bigio MR, Da Silva M, Tuor UI. Anaerobic glycolysis preceding white-matter destruction in experimental neonatal hydrocephalus. *J. Neurosurg.* 1994, **80**: 491–501.

11. Del Bigio MR. Calcium-mediated proteolytic damage in white matter of hydrocephalic rats? *J. Neuropathol. Exp. Neurol.* 2000, **59**: 946–954.

12. Del Bigio MR, Wilson MJ, Enno T. Chronic hydrocephalus in rats and humans: white matter loss and behavior changes. *Ann. Neurol.* 2003, **53**: 337–346.

13. Barkovich AJ, Edwards MS. Applications of neuroimaging in hydrocephalus. *Pediatr. Neurosurg.* 1992, **18**: 65–83.

14. Matsumoto S, Hirayama A, Yamasaki S, Shirataki K, Fujiwara K. Comparative study of various models of experimental hydrocephalus. *Child's Brain* 1975, **1**: 236–242.

15. Hochwald GM. Animal models of hydrocephalus: recent developments. *Proc. Soc. Exp. Biol. Med.* 1985, **178**: 1–11.

16. Taylor GA, Soul JS, Dunning PS. Sonographic ventriculography: a new potential use for sonographic contrast agents in neonatal hydrocephalus. *Am. J. Neuroradiol.* 1998, **19**: 1931–1934.

17. Nakayama DK, Harrison MR, Berger MS, *et al.* Correction of congenital hydrocephalus in utero. I. The model: intracisternal kaolin produces hydrocephalus in fetal lambs and rhesus monkeys. *J. Pediatr. Surg.* 1983, **18**: 331–338.

18. Flor WJ, James Jr AE, Ribas JL, Parker JL, Sickel WL. Ultrastructure of the ependyma in the lateral ventricles of primates with experimental communicating hydrocephalus. *Scan. Electron Microsc.* 1979, **3**: 47–54.

19. Hammock MK, Milhorat TH, Earle K, Di Chiro G. Vein of Galen ligation in the primate: angiographic, gross, and light microscopic evaluation. *J. Neurosurg.* 1971, **34**: 77–83.

20. Del Bigio MR. Future directions for therapy of childhood hydrocephalus: a view from the laboratory. *Pediatr. Neurosurg.* 2001, **34**: 172–181.

21. Gruneberg H. Congenital hydrocephalus in the mouse: a case of spurious pleiotropism. *J. Genet.* 1943, **45**: 1–21.

22. McLone DG, Bondareff W, Raimondi AJ. Brain edema in the hydrocephalic *hy-3* mouse: submicroscopic morphology. *J. Neuropathol. Exp. Neurol.* 1971, **30**: 627–637.

23. Berry RJ. The inheritance and pathogenesis of hydrocephalus-3 in the mouse. *J. Pathol. Bacteriol.* 1961, **81**: 157–167.

24. Robinson ML, Davy BE, Elliot C, *et al.* A new allele of an old mutation: genetic mapping of an autosomal recessive, hydrocephalus-inducing mutation in mice. In *Society for Research into Hydrocephalus and Spina Bifida, 44th Annual Scientific Meeting,* Atlanta, GA, 21–24 June 2000.

25. Robinson ML, Allen CE, Davy BE, *et al.* Genetic mapping of an insertional hydrocephalus-inducing mutation allelic to *hy3. Mamm. Genome* 2002, **13**: 625–632.

26. Davy BE, Robinson ML. Congenital hydrocephalus in *hy3* mice is caused by a frameshift mutation in *Hydin,* a large novel gene. *Hum. Mol. Genet.* 2003, **12**: 1163–1170.

27. Bronson RT, Lane PW. Hydrocephalus with hop gait (*hyh*): a new mutation on chromosome 7 in the mouse. *Devel. Brain Res.* 1990, **54**: 131–136.

28. Hong HK, Chakravarti A, Takahashi JS. The gene for soluble *N*-ethylmaleimide sensitive factor attachment protein alpha is mutated in hydrocephaly with hop gait (*hyh*) mice. *Proc. Natl Acad. Sci. USA* 2004, **101**: 1748–1753.

29. Chae TH, Allen KM, Davisson MT, Sweet HO, Walsh CA. Mapping of the mouse *hyh* gene to a YAC/BAC contig on proximal chromosome 7. *Mamm. Genome* 2002, **13**: 239–244.

30. Chae TH, Kim S, Marz KE, Hanson PI, Walsh CA. The *hyh* mutation uncovers roles for alpha SNAP in apical protein localization and control of neural cell fate. *Nature Genet.* 2004, **36**: 264–270.

31. Wagner C, Batiz LF, Rodriguez S, *et al.* Cellular mechanisms involved in the stenosis and obliteration of the cerebral aqueduct of *hyh* mutant mice developing congenital hydrocephalus. *J. Neuropathol. Exp. Neurol.* 2003, **62**: 1019–1040.

32. Kenwrick S, Watkins A, De Angelis E. Neural cell recognition molecule L1: relating biological complexity to human disease mutations. *Hum. Mol. Genet.* 2000, **9**: 879–886.

33. Kenwrick S, Jouet M, Donnai D. X-linked hydrocephalus and MASA syndrome. *J. Med. Genet.* 1996, **33**: 59–65.

34. Itoh K, Cheng L, Kamei Y, *et al.* Brain development in mice lacking L1-L1 homophilic adhesion. *J. Cell Biol.* 2004, **165**: 145–154.

35. Van Camp G, Vits L, Coucke P, *et al.* A duplication in the L1 CAM gene associated with X-linked hydrocephalus. *Nature Genet.* 1993, **4**: 421–425.

36. Jacob J, Haspel J, Kane-Goldsmith N, Grumet M. L1 mediated homophilic binding and neurite outgrowth are modulated by alternative splicing of exon 2. *J. Neurobiol.* 2002, **51**: 177–189.

37. Dahme M, Bartsch U, Martini R, *et al.* Disruption of the mouse L1 gene leads to malformations of the nervous system. *Nature Genet.* 1997, **17**: 346–349.

38. De Angelis E, Watkins A, Schafer M, Brummendorf T, Kenwrick S. Disease-associated mutations in L1 CAM interfere with ligand interactions and cell-surface expression. *Hum. Mol. Genet.* 2002, **11**: 1–12.

39. Demyanenko GP, Tsai AY, Maness PF. Abnormalities in neuronal process extension, hippocampal development, and the ventricular system of L1 knockout mice. *J. Neurosci.* 1999, **19**: 4907–4920.

40. Galbreath E, Kim SJ, Park K, Brenner M, Messing A. Overexpression of TGF-beta 1 in the central nervous system of transgenic mice results in hydrocephalus. *J. Neuropathol. Exp. Neurol.* 1995, **54**: 339–349.

41. Wyss-Coray T, Feng L, Masliah E, *et al.* Increased central nervous system production of extracellular matrix components and development of hydro-cephalus in transgenic mice overexpressing transforming growth factor-beta 1. *Am. J. Pathol.* 1995, **147**: 53–67.

42. Cohen AR, Leifer DW, Zechel M, *et al.* Characterization of a model of hydro-cephalus in transgenic mice. *J. Neurosurg.* 1999, **91**: 978–988.
43. Tada T, Kanaji M, Kobayashi S. Induction of communicating hydrocephalus in mice by intrathecal injection of human recombinant transforming growth factor-beta 1. *J. Neuroimmunol.* 1994, **50**: 153–158.
44. Kohn DF, Chinookoswong N, Chou SM. A new model of congenital hydro-cephalus in the rat. *Acta Neuropathol. (Berlin)* 1981, **54**: 211–218.
45. Jones HC, Bucknall RM. Inherited prenatal hydrocephalus in the H-Tx rat: a morphological study. *Neuropathol. Appl. Neurobiol.* 1988, **14**: 263–274.
46. Cai X, McGraw G, Pattisapu JV, *et al.* Hydrocephalus in the H-Tx rat: a monogenic disease? *Exp. Neurol.* 2000, **163**: 131–135.
47. Jones HC, Carter BJ, Depelteau JS, Roman M, Morel L. Chromosomal linkage associated with disease severity in the hydrocephalic H-Tx rat. *Behav. Genet.* 2001, **31**: 101–111.
48. Jones HC, Lopman BA, Jones TW, *et al.* The expression of inherited hydro-cephalus in H-Tx rats. *Child's Nerv. Syst.* 2000, **16**: 578–584.
49. Jones HC, Lopman BA, Jones TW, Morel LM. Breeding characteristics and genetic analysis of the H-Tx rat strain. *Eur. J. Pediatr. Surg.* 1999, **9** (Suppl. 1): 42–43.
50. Jones HC, Depelteau JS, Carter BJ, Lopman BA, Morel L. Genome-wide linkage analysis of inherited hydrocephalus in the H-Tx rat. *Mamm. Genome* 2001, **12**: 22–26.
51. Jones HC, Depelteau JS, Carter BJ, Somera KC. The frequency of inherited hydrocephalus is influenced by intrauterine factors in H-Tx rats. *Exp. Neurol.* 2002, **176**: 213–220.
52. Boillat CA, Jones HC, Kaiser GL, Harris NG. Ultrastructural changes in the deep cortical pyramidal cells of infant rats with inherited hydrocephalus and the effect of shunt treatment. *Exp. Neurol.* 1997, **147**: 377–388.
53. Jones HC, Harris NG, Briggs RW, Williams SC. Shunt treatment at two postnatal ages in hydrocephalic H-Tx rats quantified using MR imaging. *Exp. Neurol.* 1995, **133**: 144–152.
54. Jones HC, Harris NG, Rocca JR, Andersohn RW. Progressive changes in cortical metabolites at three stages of infantile hydrocephalus studied by in vitro NMR spectroscopy. *J. Neurotrauma* 1997, **14**: 587–602.
55. Jones HC, Rivera KM, Harris NG. Learning deficits in congenitally hydro-cephalic rats and prevention by early shunt treatment. *Child's Nerv. Syst.* 1995, **11**: 655–660.
56. Hawkins D, Bowers TM, Bannister CM, Miyan JA. The functional outcome of shunting H-Tx rat pups at different ages. *Eur. J. Pediatr. Surg.* 1997, **7** (Suppl. 1): 31–34.
57. Sasaki S, Goto H, Nagano H, *et al.* Congenital hydrocephalus revealed in the inbred rat, LEW/Jms. *Neurosurgery* 1983, **13**: 548–554.
58. Jones HC, Carter BJ, Morel L. Characteristics of hydrocephalus expression in the LEW/Jms rat strain with inherited disease. *Child's Nerv. Syst.* 2003, **19**: 11–18.
59. Dandy WE, Blackfan KD. An experimental and clinical study of internal hydrocephalus. *J. Am. Med. Ass.* 1913, **61**: 2216–2217.
60. Dixon WE, Heller H. Experimentelle Hypertonie durch Eröhung des intraka-niellen Druckes. *Arch. Exp. Pathol. Pharmakol.* 1932, **166**: 265–275.
61. Khan OH, Enno T, Del Bigio MR. Magnesium sulfate therapy is of mild benefit to young rats with kaolin-induced hydrocephalus. *Pediatr. Res.* 2003, **53**: 970–976.

62. Hatta J, Hatta T, Moritake K, Otani H. Heavy water inhibiting the expression of transforming growth factor-beta 1 and the development of kaolin-induced hydrocephalus in mice. *J. Neurosurg.* 2006, **104** (4 suppl): 251–258.
63. Gopinath G, Bhatia R, Gopinath PG. Ultrastructural observations in experimental hydrocephalus in the rabbit. *J. Neurol. Sci.* 1979, **43**: 333–334.
64. Gonzalez-Darder J, Barbera J, Cerda-Nicolas M, *et al.* Sequential morphological and functional changes in kaolin-induced hydrocephalus. *J. Neurosurg.* 1984, **61**: 918–924.
65. Shinoda M, Olson L. Immunological aspects of kaolin-induced hydrocephalus. *Int. J. Neurosci.* 1997, **92**: 9–28.
66. Burgess WH, Maciag T. The heparin-binding (fibroblast) growth factor family of proteins. *Annu. Rev. Biochem.* 1989, **58**: 575–606.
67. Johanson CE, Szmydynger Chodobska J, Chodobski A, *et al.* Altered formation and bulk absorption of cerebrospinal fluid in FGF-2-induced hydrocephalus. *Am. J. Physiol.* 1999, **277**: R263–R271.
68. Ohmiya M, Fukumitsu H, Nitta A, *et al.* Administration of FGF-2 to embryonic mouse brain induces hydrocephalic brain morphology and aberrant differentiation of neurons in the postnatal cerebral cortex. *J. Neurosci. Res.* 2001, **65**: 228–235.
69. Alzheimer C, Werner S. Fibroblast growth factors and neuroprotection. *Adv. Exp. Med. Biol.* 2002, **513**: 335–351.
70. Wisniewski H, Weller RO, Terry RD. Experimental hydrocephalus produced by the subarachnoid infusion of silicone oil. *J. Neurosurg.* 1969, **31**: 10–14.
71. James Jr AE, Strecker E-P. Use of silastic to produce communicating hydrocephalus. *Invest. Radiol.* 1973, **8**: 105–110.
72. Del Bigio MR, Bruni JE. Periventricular pathology in hydrocephalic rabbits before and after shunting. *Acta Neuropathol. (Berlin)* 1988, **77**: 186–195.
73. Brown JA, Rachlin J, Rubin JM, Wollmann RL. Ultrasound evaluation of experimental hydrocephalus in dogs. *Surg. Neurol.* 1984, **22**: 273–276.
74. Page LK, White WP. Transsphenoidal injection of silicone for the production of communicating or obstructive hydrocephalus in dogs. *Surg. Neurol.* 1982, **17**: 247–250.
75. Johnson MJ, Ayzman I, Wood AS, *et al.* Development and characterization of an adult model of obstructive hydrocephalus. *J. Neurosci. Methods* 1999, **91**: 55–65.
76. Luciano MG, Skarupa DJ, Booth AM, *et al.* Cerebrovascular adaptation in chronic hydrocephalus. *J. Cereb. Blood Flow Metab.* 2001, **21**: 285–294.
77. Schurr PH, McLaurin RL, Ingraham FD. Experimental studies on the circulation of the cerebrospinal fluid and methods of producing communicating hydrocephalus in the dog. *J. Neurosurg.* 1953, **10**: 515–525.
78. Kim DS, Oi S, Hidaka M, Sato O, Choi JU. A new experimental model of obstructive hydrocephalus in the rat: the micro-balloon technique. *Child's Nerv. Syst.* 1999, **15**: 250–255.
79. Dandy WE. Experimental hydrocephalus. *Ann. Surg.* 1919, **70**: 129–142.
80. Sainte-Rose C, LaCombe J, Pierre-Kahn A, Renier D, Hirsch JF. Intracranial venous sinus hypertension: cause or consequence of hydrocephalus in infants? *J. Neurosurg.* 1984, **60**: 727–736.
81. Karahalios DG, Rekate HL, Khayata MH, Apostolides PJ. Elevated intracranial venous pressure as a universal mechanism in pseudotumor cerebri of varying etiologies. *Neurology* 1996, **46**: 198–202.

82. Gil Z, Specter-Himberg G, Gomori MJ, *et al.* Association between increased central venous pressure and hydrocephalus in children undergoing cardiac catheterization: A prospective study. *Child's Nerv. Syst.* 2001, **17**: 478–482.
83. Bering Jr EA, Salibi B. Production of hydrocephalus by increased cephalic-venous pressure. *Am. Med. Ass. Arch. Neurol. Psychiatr.* 1959, **81**: 693–698.
84. Hasan M, Srimal RC, Maitra SC. Bilateral jugular vein ligation-induced alterations in the ventricular ependyma: scanning electron microscopy. *Int. Surg.* 1980, **65**: 533–540.
85. Altman J, Sudarshan K. Postnatal development of locomotion in the laboratory rat. *Anim. Behav.* 1975, **23**: 896–920.
86. Egawa T, Mishima K, Egashira N, *et al.* Impairment of spatial memory in kaolin-induced hydrocephalic rats is associated with changes in the hippocampal cholinergic and noradrenergic contents. *Behav. Brain Res.* 2002, **129**: 31–39.
87. Del Bigio MR, Crook CR, Buist R. Magnetic resonance imaging and behavioral analysis of immature rats with kaolin-induced hydrocephalus: pre- and post-shunting observations. *Exp. Neurol.* 1997, **148**: 256–264.
88. Wolfson BJ, McAllister JP II, Lovely TJ, *et al.* Sonographic evaluation of experimental hydrocephalus in kittens. *Am. J. Neuroradiol.* 1989, **10**: 1065–1067.
89. Donauer E, Wussow W, Rascher K. Experimental hydrocephalus and hydrosyringomyelia: computer tomographic studies. *Neurosurg. Rev.* 1988, **11**: 87–94.
90. Yamada H, Yokota A, Furuta A, Horie A. Reconstitution of shunted mantle in experimental hydrocephalus. *J. Neurosurg.* 1992, **76**: 856–862.
91. Drake JM, Potts DG, Lemaire C. Magnetic resonance imaging of silastic-induced canine hydrocephalus. *Surg. Neurol.* 1989, **31**: 28–40.
92. Braun KPJ, de Graaf RA, Vandertop WP, *et al.* In vivo H-1 MR spectroscopic imaging and diffusion weighted MRI in experimental hydrocephalus. *Magn. Reson. Med.* 1998, **40**: 832–839.

27

Rodent models of experimental bacterial infections in the CNS

TAMMY KIELIAN

27.1 Introduction

The purpose of this chapter is to provide a brief synopsis of bacterial meningitis and brain abscess and the animal models used to study these diseases and evaluate potential therapeutic modalities. The reader is encouraged to consult the selected references for more detailed information.

27.2 Bacterial meningitis

Despite advances made in vaccination and treatment strategies, bacterial meningitis remains associated with a significant mortality rate and incidence of neurological sequelae, particularly in very young and elderly patients. Approximately 1.2 million cases of bacterial meningitis are estimated to occur worldwide annually with 135 000 deaths.[1] Long-term effects resulting from meningitis include hearing loss, hydrocephalus, and sequelae associated with parenchymal brain damage including memory loss, cerebral palsy, learning disabilities, and seizures.[2,3] Organisms that colonize the mucosal membranes of the nasopharynx include *Neisseria meningitidis*, *Streptococcus pneumoniae*, and *Haemophilus influenzae* which are the leading etiologic agents of community-acquired meningitis. Recurring bacterial meningitis epidemics, the emergence of antimicrobial resistance among many meningeal pathogens, and the failure to introduce the *H. influenzae* conjugate vaccines (Hib) into many developing countries all contribute to bacterial meningitis remaining a serious global health problem.

Bacterial meningitis elicits a complex myriad of pathophysiological changes that present numerous obstacles when considering the design of therapeutic strategies. For example, besides the direct damage induced by pathogens, the host antibacterial response elicited during the acute phase of bacterial

Handbook of Experimental Neurology, ed. Turgut Tatlisumak and Marc Fisher. Published by Cambridge University Press. © Cambridge University Press 2006.

meningitis can be detrimental to neurons and other glia in the central nervous system (CNS) due to the toxic effects of cytokines, chemokines, proteolytic enzymes, and oxidants produced locally at the site of infection.[4,5] In addition, studies have shown that the inflammatory host response to bacterial products continues after organisms have been killed by antibiotics, revealing that the therapeutic manipulation of bacterial meningitis will be challenging.[6]

The sequence of events leading to the establishment of bacterial meningitis includes: (1) nasopharynx colonization by the pathogen, (2) microbial invasion and replication in the bloodstream, (3) penetration of bacteria across the blood–brain barrier (BBB), and (4) survival and replication of organisms in the subarachnoid space.[5] The presence of multiplying pathogens elicits the host inflammatory response which, in part, leads to the onset of clinical symptoms and the sequelae of bacterial meningitis. The major complications arising from bacterial meningitis include brain edema, hydrocephalus, increased intracranial pressure, disturbances in normal cerebrospinal fluid (CSF) and blood flow, focal CNS necrosis, and neuronal loss. These pathogenic changes in humans can be accurately recapitulated using the various rodent models of experimental meningitis described below.

27.3 Experimental models of bacterial meningitis in the infant rat

Since adult animals do not reliably develop meningitis following intranasal or intraperitoneal challenge with live bacteria without additional manipulation, infant rodents have classically been used to study both host and bacterial factors that dictate pathogen entry into the bloodstream and CNS. Infant rat experimental meningitis models have utilized three routes of infection, namely intranasal, intracisternal, and intraperitoneal.

A well-established system for studying the pathogenesis of bacterial meningitis is the *H. influenzae* infant rat model.[7] Prior to the routine vaccination of human infants against Hib, this organism was a leading cause of bacterial meningitis; however, it remains a prevalent pathogen in non-developed countries due to the relatively high cost of the Hib vaccine. The experimental model uses 5-day-old Sprague-Dawley COBS/CD suckling rats housed in litters of approximately 10 per cage with their mother. Infant animals are infected atraumatically by the application of a small volume of bacteria (10–20 µl) onto one nostril that is subsequently inhaled. Depending on the inoculum and virulence of the bacterial strain, pups will develop meningitis within 48–72 hr following infection. The infant rat intranasal model accurately reflects several important aspects of meningitis in humans in that experimental infection is obtained by the same route and bacteremia is a prerequisite for disease development. An additional advantage of the intranasal model is that the incidence of clinical meningitis is nearly 100% depending on the inoculum size and virulence of the pathogen. However, a disadvantage of the model is its variable time course of disease development. Nonetheless, the infant rat intra-nasal model remains an important research tool to investigate the events occurring during the initial stages of bacterial meningitis development, which cannot be easily addressed in many adult rodent models.

As an alternative to intranasal inoculation, infant rats can also be infected via an intraperitoneal (i.p.) route.[8,9] In this model, nursing 5–7-day-old Sprague-Dawley rat pups receive an inoculum of *H. influenzae* i.p. in 100 µl of phosphate buffered saline PBS using a 30-gauge ½ inch needle. This approach results in non-fatal meningitis typified by the polyclonal activation of lymphoid cells and elevated CSF leukocyte counts which can be studied over a protracted time interval. In addition, bacteremia and subsequent colonization of the subarachnoid space occur in this model, making this route of infection appropriate for examining hematogenous meningitis. However, the i.p. inoculation of organisms does not mimic the initial stages of natural infection since nasopharynx colonization and subsequent local penetration into the bloodstream are bypassed, which represents a limitation of this model.

Following introduction of the Hib conjugate vaccine in developed countries, group B streptococci (GBS) has become a leading cause of bacterial meningitis in infants. An intracisternal model of GBS has been developed to examine factors that contribute to neuronal injury associated with meningitis.[10] In this model, nursing Sprague-Dawley rat pups are infected around postnatal day 10 to 14 by the direct intracisternal inoculation of a GBS suspension (10 µl) using a 32-gauge needle. Pups are typically examined for signs of meningitis and specimen collection 18–20 hr following bacterial challenge. CSF is collected from the cisterna magna (10 µl) and quantitatively cultured to determine bacterial titers and evaluated for leukocyte counts. A limitation of this model is its inability to accurately mimic the natural course of meningitis development in humans since direct intracisternal inoculation bypasses naso-pharynx colonization, entry and replication of bacteria in the bloodstream, and invasion of organisms through the BBB into the subarachnoid space. However, the model is advantageous for studying factors that contribute to neuron cell death during the course of meningitis since two forms of neuronal injury can be distinguished, namely cortical neuronal necrosis and apoptosis of neurons in the dentate gyrus of the hippocampus.[11] Therefore, the intracister-nal infection model allows for the assessment of various therapeutic modalities on neuronal survival during the course of experimental meningitis.

Clinical signs of meningitis common to all infant rat experimental models include increased respiratory rate, cyanosis, and failure to nurse. The parameters typically evaluated during the course of disease to assess the therapeutic efficacy of treatment regimens include: (1) the collection of CSF and blood for quantitation of bacterial burdens and pro-inflammatory mediators which have been attributed to the pathophysiological changes accompanying meningitis, (2) evaluation of CSF lactate and glucose levels along with leukocyte counts, and (3) histopathological changes in brain tissue. In the infant rat, CSF (5–10 µl) is collected by direct puncture of the cisterna magna through the fontanella using a 30-gauge ½ inch needle while the head is held in flexion. Subsequently, CSF is recovered from the needle hub into a small glass capillary tube. Despite the advantages of the infant rat meningitis models alluded to above, one obvious disadvantage of these approaches is the limiting volumes of CSF and blood recovered due to small animal size. In addition, caution must be exercised when extending the findings obtained in infant meningitis models to adults since the immune response is not fully developed in neonates. Specifically, neonatal animals and humans have been shown to have impaired host defense mechanisms including diminished levels of complement, profound abnormalities in phagocytic function, and deficiency in some immunoglobulin classes.[3,6,9] Nonetheless, universal advantages of these models include the fact that infant rats, like humans, display preferential susceptibility to *H. influenzae* and *S. pneumoniae* coupled with the fact that bacteremia is a prerequisite for meningitis development, making them useful tools to dissect the efficacy of treatment strategies for meningitis in human infants.

27.4 Experimental meningitis models in adult rodents

In adult rodents, experimental bacterial meningitis models have been developed using three basic routes of infection, namely direct intracerebral or intracisternal injection or the inoculation of organisms via the intranasal route, each having their own distinct advantages and disadvantages.[7,12,13]

27.4.1 Intracisternal route of infection

The administration of bacteria into the cisterna magna is a common route of inoculation in many rat meningitis models.[14,15] In the intracisternal model described by Pfister and colleagues, animals are maintained under anesthesia to assess changes in regional cerebral blood flow, intracranial pressure, and brain edema formation during the acute phase of meningitis.[14,16] Adult Wistar rats weighing 250–350 g are anesthetized, tracheotomized, and artificially ventilated using a small animal ventilator. Polyethylene tubing is placed into the femoral artery and vein to measure arterial blood pressure and gases. Saline is infused via the femoral vein throughout the duration of the study (10 ml over the 6-hr period) to maintain blood volume and a rectal thermometer-controlled heating pad is used to maintain the animal's temperature at 38 °C. A catheter is inserted into the cisterna magna of the anesthetized rat placed in a stereotaxic frame by drilling a burr hole at the angle where the sagittal and lambda sutures intersect. Intracranial pressures are recorded using a pressure transducer and regional cerebral blood flow is evaluated by laser-Doppler flowmetry. Following these manipulations, cerebral blood flow and intracranial pressures are allowed to stabilize for 30 min prior to bacterial injection. A total of 75 μl of CSF is removed via the intracisternal catheter and meningitis is induced by the intracisternal administration of 75 μl of *S. pneumoniae* (10^7 colony-forming units (CFU)). Rats are maintained under anesthesia for the 6-hr duration whereupon animals are sacrificed by exsanguination. A disadvantage of this model is that great consideration must be taken when selecting anesthetic agents that may alter many of the physiologic parameters described above and interfere with the host antibacterial immune response. In addition, the continuous monitoring of animals precludes the evaluation of more chronic stages of meningitis.

Another intracisternal infection model, in which animals are allowed to emerge from anesthesia to evaluate pathogenic changes at later time points, has been utilized and modified by several groups.[9,15,17] In general, adult rats are anesthetized, whereupon a volume of CSF is removed via cisterna magna puncture (50–75 μl) using a micromanipulator fitted with a 25-gauge butterfly needle. Following CSF removal, an equal volume of phosphate buffered saline containing either *S. pneumoniae* or *H. influenzae* (both at 10^6–10^7 CFU) is injected intracisternally. Following recovery from anesthetic, animals are assessed at regular intervals for changes in body weight and temperature post-infection. Meningitis is allowed to proceed for various time points up to 24 hr, whereupon animals can be prepared for monitoring the physiological parameters described above[17] or immediately sacrificed to collect CSF, blood, and tissue samples for analysis.

Recently, the rat intracisternal model of *S. pneumoniae* meningitis has been modified for use in mice,[18] allowing investigators to study the importance of various mediators in the pathogenesis of disease using genetically engineered transgenic and knockout animals. In this approach, mice are subjected to short-term anesthesia during which meningitis is induced by the transcutaneous injection of *S. pneumoniae* into the cisterna magna (15 μl at 1×10^7 CFU/ml). Following emergence from anesthesia, animals are placed in cages, allowed to recover, and weighed. At different time points following infection, mice are anesthetized and a catheter is inserted into the cisterna magna via a burr hole in the occipital bone to collect CSF for bacterial quantitation and leukocyte counts. BBB permeability can also be evaluated in mice following an i.p. injection of 0.5 ml of 2% (w/v) Evans blue 45 min prior to sacrifice. After this time period, animals are transcardially perfused with 15 ml of cold phosphate buffered saline to remove any remaining Evans blue from the circulation. To determine cerebellar bacterial titers, the cerebellum is removed immediately following sacrifice, homogenized in sterile saline, and serial dilutions plated onto blood agar plates for quantitative cultures.

One major limitation of the intracisternal delivery route relates to its inability to completely mimic the natural course of infection since the pathogen bypasses its natural dissemination from the nasopharynx into the CNS and does not encounter the nascent cell types that would be normally engaged during colonization of the subarachnoid space. However, the intracisternal models have distinct advantages over other routes of bacterial inoculation in that meningitis is highly reproducible with a 100% incidence of clinical disease. In addition, the intracisternal models allow not only for the examination of live but also heat-killed organisms and purified bacterial products. Importantly, the study of heat-inactivated organisms can reveal the relative importance of bacterial-derived virulence factors that are not produced by killed cells.

27.4.2 Intracerebral administration of bacteria

Recently, mouse models have utilized a direct intracerebral inoculation to introduce bacteria into the brain.[19] Mice 2 months of age are injected with *S. pneumoniae* (10^3–10^4 CFU) into the right forebrain using a 27-gauge needle. Without any antibiotic intervention, the majority of animals succumb to fatal meningitis within 60 hr following infection. The signs accompanying meningitis in this model include lethargy, opisthotonus (rigid spasm of the body with back fully arched and the heels and head bent back), and seizures, which are described using a clinical scoring scale developed to characterize disease severity.[20] Histological examination of the injection site reveals a small intraparenchymatous infiltrate that lacks a capsule. Bacterial titers associated with the CSF, blood, cerebellum, and spleen are evaluated 36 hr following infection. Not unlike the intracisternal route, intracerebral infection bypasses the majority of steps required to establish natural disease including pathogen invasion and replication in the bloodstream, penetration of the BBB, and entry into the subarachnoid space. However, the major strength of this approach is the utility of examining meningitis development in genetically engineered knock-out or transgenic mouse strains to identify mediators that play a critical role in disease pathogenesis. The use of genetic mouse knockout models of meningitis alleviates the need for the pharmacological inhibition of target compounds, which can be problematic (i.e., ineffective neutralization of specific mediators and potential side effects of drugs).

27.4.3 Intranasal model of bacterial meningitis in the adult mouse

A newly developed intranasal model of experimental pneumococcal meningitis accurately recapitulates all of the steps required for bacterial colonization into the subarachnoid space and is perhaps the most physiologically relevant.[13] Hyaluronidase is administered along with the infectious pathogen to facilitate bacterial invasion into the bloodstream following nasopharynx colonization. In this model, mice are anesthetized and a 50 μl suspension of *S. pneumoniae* (8×10^4 CFU) with hyaluronidase (180 U) is applied to one nostril. Clinical illness is evaluated using a defined scale to document the extent of disease.[21] Mice are anesthetized at 24, 48, or 72 hr post-infection, whereupon blood and CSF are collected via cardiac puncture and a cisterna magna tap, respectively. These time points have been demonstrated to accurately represent the early phase of meningitis.[13] Samples are then processed for quantitation of bacterial burdens and leukocyte counts. Brain tissue is processed for histology and can also be homogenized for quantitation of cytokines/chemokines within the parenchyma. Importantly, this model utilizes adult mice instead of infant animals, allowing an accurate assessment of the host antibacterial immune response which is immature and not fully functional in infants. However, one limitation of this model is that only approximately 50% of infected animals progress to develop clinical disease, which necessitates the use of large sample sizes. In addition, it is not clear whether this approach can be used to examine meningitis pathogenesis caused by other bacterial strains.

27.4.4 Assessing therapeutic modalities for the potential treatment of bacterial meningitis

The parameters used to evaluate the efficacy of novel modalities for the clinical management of bacterial meningitis in the various animal models include but are not limited to: (1) monitoring of bacterial burdens in the CSF and blood, (2) quantitation of pro-inflammatory mediators such as cytokines/chemokines and proteolytic enzymes that have been implicated in mediating the patho-physiological changes associated with meningitis, (3) the effects on CSF pleiocytosis, and (4) changes in the degree of meningeal inflammation and/or neuronal apoptosis at the histological level.

There are several important points to consider when designing therapeutic interventions for bacterial meningitis. Firstly, whether the treatment itself will affect the host's basic physiologic functions that are inherently compromised during the course of bacterial meningitis (i.e., blood pressure, core body temperature, and respiratory rate). It would be counterproductive to administer a drug that would compound these deficits. Secondly, the effects of the therapeutic compound on the penetrance of antibiotics into the CSF must be evaluated. Thirdly, the therapeutic window of drug delivery should be examined and the timing of its administration relative to antibiotic treatment should be considered. The animal models described above provide excellent tools to evaluate the potential of various compounds for the clinical management of bacterial meningitis. Due to the complexity of the disease, effective treatment regimens will likely target several divergent pathophysiologic pathways.

27.5 Brain abscess

Brain abscess represents a significant medical problem, accounting for 1 in every 10 000 hospital admissions in the USA, and remains a serious condition despite recent advances made in detection and therapy.[22] Following infection, the potential sequelae of brain abscess include the replacement of the abscessed area with a fibrotic scar, loss of brain tissue by surgical excision, or abscess rupture and death. Indeed, if not detected early, an abscess has the potential to rupture into the ventricular space, a serious complication with an 80% mortality rate. In addition, the emergence of multi-drug-resistant strains of bacteria has become a confounding factor. The leading etiologic agents of brain abscess are the strains of *Streptococcus* and *Staphylococcus aureus*, although a myriad of other organisms have also been reported.[22,23] The most common sources of brain abscess are direct or indirect cranial infection arising from the paranasal sinuses, middle ear, and teeth. Other routes include seeding of the brain from distant sites of infection in the body (i.e., endocarditis) or penetrating trauma to the head. Following brain abscess resolution patients may experience long-term effects including seizures, loss of mental acuity, and focal neurological defects that are dependent on the lesion site.

Our laboratory has developed an experimental brain abscess model in the mouse using *S. aureus*, providing an excellent model system to study immunological pathways influencing abscess pathogenesis and the effects of therapeutic agents on disease outcome.[24,25] This model was originally established in the rat[26] but has been modified to examine the pathogenesis of brain abscess in the mouse allowing for the study of transgenic and knockout animals. The rodent brain abscess model closely mimics human disease, in that the abscess progresses through a series of well-defined stages. The early stage, or early cerebritis, occurs from day 1–3 and is typified by neutrophil accumulation, tissue necrosis, and edema. Microglial and astrocyte activation is also evident at this stage and persists throughout abscess development. The intermediate, or late cerebritis stage, occurs between days 4 and 9 and is associated with a predominant macrophage and lymphocytic infiltrate. The final or capsule stage occurs from day 10 onward and is associated with the formation of a well-vascularized abscess wall, in effect sequestering the lesion and protecting the surrounding normal brain parenchyma from additional damage. In the experimental model, abscesses are induced by the stereotactic inoculation of live *S. aureus* encapsulated in agarose beads into the caudate putamen as described in detail below. The use of agarose beads prevents the efflux of bacteria through the needle tract created during stab wound injections, allowing organisms to be focally deposited deep within the brain parenchyma. This step is critical to minimize the possibility of developing meningitis, a precaution that has not been used in other published rodent models of experimental brain abscess.[27,28] In our experience, all of the mouse strains examined to date using this model have qualitatively similar inflammatory profiles following bacterial challenge, a distinct advantage when using genetically engineered transgenic and knockout animals. In addition, the consequences of *S. aureus* infection do not appear to be influenced by gender since the responses of female and male mice are similar, another advantage when performing studies with knockout or transgenic mice where animal numbers are often limiting. However, we have found that certain mouse strains (i.e., C57/Bl/6) are exquisitely sensitive to *S. aureus* and require extensive dose–response studies prior to their use in experiments to avoid high mortality rates during the acute stages of disease.

27.5.1 Induction of experimental brain abscess in the mouse

Live *S. aureus* (or other pathogens) are encapsulated in agarose beads prior to implantation in the brain as previously described.[29,30] For brain abscess induction, mice are anesthetized and a 1-cm longitudinal incision is made along the vertex of the calvarium extending from the ear to the eye exposing the frontal sutures. A rodent stereotaxic apparatus equipped with a Cunningham mouse and neonatal rat adaptor is used to implant *S. aureus*-encapsulated beads into the caudate putamen using the following co-ordinates relative to bregma: +1.0 mm rostral, +2.0 mm lateral, and −3.0 mm deep from the surface of the brain. These co-ordinates avoid the possibility of introducing bacteria directly into the ventricles and inducing meningitis. A burr hole is made and a 5-µl Hamilton syringe fitted with a 26-gauge needle is used to slowly deliver *S. aureus*-encapsulated beads ($1 - 2 \times 10^4$ CFU in 2 µl) into the brain parenchyma. The needle remains in place for 2.5 min following injection to minimize bead efflux into the subarachnoid and/or subdural spaces. Control animals are inoculated with 2 µl of sterile agarose beads to ensure that the stab wound created during injections or deposition of agarose beads does not influence the parameters evaluated. Following injection, the burr hole is sealed with bone wax and the incision closed using surgical glue. Animal weights are recorded at regular intervals to compare differences between *S. aureus*-injected and control mice. Clinical signs of disease in *S. aureus*-infected animals include hunched posture, ruffled fur, lethargy, and precipitous weight loss.[25] Animals are sacrificed at regular intervals following infection to collect abscesses for quantitative bacterial culture, protein and RNA extraction, and immunohistochemical processing as indicated below.

Although our mouse experimental brain abscess model closely mimics human disease in that both progress through a series of well-defined histo-logical stages, the direct inoculation of bacteria into the brain parenchyma in the experimental model only represents the natural course of infection follow-ing a stab wound injury in humans. The remainder of brain abscesses arise from the direct perforation of thin sinus bones or BBB penetration by bacteria, routes of infection that are not recapitulated in our experimental model. We are currently examining other routes of bacterial inoculation that would more closely mimic these natural avenues of infection; however, it is likely that the incidence of brain abscess development using these alternative routes would be low making the utility of these models problematic. A distinct advantage of the mouse brain abscess model is that pathogenesis can be studied using transgenic and knockout mice in order to gain a better understanding of the host mediators that play a pivotal role in the disease process.

27.5.2 Experimental brain abscess models in the rat

Numerous other models of *S. aureus*-induced experimental brain abscess have been described in the rat.[26–28,31] Flaris and Hickey established a novel model of experimental brain abscess,[26] which we have recently modified for use in the mouse. In anesthetized rats, a small longitudinal incision is made lateral to midline between the ear and eye and a burr hole is drilled above the temporalis muscle lateral to the coronal suture. A microsyringe fitted with a 21-gauge needle is used to manually deliver *S. aureus*-laden agarose beads (20–40 µl)

5 to 6 mm deep into the brain parenchyma over a 15-s period. Bacteria-laden beads are placed deep in an attempt to minimize their reflux into the subarachnoid or subdural space. Following injection, the skin is sutured and animals are allowed to recover and closely monitored for signs of disease. Like our mouse model, a major advantage of this approach compared to the other rat models described below is that the formation of a solitary abscess is favored due to bacterial encapsulation in agarose beads.

In a model described by Lo and colleagues,[28] Sprague-Dawley rats weighing 250–380 g are anesthetized and injected with 1 μl (10^7 CFU) of bacteria into the middle right cerebral hemisphere posterior to the frontoparietal suture using a microsyringe connected to a micromanipulator 2.5 mm below the cortical surface. This location establishes an abscess at the gray–white matter junction in the parietal cortex. Nathan and Scheld have recently described another experimental brain abscess model in the rat using *S. aureus*.[27] Wistar rats weighing 275–300 g are anesthetized and placed in a stereotaxic frame. A 2-mm burr hole is made using a carbide drill just posterior to the coronal suture and 4 mm lateral to the midline. A total of 10^5 CFU of bacteria is delivered in a 1-μl volume using a Hamilton syringe over the course of 70 min. A limitation of this model is that only a few animals can be infected on a given day due to the long duration of injections. In addition, organisms are inoculated into the brain parenchyma in phosphate buffered saline, which due to the inherently high intracranial pressure increases the likelihood that bacteria will reflux out through the needle tract created during stab wound injections leading to the establishment of meningitis. Overall, the numbers of questions that can be addressed using the rat experimental brain abscess models are restricted by the lack of transgenic and knockout animals and limiting immunological reagents available to study the host immune response to infection.

27.5.3 Citrobacter koseri-*induced experimental brain abscess*

Another interesting model of rodent brain abscess has been described using the Gram-negative pathogen *Citrobacter koseri*.[32–34] In human infants, *C. koseri* induces meningitis whereupon approximately 77% of infected individuals develop multifocal brain abscesses. This disease etiology is intriguing since it involves both a meningitis and brain abscess component. Models of *C. koseri* infection have been established in infant rats[32,33] and mice[34] using a combined intraperitoneal/intranasal infection or intracerebral inoculation route, respectively. The infection is age-dependent in both models, in that 2-day-old animals are susceptible to brain abscess development whereas 5-day-old rodents are resistant. In addition, both routes of pathogen delivery result in similar patterns of disease progression initiated by bacteremia and leptomeningitis, followed by ventriculitis and direct extension of the infection into the periventricular brain parenchyma. It has been shown that *C. koseri* can survive and replicate in macrophages in the brain providing a mechanism for the establishment of chronic CNS infection such as brain abscesses.[33]

In the model originally described by Kline *et al.*,[32] 2-day-old rats are anesthetized and inoculated both intraperitoneally (100 μl) and intranasally (10 μl) with 4×10^5 CFU of *C. koseri*. Intranasal inoculations are administered using a P-20 Pipetman fitted with a round gel loading tip into one nostril with the head held back at a 70° angle. In this model, bacteremia occurs within 24 hr and ventriculitis is evident within the brain parenchyma 72 hr following infection. Brain abscesses are well established between 8 and 10 days after the initial bacterial challenge. At various time points following infection, blood and CSF samples are taken from anesthetized animals via intracardiac and intracisternal punctures, respectively. The advantages of this model include the fact that the routes of pathogen delivery and subsequent disease progression closely mimic those involved in natural infection in human infants, making it an attractive candidate to examine host–pathogen interactions and the efficacy of potential therapeutic regimens. However, this model has been shown to require large numbers of animals to demonstrate statistically significant differences between the virulence of different *C. koseri* strains and high bacterial inoculums to establish infection. In addition, another limitation of the rat model is the difficulty in evaluating the potential role of specific host factors since transgenic and knockout strains are not available.

A second model of *C. koseri* brain abscess has been described by Soriano *et al.*[34] using an intracerebral route of injection in infant mice. Two-day-old CD-1 mice receive an intracranial injection of bacteria (100 μl; optimal inoculum determined by dose–response studies) intracranially into the right parietal lobe by penetrating the skull with a 27-gauge needle fitted with a 1-ml tuberculin syringe. The site of inoculation is 3 mm distal to the right orbit and 2 mm lateral to the sagittal suture. The development of bacteremia is dependent upon the strain of *C. koseri* tested, where animals progress to develop purulent ventriculitis and adjacent parenchymal abscesses similar to the infant rat model discussed above, even though the mouse model uses a direct intracerebral route of infection. One obvious advantage of the infant mouse model is the potential to define the relative importance of various host immune factors in the pathogenesis of disease using transgenic or knockout mice.

27.5.4 *Assessing therapeutic modalities for the potential treatment of brain abscess*

The parameters utilized to evaluate the efficacy of novel modalities for the clinical management of brain abscess in the various experimental models include: (1) monitoring bacterial burdens in the brain parenchyma, (2) quantitating changes in pro-inflammatory mediator expression, (3) measuring BBB permeability changes, (4) evaluating differences in peripheral immune cell infiltrates and glial activation within the abscess and surrounding tissue, (5) histopathological examination of the abscess and degree of tissue involvement, and (6) changes in cerebral blood flow and other physiologic parameters. Several challenges become apparent when considering potential therapeutic interventions for brain abscess. Firstly, similar to the situation in bacterial meningitis, many brain abscess pathogens have developed antibiotic resistance. Secondly, we have recently suggested that besides infection containment, the host immune response that is an essential part of abscess formation likely also contributes to the destruction of surrounding normal brain parenchyma, which can have detrimental consequences. Thirdly, it appears likely that the host antibacterial immune response remains active even following the effective elimination of organisms by antibiotics due to the continued presence of potent immunostimulatory bacterial antigens. Therefore, interventive therapy with anti-inflammatory compounds subsequent to sufficient bacterial neutralization may be an effective strategy to minimize damage to surrounding brain parenchyma during the course of brain abscess development, leading to improvements in cognition and neurological outcomes.

27.6 Conclusions and perspectives

Due to the emergence of multi-drug-resistant strains and the ubiquitous nature of bacteria, the occurrence of bacterial meningitis and brain abscess are likely to persist. Therefore, animal models of both diseases represent the best tools to decipher the pathogenesis of infection and possible treatment strategies. The use of mouse models allow for the dissection of key host mediators of disease through the use of transgenic and knockout animals, which may reveal novel mechanisms to target for therapy. Due to the complexity in the host response to infection, effective therapies will most likely incorporate strategies that interfere with several pathophysiological mechanisms of disease.

References

1. Scheld WM, Koedel U, Nathan B, Pfister HW. Pathophysiology of bacterial meningitis: mechanism(s) of neuronal injury. *J. Infect. Dis.* 2002, **186** (Suppl. 2): S225–S233.

2. Merkelbach S, Sittinger H, Schweizer I, Muller M. Cognitive outcome after bacterial meningitis. *Acta Neurol. Scand.* 2000, **102**: 118–123.

3. Grimwood K, Anderson P, Anderson V, Tan L, Nolan T. Twelve-year outcomes following bacterial meningitis: further evidence for persisting effects. *Arch. Dis. Childh.* 2000, **83**: 111–116.

4. Nau R, Bruck W. Neuronal injury in bacterial meningitis: mechanisms and implications for therapy. *Trends Neurosci.* 2002, **25**: 38–45.

5. Koedel U, Scheld WM, Pfister HW. Pathogenesis and pathophysiology of pneumococcal meningitis. *Lancet Infect. Dis.* 2002, **2**: 721–736.

6. van der Flier M, Geelen SP, Kimpen JL, Hoepelman IM, Tuomanen EI. Reprogramming the host response in bacterial meningitis: how best to improve outcome? *Clin. Microbiol. Rev.* 2003, **16**: 415–429.

7. Tauber MG, Zwahlen A. Animal models for meningitis. *Methods Enzymol.* 1994, **235**: 93–106.

8. Smith AL, Smith DH, Averill Jr DR, Marino J, Moxon ER. Production of *Haemophilus influenzae* b meningitis in infant rats by intraperitoneal inoculation. *Infect. Immun.* 1973, **8**: 278–290.

9. Diab A, Abdalla H, Li HL, *et al.* Neutralization of macrophage inflammatory protein 2 (MIP-2) and MIP-1 alpha attenuates neutrophil recruitment in the central nervous system during experimental bacterial meningitis. *Infect. Immun.* 1999, **67**: 2590–2601.

10. Kim YS, Sheldon RA, Elliott BR, *et al.* Brain injury in experimental neonatal meningitis due to group B streptococci. *J. Neuropathol. Exp. Neurol.* 1995, **54**: 531–539.

11. Bogdan I, Leib SL, Bergeron M, Chow L, Tauber MG. Tumor necrosis factor-alpha contributes to apoptosis in hippocampal neurons during experimental group B streptococcal meningitis. *J. Infect. Dis.* 1997, **176**: 693–697.

12. Koedel U, Pfister HW. Models of experimental bacterial meningitis: role and limitations. *Infect. Dis. Clin. N. Am.* 1999, **13**: 549–577, vi.

13. Zwijnenburg PJ, van der Poll T, Florquin S, *et al.* Experimental pneumococcal meningitis in mice: a model of intranasal infection. *J. Infect. Dis.* 2001, **183**: 1143–1146.

14. Pfister HW, Koedel U, Haberl RL, *et al.* Microvascular changes during the early phase of experimental bacterial meningitis. *J. Cereb. Blood Flow Metab.* 1990, **10**: 914–922.

15. Quagliarello VJ, Long WJ, Scheld WM. Morphologic alterations of the blood–brain barrier with experimental meningitis in the rat: temporal sequence and role of encapsulation. *J. Clin. Invest.* 1986, **77**: 1084–1095.

16. Koedel U, Bernatowicz A, Paul R, *et al.* Experimental pneumococcal meningitis: cerebrovascular alterations, brain edema, and meningeal inflammation are linked to the production of nitric oxide. *Ann. Neurol.* 1995, **37**: 313–323.

17. Koedel U, Pfister HW. Protective effect of the antioxidant *N*-acetyl-L-cysteine in pneumococcal meningitis in the rat. *Neurosci. Lett.* 1997, **225**: 33–36.

18. Winkler F, Koedel U, Kastenbauer S, Pfister HW. Differential expression of nitric oxide synthases in bacterial meningitis: role of the inducible isoform for blood–brain barrier breakdown. *J. Infect. Dis.* 2001, **183**: 1749–1759.

19. Nau R, Wellmer A, Soto A, *et al.* Rifampin reduces early mortality in experimental *Streptococcus pneumoniae* meningitis. *J. Infect. Dis.* 1999, **179**: 1557–1560.

20. Wellmer A, Gerber J, Ragheb J, *et al.* Effect of deficiency of tumor necrosis factor alpha or both of its receptors on *Streptococcus pneumoniae* central nervous system infection and peritonitis. *Infect. Immun.* 2001, **69**: 6881–6886.

21. Zwijnenburg PJ, van der Poll T, Florquin S, *et al.* Interleukin-18 gene-deficient mice show enhanced defense and reduced inflammation during pneumococcal meningitis. *J. Neuroimmunol.* 2003, **138**: 31–37.

22. Townsend GC, Scheld WM.. Infections of the central nervous system. *Adv. Intern. Med.* 1998, **43**: 403–447.

23. Mathisen GE, Johnson JP. Brain abscess. *Clin. Infect. Dis.* 1997, **25**: 763–779; quiz 780–761.

24. Kielian T, Bearden ED, Baldwin AC, Esen N. IL-1 and TNF-alpha play a pivotal role in the host immune response in a mouse model of *Staphylococcus aureus*-induced experimental brain abscess. *J. Neuropathol. Exp. Neurol.* 2004, **63**: 381–396.

25. Baldwin AC, Kielian T. Persistent immune activation associated with a mouse model of *Staphylococcus aureus*-induced experimental brain abscess. *J. Neuroimmunol.* 2004, **151**: 24–32.

26. Flaris NA, Hickey WF. Development and characterization of an experimental model of brain abscess in the rat. *Am. J. Pathol.* 1992, **141**: 1299–1307.

27. Nathan BR, Scheld WM. The efficacy of trovafloxacin versus ceftriaxone in the treatment of experimental brain abscess/cerebritis in the rat. *Life Sci.* 2003, **73**: 1773–1782.

28. Lo WD, Wolny A, Boesel C. Blood–brain barrier permeability in staphylococcal cerebritis and early brain abscess. *J. Neurosurg.* 1994, **80**: 897–905.

29. Kielian T, Barry B, Hickey WF. CXC chemokine receptor-2 ligands are required for neutrophil-mediated host defense in experimental brain abscesses. *J. Immunol.* 2001, **166**: 4634–4643.

30. Kielian T, Cheung A, Hickey WF. Diminished virulence of an alpha-toxin mutant of *Staphylococcus aureus* in experimental brain abscesses. *Infect. Immun.* 2001, **69**: 6902–6911.

31. Kielian T, Hickey WF. Proinflammatory cytokine, chemokine, and cellular adhesion molecule expression during the acute phase of experimental brain abscess development. *Am. J. Pathol.* 2000, **157**: 647–658.

32. Kline MW, Kaplan SL, Hawkins EP, Mason Jr EO. Pathogenesis of brain abscess formation in an infant rat model of *Citrobacter diversus* bacteremia and meningitis. *J. Infect. Dis.* 1988, **157**: 106–112.

33. Townsend SM, Pollack HA, Gonzalez-Gomez I, Shimada H, Badger JL. *Citrobacter koseri* brain abscess in the neonatal rat: survival and replication within human and rat macrophages. *Infect. Immun.* 2003, **71**: 5871–5880.

34. Soriano AL, Russell RG, Johnson D, *et al.* Pathophysiology of *Citrobacter diversus* neonatal meningitis: comparative studies in an infant mouse model. *Infect. Immun.* 1991, **59**: 1352–1358.

28

Experimental models of motor neuron disease/ amyotrophic lateral sclerosis

RUTH DANZEISEN, BIRGIT SCHWALENSTÖCKER, AND ALBERT C. LUDOLPH

28.1 Introduction

Amyotrophic lateral sclerosis (ALS) is the most common motor neuron disorder in adults. The disease is characterized by the progressive loss of both upper and lower motoneurons, and is invariably fatal. Symptoms at the beginning of the disease include fatigue, cramps, muscular atrophy, weakness and wasting of one or more limbs or fasciculation of the tongue. As the disease progresses, patients become paralyzed and ultimately die from respiratory failure, typically within 1–3 years after diagnosis. The only medication approved for treatment of ALS is Rilutec® (Riluzole, a glutamate antagonist). However, ALS can currently not be cured and the available therapy offers only limited success, with a life extension of 3–4 months depending on the initiation of treatment. Famous ALS patients, such as the British physicist Stephen Hawking, the US baseball player Lou Gehrig (after whom the disease is named in the US), as well as the recent high incidence of ALS in soccer players especially in Italy have generated an increased public interest into this disease.

The emotional, social, and physical burdens of ALS are evident. Disease management requires sustained effort by patients, their families, caregivers, and healthcare professionals. Further, the economic impact of this disease is enormous. As the diagnosis of ALS is usually reached by exclusion, patients at the beginning of their disease generally undergo a series of arduous tests (magnetic resonance imaging (MRI), electrophysiologic studies, muscle biopsies, and blood studies). US patients often report to have spent approximately $20 000 on advanced diagnostic testing, without ever receiving a diagnosis.[1] The average length of hospitalization is longer (mean length of stay 8.4 ± 15.6 days vs. 5.4 ± 13.6 days) and more costly (mean total changes $19 810 \pm 42 589 vs. $11 924 \pm 37 114) for patients with ALS than for non-ALS patients. This

Handbook of Experimental Neurology, ed. Turgut Tatlisumak and Marc Fisher. Published by Cambridge University Press. © Cambridge University Press 2006.

can be explained by the prevalent co-morbidity (dehydration and malnutrition, acute respiratory failure, aspiration pneumonitis, and pneumonia), requiring procedures such as percutaneous endoscopic gastrostomy, mechanical ventilation, and tracheostomy.[2] Finally, home care of an ALS patient is costly, with an estimated \$200 000/year per patient (USA).[1]

The reports on ALS crude prevalence range from 1–3 to 4–6/100 000. Prevalence increases with age, reaching a peak in the 60–75 age group (33/100 000 for men, 14/100 000 for women), with a general average male preponderance of 1.5 : 1 only within the non-familial cases.[3]

Several ALS-related gene loci have been reported to date; from these, three major genes have been pinpointed. Superoxide dismutase 1 (SOD1) at 21q22 was the first ALS-related gene to be recognized;[4] it is also referred to as ALS1. ALS2 (ALSin at 2q33–34) was identified in Kuwaiti and Tunisian families; mutations cause a juvenile form of ALS, with a relatively mild phenotype. ALS can also be part of a multisystem neurodegeneration associated with tauopathies and combination of ALS with Parkinsonism. Mutations in the tau gene (17q) were first recognized in a syndrome called frontotemporal and dementia Parkinsonism (FTDP) complex. Tau mutations are characterized by large phenotypic variation, and amyotrophy may occur late in the clinical course of a tauopathy (for both ALS2 and FTDP see reference 3 and references therein). In addition, a range of susceptibility genes is known; these include neurofilament light and heavy chain, glutamate receptor (AMPA) and transporter (EAAT), mitochondrial DNA (COX gene), or manganese superoxide dismutase, to mention only some examples.[3]

ALS occurs predominantly in sporadic forms (90%), the remaining cases being familial. Mutations in SOD1 are responsible for about 20% of the familial ALS cases; most of them are inherited in an autosomal dominant fashion. Eukaryotic SOD1 is a 32 kDa homodimer, acts as an antioxidant enzyme, and locates to the cytoplasm and the mitochondrial intermembrane space. About 100 different ALS-causing mutations (mainly point-mutations) are known.[5] On a molecular level, each mutation affects the SOD1 protein in very different ways. Despite this, all mutations cause the ALS phenotype, with some differences in prognoses and clinical decline. Although it is a ubiquitous enzyme, SOD1 mutation results in the selective loss of motoneurons.

In recent years it is becoming clear that ALS is the paradigm of a multifactorial disease, possibly involving several genes and environmental factors (and probably a complex interaction therein). This complexity cannot easily be represented in a biological model. However, single causes of ALS (for example gene mutations) have given rise to models that mirror the clinical symptoms of the disease in an amazingly close fashion.

In this chapter, we give an overview of the genetic animal models for motor neuron disease, briefly mentioning non-SOD1 models of ALS. We then present a selection of published mSOD1 mouse models, with focus on the most prevalent model, the mutant human *SOD1* (G93A) expressing mouse, established in 1994 by Gurney *et al.*[6] This section includes practical advice from our and others experiences in working with that mouse strain. Finally, the more recent rat model of ALS is briefly introduced.

28.2 Late-onset non-SOD1 genetic mouse models for motor neuron disease

28.2.1 Mice overexpressing dynamitin

Overexpression of dynamitin causes disruption of the dynein/dynactin complex in postnatal motoneurons, resulting in an inhibition of retrograde axonal transport. Mice overexpressing dynamitin demonstrate late-onset (17 months of age) progressive motor neuron degeneration, resembling closely the symptoms observed in ALS patients. This mouse model confirms a critical role of disrupted axonal transport in the pathogenesis of motor neuron disease.[7]

28.2.2 Cra/Cra and Loa/Loa mice

Missense point mutations in cytoplasmic dynein heavy chain are present in Cramping 1 (*Cra1*) and Legs at odd angles (*Loa*) mice. These mutations perturb exclusively the neuron-specific function of dynein. Both mouse strains were generated by mutagenesis experiments in ENU (*N*-ethyl-*N*-nitrosourea) treated C3H male mice. There is late onset of motoneuron degeneration (16–19 months of age).[8]

28.2.3 Mice expressing human midsized neurofilament

Accumulation of neurofilaments is a reported feature of many neurodegenerative diseases, including ALS. Based on this observation, mice harboring a bacterial artificial chromosome (BAC) transgene containing the human midsized neurofilament subunit (NF-M) gene have been engineered. These mice develop a progressive hindlimb paralysis associated with neurofilamentous accumulations in ventral horn motor neurons and axonal loss in ventral motor roots, arguing that the human protein may be toxic to some mouse neurons.[9]

28.2.4 Mice expressing mutant (P301L) tau protein

Expression of a common human tau mutant (P301L) results in motor and behavioral deficits in transgenic mice, with age- and gene-dose-dependent development of neurofibrillary tangles. In these mice, the phenotype occurs at 6.5 months in hemizygous and at 4.5 months in homozygous animals. Neurofibrillary tangles and Pick-body-like neuronal lesions are present in various areas of the brain, with tau-immunoreactive pre-tangles in the cortex, hippocampus, and basal ganglia. Areas with the highest presence of neurofilbrillary tangles have reactive gliosis. The spinal cord shows axonal spheroids, anterior horn cell loss, and axonal degeneration in anterior spinal roots. Mice present with peripheral neuropathy and neurogenic atrophy in skeletal muscle. Brain and spinal cord contains insoluble tau that co-migrates with insoluble tau from brains of patients with Alzheimer's disease or frontotemporal dementia and Parkinsonism complex (FTDP-17). The phenotype of mice expressing P301L mutant tau mimics features of human tauopathies and provides a model for investigating the pathogenesis of diseases with neurofibrillary tangles.[10]

28.2.5 Mice expressing mutant SOD1

The SOD1 model of ALS, in our view, represents many advantages: the toxic effects of the mutant protein have been studied intensely in vitro (yeast and mammalian cells), providing a basis for interpretation of the results obtained from the matching animal model. Especially the SOD1(G93A) mouse model is used by many researchers to study mechanism of pathogenesis as well as efficacy of drugs, allowing to view and compare own data in a general context. Its characteristics are well-described and the mutation exists in several genetic backgrounds (Table 28.1). Finally and importantly it is maintained and available to all laboratories worldwide through Jackson Laboratories.

28.3 Which mouse strain to choose

SOD1(G93A) has been expressed in several genetic backgrounds, and it can be difficult to decide which strain may serve best for the individual need.

28.3.1 Inbred strains

Inbred mice are homozygous at all non-selective loci. This means that they offer a very homogeneous genetic background and hence little variation in

Table 28.1. *Overview of transgenic mice expressing mutant superoxide dismutase (SOD1)*

Mutation[a]	Genetic background of ova used for injection	Backcrossing (if injection was made into hybrid background)	Line name	Transgene copy number	SOD1 levels in CNS relative to control/endogenous SOD1	Age at disease onset	Duration of symptoms[b]	References
hG37R	(C57/Bl/6J × C3H/HeJ) F_2	Backcrossed to C57/Bl/6[9]	Line 42		14.5	3, 4–5 months	ND	11
			Line 9		9.0	5–6 months	ND	
			Line 106		7.2	5, 5–7 months	ND	
			Line 29		7.0	6–8 months	ND	
hG85R	(C57/Bl/6J × C3H)11	Backcrossed to C57/Bl/6[11]	Line 148		1.0	8–10 months	7–14 days	12
			Line 74		0.2	12–14 months	7–14 days	
mG86R	FVB/N	–	M1	20[13]	1.0	3–4 months	3 days to <1 month	13
hG93A	(C57/Bl/6 × SJL) F_1	Backcrossed to C57/Bl/6	G1	18		90 days	Death before day 187	6
			G5	4		ND		14
			G12	2.2		ND		
			G20	1.7		>300 days	survival until 343 days	
hG93A	(C57/Bl/6 × SJL) F_1	Backcrossed to C57/Bl/6	Homozygous G5/G5 (10 copies)			300 days, only mild symptoms	Survival until >400 days	15

[a] h, human; m, mouse.
[b] ND, not described.

Source: Shibata 2001 (reference 16).

phenotype. This is generally beneficial if small changes are anticipated. These can be changes in levels of a protein suspected to contribute to pathogenesis, or for example an anticipated drug effect. Further advantages are easy comparability to the literature, for example if meta-studies are desired. Finally, the genome of the most commonly used inbred strain, C57/Bl/6J, was the first mammalian genome to be sequenced. It is relatively well characterized, and can be accessed online.[17] The main disadvantage is the diminished viability of inbred strains. Unwanted side effects such as eye infections may occur more often, causing increased and unpredictable exclusion (euthanasia) of animals from a study. Also, it has to be considered that each line of inbred mice may respond to a drug differently, due to genetic susceptibility (in practice, this could for example be a strain-specific major histocompatibility complex (MHC) profile or cytokine profile). Therefore, a drug effect may be apparent in one inbred strain but not another. This makes data from inbred strains more difficult to extrapolate.

Inbred transgenic animals may be used for further breeding. We recommend backcrossing to freshly bought-in non-transgenic animals of that particular strain (e.g., C57/Bl/6J from Jackson Laboratories) in each generation, to avoid genetic drift at all cost.

28.3.2 *F₁ hybrids*

These are first-cross (F_1) offspring of two inbred parents of different inbred strains. They still represent a defined genetic background, as they are 50% strain 1 (e.g., C57/Bl/6) and 50% strain 2 (e.g., SJL). Due to the high level of heterozygosity, compared to inbred animals, F_1 hybrids are much more vigorous and robust. For example, we usually have no loss of hybrid animals included in drug studies due to eye infections or other co-morbidity. F_1 hybrid ova are often used for the injection of DNA in the generation of a new transgenic mouse, as hybrid females hyperovulate more easily than females of most inbred strains.

Elevated heterozygosity causes a larger variation in phenotype, meaning that small effects of a drug may be blurred in the wide range of survival times, or that small changes in disease-related protein expression may be undistinguishable from the normal inter-individual changes. However, exactly this disadvantage makes a population of offspring from F_1 hybrids a better and closer model to a human population. In our laboratory, first-generation offspring of F_1 hybrids is currently used for drug trials; efficacy is judged by motor performance and survival time. Usually group sizes of more than 20 animals are needed to obtain meaningful, statistically interpretable results.

The survival time of control mice (transgenic, vehicle-treated animals) within one study can range overall from 114 days to 150 days (in this particular study, female mice had an average survival time of 133 days, $n = 10$, while males lived on average 129 days, $n = 9$).

28.3.3 Overview of mice available from Jackson Laboratories[18]

Strain name B6.Cg-Tg (SOD1-G93A)1Gur/J (Jackson Laboratories stock number 004435)

This is a "high copy number" strain derived from Gurney's original mutant.[6] These mice carry a high copy number of the mutant allele human *SOD1* containing the Gly93 → Ala (G93A) substitution, driven by its endogenous human promoter. The integration site is unknown. Hemizygous carriers become paralyzed in one or more limbs and die usually after 19–23 weeks. Paralysis is due to loss of motor neurons from the spinal cord.

This is a congenic strain, meaning that the mutation was transferred from one genetic background to another. Here, the construct containing the mutant human G93A-*SOD1* gene was injected into fertilized B6SJLF1 mouse eggs and founder animals were obtained.[6] These were backcrossed to C57/Bl/6 J for 10 generations. Congenic strains are considered identical to the inbred strain used for backcrossing at all loci except for the transferred locus and a linked segment of chromosome. Therefore, a non-transgenic litter-mate from the colony, or any other C57/Bl/6 J mouse (Jackson Laboratories stock number 000664) may be used as a control. Additionally, C57/Bl/6 J mice overexpressing human wtSOD1 may be the appropriate control, depending on the aim of the experiment.

Strain name B6.Cg-Tg (SOD1-G93A)^{dl}1Gur/J (Jackson Laboratories stock number 002299)

A "low copy number" strain, with similar properties to the preceding strain; congenic (transfer from B6SJLF1 to B57/Bl/6, backcrossed five times), site of integration unknown. In this strain, onset of the ALS phenotype is delayed due to a reduction in transgenic copy number. The corresponding mice on the B6SJL background (Jackson Laboratories stock number 002300, see below) become paralyzed in one or more limbs beginning around 6–7 months of age. Life expectancy is normally 4–6 weeks beyond onset of symptoms. The ALS phenotype on this genetic background has not been characterized by Jackson Laboratories or by any other investigator; however, the onset of the ALS phenotype does not appear to be accelerated[19] in comparison to the same copy number in a hybrid background.

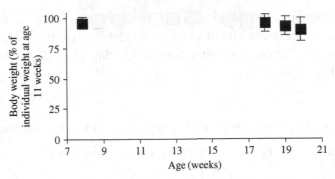

Figure 28.1. Body weight of B6SJL-Tg (G93A)1Gur/J mice (16 animals; 8 male, 8 female). Body weight (mean ± SD) is expressed as a percentage of individual weight at 11 weeks of age.

Strain name B6SJL-Tg (SOD1-G93A)1Gur/J (Jackson Laboratories stock number 002726)

A "high copy number" strain. Here, mutant SOD1 is expressed in a hybrid background (non-inbred genetic background) B6SJL; ova from this strain were used for original ova injection. This line of mice is maintained by Jackson Laboratories by backcrossing hemizygous transgenic mice to B6SJL F_1 hybrids (non-transgenic). The transgene carries a high copy number of a mutant human *SOD1* with the G93A mutation; the incorporation site is unknown. Hemizygous transgenic mice become paralyzed in one or more limbs and die by 4–5 months of age (according to Jackson Laboratories[19]). Paralysis is due to loss of motor neurons from the spinal cord. Typical motor performance, onset of symptoms, and further data in this strain (as measured in our laboratory) are shown in Figs. 28.1–28.4.

For our drug studies, we obtain hemizygous transgenic males and breed them to non-transgenic B6SJL females. We use original animals (Jackson Laboratories) for each study, to avoid inadvertently establishing sub-lines. We only use the first generation obtained from these breeding pairs. In their first-generation offspring, genetic heterogeneity is obvious, manifesting itself in multiple coat colors and in a wide range of survival times. Therefore, we recommend not to use these animals for further breeding. The advantages and disadvantages of using these mice for drug trials are outlined above (see Section 28.3.2).

Strain name B6SJL-Tg (SOD1-G93A)^{dl}1Gur/J (Jackson Laboratories stock number 002300)

A "low copy number" strain. As in the preceding strain (002726), the mutant SOD1 is expressed in the F_1 hybrid background (non-inbred genetic

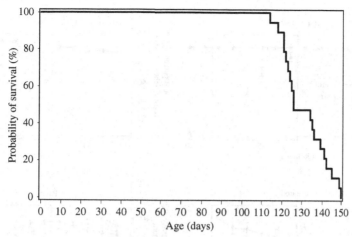

Figure 28.2. Kaplan–Meyer plot of survival in B6SJL-Tg (SOD1-G93A)1Gur/J mice. Data were obtained from 19 mice (9 male, 10 female).

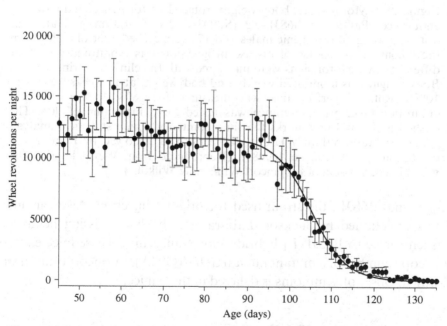

Figure 28.3. Running-wheel performance of B6SJL-Tg (SOD1-G93A)1Gur/J mice. Activity of 16 mice (8 males, 8 females) was measured for 12 hr each day (in the dark period 20:00–8:00). Mean ± SD for each day are given.

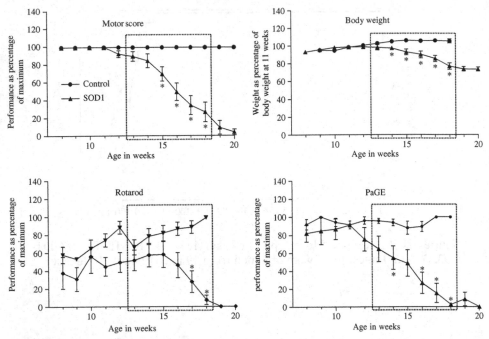

Figure 28.4. Motor score, body weight, rotarod performance, and paw grip endurance (PaGE) in B6SJL-Tg (SOD1-G93A)1Gur/J mice. Data was obtained using 10 transgenic males and 17 age-matched control males from the colony. Time course of disease progression was monitored with four different tests. Motor signs were measured with the clinical scoring system. Body weight was monitored weekly and bodyweight at 11 weeks was set as 100%. Rotarod performance was measured for 180 s. In the paw grip endurance task, grip endurance was tested for a maximum of 90 s. The dashed horizontal box marks the time points for which statistical analysis using the Mann–Whitney U-test was performed, followed by Bonferroni's correction ($p < 0.05/6$, i.e. 0.0083). (Reproduced from Weydt *et al.* 2003, with kind permission of Lippincott Williams & Wilkins.)

background) B6SJL, the strain used for original injection. Also this line of mice is maintained by Jackson Laboratories by backcrossing hemizygous transgenic mice to B6SJL F_1 hybrids (non-transgenic). These mice express a lower copy number of a mutant human *SOD1*(G93A); the incorporation site is unknown. Onset of symptoms is delayed in these mice.

28.4 Practical considerations

28.4.1 Assessment of disease onset and progression

The clearest end point is time of death, hence a simple documentation of time of death, or measurement of life extension when a drug is applied, is the easiest possible method. However, clearly it is of interest whether a drug can not only extend lifespan but also improve and preserve motor performance, or delay onset of disease. Many measurements of motor performance can be blurred by experimentator's bias. Also, in our hands, mice can display inconsistencies in apparent performance, meaning that a mouse that was predicted to die within the next 24 hr may be mobile again on the following day. These inconsistencies have prompted us to use a completely objective and long-term measure of motor performance. In order to measure the activity of each animal, mice are housed singly in a cage containing a running wheel of 11 cm diameter, attached to the roof of the cage, leaving a 1 cm distance to the cage floor. Two magnets are attached to each wheel, feeding two signals per revolution into a computer system (LMTB, Berlin). We monitor mouse activity daily throughout the whole dark period between 20:00 and 08:00 hours. Mice are removed from the breeding cage and moved into these cages at day 40 of age, to give them time to adapt. We have observed that the number of revolutions per night varies between the mice. In the pre-symptomatic stage (day 50–80, vehicle-treated animals) some mice produce as many as over 23 000 revolutions per night, whereas others are more "lazy" and produce about 2300 revolutions per night (mean 12 489, SD $\pm$ 6509, $n=$ 16). Especially when using hybrid mice, we would like to emphasize the need to use each individual mouse's base-line (before the onset of symptoms), and express loss of motor function as deviation from each individual animal's base-line.

The running wheel system, while being completely objective and time-saving for the experimentator, is costly to obtain and maintain, and may not be widely available. We therefore would like to outline reliable and objective alternative ways to assess disease progression in ALS mice.

Alternatives for measurement of motor performance, if no running wheel is available, are the rotarod test, motor score (observation and tail-suspension with scoring according to a 4-point system, outlined below), body weight, and paw grip endurance. These methods have recently been evaluated system-atically for suitability and objectivity in the measurement of disease progres-sion in ALS mice.[20] Male SOD1(G93A) mice in a hybrid background (B6SJL-Tg (SOD1-G93A)1Gur/J) were used, with non-transgenic age- and gender-matched controls. Starting at day 55 of age, animals were assessed weekly with three behavioral tests in randomized order by an observer blinded to the genotype. The results of this study are shown in Fig.28.4.

Motor score

A 4-point scoring system was used: 4 points if the animal appears normal (no sign of motor dysfunction), 3 points if hindlimb tremors are evident when animal is suspended by the tail, 2 points if gait abnormalities are present, 1 point for dragging of at least one hindlimb, 0 points for inability of the animal to right itself within 30 s. A score of <4 for 2 consecutive weeks was defined retrospectively as "disease onset."

Rotarod

Each animal was placed on a cylinder, rotating at a constant speed of 15 rpm. Animals were given three attempts to remain on the cylinder, and the longest latency to fall was recorded; 180 s was chosen as arbitrary cut-off time.

Paw grip endurance

Each animal was placed on the wire-mesh lid of a conventional housing cage. The lid was gently shaken to prompt the mouse to hold on to the wire grid. Then the lid was swiftly turned upside down. The latency until the mouse let go with at least both hindlimbs was timed; the arbitrary maximum was 90 s. Each mouse was given three tries and the longest latency was recorded.

In parallel to our observation in running wheel performance, inter-individual variation in the rotarod and the paw grip endurance test is large. Therefore, all data were normalized to the maximal value of each individual mouse (irrespective of when it occurred). Deviation from the maximal value is represented in the graph.

Body weight

The weight of each mouse was recorded and normalized to weight at 11 weeks of age. Note that body weight in our laboratory in Ulm is not such a clear indicator (Fig. 28.1), possibly due to the fact that we use a mixed (50% male, 50% female) population (see also Section 28.4.2 below).

The authors report that the first detectable sign of motor neuron disease are fine hindlimb tremors, which can best be observed when the mouse is suspended by its tail.[20] These tremors were reported to occur around day 85 (slightly before running wheel performance declines, which is after day 90). Weight loss in ALS mice becomes evident around day 90. ALS mice perform consistently worse in the rotarod test than non-transgenic mice, but the difference is not always statistically significant. Importantly, mice go through a learning phase during the first 4 weeks of observation, where both groups show an improvement of rotarod performance. Paw grip endurance of ALS mice declines slowly from around day 85, reaching significance by day 100.

In conclusion, motor score and paw grip endurance are the most sensitive methods to detect disease progression in ALS mice. However, assessment of tremors in the early phase is somewhat subjective, and requires experience and training of the observer. The paw grip endurance test, in contrast, is objective and reliable, while requiring no special equipment (conventional cage-lids are used) or training of the animals (no learning phase is required, as mice master this test almost immediately). The only disadvantage is the fact that this test is time-consuming for the observer and may not be realistic for large animal trials.

28.4.2 *Gender effects*

Gender effects in ALS mice have been reported in the literature (delayed onset in females).[21] In our laboratory, we find a trend towards better running wheel performance and towards longer survival in female mice, but in our hands these effects are not statistically significant. Gender effects may be observed in response to compounds. Therefore, we recommend to include gender as a block (i.e. to have 50% males and 50% females in each group).

28.4.3 *Housing and breeding*

Always keep the breeding room and the experimental room separate. We breed one transgenic male to two non-transgenic females of the same genetic background. Offspring are separated from the mothers at the age of 21 days, and the females can be mated again.

We usually obtain from one breeding cage (one male, two females) a maximum of four litters (approximately 48 offspring). The female : male ratio and the transgenic : non-transgenic ratios are normally 50 : 50. In practical terms this means that one breeding cage generates a maximum of 12 transgenic females and 12 transgenic males.

28.4.4 *Genotyping*

We genotype animals by tail biopsy between days 22 and 30. Genomic DNA is isolated and polymerase chain reaction (PCR) is performed according to the method described on the Jackson Laboratories home page.[18]

28.4.5 *Late-stage animals*

The time point of euthanasia is defined by the following criteria: inability to rise within 30 s, eye infection, loss of more than 20% of pre-onset body weight. When caring for late-stage animals, it is crucial to offer gel-food on the cage floor and/or wet pellets as some mice may not be able reach the food and water-bottle any more. We have, however, observed that even moribund animals may still consume significant amounts of water from the bottle. Our measurements indicate an average drinking water consumption of 7.6 ml/day/ mouse (SD ± 2.36), and we recommend to allow at least 12–15 ml (bottle) per day for each animal until death.

28.4.6 Timescale

It is important to remember that subclinical changes in ALS mice and patients occur a long time before symptoms can be observed.[22] In mice, morphological changes (fragmentation of the Golgi apparatus) have been reported as early as day 30. When ALS symptoms occur, 50% of motor neurons are already lost. When testing a drug for potential use in humans, it is also important to consider that application in humans is typically *after* onset of symptoms. Finally, depending on the method chosen for assessment of disease progression, it is crucial to allow time for learning and adaptation (we usually place mice into the running wheel before day 40).

A timescale of the pre-symptomatic and symptomatic changes in the SOD1(G93A) mice is shown in Fig. 28.5.

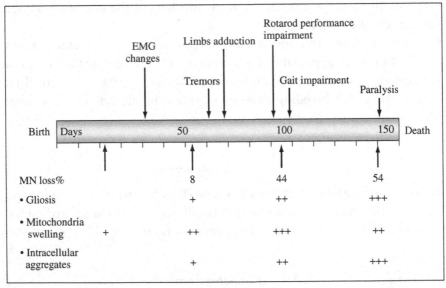

Figure 28.5. Graphic representation of the behavioural and neuropathological progression of the disease in high-expressor SOD1(G93 A transgenic) mice. EMG, electromyograph; MN, motor neuron. (Reproduced from Bendotti and Carri 2004, with kind permission of Elsevier.)

28.4.7 Copy number

The number of copies of the transgene is the major factor influencing the lifespan of ALS mice. Anecdotal reports of loss of copies, or a decrease in copy number with increasing generations, are difficult to explain. However, it is imperative never to cross two hemizygote transgenic mice to avoid the (albeit unlikely) event of hybridization between the two transgenes. A possible delay of phenotype in some colonies is more likely due to genetic drift over the generations, and the involuntary "in-house" breeding and selecting for longer survival.

28.4.8 Controls

For drug trials, the appropriate controls are vehicle-treated transgenic mice from the same litter (s) as used for the drug treatment. For mechanistic studies on factors influencing disease progression, ALS mice need to be compared to "healthy" mice. In most cases, as controls, wild-type (non-transgenic) mice from the colony may be used. If specific effects in relation to the SOD1 mutation are of interest, each investigator should consider whether a better (or additional) control is the B6SJL-TgN(SOD1)2Gur transgenic strain carrying the wild-type *SOD1* human gene (Jackson Laboratories stock number 002297).

28.5 ALS rat model

The abundant mouse model (s) for ALS have recently been complemented by the first report of a successful introduction of mSOD1 into rats (Table 28.2).[23] Sprague-Dawley rats expressing the G93A and the H46R mutation of human *SOD1* develop striking motor neuron degeneration and paralysis, due to selective loss of motor neurons in the spinal cord. Only rats expressing high copy

Table 28.2. *Transgenic rats expressing human mSOD1*

Line	Copy number	Relative SOD1 protein levels in spinal cord (human/rat)	SOD activity relative to control	Age of onset (days)	Duration (days)
H46R-4	25	6.0	0.21	145	24
G93A-39	10	2.5	3	123	8

Source: Nagai *et al.* 2001 (reference 23).

numbers (=10) of mSOD1 develop motor neuron disease. This rat model offers further support for the notion that motor neuron death in SOD1-related ALS is a consequence of one or more gain-of-function, neurotoxic properties of mSOD1 protein. The main advantage of this model is its larger size compared to mice, facilitating studies requiring sampling or manipulation of spinal fluid and spinal cord, mainly direct administration of viral- and cell-mediated therapies.

References

1. Klein LM, Forshew DA. The economic impact of ALS. *Neurology* 1996, **47**(4 Suppl. 2): S126–S129.
2. Lechtzin N, Wiener CM, Clawson L, Chaudhry V, Diette GB. Hospitalization in amyotrophic lateral sclerosis: causes, costs, and outcomes. *Neurology* 2001, **56**: 753–757.
3. Majoor-Krakauer D, Willems PJ, Hofman A. Genetic epidemiology of amyotrophic lateral sclerosis. *Clin. Genet.* 2003, **63**: 83–101.
4. Rosen DR, Siddique T, Patterson D, *et al.* Mutations in Cu/Zn superoxide dismutase gene are associated with familial amyotrophic lateral sclerosis. *Nature* 1993, **362**: 59–62.
5. See http://www.alsod.org.
6. Gurney ME. Transgenic-mouse model of amyotrophic lateral sclerosis. *New Engl. J. Med.* 1994, **331**: 1721–1722.
7. LaMonte BH, Wallace KE, Holloway BA, *et al.* Disruption of dynein/dynactin inhibits axonal transport in motor neurons causing late-onset progressive degeneration. *Neuron* 2002, **34**: 715–727.
8. Hafezparast M, Klocke R, Ruhrberg C, *et al.* Mutations in dynein link motor neuron degeneration to defects in retrograde transport. *Science* 2003, **300**: 808–812.
9. Gama Sosa MA, Friedrich Jr VL, DeGasperi R, *et al.* Human midsized neurofilament subunit induces motor neuron disease in transgenic mice. *Exp. Neurol.* 2003, **184**: 408–419.
10. Lewis J, McGowan E, Rockwood J, *et al.* Neurofibrillary tangles, amyotrophy and progressive motor disturbance in mice expressing mutant (P301L) tau protein. *Nature Genet.* 2000, **25**: 402–405.
11. Wong PC, Pardo CA, Borchelt DR, *et al.* An adverse property of a familial ALS-linked SOD1 mutation causes motor neuron disease characterized by vacuolar degeneration of mitochondria. *Neuron* 1995, **14**: 1105–1116.
12. Bruijn LI, Becher MW, Lee MK, *et al.* ALS-linked SOD1 mutant G85R mediates damage to astrocytes and promotes rapidly progressive disease with SOD1-containing inclusions. *Neuron* 1997, **18**: 327–338.
13. Ripps ME, Huntley GW, Hof PR, Morrison JH, Gordon JW. Transgenic mice expressing an altered murine superoxide dismutase gene provide an animal model of amyotrophic lateral sclerosis. *Proc. Natl Acad. Sci. USA* 1995, **92**: 689–693.
14. Dal Canto MC, Gurney ME. Neuropathological changes in two lines of mice carrying a transgene for mutant human Cu, Zn SOD, and in mice overexpressing wild-type human SOD: a model of familial amyotrophic lateral sclerosis (FALS). *Brain Res.* 1995, **676**: 25–40.

15. Dal Canto MC, Gurney ME. A low-expressor line of transgenic mice carrying a mutant human Cu, Zn superoxide dismutase (SOD1) gene develops pathological changes that most closely resemble those in human amyotrophic lateral sclerosis. *Acta Neuropathol. (Berlin)* 1997, **93**: 537–550.
16. Shibata N. Transgenic mouse model for familial amyotrophic lateral sclerosis with superoxide dismutase-1 mutation. *Neuropathology* 2001, **21**: 82–92.
17. See http://www.ncbi.nlm.nih.gov/genome/guide/mouse/.
18. All information has been summarized from http://www.jaxmice.jax.org.
19. Data from Jackson Laboratories, March 1996.
20. Weydt P, Hong SY, Kliot M, Moller T. Assessing disease onset and progression in the SOD1 mouse model of ALS. *NeuroReport* 2003, **14**: 1051–1054.
21. Veldink JH, Bar PR, Joosten EA, *et al.* Sexual differences in onset of disease and response to exercise in a transgenic model of ALS. *Neuromusc. Disord.* 2003, **13**: 737–743.
22. Bendotti C, Carri MT. SOD-linked fALS: what models have told us. *Trends Mol. Med.* 2004, **10**: 393–400.
23. Nagai M, Aoki M, Miyoshi I, *et al.* Rats expressing human cytosolic copper-zinc superoxide dismutase transgenes with amyotrophic lateral sclerosis: associated mutations develop motor neuron disease. *J. Neurosci.* 2001, **21**: 9246–9254.

29

Animal models for sleep disorders

SEIJI NISHINO AND NOBUHIRO FUJIKI

29.1 Introduction

We spend a significant part (about a third) of our lives sleeping, which is essential to our physical and psychological well-being. Sleep, however, is a fragile state that can easily be impaired by psychological stress or physical illness. For up to 10% of the general population, difficulty falling and/or maintaining sleep occurs several times a week (i.e., chronic insomnia).[1] Some of these problems may be due to existences of obstructive sleep apnea syndrome, a condition that affects over 10% of the population,[2] or due to restless leg syndrome (RLS)/periodic leg movement syndrome (PLMS), sleep-related involuntary leg movements often associated with an abnormal sensation in legs.[3] Excessive daytime sleepiness (EDS), parasomnia, and sleep problems associated with medical/psychiatric conditions are also common. Narcolepsy is a primary EDS disorder affecting about 0.05% of the population.[4] EDS is also often secondary to a severe insomnia associated with obstructive sleep apnea.[2]

Many different pathophysiological/etiological mechanisms for these sleep disorders are considered, and the International Classification of Sleep Disorders (ICSD) lists over 84 different types of disorders (Table 29.1).[5] These sleep-related problems are often chronic and negatively affect the subject's quality of life. In a 24-hr society that encourages sleep deprivation, daytime sleepiness is also an emerging issue even in healthy subjects. Accidents due to sleepiness are now well recognized as a major public hazard. The emergence of clinical sleep medicine has proceeded rapidly during the last 30 years with the awareness of these sleep problems. The evolution of sleep medicine into a distinct specialty has also played a pivotal role in the expansion of neuroscience research aiming to unravel the mechanisms underlying normal and abnormal sleep.

Progress in understanding of basic sleep physiology is largely owed to animal experiments in which various invasive techniques, such as in vivo/in vitro electrophysiology, brain lesion/transection, and functional neurochemical/anatomical experiments, have been applied. Animal models are also recently available of

Handbook of Experimental Neurology, ed. Turgut Tatlisumak and Marc Fisher. Published by Cambridge University Press. © Cambridge University Press 2006.

Table 29.1. *Classification of sleep disorders (adapted from (5))*

1. Dyssomnias
Intrinsic – e.g., psychophysiological insomnia, narcolepsy, idiopathic hypersomnia, recurrent hypersomnia, obstructive sleep apnea syndrome, central sleep apnea syndrome, periodic limb movement disorder, restless legs syndrome (RLS)
Extrinsic – e.g., inadequate sleep hygiene, insufficient sleep syndrome, environmental sleep disorder
Circadian rhythms sleep disorders – e.g., jet lag syndrome, shift-work sleep disorder, advanced sleep phase syndrome, delayed sleep phase syndrome

2. Parasomnias
Arousal disorders – e.g., confusional arousals, sleep terrors, sleepwalking
Sleep–wake transition disorders – e.g., rhythmic movement disorder, sleep starts
Parasomnias usually associated with rapid eye movement (REM) sleep – e.g., nightmares, sleep paralysis, REM sleep behavior disorder
Other parasomnias – e.g., enuresis, bruxism

3. Sleep disorders associated with:
Mental disorders – e.g., psychoses, mood disorders, anxiety disorders, alcoholism
Neurological disorders – e.g., Parkinsonism, sleep-related epilepsy, sleep-related headaches
Medical disorders – e.g., nocturnal cardiac ischemia, sleep-related asthma, sleep-related gastroesophageal reflux

4. Proposed sleep disorders – e.g., short sleeper, long sleeper, fragmentary myoclonus, sleep hyperhidrosis, pregnancy-associated sleep disorder

Source: Adapted from American Sleep Disorders Association 2001 (reference 5).

various sleep disorders that occur both spontaneously and when produced by genetic engineering (gene targeting and transgenic). With both forward genetic and reverse genetic approaches, genes responsible for narcolepsy in dogs and mice have recently been identified.[6,7] Subsequently, it has been found that a deficiency in the same neurotransmitter system (hypocretin/orexin) found in the animal models is indeed involved in human narcolepsy,[8–10] stressing the usefulness of validated animal models. Some physiological and pathophysiological aspects of sleep mechanisms can also be investigated in much simpler animals, such as zebra fishes or fruit flies, with various molecular and genetic approaches.

In this chapter, available animal models for sleep disorders and some of the major progresses in these models are introduced. Prospects of research using these models are also discussed.

29.2 Current classification of sleep disorders

The ICSD divides sleeping problems into four general classifications: dyssomnias, parasomnias, medical/psychiatric problems, and proposed disorders

(Table 29.1).[5] The proposed disorders are not yet established disorders that are under investigation. A dyssomnia is a disruption of the body's natural resting and waking patterns. Dyssomnias may be extrinsic (having an external cause) or intrinsic (having their cause in the body). A dyssomnia may also be caused by problems with a person's circadian rhythm, or internal clock. Parasomnias are conditions that interrupt sleep. They are caused by difficulties with arousal or sleep stage transitions. Sleepwalking, nightmares, bedwetting and RLS/ PMLS are all common parasomnias. It is also known that medical or psychological conditions, such as alcoholism, ulcers, asthma, and anxiety disorders, can cause rest-related disturbances. Characteristics of some common sleep disorders are summarized briefly.

29.2.1 Insomnias

Insomnia is very common and 9–15% of the general adult population suffers from chronic insomnia, and an additional 15–20% of the adult population complains of occasional sleep difficulties.[1,11] Insomnia is a very heterogeneous disease entity, and it can be caused intrinsically and extrinsically with various mechanisms. Insomnia can be subdivided into initial, midterm, and terminal insomnias, respectively characterized by difficulties falling asleep, maintaining sleep throughout the night, or awakening early in the morning.[12] The insomnias can be also classified according to the duration of symptoms as transient, short-term, medium-term, and persistent or chronic insomnias.[12] However, mechanisms involved in most insomnias are largely unknown.

29.2.2 Hypersomnias

Narcolepsy–cataplexy syndrome affects 0·02–0·06% of the general population in the USA and Western European countries.[4] Narcolepsy is characterized by excessive daytime sleepiness, cataplexy (sudden loss of muscle tone in response to strong emotion), hypnagogic hallucinations (dream-like experiences occurring at sleep onset), and sleep paralysis (the inability to move while falling asleep or on awakening).[4] Narcoleptic subjects feel refreshed after a short nap, but this does not last long and the patients become sleepy again within a few hours. Narcolepsy may therefore consist of an inability to maintain wakefulness combined with intrusion of rapid-eye-movement (REM)-sleep-associated phenomena (hallucinations, sleep paralysis, and possibly cataplexy) into wakefulness. Less common forms of hypersomnia include the idiopathic and recurrent hypersomnias.[13] Idiopathic hypersomnia is marked by excessive nocturnal sleep of good quality and by EDS which is not as severe as in the narcoleptic patients (but no refreshing after naps) and which is not REM sleep related. The best-characterized recurrent hypersomnia is the Kleine–Levin syndrome (KLS), a pervasive functional disorder of the hypothalamus characterized by hypersexuality, binge eating, and irritability associated with periods of EDS and sleep periods as long as 18–20 hours.

29.2.3 Movement disorders

RLS and PLMS are very common sleep disorders (2–5% in the general population).[3] The periodic movements occur during Non-REM sleep (NREM) and the continuous arousals impede the patients from entering deeper stages of sleep. In RLS, uncomfortable sensations in the limbs occur during the first part of the night and prevent a normal transition from wakefulness to sleep.[3] RLS and PLMS often occur together and they can be responsible for poor sleep at night and for subsequent EDS and can hence be present as causes of insomnia or EDS. The prevalence of RLS/PLMS increases with aging, and RLS/PLMS are also associated with various physical conditions, such as renal failure or iron deficiency.[3] Dopaminergic agonists, especially dopamine autoreceptor (D2/D3) agonists, have been recently found effective in RLS/PLMS.[3]

29.2.4 Sleep apnea syndromes

Sleep apnea or sleep disordered breathing is the second most common sleep disorder (after insomnia).[14] In contrast to the more frequent group of insomnias, sleep apnea is an often severe, potentially life-threatening disorder characterized by impaired patency of the upper airway during sleep.[14] There are two types of sleep apnea, obstructive and central.[14] In the latter, which is far less common, the absence of ventilatory effort parallels the collapse of the upper airway with consequent lack of airflow. Associated nocturnal symptoms include restlessness, excessive salivation and sweating, nocturia, and gastroesophageal reflux.[14] Risk factors are male gender, middle age, overweight, and facial bone abnormalities. As a consequence of chronic nocturnal hypoxemia and its attendant baroreceptor stimulation, sleep apnea patients go on to develop hypertension and cardiac arrhythmias and become more prone to the occurrence of myocardial infection, to left and right heart failure, and to cerebrovascular accidents.[14]

29.2.5 Parasomnias

Among parasomnias, three disorders are common: sleepwalking, sleep terrors, and nightmares.[15] Sleepwalking and sleep terrors are considered to be disorders of arousal, as subjects struggle to awaken from deep slow-wave sleep. They are usually age-dependent conditions being fairly common in children (about 10%) with a positive family history. Nightmares are frightening dreams occurring in REM but they do not evince the autonomic driving seen in sleep terrors.[15]

REM sleep behavior disorder (RBD) is a dramatic condition, which reflects the acting out of dream content due to a loss of the physiological muscle tone inhibition of normal REM.[16] The disorder can be idiopathic but is often associated with brainstem degenerative diseases such as the Shy Drager syndrome, olivo-ponto-cerebellar degeneration, or bilateral thalamic lesions.

29.2.6 *Circadian rhythm sleep disorders*

Intrinsic circadian rhythm sleep disorders are not common, but display scientific interests. Advanced-sleep-phase syndrome (ASPS) is a rare disorder characterized by very early sleep onset (19:00) and very early waking (04:30).[17] The opposite of advanced-sleep-phase syndrome, delayed sleep-phase syndrome (DSPS), is associated with delayed bedtime and delayed wake time.[17]

29.3 Physiology of sleep

Sleep is a complex state whose physiological function remains as one of the great mysteries in neurobiology. Although it is established that sleep and wakefulness reflect states of underlying brain activity, this concept was only established in the last half century through brain electrical activity monitoring (1920s) and the discovery of active "REM" sleep (1950s).

Sleep in the mammals is currently classified into NREM/REM sleep using three physiological measurements: (1) electroencephalography (EEG) (2) electromyography (EMG, muscle activity), and (3) electrooculography (EOG, eye movement activity).[18] With sleep onset, the EEG frequency slows, the EEG amplitude increases, and the EMG amplitude decreases (Fig. 29.1A). The subject enters NREM sleep. NREM sleep is divided into stages 1–4 in humans as increasing amounts of low-frequency, high-amplitude EEG activity (also known as delta activity) are observed. REM sleep follows NREM sleep 90–120 min (30–40 min in dogs and cats) after sleep onset (Fig. 29.1B). It is characterized by low-amplitude, high-frequency mixed EEG, the occurrence of intermittent REMs, skeletal muscle atonia, irregular cardiac/respiratory activity, and penile erection. Since REM sleep is associated with an EEG pattern that resembles the waking state, it is also called paradoxical sleep.

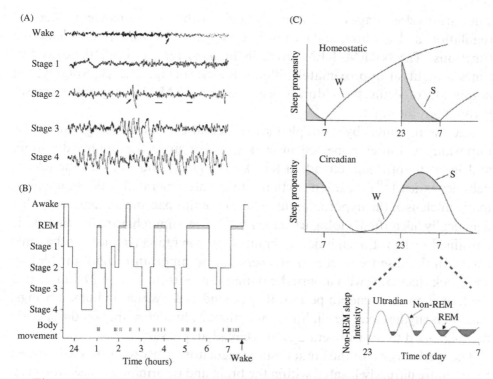

Figure 29.1. (A) The electroencephalographic (EEG) patterns associated with wakefulness and the stages of sleep. During wakefulness, there is a low-voltage fast EEG pattern, often with alpha waves, as shown here. At the arrow, there is a transition to stage 1 sleep, with the loss of the alpha rhythm and the presence of a low-voltage fast EEG. As sleep deepens, the EEG frequency slows more and more. Stage 2 is characterized by the presence of K complexes (arrow) and sleep spindles (underlined). During stage 3, delta waves (0.5–4 Hz) appear, and in stage 4, they occur more than 50% of the time. (B) The time course of sleep stages during a night's sleep in a healthy young man. During rapid eye movement (REM) sleep (shaded bars), the EEG pattern returns to low-voltage fast patterns. The percentage of time spent in REM sleep increases with successive sleep circles, and the percentage of stages 3 and 4 decreases. The EEG segments were recorded over parietal lobes (C3) except in waking, where occipital recording (O2) was used to show the alpha rhythm most clearly. (Adapted from reference 18). (C) The three main processes involved in the regulation of sleep. Homeostasis maintains the duration and intensity of sleep, the circadian rhythm determines the timing of the propensity to sleep and ultradian mechanisms underlie the NREM–REM sleep cycle. As the sleep episode progresses, the intensity of NREM sleep declines and the duration of successive REM sleep intervals increase (see also Fig. 29.3). W, awake states; S, sleep. (Adapted from reference 19.)

The various sleep stages are intimately linked with specific changes in thermo-regulation and cardiovascular, respiratory, gastrointestinal, and endocrine functions. The NREM–REM cycle in humans repeats itself three to five times a night, at approximately 90-min intervals (Fig. 29.1A). Notably, the amplitude of delta sleep during successive NREM sleep cycles decreases throughout the night.

Sleep is regulated by a coupled set of neural oscillators/cell groups. Two important and interconnected mechanisms determine the timing, duration, and intensity of sleep: circadian (clock-dependent) and homeostatic (sleep-debt dependent).[20] Circadian rhythms are mainly generated in the suprachiasmatic nucleus of the hypothalamus, which contains pacemaker neurons with a genetically identified biological clock.[21–23] The suprachiasmatic nucleus is entrained by light through neural inputs from the retina (retinohypothalamic tract). In the absence of cues (zeitgebers), most importantly light, the biological clock fluctuates with a periodicity that ranges from 23.8 to 27.1 hr, called the free-running circadian period. Recent studies show that in human beings, circadian rhythm may be slightly longer than 24 hr, depending on the specific protocol used to measure endogenous circadian phase.[24]

The mechanisms for the homoeostatic regulatory process (also called process S) are more diffusely located within the brain and determine the need for sleep after sleep deprivation (Fig. 29.1C).[20] The neuroanatomical, genetic, and neurochemical mechanisms involved in this process are largely unknown. Slow-wave sleep and EEG slow-wave activity during NREM sleep have classically been used as markers of the sleep homeostatic process. Slow-wave activity is most probably brought about by the regulation of established thalamocortical circuits.[25] Although the slow-wave process and resulting EEG phenotype might be generated through these circuits, other findings indicate the importance of other brain regions such as the hypothalamus, the basal forebrain, and the brainstem in the generation of sleep.[26–28] The importance of the pontine brainstem for generating REM is relatively well established; the brainstem aminergic neurons, such as the adrenergic locus coeruleus and serotonergic raphe neurons, are shut off during REM sleep, while a subset of cholinergic neurons are specifically active (i.e., reciprocal interactions).[26] Lesions in the brainstem in animals can produce various dissociated manifestations of REM sleep phenomena (such as REM sleep without atonia).[29,30] As mentioned earlier, occurrences of REM–NREM sleep cycles are under the ultradian regulation (i.e., cycles shorter than 24 hr) (Fig. 29.1C), and recent studies also emphasize the importance of the hypothalamus for this switching.[31]

Since these central oscillators/neuronal groups modulate the entire brain, precise synchronization and balance in the recruitment of their multiple outputs, including thermo, motor, autonomic and neuroendocrine functions, is critical to normal sleep. Many sleep disorders can thus be understood as deregulations of neuronal synchronicity and balance, possibly by intrinsic and extrinsic mechanisms.

29.4 Overview of sleep disorders with genetic backgrounds

Although most sleep disorders occur sporadically, relatively a large number of sleep disorders also run in families suggesting the importance of genetic factors in these conditions. In addition, contributions of genetic components to the pathology of sleep disorders in non-familial cases are also increasingly recognized as important. Narcolepsy is a good example; both familial (about 5%) and sporadic cases (about 95%) exist, and sporadic narcoleptic cases are also tightly associated with human leukocyte antigens (HLA) genes, genetic markers associated with immune responses.[4] Details of recent progress in narcolepsy research are discussed below. The discovery of genes/mechanisms involved in narcolepsy was achieved by forward (disease to gene) and reverse (gene to functions/diseases) genetics using instructive animal models. Thus it is likely that genetic approaches will be more central in sleep medicine, and various animal models are likely to play significant roles.

A series of experimental evidence has also suggested involvements of specific genes in several other sleep disorders. The first sleep disorder for which a single major gene mutation has been identified is fatal familial insomnia (FFI), first described by Lugaresi and colleagues in 1986.[32] This rare neurodegenerative disorder is caused by a point mutation in the prion-protein gene and is responsible for a degeneration of specific thalamic nuclei, and prion-protein gene knockout mice are also available.[33] Genetic studies in *Drosophila* and mice have recently identified major genes, such as *Clock* and *Period* genes (*Per1* and *Per2*) important in the regulation of circadian rhythms, which in turn determine the time of sleep onset and waking.[21] It has been recently shown that ASPS can be highly familial with an autosomal dominant mode of inheritance. A point mutation in a casein kinase-epsilon phosphorylation site of the *Per2* gene has been found in an ASPS family.[34] In a significant number of RLS families presents an autosomal dominant mode of transmission even if its expressivity may be variable. A positive association between female RLS subjects and the monoamine oxidase (MAO)-A gene has been recently reported.[35] This result may be consistent with the theory of an involvement of central dopaminergic system for this condition. The sleep apnea syndromes are very common but complex disorders. However, a familial trend has been identified in a few sleep apnea cases. Familial clustering of sleepwalking has been repeatedly reported by several authors, but its mode of transmission remains unknown. A recent study also reported a tight association of sleep-walking with HLA gene, DQB1*0501.[36] Due to the high diversity of HLA gene alleles, HLA genes are often chosen for genetic association studies. Two other sleep disorders have also been found to be associated with HLA genes. In a single study, REM-sleep disorder behavior (RBD) has been associated with the HLA-DQ1 (B1*05 or *06).[37] The KLS is a highly rare disorder mainly affecting adolescent boys, and combines a severe periodic hypersomnia and behavioral abnormalities. Although the condition is not familial, many symptoms of KLS are consistent with an underlying autoimmune disorder and thus might involve genetic factors, and an association with HLA-DQB1*0201 in 30 unrelated KLS patients has been reported.[38] Together with narcolepsy, so far at least four sleep disorders have been associated with polymorphisms in the HLA gene complex. These results may suggest a close interaction at the molecular level between sleep and the immune system.

29.5 Animal models of sleep disorders

29.5.1 Spontaneous occurring models

Classical sleep studies mostly used spontaneous occurring disease models; these include the canine models of narcolepsy (see below). Spontaneous occurrences of narcolepsy-like symptoms were also reported in bulls and horses.[39] Interestingly, it was recently found that canine narcolepsy exhibit PLMS-like involuntary movements during sleep, a condition often associated with human narcolepsy.[40] Violent movements during REM sleep (i.e., RBD) have been reported in both cats and dogs.[41] These movements range from spasmodic limb motions to more complex behaviors. Affected dogs may bark or growl during sleep, and may suddenly rise and start biting, either at the air, at another dog present, or at furniture or bedding. This disorder is differentiated from other movement disorders by the exclusivity of symptoms to REM sleep. The disease is most likely caused by a disturbance in brain pathways, which are responsible for inducing muscle atonia during REM sleep (loss of muscle tone during sleep that prevents the "acting out" of dreams). The occurrence of sleep apnea is reported in the English bulldog, possibly due to the shape of the face, which often impairs proper breathing during sleep.[42] The affected dogs may snore, choke sounds during sleep, exhibit prolonged periods without breathing during sleep, and have frequent arousal from sleep. English bulldogs were also used for some pharmacological studies and it is reported that modafinil (non-amphetamine wake-promoting compound) can improve sleep apneas.[43] The affected dogs may also undergo surgery that alleviates the blocked upper airway.[42] Normal dogs have also been used to study the basic sleep breathing mechanisms, especially respiratory mechanoreceptor stimuli in the arousal response. In these experiments, the dogs breathed through a cuffed endotracheal tube inserted and isocapnic progressive hypoxia was induced by rebreathing and arterial O_2 saturation and arousal from sleep and was monitored.[44]

Rat models of chronic intermittent hypoxia induced by modifying the composition of the breathing gas have also been used to investigate the effects of periodic oxygen desaturation in arousal.[45–47] It is also reported that wild-type rats and mice developed two types of central sleep apneas, that is, post-sigh (which are preceded by an augmented breath) and spontaneous apneas with higher incidence during sleep, as in normal humans.[48,49] Carley and Radulovacki extensively used the rat sleep apnea model to conduct physiological and pharmacological experiments to study the basic mechanisms of the central sleep apnea.[48,50] Several authors also argue that post-sigh apnea model may be useful to study the mechanisms of sudden infant death syndrome, since this type of apnea is frequently observed in neonates or infants.[49]

Since prevalence of many sleep disorders, such as insomnia and RLS/PLMS, increases with aging, aged animals are often used for sleep studies.[51]

29.5.2 Remarks on recent progress in narcolepsy research using animal models

Narcolepsy is the best-studied animal model of sleep disorders and substantial progress has recently been made owing to a valuable canine model. In humans, several cases of familial narcolepsy have been reported, and first-degree relatives of patients with narcolepsy have a 10–40 times greater-than-normal risk of developing narcolepsy–cataplexy.[4] However, narcolepsy is not a simple genetic disorder. No more than one-third of monozygotic twins are concordant for narcolepsy. Therefore, non-genetic factors must also play a major part. Human narcolepsy is caused by interplay of genetic and environmental factors. It shows a tight association with HLA-DR2 and HLA-DQB1*0602.[4] Interestingly, these HLA haplotypes are less tightly associated with familial narcoleptic cases, suggesting an involvement of non-HLA gene(s) in these cases.

Canine narcolepsy

Canine narcolepsy, initially found in small breeds (such as in beagles or dachshunds), was not familial, but the disease in Dobermans and Labradors exhibit familial occurrence; narcolepsy in these breeds is transmitted with a single

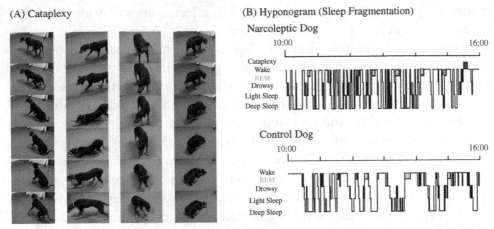

Figure 29.2. (A) Cataplectic attacks in Doberman pinschers. Emotional excitations, appetizing food, or playing easily elicit multiple cataplectic attacks in these animals. Most cataplexy attacks are bilateral (97.9%). Atonia initiated partially in the hind legs (79.8%), front legs (7.8%), neck/face (6.2%), or whole body/complete attacks (6.2%). Progression of attacks was also seen (49% of all attacks).[19] (B) The sleep/wake pattern of narcoleptic dogs (upper graph, vs. normal dog, lower graph) is very fragmented. Narcoleptic dogs also change their sleep states more frequently than they change their vigilance states.

autosomal recessive gene (*canarc-1*) with 100% penetrance (all homozygous animals develop narcolepsy before 6 months of age).[4] This made it possible to effectively carry out linkage and positional cloning studies of the susceptible gene. Canine narcolepsy in Dobermans is not linked with the dog leukocyte antigen (DLA) system as also shown in some familial cases of human narcolepsy.[4]

Affected dogs, regardless of sporadic or familial cases, exhibit very pronounced attacks of cataplexy which are mainly triggered by positive emotional experiences, such as being fed a favorite food or engaging in play. Cataplectic attacks in dogs often begin as a buckling of both hind legs, and are often accompanied by a drooping of the neck (Fig. 29.2A). The dog may collapse to the floor and remain motionless for a few seconds or several minutes. In contrast to some forms of epilepsy, excess salivation or incontinence are not observed during cataplectic attacks. During long cataplectic attacks (REM) muscle twitching may occur. These phenomena are related to the active phase of REM sleep. The muscle is always flaccid, never stiff, during cataplectic attacks, which is also different from most forms of seizure attacks. Dogs usually remain conscious (especially at the beginnings of the attacks), with eyes open and are capable of following moving objects with their eyes. If the attack lasts for an appreciable length of time (usually longer than 1–2 min), the dog may transition into sleep (often REM sleep). Dogs are often easily aroused out of an attack either by a loud noise or by being physically touched. Like narcoleptic humans, narcoleptic dogs are sleepier (fall asleep much more quickly) during the day. However, this was not noticeable in usual circumstances, because even normal dogs take multiple naps during the daytime.

A series of polygraphic studies clearly demonstrated that the dogs' sleep/wake patterns are very fragmented and their wake/sleep bouts are much shorter than that of age- and breed-matched dogs (Fig 29.2B). Narcoleptic dogs change their sleep states more frequently than they change their vigilance states.[52,53] In other words, narcoleptic subjects could not maintain long bouts of wakefulness and sleep. By systematic polygraph assessments with multiple daytime nap tests, it was objectively demonstrated that narcoleptic Dobermans showed shortened sleep latency and reduced latency to REM sleep during daytime,[52] suggesting that these dogs have very similar phenotype to those in human narcolepsy.

Identification of narcolepsy genes

After 15 years of work, Mignot and colleagues at Stanford Center for Narcolepsy identified *canarc-1*: narcolepsy in Dobermans and Labradors was found to be caused by a mutation in the hypocretin-2 receptor gene (hypocretin receptor 2 (*hcrtr2*), also called orexin type II receptor (*OxR2*)).[6] Hypocretin-1/orexin-A and hypocretin–2/orexin-B are hypothalamic neuropeptides acting on two receptor subtypes and here first found to be involved in feeding behavior.[54,55] The mutations in Dobermans and Labradors were found in the same gene, *hcrtr2*, but at different loci; both mutations cause exon skipping deletions in the *hcrtr2* transcripts and the loss of function of Hcrtr2, thus impairing postsynaptic hypocretin neurotransmission (Fig. 29.3).[6] Therefore, it appears that these mutations occur independently in both breeds.

Almost simultaneously along with the discovery of the canine narcolepsy gene, a report made by a group led by Yanagisawa showed that preprohypocretin (preproorexin) knockout mice also exhibited a narcolepsy-like phenotype, including sleep fragmentation and episodes of behavioral arrest similar to cataplexy in canine narcolepsy.[7]

Hypocretin-deficient human narcolepsy

Considering how similar human and canine narcolepsy are at the phenotypic level, it was thought that abnormalities in the hypocretin system were likely to be involved in some human narcolepsy cases, either at the functional or the genetic level. However, a large scale of screenings for mutations in human narcoleptic subjects, even in high-risk cases (familial, HLA negative, and early

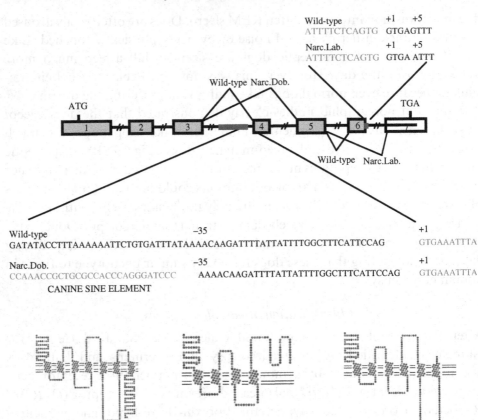

Figure 29.3. Genomic organization of the canine Hcrt2 receptor locus. The *hcrtr2* gene is encoded by seven exons. Sequence of exon–intron boundary at the site for the deletion of the transcript revealed that the canine short interspersed nucleotide element (SINE) was inserted 35 bp upstream of the 5′ splice donor site of the fourth encoded exon in narcoleptic Doberman pinschers. This insertion falls within the 5′ flanking intronic region needed for pre-mRNA lariat formation and proper splicing, causing exon 3 to be spliced directly to exon 5, and exon 4 to be omitted. This mRNA potentially encodes a non-functional protein with 38 amino acids deleted within the fifth transmembrane domain, followed by a frameshift and a premature stop codon at position 932 in the encoded RNA. In narcoleptic Labradors, the insertion was found 5 bp downstream of the 3′ splice site of the fifth exon, and exon 5 is spliced directly to exon 7, omitting exon 6.

onset), have shown that the mutation of hypocretin-related genes are very rare: among 14 polymorphisms identified in genes encoding the preprohypocretin and its two receptors, none segregates with human narcolepsy.[9] Only a single atypical patient (HLADQB1*0602 negative, very young age at onset, and severely affected) was identified with a G-to-T substitution resulting in a Leu-to-Arg change in the signal peptide of the preprohypocretin gene, suggesting that almost all narcoleptic humans are not caused by mutations in the highly penetrant hypocretin-related genes.[9]

However, neurochemical screening in human narcolepsy revealed that the hypocretin system has also been implicated in the etiology of human narcolepsy; narcoleptics have undetectable hypocretin-1 levels in their cerebrospinal fluid (CSF) and in a small number of post mortem cases a dramatic reduction in the number of hypocretin containing neurons is observed in the hypothalamus.[8-10] Low CSF hypocretin levels are very specific to narcolepsy compared to other sleep and neurological disorders,[56,57] and the CSF hypocretin measures will be included as one of the biological tests for the second revision of ICSD. Taken together with the fact that the disease is tightly associated with the HLA antigens, the most likely cause of hypocretin deficiency in narcolepsy is an autoimmune process resulting in acute or progressive degeneration of hypocretin-containing neurons. It has also been found that CSF and brain hypocretin levels in sporadic narcoleptic dogs are undetectably low, like most humans, suggesting they share common pathophysiological mechanisms.[58] Also transgenic mice carrying the promoter of the human prepro-hypocretin gene ligated to a truncated human ataxin-3, a gene with CAG repeat from a person affected with Machado–Joseph disease, develop narcolepsy.[59] This narcoleptic mice model is transgenic, but cell-targeting and the transgene can induce postnatal cell death of hypocretin-containing neurons.[59] Interestingly, these transgenic mice present symptoms similar to hypocretin ligand knockout mice (and human narcolepsy), but the onset of the symptoms was later than that of knockout mice.[7,59] This result is consistent with the postnatal cell death hypothesis for human narcolepsy. Because over 90% of narcoleptics have no family history of narcolepsy and monozygotic twins are mostly discordant, environmental factors might play an important role. The environmental factors might trigger narcolepsy by inducing an autoimmune reaction that targets hypocretin neurons. The precise mechanisms of the hypocretin cell death should be determined to prevent and/or rescue the disease.

Continuing animal studies in narcolepsy research

Since the lack of hypocretin ligand is the major pathophysiology in most human subjects,[56,60] supplements of hypocretin may be a promising approach for treatment. For these experiments, various animal models of narcolepsy are also informative. Hypocretin replacement therapy in ligand deficient sporadic dogs revealed that peripheral administration of hypocretin peptide is ineffective,[61,62] suggesting the necessity of developments of small molecular (i.e., non-peptide) hypocretin agonists that penetrate to the central nervous system (CNS). Using narcoleptic mice, Mieda *et al.* also demonstrated that central administration (intracerebroventricular) of the hypocretin peptide as well as gene therapy by crossing the ectopic expression (with beta-actin pro-motor) of hypocretin transgenic mice with hypocretin/ataxin-3 mice rescue the narcolepsy phenotype.[63] These results suggest that hypocretin replace-ment therapies, including by cell transplantation and gene therapy, may be the most promising new therapeutic options for the human disease.

Although these new developments revolutionized our understanding of both human and canine narcolepsy, a great gap still needs to be bridged between the hypocretin system and what we know about the neurochemistry, pharmacology, and genetics of narcolepsy.

PLMS associated with narcolepsy

We recently observed that *hcrtr2*-mutated narcoleptic Dobermans exhibit periodic movements during sleep resembling human PLMS, suggesting that the narcoleptic dog animal model can also be used for PLMS. PLMS, a prevalent sleep-related movement disorder of unknown etiology, is often asso-ciated with various neurological conditions, such as narcolepsy,[64,65] central and obstructive sleep apnea, lumbosacral narrowing, and, most recently, with attention-deficit hyperactivity disorder (ADHD).[3,65,66] Regarding the associa-tion with narcolepsy, it is reported that as many as 25–50% of narcoleptic patients have PLMS.[64,65] Furthermore, it is also known that only one identified human narcolepsy case with preprohypocretin gene mutation also exhibits severe PLMS.[9] Although RLS, first described by Ekbom,[67] is likely to be distinct from PLMS, a great majority of patients with RLS also experience PLMS. Interestingly, RLS is relatively rare in narcoleptic subjects suggesting a co-morbidity of narcolepsy with pure motor component of RLS/PLMS.

The PLMS-like movements of narcoleptic dogs are jerky, unilateral or bilateral slow leg movements during quiet wakefulness, drowsiness and light sleep, and less often during deep sleep and REM sleep.[40] This movement is characterized by repetitive dorsiflexions of the ankle with occasional flexion of the knee and hip. Movement lasts 0.5–1.5 s and occurs repeatedly (4 to 20 times) with regular intervals of 3–10 s. Higher incidence of these movements was observed in narcoleptic dogs compared to control dogs, and these were easily distinguishable from other involuntary movement during sleep such as shivering (occurs during the light and deep sleep stages at low recording temperature and is usually accompanied by large movements around the shoulders and neck) and muscle twitching during REM sleep (occurs in any part of the body, including neck muscles (short duration of <0.2 s), often accompanying other phasic REM sleep phenomena such as REMa).

We also observed that selective D2/D3 agonists, including compounds used for the treatment of human PLMS such as pramipexole and ropinirole, significantly aggravate cataplexy in narcoleptic dogs, but also alleviate PLMS-like movements.[68] This suggests that dopaminergic D2/D3 mechanisms are involved in the occurrence of both cataplexy and PLMS. These results, taken together with the finding that narcoleptic dogs are very sensitive to D2/D3 compounds,[69] suggest that "dysregulation" of the dopaminergic system may exist in canine narcolepsy, and that this may be specifically involved both in sleep-related motor inhibition (cataplexy) and activation (PLMS).

29.5.3 Brain lesion models

From the mid-1950s, the neural control of sleep, especially REM sleep generation, has been intensively studied. Using the technique of surgical separation of the neuraxis at different levels of the brain stem, investigators have isolated the neural control of REM sleep to the pontine brain stem.[26,70] Additionally, finely placed lesions and focal brain stimulation within the pons and adjacent regions have revealed the cell groups responsible for a number of the components of REM sleep. Another prominent component of REM sleep is the profound paralysis of skeletal muscles (REM sleep atonia). REM sleep paralysis has been shown to be due to a small region of the dorsal pons, the nucleus subcoeruleus. A lesion to this nucleus abolishes the REM sleep paralysis. A very dramatic observation is that during REM sleep, cats with such lesions became very active and agitated, as if they were acting out an emotionally charged dream episode.[29,30]

Similarly lesions in the hypothlamic structures induce insomnia and hypersomnia depending on the brain structure and method used.[71,72] These results may mirror the earlier neuropathological observation by von Economo,[73] who observed that lesions (associated with encephalitis lethargica) in the anterior hypothalamus induce insomnia, while those in the posterior hypothalamus induce hypersomnia. Recently a group of neurons was discovered that selectively activate during slow-wave sleep in the ventrolateral peroptic area (VLOP),[74] and the lesion in the VLOP induces insomnia; it is proposed that this model may be useful as an animal model of insomnia.[75]

In most studies, lesions induced by heating or kanic acid were used, but these techniques also damage the fibers, so ibotenic acid was used to more selectively damage neurons.[71,72,75]

More recently immunolesions (conjugated with antibodies[76]) and with neurotoxins conjugated to neurotransmitters (such as hypocretin-2 saporin[77]) have been introduced. It is known that injections such as hypocretin-2 saporin in the lateral hypothalamus selectively kill hypocretin neurons (assuming that hypocretin-2 saporin binds to hypocretin autoreceptors) and induce narcolepsy phenotype in rats.[77] This technique is also used to selectively destroy histamine neurons in the transcranial magnetic stimulation (TMS) that express hypocretin receptor-2.[78]

Most elegantly, as mentioned above, postnatal hypocretin cell death was induced in transgenic mice of triplet repeat ataxin-3 gene with preprohypocretin promotor, and these transgenic mice developed narcolepsy phenotype.[59]

Although selectivity and specificity of lesions made with these new technique still need to evaluated, less selective chemical/thermal lesion techniques are now outmoded.

29.6 Forward genetics

29.6.1 Random mutagenesis

One of the most important discoveries in neuroscience in the twentieth century was the identification and cloning of the clock genes in mammals. Since circadian behavior is precisely defined and easily quantified, it is well suited for genetic manipulation and screening. Treatment of mice with *N*-ethyl-*N*-nitrosourea (ENU), a mutagene, and screening for changes in the circadian rhythmicity resulted in the discovery of a semidominant, autosomal mutation, named *clock*. Mice mutant for *clock* exhibited significantly longer circadian periods when kept in constant darkness and over time they became arrhythmic.[79] Both heterozygous and homozygous mutant mice showed reduced total sleep time but little difference from wild-type in the compensatory sleep rebound or changes in delta power in NREM sleep following sleep deprivation.[80] Linkage analyses mapped the *clock* mutation to chromosome 5 and allowed positional cloning of the *clock* gene.[81] These discoveries led to the understanding of the molecular mechanisms involved in the circadian clock of mammals,[22,23] and an extraordinary example of the power of chemical mutagenesis and its applicability.

The mutagenesis approach is straightforward: mutation occurs at random in the whole genome; this is followed by high-throughput screening of all mutant offspring to detect a major effect on a given phenotype. Both dominant and recessive mutations can be screened in the same way as a single gene mutation in a pathological condition. Once the mutated gene is localized, candidate gene or positional cloning approaches are used for its identification, and ultimately its functional analysis can be performed by gain or loss of function. Thus, it is likely this approach may also be useful in generating a number of "sleep" mutants. However, genetic screens in this approach are for fully penetrant dominant and recessive mutations and therefore may not able to identify small-effect sequence variations that may turn out to be essential for some aspects of the phenotype. In addition, with currently available technologies, recording and analyzing sleep of thousands of mice in a mutant screen does not seem feasible, at least not in a single academic laboratory. However, this limitation can be overcome by the large-scale mutagenesis and the high-throughput screening programs[82] or mutagenesis in simple animal models, such as fruit fly (see below).

29.6.2 Sleep phenotype variations and quantitative trait loci

Multiple genes are likely involved in natural variations in complex traits, including sleep phenotype, and effects of each gene may have only subtle effects. The quantitative trait loci (QTL) method is one of the genome-wide approaches used to detect all genes with variable effects on the trait, and it has been extensively used to analyze natural polygenic traits.[83,84]

The QTL is based on the idea of interval mapping. Mapping uses DNA marker information to estimate the genotype and likely QTL at every point in the genome by calculating the maximum-likelihood linkage score.[85] The approach to analyzing complex genetic traits by QTL is facilitated by the availability of advanced animal crosses, high-density linkage maps, and powerful analytical tools.[85–87]

A significant phenotypic variability of sleep observed between different inbred mice strains suggested complex interactions between a number of genes,[88–90] although a single gene mode of inheritance of some sleep-related genes, such as the gene responsible for the frequency of the theta rhythm during REM sleep, are also known (see below).[91]

QTL analysis was therefore applied in various inbred mice to dissect sleep-related genes. A provisional QTL for the amount of REM sleep was originally assigned to chromosomes 4, 5, 7, 12, 16, and 17.[92,93] However, a high level of significance was reached for markers on chromosome 1 using C57/Bl/6 × DBA/2 (B × D), i.e., when different recombinant inbred strains of mice were studied.[90] These observations suggest that there are a number of genes that interact with each other to determine the amount of sleep in mice and the outcome of these interactions (i.e., sleep phenotype) depend on the genetic background.[94] This is a general issue for QTL studies such as these in mice.

Quantitative analyses of EEG power spectra also showed that sleep EEG components differ significantly between different inbred strains of mice.[88,89] The homeostatic drive, which is related to the duration of prior wakefulness (see Fig. 29.1A),[20] is also strongly influenced by the genotype of the mouse.[88,95] Thus, delta power rebound after sleep deprivation in B × D recombinant inbred strains was used in QTL analyses to map genes underlying this phenotype.[88] A significant QTL was identified on chromosome 13 that was responsible for 50% of the genetic variance in this trait.[88] This region contains the gene encoding the receptor for the brain-derived neurotrophic factor (BDNF) that increases in the brain following sleep deprivation.[96] In addition, a suggestive QTL has been located on chromosome 2, which comprises a number of genes, including glycogen phosphorylase,[97] adenosine deaminase,[98] growth-hormone-related hormone (GHRH), and somatostatin,[99] that relate to mechanisms proposed to be involved in the regulation of sleep and wakefulness. Attempts to identify other sleep QTL in rodents, however, resulted in major discrepancies between different laboratories;[92,93] it is likely that the inconsistencies were due to the lack of strictly defined phenotypes, the limited number of experimental animals, and the differences in recombinant inbred strains. Despite the fact that QTL requires significant amounts of phenotype and genotype tests, a QTL for a specific trait generally remains crudely localized (usually between 20 and 30 centimorgans). These large regions may contain a single major gene or several genes with small effects. Also, QTLs may interact with each other (epistasis), an effect that is difficult to detect in QTL mapping experiments. Once the QTL region is verified, the next step is to finely map the QTL down to the smallest chromosomal region,[100] amenable to candidate gene analysis. The final identification of functional QTNs (sequence variants) is the most difficult part, since QTNs may be found every few kilobases. Therefore, a combination of several approaches is necessary for mapping and candidate gene analysis. High-resolution QTL mapping in conjunction with future developments in high-throughput phenotyping and genotyping and the availability of whole genome sequences of several major mouse strains should identify candidate genes to be investigated. Finally, all of those candidate genes must then be mutated either by classical homologous recombination (knockout) or by the serial nested chromosomal deletions[101] to examine if the identified genes are responsible for the observed phenotype variations. Because most QTNs will probably be involved in gene regulation rather than being mutations affecting the protein function, further gene expression profiling with high-throughput genotyping technologies (e.g., microarray or TaqMan) and gene translation and posttranslational protein analyses should be used to uncover the molecular mechanisms involved.

Despite these strategic concerns, Tafti and colleagues identified a gene underlying a sleep-related trait using QTL; a deficiency in short-chain acyl-coenzyme A dehydrogenase (encoded by *Acad*) in mice causes a marked slowing in theta frequency during paradoxical sleep. Inbred strains vary greatly in their frequency of EEG theta oscillations (5–9 Hz) during REM sleep.[91] The frequency difference amounts to 1 Hz between inbred strains with slow (5.75–6.25 Hz) and strains with fast theta oscillations (6.75–7.75 Hz). The segregation of this trait was followed in intercross and backcross and recombinant inbred (RI) panels between BALB/cByJ (slow theta) and C57/Bl/6 J (fast theta). With the QTL approach one single gene was identified on chromosome 5 that was tightly linked to theta frequency (logarithm of the odds (LOD) score >30). The gene was finally identified to be *Acad*. *Acad*'s expression in brain regions is involved in theta generation, notably the hippocampus. Microarray analysis of gene expression in mice with mutations in *Acad* indicates overexpression of Glo1 (encoding glyoxylase 1), a gene involved in the detoxification of metabolic by-products. Administration of acetyl-L-carnitine (ALCAR) to mutant mice significantly recovers slow theta and Glo1 overexpression.[91] Thus, an underappreciated metabolic pathway involving fatty acid beta-oxidation also regulates theta oscillations during sleep. Functional importance of this sleep-related gene and trait variation still needs to be investigated further. This example proves that QTL analysis can be successful in identifying new genes underlying sleep and EEG traits although in this particular case the trait difference between the progenitor strains was found to be a single gene effect.

29.7 Candidate gene approach

29.7.1 Transgenic and gene targeting in mice

As opposed to the forward genetic approaches described above, reverse genetic approaches evaluate influences of alteration of known genes in the expression of a trait of interest. Reverse genetics has been made possible by the development of gene targeting and transgenic animals. By homologs recombination in embryonic stem cells, an altered gene construct can replace the existing gene.[102] If the inserted gene-construct translates into a non-functional protein, the animals homozygous for this construct are often referred to as knockout animals. With non-homologs (illegitimate) recombination one or more gene copies are inserted into the genome at undefined locations.[103] Animals carrying these constructs are often referred to as transgenic animals. Animals produced with this transgenic method often are gain-of-function mutants since they express a novel gene product or overexpress a normal gene. With both techniques, one can create animal models to study the effects of change in protein levels on sleep (from overexpression in transgenics, to non-functional protein in knockouts), altered, or novel proteins (knockin, transgenic). These animal models are also useful in confirming the role of genes that were identified by forward genetic approaches.[104]

Since large numbers of knockout and transgenic animals have been used in the sleep research field, a list of published studies in which sleep was recorded was generated (Table 29.2). The first sleep studies using genetically engineered mice appeared in 1996.[105,106] Since altered prion protein plays a major role in the prion diseases, including fatal familial insomnia, sleep pattern with prion knockout mice was examined.[105] Beside this study, most studies focused on pathways already known to be involved in sleep regulation. For example, the monoamines including serotonin, dopamine, histamine, and gamma-aminobutyric acid (GABA) were among the first neurotransmitters to have been suggested as playing a role in sleep regulation[27] and knockout models for their receptors and transporters have been studied.[107–114] Another pathway studied and implicated in sleep is the cytokine pathway, since several research groups have shown the involvement of cytokines in sleep regulation[115] and since several sleep disorders are associated with certain HLA haplotypes. Knockout mice for this pathway include interleukin (IL)-1 type I receptor, IL-10, tumor necrosis factor (TNF), and the TNF receptors-1 and -2 (116–118). Knockout mice for genes that are regarded as canonical circadian genes (*clock*, period-1 and -2 (*Per1, Per2*),[119] and cryptochrome-1 and -2 (*Cry1, Cry2*)[120]) and genes known to alter circadian rhythms (albumin-D-binding protein (DBP)[121] and ras-associated binding protein 3a (Rab3a)[122]) were also generated and sleep phenotype was studied. Finally, hypocretin-related genes (pre-prohypocretin, hyprocretin receptor-1 and -2, and double receptor knockout mice) were generated to study the roles of hypocretin neurotransmission in narcolepsy and for sleep regulation.[7,123]

As also described in the QTL section, in order to identify genes that are involved in the homeostatic regulation of sleep, studies were performed in which sleep deprivations and rebound sleep was monitored in various genetically engineered mice. Mice lacking functional genes for the serotonin 2C receptor,[114] Cry1 and Cry2,[120] and Rab3a[122] all were reported to have an altered NREM sleep rebound after sleep deprivation.

Changes in REM sleep homeostasis have also been observed in several knockout models. In mice lacking serotonin 1A or 1B receptors,[111,113] DBP,[121] Cry1, and Cry2,[120] and in *clock* mutant mice,[80] loss of REM sleep was followed by a compensatory increase in REM that was smaller than in wild-type animals or lacking altogether. Apart from the serotonin 1A and 1B receptor knockout mice that displayed increased REM sleep during base-line,[111,113] these changes in the REM sleep response after sleep deprivation could not be attributed to genotype differences in REM sleep during base-line.

Table 29.2. *Animal models of human sleep disorders*

Models	Main phenotype/effect	References
Spontaneously occurring		
Narcolepsy (dog, horse, bull)	Cataplexy (dog, bull), sleep fragmentations (dog), sleep attacks (horse)	4, 39
Obstructive sleep apnea (English bulldog)	Snore, choke sounds during sleep, prolonged periods without breathing during sleep	42
Central sleep apnea (rat, mice)	Post-sigh and spontaneous apneas	48, 49
REM sleep behavior disorder (dog, cat)	Violent movements during REM sleep	41
PLMS (narcoleptic Dobermans)	Unilateral or bilateral slow leg movements during sleep	40
Genetic engineering (effects of gene manipulation on sleep in mice)		
Mutagenesis		
clock	Decreased NREM sleep, no REM sleep increase after sleep deprivation	80
earlybird (Rab3a)	Reduced response to sleep deprivation in NREM sleep 101	179
Point mutation		
GABA-A receptor α1	No effect on diazepam-induced sleep changes	124
Transgenic		
Beta-amyloid precursor protein	Decreased REM sleep, increased sleep fragmentation	172
Growth hormone	Tyrosine hydroxylase-hGH transgenic dwarf mice with a endogenous somatotropic deficiency Decreased NREM sleep in mice	106
	Increased REM sleep when overexpressed	173
Insulin	Non-specific background effect	174
Hypocretin/ataxin-3 (hypocretin-neuron targeted apoptosis)	Narcolepsy	59
Prostaglandin D synthase	Increased NREM sleep after tail clipping	175
Knockout		
Period-1, Period-2	Altered distribution of sleep amount in base-line, reduced response to sleep deprivation in frontal EEG delta power	119
Rab3a	Increased NREM sleep, reduced response to sleep deprivation in NREM sleep amount	122

Table 29.2. (*cont.*)

Models	Main phenotype/effect	References
Cryptochromes-1 and -2	Increased NREM sleep consolidation, amount, and EEG delta power, decreased response to sleep deprivation in these variables	120
Albumin-D-binding protein (DBP)	Decreased sleep continuity, decrease daily amplitude in EEG delta power, no increase in REM sleep after sleep deprivation	121
Dopamine transporter	Sleep fragmentation, no response to amphetamines and modafinil	107
Dopamine beta-hydroxygenase deficiency	No change in sleep at the base-line, but shorter sleep latency under various conditions	127
Gamma aminobutyric acid (GABA)-A receptor β3	No response to oleamide	112
Histidine-decarboxylase	Increased REM sleep, decreased wakefulness at dark onset, NREM sleep EEG power redistributed to faster frequencies	108
Histamine H1 receptor	No response to hypocretin 1 (to promote wakefulness)	109
Histamine H3 receptor	Decrease in overall locomotor activity	110
Serotonin 1A receptor	Increased REM sleep, no REM sleep increase after sleep deprivation	111
Serotonin 1B receptor	Increased REM sleep, no REM sleep increase after sleep deprivation	113
Serotonin 2C receptor	Less NREM sleep at base-line, increased rebound in NREM sleep and EEG delta power after sleep deprivation	114
Prepro-hypocretin	Narcolepsy	7
Hypocretin receptor 1	Subtle sleep abnormality	123
Hypocretin receptor 2	Milder phenotype (cataplexy and sleep fragmentation) than ligand knockout	123
Double receptors	Narcolepsy, phenotype similar to ligand knockout	123
Interleukin-1 type I receptor	Decreased total sleep time (TST) during the dark period, no response to interleukin-1 beta	116
Interleukin-10	Increased NREM sleep during the dark period, altered response to lipopolysaccharide challenge	117
Tumor necrosis factor (TNF) receptor-1	Decreased total sleep time (TST) in light period, no response to TNF alpha, no change in total sleep time (TST)	118, 176

Table 29.2. (*cont.*)

Models	Main phenotype/effect	References
TNF receptor-2	Decreased REM sleep in light period	118
TNF/lymphotoxin-α	Decreased REM sleep in light period, increased NREM sleep consolidation and EEG delta power	118
Prion protein	Non-congenic line: decreased sleep continuity, longer-lasting EEG delta power increase after sleep deprivation	105
	Congenic line: longer-lasting EEG delta power increase after sleep deprivation	33
Voltage-gated K-channel	Decreased "high" EEG delta power	177
c-Fos	Increased wakefulness, decreased NREM sleep	178
Fos B	Decreased REM sleep	178

Knockout mice can also be used for pharmacological experiments, such as to evaluate the modes of action of stimulants and hypnotics. For example, the experiments using dopamine transporter (DAT) knockout mice have shown that DAT is a critical molecular mediating the wake-promoting effects of amphetamine and modafinil.[107] Similarly, mice with point mutations of GABA-A receptor α1 were used to dissect the molecular mechanisms of the hypnotic action of benzodiazepines.[124] Furthermore it has been shown that wake-promoting effect of central administration of hypocretin-1 is abolished in histamine H1 receptor knockout mice.[109]

29.7.2 General considerations for interpreting the results using knockout and transgenic mice

Genetic background can significantly affect behavioral measures. The majority of knockout mice are crosses between the 129SV strain used to obtain embryonic stem cells and different inbred mouse strains. As explained in the QTL section, sleep phenotypes significantly vary among mice with different genetic backgrounds. Therefore, it is possible that genetic background segregates in mutants independently of the mutation itself, and the behavioral data must be interpreted cautiously.[125] Most researchers are now aware of this concern, but it takes a long time to generate the congenic mouse line to match the genetic background between knockout and wild type mice. Although most investigators desire to publish initial results quickly, they usually confirm the initial findings using the congenic mice line at later stages to exclude the background influence.[33,105] As emphasized repeatedly, sleep is fundamentally physiological and is essential for survival, and multiple systems are involved in its regulation. Therefore if the congenital knockout/trangenic mice do not develop lethal phenotypes, developmental compensation (e.g., other molecules could compensate for the lacking protein[104]) are likely to have occurred. Good examples of this are dopamine beta-hydoxygenase (DBH) deficiency cases. No one appears to disagree with the importance of the norepinephrine in the regulation of vigilance. However, sleep in patients with DBH deficiency (i.e., norepinephrine deficiency) is not significantly altered, and only orthostatic hypotension appears as the major symptoms of the DBH deficiency.[126] Similarly, no differences were found in any sleep parameters between the DBH-deficient mice and wild-type mice under base-line conditions, but DBH-deficient mice showed a significantly shorter latency to sleep under certain conditions,[127] meaning that other mechanisms (such as dopamine) likely compensate for most functions where norepinephrine is involved.

Some of these issues could be overcome by developing (tissue-specific) conditional or inducible knockout models where the acute effects of loss of function can be studied in structures of interest.[128] The hypocretin cell targeting transgenic narcoleptic mice by postnatal ablation of hypocretin with ataxin-3/polyglutamete transgene discussed earlier is also another new example (see also below).

29.7.3 *Functional genomics in rats*

Although sleep studies using knockout rats are not yet available, Beuckman and colleagues recently produced narcoleptic transgenic rats carrying the promoter of the human prepro-hypocretin gene ligated to a truncated human ataxin-3.[129] Similar to the results reported in mice, rats exhibit cataplexy-like behavior and fragmented vigilance states, a decreased latency to rapid REM sleep, and direct transitions from wakefulness to REM sleep, suggesting that hypocretin/ataxin-3 transgenic rats could provide a useful model of human narcolepsy. When compared to mice, rats are better suited for sleep research because their larger size facilitates experimental manipulation and also because more is known about their brain neuronal circuitry. The usefulness of the rat as a model system has been strengthened by rapid progress of the Rat Genome Project, which has a goal of identifying unique rat genes by extensive mapping efforts, as well as availability of numerous inbred and recombinant rat strains.[130] Therefore rat functional genomics holds great potential and promise in future sleep research.

29.7.4 Antisense targeting

Another strategy that qualifies as a reverse genetic strategy is antisense targeting. With this strategy one can selectively, locally, and transiently downregulate the expression of a gene product at the level of the RNA (single- or double-stranded RNA) or DNA.[131] The basic idea is to induce translational arrest through sequence specific hybridization of the mRNA to synthetic oligodeoxynucletides. This technique has been applied to study the effects on sleep of c-Fos protein expression in the medial preoptic area,[132] of glutamic acid decarboxylase,[133] and hypocretin-2 receptor[134] in the pontine reticular formation, adenosine A1 receptor in the basal forebrain,[135] and of the serotonin transporter in the dorsal raphe nucleus.[136] This approach can apply to both mice and rats, as the sequence information of genes of interest becomes available.

29.8 Simpler animal models

Although discussion in this chapter has been mostly based on mammalian animal models for sleep disorders, molecular biology and other technical advances are most efficiently applied to large numbers of rapidly reproducing, inexpensive, small organisms, including prokaryotes and invertebrates as well as simple vertebrates, to study complex behaviors, such as circadian rhythms and long-term memory consolidation. Furthermore, the information gained can often be shown to be relevant to humans by demonstrating that the genes and their products are evolutionarily conserved (see a recent review in reference 137).

Progress in the field of circadian rhythm research has special relevance for sleep research. Firstly, mammalian sleep is at least partly regulated as an output of the biological clock, although a homeostatic regulatory mechanism is also important in the onset and duration of sleep.[138] Secondly, it is a reasonable proposal that sleep evolved from a simpler circadian rest state. While the existence of sleep across the animal kingdom has been a matter of great dispute, no one appears to disagree that rest occurs throughout the animal kingdom.

The field of chronobiology proceeded from the parsimonious expectation that common mechanisms regulate diverse circadian phenomena. This prediction has proved true for parameters ranging from metabolic processes in prokaryotes,[139] to eclosion and locomotion in populations of insects[140] to endocrine rhythms, body temperature, and cognitive function in mammals.[141] Once these rhythms were well described, appropriate parameters were chosen as assays to screen for mutants with aberrant circadian rhythms. Large-scale screens identified mutations in genes required for circadian rhythms, termed "clock genes." These mutants then provided material for the efficient application of modern molecular genetic techniques.

The discovery of the first clock gene, *period* (*per*), in *Drosophila melanogaster* has been followed by the identification of further genes in *Drosophila*,[142] cyanobacteria,[143] the bread mold *Neurospora*,[144] and mammals including hamsters, mice, and humans.[145-147] Both *per* mRNA and its protein product, PERIOD (PER), cycle with a circadian period in cells including neural and retinal cells. One fundamental property of these molecular clocks is that their transcription is regulated by autoregulatory feedback loops.[21-23] Many components of clock molecular mechanisms are now understood and known to be common to fruit flies and mammals. This may also suggest that sleep-like states in simple animal models can also be broadly relevant.

In 1984, Campbell and Tobler reviewed over 100 studies in over 150 species seeking evidence for sleep from invertebrates to primates, using behavioral criteria. The behaviors required were: (1) a stereotypic or species-specific posture, (2) behavioral quiescence, (3) an elevated arousal threshold, and (4) state reversibility with stimulation.[148] Using these criteria to review previous laboratory and field studies, the authors concluded that there is evidence for sleep-like states in 19 species of fish, 16 reptiles, and 9 amphibians, as well as several invertebrates (cockroaches, bees, and octopuses). Hendricks *et al.* had augmented Tobler's criteria by explicitly stating and clarifying some features of "sleep" that seem intuitive, and they include a requirement for state-related neural functional changes.[137] The neural changes need not resemble the specific state-related EEG patterns used to characterize mammalian and avian sleep. In simple animals, molecular or neurochemical techniques might be more suitable than electrophysiology in some systems to provide evidence that neuronal activity is altered in a state-related fashion.[137]

The candidate species should be a common, inexpensive, plentiful animal. In addition, it would be ideal if sufficient molecular genetics information was readily available. An accessible CNS with anatomical analogies to the mammalian system would be helpful in allowing extrapolation to mammals. Sleep studies in *Drosophila melanogaster* (invertebrates) and *Danio rerio* (vertebrates) are discussed below.

29.8.1 Drosophila melanogaster

The fruit fly *Drosophila melanogaster* is a particularly attractive subject for molecular neurobiology because behavioral studies of the intact organism can complement the molecular genetic approach and has been well justified and used for the genetic basis of behaviors including circadian rhythms.[149]

The small size, prolific reproduction rates, small gene number, and short life cycle of the fruit fly combine to make studies efficient, inexpensive, and easily replicated. Extensive literature and databases of genetic and CNS information are also available; the creation and maintenance of transgenics are also well established[150] and the experimenter can manipulate both the temporal and spatial features of transgene expression.[151,152]

However, the small size and rigid exoskeleton of *Drosophila* represent technical challenges for access to the central brain of the intact animal. Another limitation is that the insect CNS lacks analogous anatomical structures to those of mammals. Nonetheless, many of the neurotransmitters, receptors, and transport systems are evolutionarily conserved, including most of those related to sleep control in mammals: serotonin, dopamine, histamine, and acetylcholine.[153–155]

Similar to the observation in other insects,[156] inactive episodes of rest of *Drosophila melanogaster* may be considered as sleep, based on the following observations.[149] During periods of rest, a stronger sensory stimulus is required to elicit an orienting response. This is comparable to sleep, as we know it, during which a stronger stimulus is necessary to elicit a response. Furthermore, if fruit flies are prevented from entering their resting state for a period of time and then permitted to do so, the insects will show an increased amount of time in the quiet state. This is comparable to the rebound of sleep time after a period of sleep deprivation has been imposed in mammals. Moreover, periods of rest in *Drosophila* occur mainly during the dark phase of the 24-hr day, which reveals a circadian rhythm comparable to the sleep–waking pattern seen in diurnal vertebrate species. Recently, Nitz *et al.* were able to obtain prolonged recordings of local field potentials (LFPs) from the medial part of the fly brain, between the mushroom bodies.[157] They found that LFPs from awake, moving fruit flies are dominated by spike-like potentials and that these spikes largely disappear during the quiescent state when arousal thresholds are increased. Targeted genetic manipulations demonstrated that LFPs had their origin in brain activity and were not merely an artifact of movement or electromyographic activity. Thus, like in mammals, wakefulness and sleep in fruit flies are accompanied by different patterns of brain electrical activity.

Fly sleep behavior was first monitored using visual observation and an ultrasound activity monitoring system, but these methods are impractical for evaluating sleep–waking parameters in a large-scale project. A recent automatic infrared system (Drosophila Activity Monitoring System (DAMS), Trikinetics, Waltham, MA) was designed to monitor hundreds or thousands of flies simultaneously. One DAMS monitor contains 32 glass tubes, each housing a single fly and enough food for 1 week of recording. Using these devices and by visual observations, it was shown that flies are mostly active and moving around during the day, while during the night they show long periods of immobility that can last several hours.

Gene expression profiling and mutagenesis screening are now also used in sleep research in flies.[158] Although no mutation has been identified that can produce a non-sleeping fly, the daily sleep quota differs among mutant lines, though very few mutations can shorten sleep time to less than 300 min/day. Furthermore, in flies, even fewer mutations can disrupt the homeostatic regulation of sleep, i.e., few can abolish the ability of a fly to recover some of the sleep lost during sleep deprivation.[158] It is thus conceivable that the characterization of the sleep mutant lines should help in identifying crucial cellular pathways involved in the regulatory mechanisms of sleep and/or in its functional consequences.

29.8.2 Danio rerio

The zebrafish has also recently become a popular organism for studying biological processes. As well as reproducing rapidly, the larval zebrafish is a particularly attractive organism in which to study developmental gene expression or cell–cell interactions because it is transparent, permitting direct visualization of the internal organs including the CNS.[159,160] The piscine nervous system has considerable analogy to the mammalian regarding brainstem systems implicated in vigilance control, including, for example, a serotonergic raphe,[161] a noradrenergic locus coeruleus,[162,163] and histaminergic tuberomammillary body.[164] Calcium-sensitive dyes injected in the CNS are taken up by axons and transported retrograde to the neural soma, where the dye changes in response to calcium influx and can be studied for at least several days.[159,160] This method can be used to visualize state-related changes in neural activity in single neurons or in functionally or developmentally related groups of neurons in the living animal. Similarly, one might be able to directly visualize state-related gene expression by linking luciferase to the relevant promoters.[165]

Sleep-like behaviors in zebrafish were recently characterized using classical behavioral criteria and an automatic infrared video recording system.[166] Video recordings showed the occurrence of a clear, prolonged state of immobility in all zebrafish individuals. A characteristic posture (tailfin pointed downward) and preferred tank position (either at the surface or the bottom of the recording chamber) was consistently observed during these immobility periods. Rhythmic locomotor activity was evident in both light–dark and dark–dark conditions, with the immobile periods typically occurring during the biological night. Furthermore, electrical stimulation was able to immediately reverse the sleep-like state into an active state. Thus, this sleep-like state in zebrafish has similarity to mammalian or *Drosophila* sleep and awaits further characterization. Pharmacological experiments using hypnotics, barbiturates, benzodiazepines, and antihistaminics are also in progress.[167]

Although the depth of genetic data still lags far behind that of *Drosophila*, sleep-related gene profiling and molecular biological studies have also been initiated. The preprohypocretin gene and receptor have also been cloned in zebrafish and pufferfish.[168,169] Attempts to create several lines of transgenic, sleep-related genes (including postnatal ablation of hypocretin neurons, and visualization of neurotransmitter systems) in zebrafish are also in progress.[170]

Thus zebrafish are likely to be useful for new genome-wide genetic screens for sleep-related genes the study of various neuronal projections and cellular mechanisms and possibly sleep phenotypic rescue.

29.9 Conclusions

Spontaneous occurring animal models for sleep disorders are indispensable, but availability of these models is very limited. Sleep research using animals has also been shifted from the classical brain transection and lesions experiments in cats and rats to neurochemical, molecular, and genetic approaches in mice and other simple animal species.

A picture emerges that in order to progress, multiple approaches using different animal models and genetic techniques have to be used in parallel, especially since most sleep disorders are genetically influenced. The successful identification of a mutation in the hypocretin-2 receptor underlying canine narcolepsy is the single best example of the feasibility of this approach. The study of an animal model of human narcolepsy began at Stanford University 20 years ago. Initial efforts were focused at the pharmacology of cataplexy and sleep but true progress was made using the genetic approach that culminated with the discovery of the responsible mutation. Involvement of neuronal pathways was also confirmed almost simultaneously by experiments using genetically engineered mice models. Once the pathway was identified in these animals, its implication in human narcolepsy was quickly demonstrated by the discovery of hypocretin deficiency. Future breakthroughs in the hunt for the discovery of "sleep genes" and novel sleep regulatory mechanisms are likely to come from the parallel use of mice as well as simple animals, such as fruit fly and zebrafish models. Thousands of mutant strains in these species await sleep phenotyping, and these numbers are rapidly increasing, possibly saturating the genome within the decade. Considering the fact that we still know very little about the molecular basis of sleep and how ineffective the current treatments for common sleep disorders such as insomnia or hypersomnia are, molecular genetic approaches become more important for developing better therapies and uncovering sleep functions and disorders. However, it should be also emphasized that discovery of narcoleptic dogs was due to the careful observation of the phenotype (i.e., differentiation from seizure or syncope). Similarly, a link between hypocretin ligand deficiency and narcolepsy in preprohypocretin knockout mice could not have been made without excellent scientific acumen combined with a modicum of luck, especially since cataplexy in mice mainly occurs in the dark period. These tenacious efforts, together with application of modern technologies, have given an excellent example in timely manner.

Acknowledgment

Part of the study was supported by National Institutes of Health grant NS 23724 and an RLS research award.

References

1. Mellinger GD, Balter MB, Uhlenhuth EH. Insomnia and its treatment: prevelance and correlates. *Arch. Gen. Psychiatr*. 1985, **42**: 225–232.
2. Young T. Sleep-disordered breathing in older adults: is it a condition distinct from that in middle-aged adults? *Sleep* 1996, **19**: 529–530.
3. Allen RP, Earley CJ. Restless legs syndrome: a review of clinical and pathophysiologic features. *J. Clin. Neurophysiol*. 2001, **18**: 128–147.
4. Nishino S, Mignot E. Pharmacological aspects of human and canine narcolepsy. *Progr. Neurobiol*. 1997, **52**: 27–78.
5. American Sleep Disorders Association. *International Classification of Sleep Disorders: Diagnostic and Coding Manual*. Rochester, MN: American Academy of Sleep Medicine, 2001.
6. Lin L, Faraco J, Li R, *et al*. The sleep disorder canine narcolepsy is caused by a mutation in the hypocretin (orexin) receptor 2 gene. *Cell* 1999, **98**: 365–376.
7. Chemelli RM, Willie JT, Sinton CM, *et al*. Narcolepsy in orexin knockout mice: molecular genetics of sleep regulation. *Cell* 1999, **98**: 437–451.
8. Thannickal TC, Moore RY, Nienhuis R, *et al*. Reduced number of hypocretin neurons in human narcolepsy. *Neuron* 2000, **27**: 469–474.
9. Peyron C, Faraco J, Rogers W, *et al*. A mutation in a case of early onset narcolepsy and a generalized absence of hypocretin peptides in human narcoleptic brains. *Nature Med*. 2000, **6**: 991–997.
10. Nishino S, Ripley B, Overeem S, Lammers GJ, Mignot E. Hypocretin (orexin) deficiency in human narcolepsy. *Lancet* 2000, **355**: 39–40.
11. Ford DE, Kamerow DB. Epidemiologic study of sleep disturbances and psychiatric disorders: an opportunity for prevention? *J. Am. Med. Ass*. 1989, **262**: 1479–1484.

12. Nishino S, Dement WC. Neuropharmacology of sedative-hypnotics and CNS stimulants in sleep medicine. In *Psychiatric Clinics of North America: Annual Drug Therapy*. Philadelphia, PA: W. B. Saunders, 1998, pp. 85–144.
13. Black JE, Brooks SN, Nishino S. Narcolepsy and syndromes of primary excessive daytime somnolence. *Semin. Neurol.* 2004, **24**: 271–282.
14. Guilleminault C. Clinical features and evaluation of obstructive sleep apnea. In Kryger MH, Roth T, Dement WC (eds.) *Principles and Practice of Sleep Medicine*, 2nd edn. Philadelphia, PA: W. B. Saunders, 1994, pp. 667–677.
15. Guilleminault C, Anders TF. The pathophysiology of sleep disorders in pediatrics. II. Sleep disorders in children. *Adv. Pediatr.* 1976, **22**: 151–174.
16. Mahowald MW, Schenk CH. *REM Sleep Behavior Disorder*, 2nd edn. Philadelphia, PA: W. B. Saunders, 1994.
17. Roehrs T, Roth T. *Chronic Insomnia Associated with Circadian Rhythm Disorders*, 2nd edn. Philadelphia, PA: W. B. Saunders, 1994.
18. Carskadon M, Dement WC. Normal human sleep. In Kryger MH, Roth T, Dement WC (eds.) *Principles and Practice of Sleep Medicine*, 2nd edn. Philadelphia, PA: W. B. Saunders, 1994, pp. 16–25.
19. Borbéry AA. Introduction. In Borbéry AA, Hayaishi O, Sejnowski AJ, Altman JS (eds.) *The Regulation of Sleep*. Strasbourg: HFSP, 2000, pp. 17–25.
20. Borbéry AA. *Sleep Homeostatsis and Models of Sleep Regulation*, 2nd edn. Philadelphia, PA: W. B. Saunders, 1994.
21. Lowrey PL, Takahashi JS. Mammalian circadian biology: elucidating genome-wide levels of temporal organization. *Annu. Rev. Genomics Hum. Genet.* 2004, **5**: 407–441.
22. King DP, Takahashi JS. Molecular genetics of circadian rhythms in mammals. *Annu. Rev. Neurosci.* 2000, **23**: 713–742.
23. Reppert SM, Weaver DR. Molecular analysis of mammalian circadian rhythms. *Annu. Rev. Physiol.* 2001, **63**: 647–676.
24. Czeisler CA, Duffy JF, Shanahan TL, *et al.* Stability, precision, and near-24-hour period of the human circadian pacemaker. *Science* 1999, **284**: 2177–2181.
25. Steriade M, Contreras D, Curro Dossi R, Nunez A. The slow (<1 Hz) oscillation in reticular thalamic and thalamocortical neurons: scenario of sleep rhythm generation in interacting thalamic and neocortical networks. *J. Neurosci.* 1993, **13**: 3284–3299.
26. Siegel JM. Brainstem mechanisms generating REM sleep. In Kryger MH, Roth T, Dement WC (eds.) *Principles and Practice of Sleep Medicine*. Philadelphia, PA: W. B. Saunders, 2000, pp. 112–133.
27. Jones BE. Basic mechanism of sleep–wake states. In Kryger MH, Roth T, Dement WC (eds.) *Principles and Practice of Sleep Medicine*, 2nd edn. Philadelphia, PA: W. B. Saunders, 1994, pp. 145–162.
28. Nishino S, Taheri S, Black J, Nofzinger E, Mignot E. The neurobiology of sleep in relation to mental illness. In Charney DS (ed.) *Neurobiology of Mental Illness*. New York: Oxford University Press, 2004, pp. 1160–1179.
29. Sastre JP, Sakai K, Jouvet M. Persistence of paradoxical sleep in the cat after destruction of the pontine gagantocellular tegmental field with kainic acid. *C. R. Séances Acad. Sci. D* 1979, **289**: 959–964. (In French)
30. Hendricks JC, Morrison AR, Mann GL. Different behaviors during paradoxical sleep without atonia depend on pontine lesion site. *Brain Res.* 1982, **239**: 81–105.
31. Saper CB, Chou TC, Scammell TE. The sleep switch: hypothalamic control of sleep and wakefulness. *Trends Neurosci.* 2001, **24**: 726–731.

32. Lugaresi E, Medori R, Montagna P, *et al*. Fatal familial insomnia and dysautonomia with selective degeneration of thalamic nuclei. *New Engl. J. Med.* 1986, **315**: 997–1003.

33. Tobler I, Deboer T, Fischer M. Sleep and sleep regulation in normal and prion protein-deficient mice. *J. Neurosci.* 1997, **17**: 1869–1879.

34. Toh KL, Jones CR, He Y, *et al*. An hPer2 phosphorylation site mutation in familial advanced sleep phase syndrome. *Science* 2001, **291**: 1040–1043.

35. Desautels A, Turecki G, Montplaisir J, *et al*. Identification of a major susceptibility locus for restless legs syndrome on chromosome 12q. *Am. J. Hum. Genet.* 2001, **69**: 1266–1270.

36. Lecendreux M, Bassetti C, Dauvilliers Y, *et al*. HLA and genetic susceptibility to sleepwalking. *Mol. Psychiatr.* 2003, **8**: 114–117.

37. Schenck CH, Garcia-Rill E, Segall M, Noreen H, Mahowald MW. HLA class II genes associated with REM sleep behavior disorder. *Ann. Neurol.* 1996, **39**: 261–263.

38. Dauvilliers Y, Mayer G, Lecendreux M, *et al*. Kleine–Levin syndrome: an autoimmune hypothesis based on clinical and genetic analyses. *Neurology* 2002, **59**: 1739–1745.

39. Mignot EJ, Dement WC. Narcolepsy in animals and man. *Equine Vet. J.* 1993, **25**: 476–477.

40. Okura M, Fujiki N, Ripley B, *et al*. Narcoleptic canines display periodic leg movements during sleep. *Psychiatr. Clin. Neurosci.* 2001, **55**: 243–244.

41. Hendricks JC, Lager A, O'Brien D, Morrison AR. Movement disorders during sleep in cats and dogs. *J. Am. Vet. Med. Assoc.* 1989, **194**: 686–689.

42. Hendricks JC, Kline LR, Kovalski RJ, *et al*. The English bulldog: a natural model of sleep-disordered breathing. *J. Appl. Physiol.* 1987, **63**: 1344–1350.

43. Panckeri KA, Schotland HM, Pack AI, Hendricks JC. Modafinil decreases hypersomnolence in the English bulldog, a natural animal model of sleep-disordered breathing. *Sleep* 1996, **19**: 626–631.

44. Yasuma F, Kozar LF, Kimoff RJ, Bradley TD, Phillipson EA. Interaction of chemical and mechanical respiratory stimuli in the arousal response to hypoxia in sleeping dogs. *Am. Rev. Respir. Dis.* 1991, **143**: 1274–1277.

45. Bakehe M, Miramand JL, Chambille B, Gaultier C, Escourrou P. Cardiovascular changes during acute episodic repetitive hypoxic and hypercapnic breathing in rats. *Eur. Respir. J.* 1995, **8**: 1675–1680.

46. Fletcher EC, Bao G. Effect of episodic eucapnic and hypocapnic hypoxia on systemic blood pressure in hypertension-prone rats. *J. Appl. Physiol.* 1996, **81**: 2088–2094.

47. Bao G, Metreveli N, Fletcher EC. Acute and chronic blood pressure response to recurrent acoustic arousal in rats. *Am. J. Hypertens.* 1999, **12**: 504–510.

48. Carley DW, Trbovic S, Radulovacki M. Sleep apnea in normal and REM sleep-deprived normotensive Wistar–Kyoto and spontaneously hypertensive (SHR) rats. *Physiol. Behav.* 1996, **59**: 827–831.

49. Nakamura A, Kuwaki T. Sleep apnea in mice: a useful animal model for study of SIDS? *Early Hum. Devel.* 2003, **75** (Suppl.): S167–S174.

50. Carley DW, Radulovacki M. Role of peripheral serotonin in the regulation of central sleep apneas in rats. *Chest* 1999, **115**: 1397–1401.

51. Desarnaud F, Murillo-Rodriguez E, Lin L, *et al*. The diurnal rhythm of hypocretin in young and old F344 rats. *Sleep* 2004, **27**: 851–856.

52. Nishino S, Riehl J, Hong J, *et al*. Is narcolepsy REM sleep disorder? Analysis of sleep abnormalities in narcoleptic Dobermans. *Neurosci. Res.* 2000, **38**: 437–446.

53. Kaitin KI, Kilduff TS, Dement WC. Evidence for excessive sleepiness in canine narcoleptics. *Electroencephalogr. Clin. Neurophysiol.* 1986, **64**: 447–454.

54. Sakurai T, Amemiya A, Ishil M, *et al.* Orexins and orexin receptors: a family of hypothalamic neuropeptides and G-protein-coupled receptors that regulate feeding behavior. *Cell* 1998, **92**: 573–585.

55. De Lecea L, Kilduff TS, Peyron C, *et al.* The hypocretins: hypothalamus-specific peptides with neuroexcitatory activity. *Proc. Natl Acad. Sci. USA* 1998, **95**: 322–327.

56. Mignot E, Lammers GJ, Ripley B, *et al.* The role of cerebrospinal fluid hypocretin measurement in the diagnosis of narcolepsy and other hypersomnias. *Arch. Neurol.* 2002, **59**: 1553–1562.

57. Ripley B, Overeem S, Fujiki N, *et al.* CSF hypocretin/orexin levels in narcolepsy and other neurological conditions. *Neurology* 2001, **57**: 2253–2258.

58. Ripley B, Fujiki N, Okura M, Mignot E, Nishino S. Hypocretin levels in sporadic and familial cases of canine narcolepsy. *Neurobiol. Dis.* 2001, **8**: 525–534.

59. Hara J, Beuckmann CT, Nambu T, *et al.* Genetic ablation of orexin neurons in mice results in narcolepsy, hypophagia, and obesity. *Neuron* 2001, **30**: 345–354.

60. Nishino S, Ripley B, Overeem S, *et al.* Low CSF hypocretin (orexin) and altered energy homeostasis in human narcolepsy. *Ann. Neurol.* 2001, **50**: 381–388.

61. Fujiki N, Ripley B, Yoshida Y, Mignot E, Nishino S. Effects of IV and ICV hypocretin-1 (orexin A) in hypocretin receptor-2 gene mutated narcoleptic dogs and IV hypocretin-1 replacement therapy in a hypocretin ligand deficient narcoleptic dog. *Sleep* 2003, **6**: 953–959.

62. Schatzberg SJ, Barrett J, Cutter Kl, Ling L, Mignot E. Case study: effect of hypocretin replacement therapy in a 3-year-old Weimaraner with narcolepsy. *J. Vet. Internal. Med.* 2004, **18**: 586–588.

63. Mieda M, Willie JT, Hara J, *et al.* Orexin peptides prevent cataplexy and improve wakefulness in an orexin neuron-ablated model of narcolepsy in mice. *Proc. Natl Acad. Sci. USA* 2004, **101**: 4649–4654.

64. Wittig R, Zorick F, Piccione P, Sicklesteel J, Roth T. Narcolepsy and disturbed nocturnal sleep. *Clin. Electroencephalogr.* 1983, **14**: 130–134.

65. Walters AS, Picchietti DL, Ehrenberg BL, Wagner ML. Restless legs syndrome in childhood and adolescence. *Pediatr. Neurol.* 1994, **11**: 241–245.

66. Picchietti DL, England SJ, Walters AS, Willis K, Verrico T. Periodic limb movement disorder and restless legs syndrome in children with attention-deficit hyperactivity disorder. *J. Child. Neurol.* 1998, **13**: 588–594.

67. Ekbom K. Restless legs. *Acta Scand. (Suppl.)* 1945, **158**: 1–123.

68. Nishino S, Shiba T, Yoshida Y, *et al.* Hypocretin/dopaminergic interactions: pharmacological studies of cataplexy and PLMS in canine narcolepsy. *Sleep* 2003, **26** (Suppl.): A345–A346.

69. Reid MS, Tafti M, Nishino S, *et al.* Local administration of dopaminergic drugs into the ventral tegmental area modulate cataplexy in the narcoleptic canine. *Brain Res.* 1996, **733**: 83–100.

70. Jouvet M. Recherche sur les structures nerveuses et les mécanismes responsables des différentes phases du sommeil physiologique. *Arch. Ital. Biol.* 1962, **100**: 125–206.

71. McGinty DJ, Sterman MB. Sleep suppression after basal forebrain lesions in the cat. *Science* 1968, **160**: 1253–1255.

72. Sakai K, El Mansari M, Lin JG, Zhang JG, Vanni-Mercier G. The posterior hypothalamus in the regulation of wakefulness and paradoxical sleep. In Mancia

M, Marini G (eds.) *The Diencephalon and Sleep*. New York: Raven Press, 1990, pp. 171–198.

73. Economo C von. *Encephalitis Lethargica: Its Sequelae and Treatment*. London: Oxford Medical Publications, 1931.

74. Sherin J, Shiromani P, McCarley R, Saper C. Activation of ventrolateral preoptic neurons during sleep. *Science* 1996, **271**: 216–220.

75. Lu J, Greco MA, Shiromani P, Saper CB. Effect of lesions of the ventrolateral preoptic nucleus on NREM and REM sleep. *J. Neurosci*. 2000, **20**: 3830–3842.

76. Kapas L, Obal Jr F, Book AA, *et al*. The effects of immunolesions of nerve growth factor-receptive neurons by 192 IgG-saporin on sleep. *Brain Res*. 1996, **712**: 53–59.

77. Gerashchenko D, Kohls MD, Greco M, *et al*. Hypocretin-2–saporin lesions of the lateral hypothalamus produce narcoleptic-like sleep behavior in the rat. *J. Neurosci*. 2001, **21**: 7273–7283.

78. Gerashchenko D, Chou TC, Blanco-Centurion CA, Saper CB, Shiromani PJ. Effects of lesions of the histaminergic tuberomammillary nucleus on spontaneous sleep in rats. *Sleep* 2004, **27**: 1275–1281.

79. Vitaterna MH, King DP, Chang AM, *et al*. Mutagenesis and mapping of a mouse gene clock, essential for circadian behavior. *Science* 1994, **264**: 719–725.

80. Naylor E, Bergmann BM, Krauski K, *et al*. The circadian clock mutation alters sleep homeostasis in the mouse. *J. Neurosci*. 2000, **20**: 8138–8143.

81. King DP, Zhao Y, Sangoram AM, *et al*. Positional cloning of the mouse clock gene. *Cell* 1997, **89**: 641–653.

82. Nolan PM, Peters J, Vizor L, *et al*. Implementation of a large-scale ENU mutagenesis program: towards increasing the mouse mutant resource. *Mamm. Genome* 2000, **11**: 500–506.

83. Berrettini WH, Ferraro TN, Alexander RC, Buchberg AM, Vogel WH. Quantitative trait loci mapping of three loci controlling morphine preference using inbred mouse strains. *Nature Genet*. 1994, **7**: 54–58.

84. Tarricone BJ, Hingtgen JN, Belknap JK, Mitchell SR, Nurnberger Jr JI. Quantitative trait loci associated with the behavioral response of B × D recombinant inbred mice to restraint stress: a preliminary communication. *Behav. Genet*. 1995, **25**: 489–495.

85. Lander ES, Schork NJ. Genetic dissection of complex traits. *Science* 1994, **265**: 2037–2048.

86. Lindblad-Toh K, Winchester E, Daly MJ, *et al*. Large-scale discovery and genotyping of single-nucleotide polymorphisms in the mouse. *Nature Genet*. 2000, **24**: 381–386.

87. Hudson TJ, Church DM, Greenaway S, *et al*. A radiation hybrid map of mouse genes. *Nature Genet*. 2001, **29**: 201–205.

88. Franken P, Chollet D, Tafti M. The homeostatic regulation of sleep need is under genetic control. *J. Neurosci*. 2001, **21**: 2610–2621.

89. Franken P, Malafosse A, Tafti M. Genetic variation in EEG activity during sleep in inbred mice. *Am. J. Physiol*. 1998, **275**: R1127–R1137.

90. Tafti M, Chollet D, Valatx JL, Franken P. Quantitative trait loci approach to the genetics of sleep in recombinant inbred mice. *J. Sleep Res*. 1999, **8**(Suppl. 1): 37–43.

91. Tafti M, Petit B, Chollet D, *et al*. Deficiency in short-chain fatty acid beta-oxidation affects theta oscillations during sleep. *Nature Genet*. 2003, **34**: 320–325.

92. Tafti M, Franken P, Kitahama K, *et al*. Localization of candidate genomic regions influencing paradoxical sleep in mice. *NeuroReport* 1997, **8**: 3755–3758.
93. Toth LA, Williams RW. A quantitative genetic analysis of slow-wave sleep and rapid-eye movement sleep in CXB recombinant inbred mice. *Behav. Genet.* 1999, **29**: 329–337.
94. Nadeau JH, Singer JB, Matin A, Lander ES. Analysing complex genetic traits with chromosome substitution strains. *Nature Genet.* 2000, **24**: 221–225.
95. Franken P, Malafosse A, Tafti M. Genetic determinants of sleep regulation in inbred mice. *Sleep* 1999, **22**: 155–169.
96. Cirelli C, Tononi G. Gene expression in the brain across the sleep–waking cycle. *Brain Res.* 2000, **885**: 303–321.
97. Kong J, Shepel PN, Holden CP, *et al*. Brain glycogen decreases with increased periods of wakefulness: implications for homeostatic drive to sleep. *J. Neurosci.* 2002, **22**: 5581–5587.
98. Porkka-Heiskanen T, Kalinchuk A, Alanko L, Urrila A, Stenberg D. Adenosine, energy metabolism, and sleep. *Sci. World J.* 2003, **3**: 790–798.
99. Gardi J, Obal Jr F, Fang J, Zhang J, Krueger JM. Diurnal variations and sleep deprivation-induced changes in rat hypothalamic GHRH and somatostatin contents. *Am. J. Physiol.* 1999, **277**: R1339–R1344.
100. Darvasi A. Experimental strategies for the genetic dissection of complex traits in animal models. *Nature Genet.* 1998, **18**: 19–24.
101. Su H, Wang X, Bradley A. Nested chromosomal deletions induced with retroviral vectors in mice. *Nature Genet.* 2000, **24**: 92–95.
102. Capecchi MR. The new mouse genetics: altering the genome by gene targeting. *Trends Genet.* 1989, **5**: 70–76.
103. Jaenisch R. Transgenic animals. *Science* 1988, **240**: 1468–1474.
104. Williams RS, Wagner PD. Transgenic animals in integrative biology: approaches and interpretations of outcome. *J. Appl. Physiol.* 2000, **88**: 1119–1126.
105. Tobler I, Gaus SE, Deboer T, *et al*. Altered circadian activity rhythms and sleep in mice devoid of prion protein. *Nature* 1996, **380**: 639–642.
106. Zhang J, Obal Jr F, Fang J, Collins BJ, Krueger JM. Non-rapid eye movement sleep is suppressed in transgenic mice with a deficiency in the somatotropic system. *Neurosci. Lett.* 1996, **220**: 97–100.
107. Wisor JP, Nishino S, Sora I, *et al*. Dopaminergic role in stimulant-induced wakefulness. *J. Neurosci.* 2001, **21**: 1787–1794.
108. Parmentier R, Ohtsu H, Djebbara-Hannas Z, *et al*. Anatomical, physiological, and pharmacological characteristics of histidine decarboxylase knock-out mice: evidence for the role of brain histamine in behavioral and sleep-wake control. *J. Neurosci.* 2002, **22**: 7695–7711.
109. Huang ZL, Qu WM, Li WD, *et al*. Arousal effect of orexin A depends on activation of the histaminergic system. *Proc. Natl Acad. Sci. USA* 2001, **98**: 9965–9970.
110. Toyota H, Dugovic C, Koehl M, *et al*. Behavioral characterization of mice lacking histamine H(3)-receptors. *M. l. Pharmacol.* 2002, **62**: 389–397; erratum, *M. l. Pharmacol.* 2002, **62**: 763.
111. Boutrel B, Monaca C, Hen R, Hamon M, Adrien J. Involvement of 5-HT1 A receptors in homeostatic and stress-induced adaptive regulations of paradoxical sleep: studies in 5-HT1 A knock-out mice. *J. Neurosci.* 2002, **22**: 4686–4692.
112. Laposky AD, Homanics GE, Basile A, Mendelson WB. Deletion of the GABA(A) receptor beta 3 subunit eliminates the hypnotic actions of oleamide in mice. *NeuroReport* 2001, **12**: 4143–4147.

113. Boutrel B, Franc B, Hen R, Hamon M, Adrien J. Key role of 5-HT1B receptors in the regulation of paradoxical sleep as evidenced in 5-HT1B knock-out mice. *J. Neurosci.* 1999, **19**: 3204–3212.

114. Frank MG, Stryker MP, Tecott LH. Sleep and sleep homeostasis in mice lacking the 5-HT2c receptor. *Neuropsychopharmacology* 2002, **27**: 869–873.

115. Krueger JM, Takahashi S, Kapas L. Cytokines in sleep regulation. *Adv. Neuroimmunol.* 1995, **5**: 171–188.

116. Fang J, Wang Y, Krueger JM. Effects of interleukin-1 beta on sleep are mediated by the type I receptor. *Am. J. Physiol.* 1998, **274**: R655–R660.

117. Toth LA, Opp MR. Cytokine- and microbially induced sleep responses of interleukin-10 deficient mice. *Am. J. Physiol. Regul. Integr. Comp. Physiol.* 2001, **280**: R1806–R1814.

118. Deboer T, Fontana A, Tobler I. Tumor necrosis factor (TNF) ligand and TNF receptor deficiency affects sleep and the sleep EEG. *J. Neurophysiol.* 2002, **88**: 839–846.

119. Kopp C, Albrecht U, Zheng B, Tobler I. Homeostatic sleep regulation is preserved in *mPer1* and *mPer2* mutant mice. *Eur. J. Neurosci.* 2002, **16**: 1099–1106.

120. Wisor JP, O'Hara BF, Terao A, *et al.* A role for cryptochromes in sleep regulation. *BMC Neurosci.* 2002, **3**: 20.

121. Franken P, Lopez-Molina L, Marcacci L, Schibler U, Tafti M. The transcription factor DBP affects circadian sleep consolidation and rhythmic EEG activity. *J. Neurosci.* 2000, **20**: 617–625.

122. Kapfhamer D, Valladares O, Sun Y, *et al.* Mutations in *Rab3a* alter circadian period and homeostatic response to sleep loss in the mouse. *Nature Genet.* 2002, **32**: 290–295.

123. Willie JT, Chemelli RM, Sinton CM, *et al.* Distinct narcolepsy syndromes in Orexin receptor-2 and Orexin null mice: molecular genetic dissection of Non-REM and REM sleep regulatory processes. *Neuron* 2003, **38**: 715–730.

124. Tobler I, Kopp C, Deboer T, Rudolph U. Diazepam-induced changes in sleep: role of the alpha 1 GABA(A) receptor subtype. *Proc. Natl Acad. Sci. USA* 2001, **98**: 6464–6469.

125. Bucan M, Abel T. The mouse: genetics meets behaviour. *Nature Genet.* 2002, **3**: 114–123.

126. Man in 't Veld A, Boomsma F, Lenders J, *et al.* Patients with congenital dopamine beta-hydroxylase deficiency: a lesson in catecholamine physiology. *Am. J. Hypertens.* 1988, **1**: 231–238.

127. Hunsley MS, Palmiter RD. Norepinephrine-deficient mice exhibit normal sleep–wake states but have shorter sleep latency after mild stress and low doses of amphetamine. *Sleep* 2003, **26**: 521–526.

128. Lewandoski M. Conditional control of gene expression in the mouse. *Nature Genet.* 2001, **2**: 743–755.

129. Beuckmann CT, Sinton CM, Williams SC, *et al.* Expression of a poly-glutamine-ataxin-3 transgene in orexin neurons induces narcolepsy–cataplexy in the rat. *J. Neurosci.* 2004, **24**: 4469–4477.

130. Twigger S, Lu J, Shimoyama M, *et al.* Rat Genome Database (RGD): mapping disease onto the genome. *Nucleic Acids Res.* 2002, **30**: 125–128.

131. Weiss B, Davidkova G, Zhang SP. Antisense strategies in neurobiology. *Neurochem. Int.* 1997, **31**: 321–348.

132. Cirelli C, Pompeiano M, Arrighi P, Tononi G. Sleep–waking changes after *c-fos* antisense injections in the medial preoptic area. *NeuroReport* 1995, **6**: 801–805.

133. Xi MC, Morales FR, Chase MH. Evidence that wakefulness and REM sleep are controlled by a GABAergic pontine mechanism. *J. Neurophysiol.* 1999, **82**: 2015–2019.

134. Thakkar MM, Ramesh V, Strecker RE, McCarley RW. Microdialysis perfusion of orexin-A in the basal forebrain increases wakefulness in freely behaving rats. *Arch. Ital. Biol.* 2001, **139**: 313–328.

135. Thakkar MM, Winston S, McCarley RW. A1 receptor and adenosinergic homeostatic regulation of sleep–wakefulness: effects of antisense to the A1 receptor in the cholinergic basal forebrain. *J. Neurosci.* 2003, **23**: 4278–4287.

136. Fabre V, Boutrel B, Hanoun N, *et al.* Homeostatic regulation of serotonergic function by the serotonin transporter as revealed by nonviral gene transfer. *J. Neurosci.* 2000, **20**: 5065–5075.

137. Hendricks JC, Sehgal A, Pack AI. The need for a simple animal model to understand sleep. *Progr. Neurobiol.* 2000, **61**: 339–351.

138. Borbely AA, Tobler I. Sleep regulation: relation to photoperiod, sleep duration, waking activity, and torpor. *Progr. Brain Res.* 1996, **111**: 343–348.

139. Johnson CH, Golden SS, Ishiura M, Kondo T. Circadian clocks in prokaryotes. *Mol. Microbiol.* 1996, **21**: 5–11.

140. Pittendrigh CS. Circadian systems. I. The driving oscillation and its assay in *Drosophila pseudoobscura*. *Proc. Natl Acad. Sci. USA* 1967, **58**: 1762–1767.

141. Moore RY. Circadian rhythms: basic neurobiology and clinical appplications. *Annu. Rev. Med.* 1997, **49**: 253–266.

142. Sehgal A, Price JL, Man B, Young MW. Loss of behavioral rhythms and per RNA oscillations in the *Drosophilia* mutant *timeless*. *Science* 1994, **263**: 1603–1605.

143. Ishiura M, Kutsuna S, Aoki S, *et al.* Expression of a gene cluster kaiABC as a circadian feedback process in cyanobacteria. *Science* 1998, **281**: 1519–1523.

144. Garceau NY, Liu Y, Loros JJ, Dunlap JC. Alternative initiation of translation and time-specific phosphorylation yield multiple forms of the essential clock protein FREQUENCY. *Cell* 1997, **89**: 469–476.

145. Shearman LP, Zylka MJ, Weaver DR, Kolakowski Jr LF, Reppert SM. Two period homologs: circadian expression and photic regulation in the suprachias-matic nuclei. *Neuron* 1997, **19**: 1261–1269.

146. Sun ZS, Albrecht U, Zhuchenko O, *et al.* RIGUI, a putative mammalian ortholog of the *Drosophila period* gene. *Cell* 1997, **90**: 1003–1011.

147. Tei H, Okamura H, Shigeyoshi Y, *et al.* Circadian oscillation of a mammalian homologue of the *Drosophila period* gene. *Nature* 1997, **389**: 512–516.

148. Campbell SS, Tobler I. Animal sleep: a review of sleep duration across phylogeny. *Neurosci. Biobehav. Rev.* 1984, **8**: 269–300.

149. Hendricks JC. Invited review: Sleeping flies don't lie: the use of *Drosophila melanogaster* to study sleep and circadian rhythms. *J. Appl. Physiol.* 2003, **94**: 1660–1672; discussion 1673.

150. Engels WR. P elements in *Drosophila*. *Curr. Topics Microbiol. Immunol.* 1996, **204**: 103–123.

151. de Belle JS, Heisenberg M. Associative odor learning in *Drosophila* abolished by chemical ablation of mushroom bodies. *Science* 1994, **263**: 692–695.

152. Yin JC, Del Vecchio M, Zhou H, Tully T. CREB as a memory modulator: induced expression of a dCREB2 activator isoform enhances long-term memory in *Drosophila*. *Cell* 1995, **81**: 107–115.

153. Saudou F, Hen R. 5-Hydroxytryptamine receptor subtypes in vertebrates and invertebrates. *Neurochem. Int.* 1994, **25**: 503–532.

154. Nassel DR. Histamine in the brain of insects: a review. *Microsc. Res. Tech.* 1999, **44**: 121–136.

155. Nassel DR. Neuropeptides, amines and amino acids in an elementary insect ganglion: functional and chemical anatomy of the unfused abdominal ganglion. *Progr. Neurobiol.* 1996, **48**: 325–420.

156. Tobler I, Neuner-Jehle M. 24-h variation of vigilance in the cockroach *Blaberus giganteus. J. Sleep Res.* 1992, **1**: 231–239.

157. Nitz DA, van Swinderen B, Tononi G, Greenspan RJ. Electrophysiological correlates of rest and activity in *Drosophila melanogaster. Curr. Biol.* 2002, **12**: 1934–1940.

158. Cirelli C. Searching for sleep mutants of *Drosophila melanogaster. BioEssays* 2003, **25**: 940–949.

159. Cox KJ, Fetcho JR. Labeling blastomeres with a calcium indicator: a non-invasive method of visualizing neuronal activity in zebrafish. *J. Neurosci. Methods* 1996, **68**: 185–191.

160. Fetcho JR, O'Malley DM. Visualization of active neural circuitry in the spinal cord of intact zebrafish. *J. Neurophysiol.* 1995, **73**: 399–406.

161. Ekstrom P. Developmental changes in the brainstem serotonergic nuclei of teleost fish and neural plasticity. *Cell Mol. Neurobiol.* 1994, **14**: 381–393.

162. Ma PM. Catecholaminergic systems in the zebrafish. I. Number, morphology, and histochemical characteristics of neurons in the locus coeruleus. *J. Comp. Neurol.* 1994, **344**: 242–255.

163. Ma PM. Catecholaminergic systems in the zebrafish. II. Projection pathways and pattern of termination of the locus coeruleus. *J. Comp. Neurol.* 1994, **344**: 256–269.

164. Eriksson KS, Peitsaro N, Karlstedt K, Kaslin J, Panula P. Development of the histaminergic neurons and expression of histidine decarboxylase mRNA in the zebrafish brain in the absence of all peripheral histaminergic systems. *Eur. J. Neurosci.* 1998, **10**: 3799–3812.

165. Liang MR, Alestrom P, Collas P. Glowing zebrafish: integration, transmission, and expression of a single luciferase transgene promoted by noncovalent DNA-nuclear transport peptide complexes. *Mol. Reprod. Devel.* 2000, **55**: 8–13.

166. Yokogawa T, Zhang J, Renier C, Mignot E. Characterization of a sleep-like state in adult zebrafish. *Sleep* 2004, **27**(Abstract Suppl.): A84.

167. Renier CM, Rosa FM, Mignot E. Pharmacogenomics of sleep-promoting drugs in zebrafish. *Sleep* 2004, **27**(Abstract Suppl.): A389.

168. Faraco JH, Chan Y, Mignot E. Characterization of the hypocretin/orexin ligand and receptor loci in the zebrafish. *Sleep* 2003, **26**(Abstract Suppl.): A422.

169. Gaus SE, Faraco J, Mignot E. Hypocretin/orexin gene expression in the developing zebrafish. *Sleep* 2003, **26**(Abstract Suppl.): A417–418.

170. Gaus SE, Faraco J, Renier C, *et al.* Developing zebrafish through random mutagenesis. *Sleep* 2004, **27**(Abstract Suppl.): A386–387.

171. Fujiki N, Morris L, Mignot E, Nishino S. Analysis of onset location, laterality and propagation of cataplexy in canine narcolepsy. *Psychiatr. Clin. Neurosci.* 2002, **56**: 275–276.

172. Huitron-Resendiz S, Sanchez-Alavez M, Gallegos R, *et al.* Age-independent and age-related deficits in visuospatial learning, sleep-wake states, thermoregulation and motor activity in PDAPP mice. *Brain Res.* 2002, **928**: 126–137.

173. Hajdu I, Obal Jr F, Fang J, Krueger JM, Rollo CD. Sleep of transgenic mice producing excess rat growth hormone. *Am. J. Physiol. Regul. Integr. Comp. Physiol.* 2002, **282**: R70–R76.

174. Valatx JL, Douhet P, Bucchini D. Human insulin gene insertion in mice: effects on the sleep–wake cycle? *J. Sleep Res.* 1999, **8**(Suppl. 1): 65–68.

175. Pinzar E, Kanaoka Y, Inui T, *et al.* Prostaglandin D synthase gene is involved in the regulation of non-rapid eye movement sleep. *Proc. Natl Acad. Sci. USA* 2000, **97**: 4903–4907.

176. Fang J, Wang Y, Krueger JM. Mice lacking the TNF 55 kDa receptor fail to sleep more after TNF-alpha treatment. *J. Neurosci.* 1997, **17**: 5949–5955.

177. Vyazovskiy VV, Deboer T, Rudy B, *et al.* Sleep EEG in mice that are deficient in the potassium channel subunit K.v.3.2. *Brain Res.* 2002, **947**: 204–211.

178. Shiromani PJ, Basheer R, Thakkar J, *et al.* Sleep and wakefulness in c-fos and fos B gene knockout mice. *Brain Res. Mol. Brain Res.* 2000, **80**: 75–87.

179. Kapfhamer D, Valladares O, Sun Y, *et al.* Mutations in Rab3a alter circadian period and homeostatic response to sleep loss in the mouse. *Nature Genet.* 2002, **32**: 290–295.

30

Experimental models of muscle diseases

ANU SUOMALAINEN, KATJA E. PELTOLA MJOSUND,
ANDERS PAETAU, AND CARINA WALLGREN-PETTERSSON

30.1 Introduction

The body harbors a complex muscle system, in which individual muscles can be identified by their size, position, shape, function, and attachments. The skeletal muscles are striated and voluntary, highly specialized muscles, which attach to bones via tendons, have a specific anatomical position and innervation, and move the skeleton. Cardiac muscle is of a unique kind, striated and of involuntary type. The smooth muscle is also involuntary, and moves the bowel, modifies vessels, and constricts the bladder, to name just a few of its functions. By muscle diseases, one usually means diseases affecting the skeletal muscle, and experimental research on this muscle type is the focus of this chapter.

Diseases of muscle may result from a range of defects, from developmental defects to those in structural backbone proteins and energy metabolism. Research clarifying the nature of defects in muscle diseases has been a valuable source of information for understanding normal muscle function. Experimental muscle models can be created to study the normal function of a protein, or to study the effect of a gene mutation to clarify disease pathogenesis. Alternatively, interesting phenotypes may have arisen spontaneously in experimental animal lines, and their characterization may bring new knowledge of muscle function and diseases. Most experimental procedures concerning muscle diseases are common routine techniques of molecular biology and genetics. Therefore, in this chapter, we have concentrated on introducing those aspects of experimental muscle research that are specific for the tissue and its diseases.

30.2 Muscle individuality

Individual muscles are highly specialized, and differ from each other by their set of expressed proteins, for example by their structural protein variants – which may be numerous[1] – or by their energy metabolism. The muscular individualism

Handbook of Experimental Neurology, ed. Turgut Tatlisumak and Marc Fisher. Published by Cambridge University Press. © Cambridge University Press 2006.

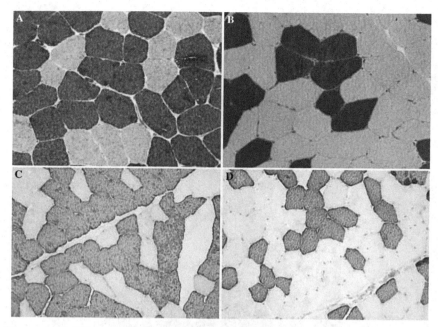

Figure 30.1. Fiber type determination. (A) Muscle fibers stained for ATPase activity in pH 10.4 with Herovici staining; dark fibers, type 2 muscle fibers. (B) ATPase in pH 4.3 with Herovici; type 1 fibers stain dark. (C) Type 2 muscle fibers immunostained with MyHC-fast antibodies. (D) Type 1 muscle fibers immunostained with MyHC-slow antibodies. Frozen sections, original magnification × 200.

is beautifully exemplified in muscle dystrophies affecting just one or few specific muscles. Isolated dystrophy of the tibialis anterior muscle of the foreleg is the feature of an inherited disorder, tibial muscular dystrophy,[2,3] caused by mutations in gene for the gigantic muscle protein titin.[3] This restricted phenotype seen in persons heterozygous for these mutations could be explained by different splice variants of the titin gene being expressed in specific muscles.[4] Interestingly, persons homozygous for these mutations have a clearly more severe muscle disorder, affecting several muscle groups. The functional impact of this specificity is still unknown. Defects affecting the late stages of fetal muscle development may result in complete lack of certain muscles.[5]

The physiological features of a specific muscle are determined by its muscle fiber types. Muscle fibers can be divided into different types based on their metabolism and contractile properties. The slow-twitch type 1 fibers contain slow isoform contractile proteins, high volumes of mitochondria, high levels of myoglobin, high capillary densities, and high oxidative enzyme capacity. The type 2 muscle fibers can be distinguished based on the myosin heavy chain (MyHC) type that they express: fast-twitch type 2A muscle fibers are

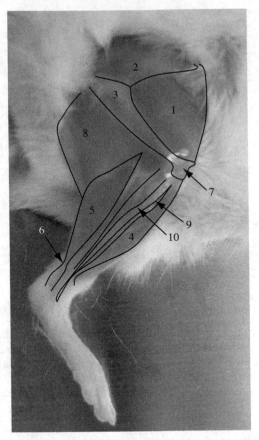

Figure 30.2. The mouse hind limb muscles frequently used for research purposes, and useful anatomical landmarks: 1, musculus quadriceps femoris; 2, m. gluteus medius; 3, m. tensor fasciae latae; 4, m. tibialis anterior; 5, m. triceps surae (consists of m. gastrocnemius caput mediale and laterale, and a small m. soleus); 6, Achilles tendon; 7, patellar tendon; 8, m. biceps femoris; 9, m. extensor digitorum longus; 10, m. extensor digitorum lateralis. M. tibialis anterior and m. extensor digitorum longus mainly consist of fast MyHC isoforms (MyHC 2B and 2X) and are thus used as models for studies of fast-twitch muscle fibers, whereas m. soleus has been used as a model for oxidative muscle, since it has a high proportion of MyHC 1.[19]

oxidative, fast-twitch type 2B fibers are glycolytic and type 2X fibers are fast-twitch, and can be either oxidative or glycolytic. MyHC 2B is not expressed in humans, but it is in mice.[6] The type 2A fibers exhibit fast contraction and high oxidative capacity, whereas fast-glycolytic fibers have high glycolytic enzyme activity and high rate of force production but low fatigue resistance. In rats, but not in humans, the type 2A fibers have higher oxidative capacity than type 1 fibers.[7,8] The traditional way of distinguishing between the types has been to stain for their ATPase activity with preincubations at different pH levels, which stain the muscle in a checkerboard pattern (Fig. 30.1), distinguishing type 1 from type 2 fibers. This has mostly been replaced by immunohistochemical detection of the different MyHC types. A small percentage of muscle fibers does not stain for any of the myosin types, and may be undergoing fiber-type transition, which probably represents adaptation of the muscle to mechanical demands.[9] A change in innervation may also modify the fiber-type composition.[10] Unlike in humans, specific limb muscles in rodents may be mostly of one type, for example the soleus muscle of Lewis rats are 96% type 1, whereas the extensor digitorum longus contains just 5% of type 1.[11] Different muscles of the mouse hind leg and their dominating fiber types are depicted in Fig. 30.2.

Some muscle diseases are also known to affect only one muscle fiber type; for example in gyrate atrophy of choroid and retina, an inborn error of metabolism, type 2 glycolytic muscle fibers are selectively atrophied and display pathological changes, whereas oxidative type 1 fibers appear normal.[12] Adult human skeletal muscle shows plasticity and can undergo conversion between different fiber types, e.g., in response to disease, exercise training, or modulation of motor neuron activity.[13–18] Importantly, it is becoming evident that not all muscle proteins change in parallel in response to cellular changes resulting from for example disease or muscle exercise. Therefore, changes in for example contractile proteins may not be paralleled by changes in proteins associated with energy metabolism, and the traditional fiber-type classification may be too simplistic to describe the phenotype.[6]

30.3 Muscle sampling and histological analysis

The target muscle for studies should be carefully chosen, and the correct muscle to be sampled depends on the specific questions: which muscle does the disease of interest affect, and what is the fiber-type distribution and metabolic nature of the muscle of interest? For example, biochemical tests can give completely different results depending on whether the sample is taken from the vastus lateralis muscle of the thigh or from the rectus muscle of the abdomen. Therefore, even though presenting as convenient, abdominal surgery is rarely an optimal source of control muscle samples.

In experimental animals, the fiber-type distribution within a given muscle does not necessarily follow the distribution in humans. In a study of MyHC isoform distributions of the soleus and tibialis anterior muscles in the mouse, rat, rabbit, and humans, the proportion of slow myosin generally increased with increasing body size.[19] For example, type 2B muscle fibers make up 77% of mouse skeletal muscle mass.[20]

Muscle samples should be taken carefully, avoiding squeezing or applying pressure to the sample, e.g., by forceps. For histological analysis, the samples should be taken on a sterile plate with a pad moisturized by physiological saline, and kept on ice. This sample is then frozen rapidly in isopentane (precooled in liquid nitrogen to $-160\,°C$), to avoid crystal formation and microstructure damage in the sample. Sample processing in the cryotome and stainings follow routine histological procedures.

30.4 Muscle satellite cells, differentiation, and muscle cell culture

Muscles contain their own repair kit, dormant satellite cells that are able to fuse with each other to form multinuclear myotubes, or with existing muscle fibers, and that underlie muscle growth and repair. Satellite cells have been programmed in the myogenic direction from the stem cell stage. These cells are the cell population, which give rise to the myoblast culture.

Myoblast culture in our group is done as previously described in detail, in culture conditions favoring myoblast but not fibroblast growth.[21] When starting from a tissue sample, the culture contains a mixture of cells, for example fibroblasts and myoblasts. When established, the myoblast fraction can be enriched utilizing an antibody targeted against a protein expressed at the surface of myoblasts, but lacking in fibroblasts. We use Miltenyi Biotec® mouse N-CAM antibody (the hybridoma cell line kindly provided by Professor H. Lochmueller). The myoblasts covered with the antibody are then mixed with magnetic beads (Miltenyi Biotec®) with anti-mouse antibody, and the bead–myoblast complexes are then captured in an iron column, the flowthrough with fibroblasts collected, and the myoblast-enriched fraction eluted from the column. The purity of the culture can be tested by shifting the cells to a serum-poor differentiation medium,[21] which will induce fusion of the confluent myoblast culture, to form multinuclear myotubes. In culture conditions, myotubes express myofibrillar structure with banding and they can contract. Muscle differentiation can be taken further by innervating the muscle culture. This involves dissection of a slice of rat spinal medulla, implanting it into a newly fused myoblast culture, and allowing the neurite outgrowth.[22] Innervation takes the muscle program to stages further than in the absence of neuromuscular junctions.

It is of importance to note, that in in vitro conditions, some pathways of mature muscle are not induced at all. Muscle variants that are only expressed in mature muscle may not be expressed even in myotubes. Several groups have taken the differentiation still one step further by for example treating a thigh of immunocompromised mice (e.g., Nude, severe combined immunodeficiency (SCID)) by irradiation and chemicals, destroying the local muscle and preventing regeneration.[23,24] This damaged tissue is then repopulated by human myoblasts which are injected into the site of the lesion. This is a technically challenging method, but when successful, produces fully differentiated human muscle fibers.[23,24] The resulting specific fiber types have not been studied in detail. Expression of human muscle structural proteins, however, has been nicely demonstrated.

Sometimes muscle is not available for study, but fibroblasts are. Fibroblasts can, however, be directed towards the muscle cell direction by overexpressing factors of the myogenic pathway, such as MyoD,[25] Myf-5,[26,27] Myogenin,[28] or MRF4.[29] These transcription factors induce the expression of many muscle-specific genes, which then can be studied in these myofibroblasts. We utilize a retrovirus, expressing murine MyoD under a viral promoter (generous gift of Dr D. A. Miller), to initiate myogenic pathways in fibroblasts. This is useful, but its limitations have to be recognized: certain muscle-specific proteins are not under the regulation of MyoD, and therefore not induced. In our experience, myofibroblasts undergo partial transdifferentiation only.

30.5 Transfection of myoblast cultures

Human and rodent myoblasts are useful tools when studying muscle diseases in cultured cells. Rodent myoblasts usually immortalize spontaneously, do not require specific growth conditions, and fuse readily. Often-used lines are mouse C2C12 cells[30] and rat L6 or L8 myoblasts.[31,32]

Myoblasts are often difficult to transfect efficiently using direct episomal plasmid transfection. The use of virus vectors avoids this problem, and high transduction efficiency can be achieved. We routinely clone the genes of interest into a retroviral vector (e.g., BMN-Ires-GFP, pLXSN, pLXSH, or BABE-puro or hygro).[33–38] High-titer virus is produced utilizing a packaging cell line, and the filtered virus is used to infect the recipient myoblast line, and to insert the gene of interest into the genome of the cell. This results in a cell line stably expressing the gene of interest. Amphotropic viruses have the capacity to infect human cells and a wide range of other species, and ecotropic viruses infect rodent cells, but not human. The protocols for retrovirus production can be found in specific handbooks, and the routine protocols also apply to the myoblast transduction. Retroviruses, however, require a specific safety level for their use, which may limit their use in some laboratories.

30.6 Genetically modified mice as models for muscle phenotypes

Cell culture systems do not allow full assessment of disease pathogenesis, and therapy-targeted studies require the development of model organisms.

Table 30.1. *Examples of promotors used to drive transgene expression in the muscle*

Promoter	Muscle expression, muscle fiber type	References
Skeletal muscle actin	Cardiac, skeletal	39
Chimeric rat alpha-actin–human embryonic globin	Cardiac, skeletal	40
Alpha cardiac actin	Cardiac and skeletal muscle, early development up to E15.5, then declining	41
Alpha skeletal actin	Cardiac and skeletal muscle, from E15.5 to mature muscle	41,43
Beta actin	Constitutive, including cardiac and skeletal muscles; enhanced slow-twitch, lower level but present fast-twitch	44
Muscle creatine kinase	Skeletal and cardiac muscle	45
Myosin light chain	Mostly fast-twitch skeletal muscle fiber types	46,47
Beta myosin heavy chain	Embryonal cardiac, adult skeletal muscle type 1 slow-twitch fibers	48
Human aldolase A	Fast-twitch skeletal muscle (2B, 2X)	49

Genetically modified mice are the most commonly used model. Transgenic overexpressing mouse models or gene inactivation by knockout or a mutation knockin are the routine approaches of choice. Again, the transgenic methods for muscle models are similar to those for any other target tissue. Therefore, in this chapter, we will focus on discussing what kind of promoters should be chosen, for overexpression or for conditional knockout models, to drive the expression of the gene of interest in muscle.

Table 30.1 summarizes various promoters used to drive expression in the muscle. Actin is a major protein component of the muscle sarcomere, and promoters of actin isoforms have frequently been used to drive transgene expression in muscle. The expression patterns of the different isoforms vary during development, specific early isoforms being changed along with muscle maturation. The human skeletal α-actin is frequently used to drive expression in the fast glycolytic muscle fibers,[41] whereas slow-twitch fiber-type expression can be driven using for example the MyHC β-promoter.[42] The human cytoplasmic β-actin is constitutively expressed, but its expression in muscle is low in oxidative type 1 fibers, and higher in type 2 fibers. It has been used to drive relatively strong overexpression, which is not regulated during development,[50] and the expression can be enhanced by including, e.g., cytomegalovirus enhancer sequences into the expression construct.[51] In our hands the pure promoter drives moderate overexpression, and reacts considerably to the transgene insertion site (A. Suomalainen and H. Tyynismaa, unpublished observation).[44,52] Many muscle-specific promoters drive expression both in the cardiac and skeletal muscle (Table 30.1). If physiological expression levels were wanted, a good option would be to utilize the original promoter and enhancers of the gene of interest. This is achieved for example by utilizing a genomic clone as the transgene, such as a P_1 artificial chromosome (PAC) or a bacterial artificial chromosome (BAC), including the region of interest.[53,54] The drawback of this approach is that the genomic clone also may contain other genes in addition to the one of interest, the phenotype might be affected by overexpression of those, and this may complicate interpretations of the effect of the transgene. However, this is the only way to study a gene under its natural physiological regulation.

Transient effects of transgenes can be studied by in vivo transfection.[55] The transgene is not inserted into the genome, but remains episomal, and is expressed over a period of time from days to weeks. The method involves injections of the transgene into a specific muscle, under anesthesia, electrical stimulation of DNA uptake, and follow-up of the expression during the following days.

30.7 Functional testing of murine muscle

Testing of intact muscle performance can only be achieved by studying functioning muscles of experimental animals. The nature of the functional tests depend on the muscle phenotype. We present here some of the frequently used test methods, but sometimes the most relevant tests have to be developed on site. The mouse genetic background may considerably affect the test results,[56] and therefore the best controls are healthy same-sex litter-mates, and if those are not available, age-matched controls of the same sex and strain.

Often a muscle defect manifests as muscle weakness or exercise intolerance. Phenotype testing can be roughly divided into two categories: testing for endurance exercise capacity and muscle strength testing. Several commercially available devices have been designed for testing a mouse muscle phenotype.

A frequently used test for mouse muscle strength is the grip strength test (Fig. 30.3). The mouse grips a bar or a grid with its forepaws, and the researcher gently pulls the mouse by the tail. The bar or the grid is connected to an isometric force transducer and the pulling force that makes the mouse release the bar is recorded.[57,58] Variations of this method, such as the rope test

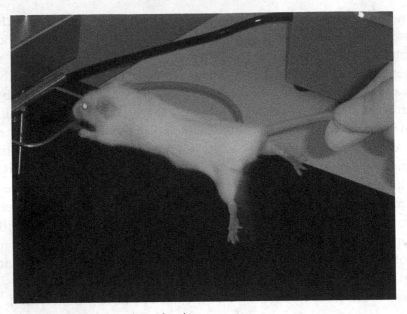

Figure 30.3. Grip strength testing in mouse.

or the coat-hanger test, also assess motor co-ordination, in addition to iso-metric muscle strength. In the rope test, the mouse climbs a rope or a wire, and the time required for climbing the distance of 20 cm, with all four paws attached, is recorded.[59] In the coat-hanger test the mouse is placed on a triangular bar setup, holding a diagonal bar with its forepaws and the horizontal bar with its hind paws. For example, the time of four paws attached to diagonal bar, snout reaching halfway or the top of the diagonal bar, and the time of falling can be recorded.[59,60] Muscle strength can also be measured by electrically stimulating intact muscle in situ and measuring the force produced. This requires anesthesia, but eliminates possible motivational and learning effects on the results.

Endurance exercise can reveal a difference between the performance of the diseased mice and the controls.[61] Furthermore, it can ameliorate the disease course, or on the contrary, induce the disease progression.[62] Endurance exercise capacity can be measured by voluntary or involuntary tests, as follows.

Voluntary wheel running utilizes a setup in which the mouse has a running wheel available in the cage, and the running activity (distance, speed, maximum speed, etc.) is recorded. This offers a useful model system for elucidating exercise capacity and the voluntary running behavior in mice. Daily running-wheel activity levels have been indicated as an indirect measure of aerobic capacity,[63] and the voluntary running speed has been suggested to be positively associated with oxygen consumption.[64] Voluntary wheel running has been shown to provide a sufficient endurance exercise stimulus to trigger significant skeletal and cardiac muscle adaptation to exercise in approximately 4 weeks.[65] The advantages of this approach are its ease and affordability. A hamster-sized running wheel can be fitted with a digital magnetic counter to monitor daily running distance, velocity, and time. It is important to utilize a wheel into which the tail of the mouse does not get trapped, and a counter that measures running in both directions. A healthy young mouse may run from 1 to 9 km per day, and the daily running-wheel activity level in mice is significantly affected by genetic background and gender.[56,66,67]

Involuntary treadmill running has been widely used in exercise testing and training of mice.[68–70] The motorized treadmill belt speed and inclination can be adjusted and various stimuli (air puff, cold water, or electrical) can be used to stimulate the running. Treadmill exercise allows training interventions and testing exercise capacity in a standardized manner. A treadmill in an enclosed space also allows measurement of, e.g., respiratory gases during exercise, which allows obtaining detailed information, and all animals can be compared in a standardized manner. However, marked compliance differences in different mouse strains in treadmill running exist. In addition to running, endurance can be tested by swimming tests.

Testing with a rotorod apparatus (e.g., Rotarod) is frequently used in mouse models for neurological disease or skeletal muscle disorders and mainly reflects motor co-ordination and muscle function. The mice try to stay on a rod that rotates at constant or accelerating speed, and the time before falling is recorded.[58]

Often the disease to be studied requires specific tests to be developed, and most often a combination of several tests has to be used in order for a consensus to be reached on the functional defect.

30.8 In vitro measurement of single fiber and skinned fiber force

A long history of muscle physiology research has been based on experiments on single or skinned fibers.[71,72] These experimental setups utilize muscle preparation and analysis in vitro as whole muscle preparations, single muscle fibers, or skinned muscle fibers, attached between a force transducer. The fibers can be exposed to various substances, and their strength and contractile characteristics are studied. For example, metabolism, length–tension, force–velocity, force–stimulation, and stiffness of the muscle or muscle fiber can be measured.[73] These approaches give an objective measure of the muscle characteristics, but require some special skills, and may not always reflect the situation of the whole animal.

30.9 Non-invasive muscle research

Muscle metabolites can be recorded non-invasively in humans and mice by nuclear magnetic resonance (NMR) spectroscopy. Accumulation of, for example, lactate can be followed over time, as well as that of phosphate compounds. NMR can be combined with exercise, such as ergometry, and the dynamics of the metabolite changes can be monitored, while simultaneously recording oxygen consumption and CO_2 production. Magnetic resonance imaging (MRI) with experimental MRI units (at least 4.7 Tesla to allow adequate resolution in rodents) enables the evaluation of muscle volume, as well as of the water and connective tissue content. Whole-body MRI also gives an overview of the complete muscle mass, and may best reveal the absence of single muscles.

30.10 Working towards specific therapies using cellular and animal models

Muscle tissue develops and differentiates during fetal life and is already highly specialized at birth. Therefore, any specific therapeutic approaches for patients affected by muscle disorders face the problem of correcting a defect that is present in all or most of the cells of this postmitotic and rather stable tissue, constituting around 40% of the body. To date, the "therapeutic successes" in, for example, Duchenne muscular dystrophy have mostly been achieved in experimental studies of cellular or animal models, and have not been directly applicable to patients.[74,75] Therefore, understanding pathogenesis, achieving safe and efficient delivery to target tissue, developing reliable ways of monitoring the clinical response, and finding the optimal time of treatment for different disorders are the major obstacles to overcome before heading into treatment trials in patients. Numerous research groups have risen to these challenges, and some of their work will be summarized below. The method of choice for each muscle disorder will depend on the nature of the causative gene and the structure, location and function of its protein product.

30.10.1 Upregulation of alternative genes

The principle of this method is to compensate for the loss or malfunction of a gene product by increasing the expression of another gene encoding a protein with related function. A major advantage of this method is that the protein in question would not be expected to cause an immune response, which is a problem when exogenous proteins are introduced. The approach requires detailed characterization of the promoter regions and of expressional regulation of the target genes. Examples of potentially useful strategies include upregulating the expression of utrophin to partially overcome the adverse effects caused by the absence of dystrophin in Duchenne muscular dystrophy,[76] and upregulating the cardiac form of actin in nemaline myopathy caused by mutations in the skeletal α-actin gene.[77,78] This applies to diseases in which gene dosage has been noted to influence disease severity, suggesting that increased production of the normal protein may be beneficial. This hypothesis has been corroborated by studies of mouse models for nemaline myopathy.[79]

30.10.2 Gene repair: antisense oligonucleotide-induced exon skipping

In diseases caused by a stop codon and premature termination of a protein, attempts can be made to repair the gene. The lost function may sometimes be partially compensated by removing the exon with the stop codon from the mRNA, resulting in the production of a shortened protein. This can be achieved by the use of specific antisense oligonucleotides, which redirect mRNA splicing to skipping the defective exon. A potentially good target is a long repetitive protein, such as dystrophin. Specific antisense oligonucleotides,[80,81] chimeric RNA/DNA oligonucleotides,[82] or inhibitory RNAs[83] have been successfully used in cell cultures and in mice to induce specific skipping of the exon harboring the mutation. Partial restoration of the membranes and their function has been achieved. Small nuclear inhibitory RNAs, carried by adeno-associated viruses, injected systemically into the bloodstream, seem to give the best results so far, with significant restoration of muscle function lasting for several weeks.[83] The underlying idea is that the replacement of dystrophin at the cell membrane by a shorter, dystrophin-like protein might turn the histological and clinical features of Duchenne muscular dystrophy into those of the milder Becker type.

30.10.3 Cell replacement

Muscle defect or damage can in principle be repaired by transplanted myoblasts or stem cells that have the capacity to fuse to form myotubes or to fuse with existing myocytes. An advantage of cell replacement therapy would be the restoration of the lost or non-functional protein independently of the nature and location of the mutation. The transplants can originate from the affected subject, or from a healthy donor. If the subject him/herself (autologous transplantation) were the cell source, the gene defect could be corrected in vitro, cells expanded, and then returned to the circulation or the muscle of the subject. Autologous transplants would escape immune response, but the protein produced by the cells might still be antigenic.[84,85] Potentially this method could also restore muscle tissue.[86,87] This would be desirable in dystrophic disease processes, in which muscle tissue is continuously destroyed, or in diseases caused by mitochondrial DNA mutations, in which the quantity of wild-type mitochondrial DNA could potentially be increased above a threshold allowing functional cell respiration.

Muscle damage initiates myoblast activation locally, but myoblast transfer could potentially be given also as injections into the muscle or into the circulation, to enhance repair. Successful results have been obtained in mice and non-human primates,[88] but results in initial human trials[89–91] have so far been discouraging. Muscle-derived stem cells have the advantage over satellite cells of being self-renewing and not committed to the myogenic or mesenchymal cell lineages.[84] Experimental work is currently focusing on solving the problems of delivery and maintenance of these cells, and exploring the use of bone-marrow-derived stem cells or vessel-derived stem cells (mesangioblasts)[92] rather than embryonic ones.

30.10.4 Gene replacement

Gene replacement is one of the first approaches suggested for gene therapy: complementation of the endogenous dysfunctional gene by expression of a wild-type copy from a gene construct. The gene of interest may be introduced into the tissue by viral vectors, often adenoviral or adeno-associated viral vectors. Gene therapy trials of muscle diseases face challenges similar to all gene therapeutic approaches: difficulties in delivery of the gene to the target tissue, immune response against the viral vectors, and transient expression. Furthermore, the size of the gene to be inserted is limited. Encouraging results have been achieved through the use of short plasmid vectors (which are neither as toxic nor as immunogenic as viral vectors) and through a "gutting" procedure reducing the antigenicity of the viral vector. These advances have been deemed promising enough for permissions to be granted for phase I trials in humans.[93–95]

References

1. Donner K, Sandbacka M, Lehtokari VL, Wallgren-Pettersson C, Pelin K. Complete genomic structure of the human nebulin gene and identification of alternatively spliced transcripts. *Eur. J. Hum. Genet.* 2004, **12**: 744–751.
2. Udd B, Partanen J, Halonen P, *et al.* Tibial muscular dystrophy: late adult-onset distal myopathy in 66 Finnish patients. *Arch. Neurol.* 1993, **50**: 604–608.

3. Hackman P, Vihola A, Haravuori H, *et al.* Tibial muscular dystrophy is a titinopathy caused by mutations in TTN, the gene encoding the giant skeletal-muscle protein titin. *Am. J. Hum. Genet.* 2002, **71**: 492–500.
4. Hackman JP, Vihola AK, Udd AB. The role of titin in muscular disorders. *Ann. Med.* 2003, **35**: 434–441.
5. Mankoo BS, Collins NS, Ashby P, *et al.* Mox2 is a component of the genetic hierarchy controlling limb muscle development. *Nature* 1999, **400**: 69–73.
6. Spangenburg EE, Booth FW. Molecular regulation of individual skeletal muscle fibre types. *Acta Physiol. Scand.* 2003, **178**: 413–424.
7. Baldwin KM, Klinkerfuss GH, Terjung RL, Mole PA, Holloszy JO. Respiratory capacity of white, red, and intermediate muscle: adaptive response to exercise. *Am. J. Physiol.* 1972, **222**: 373–378.
8. Essen B, Jansson E, Henriksson J, Taylor AW, Saltin B. Metabolic characteristics of fibre types in human skeletal muscle. *Acta Physiol. Scand.* 1975, **95**: 153–165.
9. Smerdu V, Erzen I. Dynamic nature of fibre-type specific expression of myosin heavy chain transcripts in 14 different human skeletal muscles. *J. Muscle Res. Cell Motil.* 2001, **22**: 647–655.
10. Rhee HS, Lucas CA, Hoh JF. Fiber types in rat laryngeal muscles and their transformations after denervation and reinnervation. *J. Histochem. Cytochem.* 2004, **52**: 581–590.
11. Soukup T, Zacharova G, Smerdu V. Fibre type composition of soleus and extensor digitorum longus muscles in normal female inbred Lewis rats. *Acta Histochem.* 2002, **104**: 399–405.
12. Sipila I, Simell O, Rapola J, Sainio K, Tuuteri L. Gyrate atrophy of the choroid and retina with hyperornithinemia: tubular aggregates and type 2 fiber atrophy in muscle. *Neurology* 1979, **29**: 996–1005.
13. Booth FW, Thomason DB. Molecular and cellular adaptation of muscle in response to exercise: perspectives of various models. *Physiol. Rev.* 1991, **71**: 541–585.
14. Wang YX, Zhang CL, Yu RT, *et al.* Regulation of muscle fiber type and running endurance by PPAR delta. *PLoS Biol* 2004, **2**: e294.
15. Pette D. Training effects on the contractile apparatus. *Acta Physiol. Scand.* 1998, **162**: 367–376.
16. Olson EN, Williams RS. Remodeling muscles with calcineurin. *BioEssays* 2000, **22**: 510–519.
17. Jarvis JC, Mokrusch T, Kwende MM, Sutherland H, Salmons S. Fast-to-slow transformation in stimulated rat muscle. *Muscle Nerve* 1996, **19**: 1469–1475.
18. Hood DA. Invited review: Contractile activity-induced mitochondrial biogenesis in skeletal muscle. *J. Appl. Physiol.* 2001, **90**: 1137–1157.
19. Pellegrino MA, Canepari M, Rossi R, *et al.* Orthologous myosin isoforms and scaling of shortening velocity with body size in mouse, rat, rabbit and human muscles. *J. Physiol.* 2003, **546**: 677–689.
20. Agbulut O, Li Z, Mouly V, Butler-Browne GS. Analysis of skeletal and cardiac muscle from desmin knock-out and normal mice by high resolution separation of myosin heavy-chain isoforms. *Biol. Cell* 1996, **88**: 131–135.
21. Shoubridge EA, Johns T, Boulet L. Use of myoblast cultures to study mitochondrial myopathies. *Methods Enzymol.* 1995, **264**: 465–475.
22. Martinuzzi A, Askanas V, Kobayashi T, Engel WK, Di Mauro S. Expression of muscle-gene-specific isozymes of phosphorylase and creatine kinase in innervated cultured human muscle. *J. Cell Biol.* 1986, **103**: 1423–1429.

23. Sasarman F, Karpati G, Shoubridge EA. Nuclear genetic control of mitochondrial translation in skeletal muscle revealed in patients with mitochondrial myopathy. *Hum. Mol. Genet.* 2002, **11**: 1669–1681.

24. Clark KM, Watt DJ, Lightowlers RN, *et al.* SCID mice containing muscle with human mitochondrial DNA mutations: an animal model for mitochondrial DNA defects. *J. Clin. Invest.* 1998, **102**: 2090–2095.

25. Davis RL, Weintraub H, Lassar AB. Expression of a single transfected cDNA converts fibroblasts to myoblasts. *Cell* 1987, **51**: 987–1000.

26. Edmondson DG, Olson EN. A gene with homology to the myc similarity region of MyoD1 is expressed during myogenesis and is sufficient to activate the muscle differentiation program. *Genes Devel.* 1989, **3**: 628–640.

27. Wright WE, Sassoon DA, Lin VK. Myogenin, a factor regulating myogenesis, has a domain homologous to MyoD. *Cell* 1989, **56**: 607–617.

28. Braun T, Buschhausen-Denker G, Bober E, Tannich E, Arnold HH. A novel human muscle factor related to but distinct from MyoD1 induces myogenic conversion in 10T1/2 fibroblasts. *EMBO J.* 1989, **8**: 701–709.

29. Braun T, Bober E, Winter B, Rosenthal N, Arnold HH. Myf-6, a new member of the human gene family of myogenic determination factors: evidence for a gene cluster on chromosome 12. *EMBO J.* 1990, **9**: 821–831.

30. Blau HM, Pavlath GK, Hardeman EC, *et al.* Plasticity of the differentiated state. *Science* 1985, **230**: 758–766.

31. Richler C, Yaffe D. The in vitro cultivation and differentiation capacities of myogenic cell lines. *Devel. Biol.* 1970, **23**: 1–22.

32. See http://www.lgcpromochem.com/atcc/.

33. Miller AD, Rosman GJ. Improved retroviral vectors for gene transfer and expression. *Biotechniques* 1989, **7**: 980–982, 984–986, 989–990.

34. Miller AD. Progress toward human gene therapy. *Blood* 1990, **76**: 271–278.

35. Miller AD, Miller DG, Garcia JV, Lynch CM. Use of retroviral vectors for gene transfer and expression. *Methods Enzymol.* 1993, **217**: 581–599.

36. Hitoshi Y, Lorens J, Kitada SI, *et al.* Toso, a cell surface-specific regulator of Fas-induced apoptosis in T cells. *Immunity* 1998, **8**: 461–471.

37. Nolan GP, Shatzman AR. Expression vectors and delivery systems. *Curr. Opin. Biotechnol.* 1998, **9**: 447–450.

38. See http://www.stanford.edu/group/nolan/retroviral_systems/retsys.html.

39. Gunning P, Ponte P, Blau H, Kedes L. Alpha-skeletal and alpha-cardiac actin genes are coexpressed in adult human skeletal muscle and heart. *Mol. Cell Biol.* 1983, **3**: 1985–1995.

40. Shani M. Tissue-specific and developmentally regulated expression of a chimeric actin-globin gene in transgenic mice. *Mol. Cell Biol.* 1986, **6**: 2624–2631.

41. Brennan KJ, Hardeman EC. Quantitative analysis of the human alpha-skeletal actin gene in transgenic mice. *J. Biol. Chem.* 1993, **268**: 719–725.

42. Song Q, Young KB, Chu G, *et al.* Overexpression of phospholamban in slow-twitch skeletal muscle is associated with depressed contractile function and muscle remodeling. *FASEB J.* 2004, **18**: 974–976.

43. Walsh FS, Hobbs C, Wells DJ, Slater CR, Fazeli S. Ectopic expression of NCAM in skeletal muscle of transgenic mice results in terminal sprouting at the neuromuscular junction and altered structure but not function. *Mol. Cell Neurosci.* 2000, **15**: 244–261.

44. Tyynismaa H, Sembongi H, Bokori-Brown M, *et al.* Twinkle helicase is essential for mtDNA maintenance and regulates mtDNA copy number. *Hum. Mol. Genet.* 2004.

45. Levak-Frank S, Radner H, Walsh A, *et al.* Muscle-specific overexpression of lipoprotein lipase causes a severe myopathy characterized by proliferation of mitochondria and peroxisomes in transgenic mice. *J. Clin. Invest.* 1995, **96**: 976–986.

46. Musaro A, McCullagh K, Paul A, *et al.* Localized Igf-1 transgene expression sustains hypertrophy and regeneration in senescent skeletal muscle. *Nature Genet.* 2001, **27**: 195–200.

47. Shani M. Tissue-specific expression of rat myosin light-chain 2 gene in transgenic mice. *Nature* 1985, **314**: 283–286.

48. Rindt H, Knotts S, Robbins J. Segregation of cardiac and skeletal muscle-specific regulatory elements of the beta-myosin heavy chain gene. *Proc. Natl Acad. Sci. USA* 1995, **92**: 1540–1544.

49. Salminen M, Maire P, Concordet JP, *et al.* Fast-muscle-specific expression of human aldolase A transgenes. *Mol. Cell Biol.* 1994, **14**: 6797–6808.

50. Yamashita T, Kasai N, Miyoshi I, *et al.* High level expression of human alpha-fetoprotein in transgenic mice. *Biochem. Biophys. Res. Commun.* 1993, **191**: 715–720.

51. Isoda K, Kamezawa Y, Tada N, Sato M, Ohsuzu F. Myocardial hypertrophy in transgenic mice overexpressing human interleukin 1 alpha. *J. Card. Fail.* 2001, **7**: 355–364.

52. Imai S, Kaksonen M, Raulo E, *et al.* Osteoblast recruitment and bone formation enhanced by cell matrix-associated heparin-binding growth-associated molecule (HB-GAM). *J. Cell Biol.* 1998, **143**: 1113–1128.

53. Ekstrand MI, Falkenberg M, Rantanen A, *et al.* Mitochondrial transcription factor A regulates mtDNA copy number in mammals. *Hum. Mol. Genet.* 2004, **13**: 935–944.

54. Voet T, Schoenmakers E, Carpentier S, Labaere C, Marynen P. Controlled transgene dosage and PAC-mediated transgenesis in mice using a chromosomal vector. *Genomics* 2003, **82**: 596–605.

55. Grifone R, Laclef C, Spitz F, *et al.* Six1 and Eya1 expression can reprogram adult muscle from the slow-twitch phenotype into the fast-twitch phenotype. *Mol. Cell Biol.* 2004, **24**: 6253–6267.

56. Lerman I, Harrison BC, Freeman K, *et al.* Genetic variability in forced and voluntary endurance exercise performance in seven inbred mouse strains. *J. Appl. Physiol.* 2002, **92**: 2245–2255.

57. Meyer OA, Tilson HA, Byrd WC, Riley MT. A method for the routine assessment of fore- and hindlimb grip strength of rats and mice. *Neurobehav. Toxicol.* 1979, **1**: 233–236.

58. Derave W, Van Den Bosch L, Lemmens G, *et al.* Skeletal muscle properties in a transgenic mouse model for amyotrophic lateral sclerosis: effects of creatine treatment. *Neurobiol. Dis.* 2003, **13**: 264–272.

59. Thifault S, Girouard N, Lalonde R. Climbing sensorimotor skills in Lurcher mutant mice. *Brain Res. Bull.* 1996, **41**: 385–390.

60. Lalonde R, Kim HD, Fukuchi K. Exploratory activity, anxiety, and motor coordination in bigenic APPswe + PS1/DeltaE9 mice. *Neurosci. Lett.* 2004, **369**: 156–161.

61. Hara H, Nolan PM, Scott MO, *et al.* Running endurance abnormality in mdx mice. *Muscle Nerve* 2002, **25**: 207–211.

62. Joya JE, Kee AJ, Nair-Shalliker V, *et al.* Muscle weakness in a mouse model of nemaline myopathy can be reversed with exercise and reveals a novel myofiber repair mechanism. *Hum. Mol. Genet.* 2004, **13**: 2633–2645.

63. Swallow JG, Garland Jr T, Carter PA, Zhan WZ, Sieck GC. Effects of voluntary activity and genetic selection on aerobic capacity in house mice (*Mus domesticus*). *J. Appl. Physiol.* 1998, **84**: 69–76.

64. Fernando P, Bonen A, Hoffman-Goetz L. Predicting submaximal oxygen consumption during treadmill running in mice. *Can. J. Physiol. Pharmacol.* 1993, **71**: 854–857.

65. Allen DL, Harrison BC, Maass A, *et al*. Cardiac and skeletal muscle adaptations to voluntary wheel running in the mouse. *J. Appl. Physiol.* 2001, **90**: 1900–1908.

66. Lightfoot JT, Turner MJ, Daves M, Vordermark A, Kleeberger SR. Genetic influence on daily wheel running activity level. *Physiol. Genomics* 2004.

67. Lightfoot JT, Turner MJ, Debate KA, Kleeberger SR. Interstrain variation in murine aerobic capacity. *Med. Sci. Sports Exerc.* 2001, **33**: 2053–2057.

68. Yang Q, Osinska H, Klevitsky R, Robbins J. Phenotypic deficits in mice expressing a myosin binding protein C lacking the titin and myosin binding domains. *J. Mol. Cell. Cardiol.* 2001, **33**: 1649–1658.

69. Bao S, Garvey WT. Exercise in transgenic mice overexpressing GLUT4 glucose transporters: effects on substrate metabolism and glycogen regulation. *Metabolism* 1997, **46**: 1349–1357.

70. Nair-Shalliker V, Kee AJ, Joya JE, *et al*. Myofiber adaptational response to exercise in a mouse model of nemaline myopathy. *Muscle Nerve* 2004, **30**: 470–480.

71. Hellam DC, Podolsky RJ. Force measurements in skinned muscle fibres. *J. Physiol.* 1969, **200**: 807–819.

72. Ford LE, Podolsky RJ. Intracellular calcium movements in skinned muscle fibres. *J. Physiol.* 1972, **223**: 21–33.

73. Childers MK, McDonald KS. Regulatory light chain phosphorylation increases eccentric contraction-induced injury in skinned fast-twitch fibers. *Muscle Nerve* 2004, **29**: 313–317.

74. Dubowitz V. Therapeutic possibilities in muscular dystrophy: the hope versus the hype. *Neuromusc. Disord.* 2002, **12**: 113–116.

75. Dubowitz V. Therapeutic efforts in Duchenne muscular dystrophy: the need for a common language between basic scientists and clinicians. *Neuromusc. Disord.* 2004, **14**: 451–455.

76. Perkins KJ, Davies KE. The role of utrophin in the potential therapy of Duchenne muscular dystrophy. *Neuromusc. Disord.* 2002, **12** (Suppl. 1): S78–S89.

77. Nowak KJ, Wattanasirichaigoon D, Goebel HH, *et al*. Mutations in the skeletal muscle alpha-actin gene in patients with actin myopathy and nemaline myopathy. *Nature Genet.* 1999, **23**: 208–212.

78. Agrawal PB, Strickland CD, Midgett C, *et al*. Heterogeneity of nemaline myopathy cases with skeletal muscle alpha-actin gene mutations. *Ann. Neurol.* 2004, **56**: 86–96.

79. Corbett MA, Robinson CS, Dunglison GF, *et al*. A mutation in alpha-tropomyosin(slow) affects muscle strength, maturation and hypertrophy in a mouse model for nemaline myopathy. *Hum. Mol. Genet.* 2001, **10**: 317–328.

80. Dunckley MG, Manoharan M, Villiet P, Eperon IC, Dickson G. Modification of splicing in the dystrophin gene in cultured Mdx muscle cells by antisense oligoribonucleotides. *Hum. Mol. Genet.* 1998, **7**: 1083–1090.

81. Wilton SD, Lloyd F, Carville K, *et al*. Specific removal of the nonsense mutation from the mdx dystrophin mRNA using antisense oligonucleotides. *Neuromusc. Disord.* 1999, **9**: 330–338.

82. Bertoni C, Lau C, Rando TA. Restoration of dystrophin expression in mdx muscle cells by chimeraplast-mediated exon skipping. *Hum. Mol. Genet.* 2003, **12**: 1087–1099.

83. Goyenvalle A, Vulin A, Fougerousse F, *et al.* Rescue of dystrophic muscle through U7 snRNA-mediated exon skipping. *Science* 2004.

84. Huard J, Cao B, Qu-Petersen Z. Muscle-derived stem cells: potential for muscle regeneration. *Birth Defects Res. Part C Embryo Today* 2003, **69**: 230–237.

85. Carter JE, Schuchman EH. Gene therapy for neurodegenerative diseases: fact or fiction? *Br. J. Psychiatr.* 2001, **178**: 392–394.

86. Skuk D, Goulet M, Roy B, Tremblay JP. Myoblast transplantation in whole muscle of nonhuman primates. *J. Neuropathol. Exp. Neurol.* 2000, **59**: 197–206.

87. Skuk D, Tremblay JP. Myoblast transplantation: the current status of a potential therapeutic tool for myopathies. *J. Muscle Res. Cell Motil.* 2003, **24**: 285–300.

88. Partridge TA, Morgan JE, Coulton GR, Hoffman EP, Kunkel LM. Conversion of mdx myofibres from dystrophin-negative to -positive by injection of normal myoblasts. *Nature* 1989, **337**: 176–179.

89. Gussoni E, Pavlath GK, Lanctot AM, *et al.* Normal dystrophin transcripts detected in Duchenne muscular dystrophy patients after myoblast transplantation. *Nature* 1992, **356**: 435–438.

90. Karpati G, Ajdukovic D, Arnold D, *et al.* Myoblast transfer in Duchenne muscular dystrophy. *Ann. Neurol.* 1993, **34**: 8–17.

91. Mendell JR, Kissel JT, Amato AA, *et al.* Myoblast transfer in the treatment of Duchenne's muscular dystrophy. *New Engl. J. Med.* 1995, **333**: 832–838.

92. Sampaolesi M, Torrente Y, Innocenzi A, *et al.* Cell therapy of alpha-sarcoglycan null dystrophic mice through intra-arterial delivery of mesoangioblasts. *Science* 2003, **301**: 487–492.

93. Thioudellet C, Blot S, Squiban P, Fardeau M, Braun S. Current protocol of a research phase I clinical trial of full-length dystrophin plasmid DNA in Duchenne/Becker muscular dystrophies. I. Rationale. *Neuromusc. Disord.* 2002, **12** (Suppl. 1): S49–S51.

94. Romero NB, Benveniste O, Payan C, *et al.* Current protocol of a research phase I clinical trial of full-length dystrophin plasmid DNA in Duchenne/Becker muscular dystrophies. II. Clinical protocol. *Neuromusc. Disord.* 2002, **12** (Suppl. 1): S45–S48.

95. Fardeau M. Current protocol of a research phase I clinical trial of full-length dystrophin plasmid DNA in Duchenne/Becker muscular dystrophies. III. Ethical considerations. *Neuromusc. Disord.* 2002, **12** (Suppl. 1): S52–S54.

Index

Note: page numbers in *italics* refer to figures and tables.